Pediatric and Congenital Cardiology, Cardiac Surgery and Intensive Care

Eduardo M. da Cruz • Dunbar Ivy
James Jaggers

Editors

Pediatric and Congenital Cardiology, Cardiac Surgery and Intensive Care

Volume 3

With 1377 Figures and 296 Tables

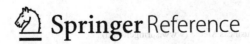

Springer Reference

Editors
Eduardo M. da Cruz
Department of Pediatric Cardiology & Intensive Care
Children's Hospital Colorado
University of Colorado School of Medicine
Aurora, CO, USA

Dunbar Ivy
Department of Pediatric Cardiology
Children's Hospital Colorado
University of Colorado School of Medicine
Aurora, CO, USA

James Jaggers
Department of Pediatric Cardiac Surgery
Children's Hospital Colorado
University of Colorado School of Medicine
Aurora, CO, USA

ISBN 978-1-4471-4618-6   ISBN 978-1-4471-4619-3 (eBook)
ISBN 978-1-4471-4620-9 (print and electronic bundle)
DOI 10.1007/978-1-4471-4619-3
Springer London Heidelberg New York Dordrecht

Library of Congress Control Number: 2013942788

Printed on acid-free paper

Springer is part of Springer Science+Business Media (www.springer.com)

To Suzanne, Esteban, Tomás and all my dear family and beloved ones
To my inspiring mentors and mentees
To all the children of the World

Eduardo M. da Cruz

To my loving and patient wife and daughters, Ellen, Madeline and Meg

Dunbar Ivy

This book is dedicated to children and families with congenital cardiac disease for whom I have been privileged to care for and to the teachers and mentors who have provided me the knowledge and skill to do so

James Jaggers

Foreword I

The last thirty years has seen some spectacular advances in the diagnosis and management of children with congenital and acquired heart disease. In the former instance, we have moved from an era of an early palliative surgical approach followed by later repair when mortality of 10 % or higher was common to the modern approach of surgical reconstruction in infancy with a mortality of less than 5 %. Underlying this success story are contributions from all the groups that are involved in the care of children with heart disease including pediatric cardiac nurses, cardiologists and cardiac surgeons, perfusionists, anesthesiologists and pediatric intensivists. They are all members of a team and teamwork is the key ingredient of high performing pediatric cardiac programmes.

My own area of intensive care medicine is an essential part of that team and has now developed into a specialty of pediatric cardiac critical care in it's own rite with an expectation that physicians should have a comprehensive knowledge of cardiac anatomy and physiology as well appropriate training in pediatric intensive care medicine. The newer generation of trainees will also be expected to have expertise in echocardiography, extracorporeal technology and mechanical support. This *Textbook of Pediatric and Congenital Cardiology, Cardiac Surgery and Intensive Care* will be source material for all this because it covers every aspect of heart disease in children and will be an invaluable resource for all team members in the pediatric cardiac programme.

Desmond Bohn, MB FRCPC,
Professor of Anesthesia and Pediatrics
Former Chief, Department of Critical Care Medicine
The Hospital for Sick Children, Toronto
University of Toronto

Foreword II

To say that this text is a monumental undertaking is an understatement. The crux of this work is in the subtitle. It is *comprehensive, interdisciplinary*, and, perhaps most importantly, *interactive*. There are several excellent existing textbooks of pediatric cardiology, most of which follow a familiar format of chapters on anatomy and embryology, structural malformations, myocardial/inflammatory diseases, and perhaps heart failure and pulmonary hypertension. None that I know of, cover such a diverse range of subjects as this text: therapeutic hypothermia and tracheal reconstruction; venous thromboembolism and trypanosomiasis; Takayasu disease and Nursing. Authorship is likewise diverse, with contributors from all across the world.

Medicine is an extremely rapidly changing field. The time, often years, between the decision to publish a textbook and the actual publication frequently means that much of what is written is out of date by the time of publication. Thus the decision of the editors and publisher to create both a print and a web version, the latter to be updated frequently and read on a peripheral mobile device help make it both current and accessible. No one carries a large textbook into the ER in the middle of the night, but everyone carries a mobile phone.

Howard P. Gutgesell, MD
Professor of Pediatrics, Emeritus
University of Virginia Medical School
Charlottesville, Virginia

Foreword III

Sixty years ago on May 6 1953 John Gibbon was the first to achieve successful repair of a congenital heart defect using a heart lung machine. What is often forgotten however is that Gibbon's subsequent five patients did not survive. Many other pioneers of cardiac surgery of that era had equally dismal results. Today the outlook for the child with congenital heart disease has improved dramatically. At the top of my list of reasons for that improvement has been the establishment of cohesive interdisciplinary teams of individuals dedicated to the care of patients with congenital heart disease. While these individuals may have expertise in an incredibly specialized area of cardiac surgery, cardiology, cardiac anesthesia, cardiac intensive care, perfusion, cardiac nursing or many of the essential ancillary healthcare support areas, their individual contribution to the successful care of a child with a complex congenital heart problem is only as good as the weakest link in the entire team. This stunning new textbook edited by Eduardo M. Da Cruz, Dunbar Ivy and James Jaggers brings together authors from all of the many components of the healthcare team devoted to care of the individual, both adult and pediatric, with congenital heart disease. The primary editors have assembled a team of specialist sub-editors who have each assembled a sub-team of contributors from around the globe. One of the great joys of working within the field of congenital heart disease is that in contrast to many other medical specialties, we are a relatively small family who have come to know each other on a global scale, symbolized by our quadrennial meeting at the World Congress of Pediatric Cardiology and Congenital Heart Surgery.

The authors have brought the reader into the new millennium of publishing by creating an electronic version of this textbook that includes access to videos demonstrating surgical technique as well as diagnostic modalities. The exhaustiveness of the coverage is truly breathtaking. Just reading the list of contents and appreciating the breadth of coverage draws attention to the very considerable care and effort that the editors have put into assembling this unique book. Whether a cardiologist, cardiac surgeon, cardiac intensivist, a cardiac anesthesiologist or a nurse in the intensive care unit or any one of the many supporting allied healthcare workers in the field of congenital cardiac care, the reader will surely not be disappointed.

Richard Jonas, MD
Professor of Pediatric Cardiac Surgery
Chief of Cardiovascular Surgery and
co-director of the Children's National Heart Institute
Children's National Medical center
Washington, DC, USA

Preface

Pediatric and congenital cardiac patients, from the fetus to the adult, remain in the current century a complex challenge in an ever evolving discipline. Successful cardiovascular programs currently deal with the most critical patients by promoting a horizontal convergence of multiple specialties. Many, if not most, programs have multidisciplinary teams available, and yet the challenge remains to make these teams operate as *interdisciplinary*. Two key goals ought to be pursued in order to achieve successful short and long term outcomes with pediatric cardiac patients. Firstly, the driving force should always be *quality improvement and safety*, and secondly good *communication* shall prevail. There are two main pillars of the latter endeavors, namely individual-based and system-based principles. Individual-based principles are quite subjective and more difficult to manage, since they depend on personalities and behavior. In a balanced environment, individuals should be able to endorse a willingness to develop exhaustive knowledge, team work, trust, self-awareness, capacity to listen, common sense and respect. System-based practices are more objective, and although requiring cultural changes, promote consistency, harmonious interaction and better outcomes. Such practices allow the development of common paths for the team to follow, whilst enhancing good communication and reducing risks, optimizing prevention of complications, better handling fluctuations and identifying outliers, and predicting likely outcomes based on accurate data. The implementation and consolidation of efficient programs require systematic audits, development of sound database platforms, development of plans to address deficiencies, implementation of simulation and quality improvement and safety programs, and the eagerness for transparency and to share the available information with staff, patients and their families in a non-repressive and constructive atmosphere. Such models are not of the realm of utopia, although they are challenging to establish, at least whilst inducing the required cultural changes and promoting the conviction of their usefulness.

The textbook of Pediatric and Congenital Cardiology, Cardiac Surgery and Intensive Care intends to achieve an ultimate objective beyond providing reliable scientific information. It endeavors to symbolize the imperative need for a cohesive and transparent interdisciplinary blend of expertise, by bringing together world renowned authors from different regions around the Globe, and representing the many specialties concerned by and involved in the management of pediatric patients with congenital and acquired cardiac diseases. We have been privileged to gather many experts from reference programs to whom we will remain forever grateful. As much as we have endeavored to remain consistent, some authors may express personal opinions and hypothesis in a constructive manner, which -as we expect- may help readers understand the many facets and complexities of patient management at different levels. Very importantly, in this project readers will be able to access a website which we see as a source of constantly updated information, including videos dedicated to diagnosis and surgical interventions, and that should evolve overtime into a more interactive tool. We sincerely hope that the Textbook of Pediatric and Congenital Cardiology, Cardiac Surgery and Intensive Care will become a useful tool in the armamentarium of those caring for such complex patients; we aim to provide updated information to help caregivers become better practitioners and human beings. If so, this textbook would have achieved its *raison d'être*.

July 2013   Eduardo M. da Cruz
                                                                          Aurora, CO, USA
                                                                               Dunbar Ivy
                                                                          Aurora, CO, USA
                                                                            James Jaggers
                                                                          Aurora, CO, USA

Acknowledgments

We would like to express our sincere gratefulness to the Section Editors, the Website Editor and to all the authors who dedicated countless hours to produce a work of outstanding quality, with the genuine aim of sharing good practice.

We also want to thank our families for their second-to-none patience and support during the three years of production.

Last but not least, we thank Springer-Verlag, particularly Grant Weston, Mansi Seth and Navjeet Kaur for their advice and collaboration.

Eduardo M. da Cruz
Dunbar Ivy
James Jaggers
Editors-in-Chief

About the Editors

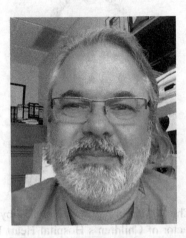

Eduardo M. da Cruz, MD, Head of Pediatric Cardiac Critical Care Program, Head of Pediatric Cardiology Inpatient Services, Director of Cardiac Intensive Care Unit, Director of Cardiac Progressive Care Unit, Children's Hospital Colorado and Professor of Pediatrics (Pediatric Cardiology & Intensive Care), University of Colorado Denver, School of Medicine, Aurora, CO, USA

Eduardo M. da Cruz is a Professor of Pediatrics (Pediatric Cardiology and Intensive Care) and the Head of the Pediatric Cardiac Critical Care Program & Inpatient Services at The Heart Institute, Department of Pediatrics, Children's Hospital Colorado, University of Colorado Denver-School of Medicine. He trained in pediatrics, pediatric cardiology and intensive care and has been an attending physician for 20 years in Europe and in the USA. He has extensive experience in the medical and perioperative management of neonates, children and young adults with complex congenital or acquired heart, including heart transplant, mechanical assistance and quality improvement and safety. He is very actively involved in clinical research and teaching in the fields of pediatric cardiology and cardiac intensive care, has delivered hundreds of international lectures and is the editor of various Cardiology and CICU reference textbooks. Eduardo M. da Cruz has published 50 book chapters and dozens of manuscripts in peer-reviewed journals. He is the founder of the Working Group on Pediatric Cardiac Intensive Care of the

Association for the European Paediatric and Congenital Cardiology (AEPC), Deputy Chair and founder of the Section on Hemodynamics and Heart Disease of the European Society of Paediatric and Neonatal Intensive Care (ESPNIC), Board Member of the Congenital Domain of the European Association for Cardio-Thoracic Surgery (EACTS), member of the Society of Pediatric Research (SPR) and of multiple international Societies, and the President of Surgeons of Hope Foundation, based in New York.

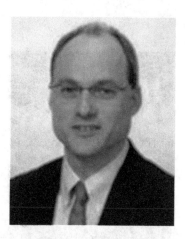

Dunbar Ivy, MD, Chief of Pediatric Cardiology, Selby's Chair of Pediatric Cardiology, Co-Director of Children's Hospital Heart Institute, Director of Pediatric Pulmonary Hypertension Program Children's Hospital Colorado and Professor of Pediatrics, University of Colorado School of Medicine Aurora, CO, USA

Dr. Dunbar Ivy began his medical career at Tulane University School of Medicine following his premedical studies at Davidson College. While at Tulane, he became excited about a career in Pediatric Cardiology under the mentorship of Dr Arthur Pickoff. He then obtained training in General Pediatrics at the University of Colorado School of Medicine in Denver, Colorado. Early mentors in Pediatric Cardiology included Drs. Michael Schaffer and Henry Sondheimer. Interest in altitude related illness and pulmonary hypertension in congenital heart disease were fostered by Dr Robert Wolfe on the clinical side and Drs Steve Abman and John Kinsella in the fetal sheep laboratory while a fellow in Pediatric Cardiology at the University of Colorado. Following fellowship, he became a research instructor under the guidance of Dr Mark Boucek, who encouraged him to pursue a career as a clinician scientist. During his time as a Bugher fellow, he obtained early grants from the March of Dimes and American Heart Association regarding the role of endothelin in the perinatal pulmonary circulation. This work transitioned into a National Institutes of Health K-08 award to continue to study molecular derangements in the endothelin pathway in models of pulmonary hypertension. In 2003 Dr Ivy took the position of Chief of Pediatric Cardiology and Selby's Chair of Pediatric Cardiology. His research focus became more clinical and translational. As Director of the Pediatric Pulmonary Hypertension Program, he began early clinical studies of medical therapy in children, including the use of intravenous epoprostenol, subcutaneous treprostinil, and oral bosentan. He began to work with Dr Robin Shandas regarding measurement of right ventricular afterload in children with pulmonary hypertension in an NIH sponsored Specialized Centers of Clinically Oriented Research grant headed by Dr Kurt Stenmark. Further work on ventricular vascular coupling has continued with NIH funding with Dr Shandas. Dr Ivy was the inaugural Chairman of the first Pediatric Pulmonary Hypertension taskforce at the World Symposium of Pulmonary Hypertension in Nice, France in 2013. Dr. Ivy is a member of multiple societies, and has published over 150 peer reviewed manuscripts.

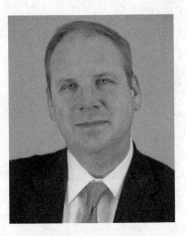

James Jaggers, MD, Barton-Elliman Chair and Chief of Pediatric Cardiac Surgery, Professor of Surgery, Children's Hospital Colorado, University of Colorado, Aurora, CO, USA

Dr. James Jaggers began his medical career at the University of Nebraska Medical Center as a medical student. He then obtained training in general Surgery at the Oregon Health Sciences University in Portland Oregon and Thoracic Surgery training at the University of Colorado Health Sciences Center in Denver. During this period he also completed a Pediatric Cardiac Surgery Fellowship at the Children's Hospital in Denver. Following this he took a faculty position at Duke University Medical Center in Thoracic and Pediatric cardiac Surgery where he rose to the rank of Associate Professor with tenure. This tenure at Duke was interrupted by a very brief position at the University of Missouri and Mercy Children's Hospital in Kansas City. Following this, he returned to Duke to assume the position of Chief of Pediatric Cardiac surgery and Director of the Duke Pediatric Heart Institute. During his time at Duke, Dr. Jaggers directed the pediatric cardiovascular surgery laboratory and mentored many research fellows. He was principal and co-principal investigator on two basic Science NIH grants and one Pediatric Heart Network NHLBI sponsored multicenter study. In 2010, Dr. Jaggers moved to the University of Colorado and Children's Hospital Colorado where he is now the Barton Elliman Chair of Congenital Cardiac Surgery and Professor of Surgery. His current research interests include Outcomes research in care of Congenital Heart Disease and investigation into the protein signaling of aortic stenosis and uncompensated cardiac hypertrophy and myocardial dysfunction. Clinical interests include complex neonatal heart surgery, cardiac transplantation and fetal intervention for cardiac defects. Dr. Jaggers is a member of multiple Societies, and has published 117 peer reviewed manuscripts, published 21 book chapters and is a reputed international lecturer with 75 invited lectures.

Section Editors

Philippe Acar Pediatric Cardiology Unit, Children's Hospital - Toulouse University Hospital, France

Carl L. Backer Division of Cardiovascular-Surgery, Children's Hospital of Chicago, Chicago, IL, USA

Paul Bakerman Critical Care Medicine, Phoenix Children's Hospital, Phoenix, AZ, USA

Lee Benson Cardiology, The Hospital for Sick Children, Cardiac Diagnostic and Interventional Unit, Toronto, ON, Canada

Robert A. Berg The Children's Hospital of Philadelphia, Department of Anesthesiology and Critical Care Medicine Division of Critical Care, Philadelphia, PA, USA

Rolf M. F. Berger Pediatric and Congenital Cardiology Beatrix Children's Hospital, University Medical Center Groningen Center for Congenital Heart Diseases, Groningen, The Netherlands

Stuart Berger Department of Pediatrics, Medical College of Wisconsin, Milwaukee, WI, USA

Donald Berry Department of Pharmacy, Children's Hospital of Pittsburgh, Pittsburgh, PA, USA

Steven Choi Montefiore Medical Center, Rosenthal Pavilion Bronx, NY, USA

Kathryn K. Collins The Children's Hospital, Section of Cardiology/B100, Aurora, CO, USA

Heidi Dalton Phoenix Children's Hospital, Phoenix, AZ, USA

Stephen R. Daniels Department of Pediatrics, Section of Cardiology, University of Colorado School of Medicine, The Children's Hospital Colorado, Aurora, CO, USA

Jean-Claude Fouron Department of Pediatrics, Centre Hospitalier Universitaire (CHU) Saint-Justine, University of Montreal, Quebec, Canada

George Hoffman Department of Pediatric Anesthesiology, Medical College of Wisconsin, Milwaukee, WI, USA

Viktor Hraska German Pediatric Heart Centre, Asklepios Clinic Sankt Augustin, Sankt Augustin, Germany

Daphne Hsu Division of Pediatric Cardiology, Children's Hospital at Montefiore, Bronx, NY, USA

Richard Ing Children's Hospital Colorado, Aurora, CO, USA

Jonathan Kaufman The Children's Hospital Cardiology, Aurora, CO, USA

Patricia Lincoln Children's Hospital Boston, Boston, MA, USA

David Moromisato Children's Hospital Los Angeles, Division of Critical Care Medicine, Department of Anesthesiology Critical Care Medicine, Los Angeles, CA, USA

Ricardo Muñoz Division of Pediatric Cardiology, Children's Hospital of Pittsburgh of UPMC, Pittsburgh, PA, USA

Steve Neish Division of Cardiology, The University of Texas Health Science Center, San Antonio, USA

Shakeel Qureshi Evelina Children's Hospital, Paediatric Cardiology, London, UK

Niurka Rivero Children's Hospital Los Angeles, Department of Anesthesiology Critical Care Medicine, Division of Critical Care Medicine, Los Angeles, CA, USA

Michael J. Rutter University of Cincinnati College of Medicine, Cincinatti, OH, USA

Lara Shekerdemian Paediatrics, Baylor College of Medicine, Houston, TX, USA

Matthias Siepe Clinic for Cardiovascular Surgery, University Hospital. Freiburg, Freiburg, Germany

Sandra Staveski Pediatric Cardiovascular Intensive Care Unit, Lucile Packard Children's Hospital, Stanford, USA

Mark D. Twite Children's Hospital Colorado Anesthesiology, Aurora, CO, USA

Ross M. Ungerleider Wake Forest University Baptist Medical Center, Medical Center Boulevard, Winston Salem, NC, USA

Carol Vetterly Department of Pharmacy, University of Pittsburgh School of Pharmacy, Children's Hospital of Pittsburgh, Pittsburgh, PA, USA

Gary Webb Cincinnati Children's Hospital Medical Center, Cincinatti OH, USA

Steven A. Webber James C. Overall Professor and Chair, Department of Pediatrics Vanderbilt University School of Medicine Pediatrician-in-Chief, Monroe Carell Jr. Children's Hospital at Vanderbilt, Nashville, TN, USA

Contents

Volume 1

Section I General Aspects **1**
Dunbar Ivy and Steve Neish

1 **Genetics of Congenital and Acquired Cardiovascular
Disease** 3
John L. Jefferies, Hugo R. Martinez, and Jeffrey A. Towbin

2 **Normal Cardiac Anatomy** 17
Robert H. Anderson, Andrew C. Cook, Anthony J. Hlavacek,
Horia Muresian, and Diane E. Spicer

3 **Chromosomal Anomalies Associated with Congenital
Heart Disease** 47
Kathryn C. Chatfield and Matthew A. Deardorff

4 **Outcomes Analysis and Quality Improvement for the
Treatment of Patients with Pediatric and Congenital
Heart Disease** 73
Jeffrey P. Jacobs

5 **Pediatric Risk Adjustment for Congenital
Heart Disease** 95
Kathy Jenkins, Kimberlee Gauvreau, Lisa Bergersen,
Meena Nathan, and Ravi Thiagarajan

6 **Transport of the Critically Ill Cardiac Patient** 105
Aaron G. DeWitt and John R. Charpie

7 **General Pre-Operative and Post-Operative
Considerations in Pediatric Cardiac Patients** 117
Heather A. Dickerson and Antonio G. Cabrera

8 **Special Considerations in the Medical and Surgical
Management of the Premature Infant** 131
S. Adil Husain

Section II Fetal Cardiology **149**
Jean-Claude Fouron

9   **Normal and Abnormal Development of the Heart** 151
    Robert H. Anderson, Antoon F. M. Moorman,
    Nigel A. Brown, Simon D. Bamforth, Bill Chaudhry,
    Deborah J. Henderson, and Timothy J. Mohun

10 **Transition from Fetal to Neonatal Circulation** 179
    Bettina Cuneo

11 **Structural Heart Disease in the Fetus** 201
    John M. Simpson and Caroline B. Jones

12 **Evaluation of Fetal Cardiovascular Physiology in
    Cardiac and Non-cardiac Disease** 227
    Anita Szwast and Jack Rychik

13 **Fetal Myocardial Mechanics** 249
    Anita J. Moon-Grady and Lisa K. Hornberger

14 **Fetal Arrhythmias** 271
    Lisa Howley and Michelle Carr

15 **Fetal Cardiac Intervention** 293
    Brian T. Kalish and Wayne Tworetzky

Section III Assessment of the Cardiac Patient **301**
Daphne Hsu

16 **Assessment of the Cardiac Patient: History and
    Physical Examination** 303
    Daphne T. Hsu and Welton M. Gersony

17 **Assessment of the Newborn** 317
    William Mahle

18 **Assessment of the Athlete for Sports Participation** 327
    Joshua Kovach and Stuart Berger

19 **Assessment of the Adult with Congenital
    Heart Disease** 339
    George Lui

20 **Basics of Pediatric Electrocardiography and Invasive
    Electrophysiology: Principles of Cardiac Testing** 349
    Robert H. Pass and Scott R. Ceresnak

21 **Echocardiographic Assessment of Cardiac Disease** 375
    Sarah Chambers and Leo Lopez

22 **Exercise Testing in the Assessment of the Cardiac
    Patient** 399
    Jonathan Rhodes

23   Cardiac Catheterization: Basic Hemodynamics and
     Angiography 409
     Diego Porras, Lisa Bergersen, and Jeff Meadows

24   Basics of Cardiac MRI in the Assessment of Cardiac
     Disease 429
     Nadine Choueiter

25   Assessment of the Pediatric Patient with Chest Pain 443
     Devyani Chowdhury

26   Assessment of the Patient with Syncope 449
     Christine A. Walsh and Myles S. Schiller

Section IV   Preventive Cardiology   461
Stephen Daniels

27   Promoting Cardiovascular Health 463
     Stephen R. Daniels

28   Arterial Hypertension: Evaluation
     and Management 481
     Joseph T. Flynn

29   Obesity, Metabolic Syndrome and Type 2 Diabetes 499
     Julia Steinberger and Aaron S. Kelly

30   Hypercholesterolemia and Dyslipidemia 509
     Elizabeth Yeung and Robert Eckel

31   Non-invasive Assessment of Arterial Structure
     and Function 531
     Michael R. Skilton and David S. Celermajer

32   Echocardiography in the Assessment of Cardiovascular
     Disease Risk 547
     Thomas R. Kimball

Volume 2

Section V   Cardiovascular Anesthesia   557
Mark D. Twite and Richard J. Ing

33   Anesthetic Agents and Their Cardiovascular Effects 559
     Dean B. Andropoulos

34   Operative Preparation of the Patient for Heart
     Surgery: Airway and Ventilation, Vascular Access
     and Monitoring 573
     Sana Ullah and Luis M. Zabala

35   Anesthetic Techniques for Specific Cardiac
     Pathology 625
     Richard J. Ing, Steven P. Goldberg, and Mark D. Twite

36 Intra-operative Anticoagulation, Hemostasis and Blood
     Conservation 659
     Philip Arnold and Prem Venugopal

37 Transport and Transfer of Care of Critically-Ill
     Children 683
     Mark D. Twite and Richard J. Ing

38 Fast-Tracking and Regional Anesthesia in Pediatric
     Patients Undergoing Congenital Heart Surgery 691
     Alexander Mittnacht and Cesar Rodriguez-Diaz

39 Post-Operative Sedation and Analgesia 705
     Ellen Rawlinson and Richard F. Howard

40 Anesthesia in the Cardiac Catheterization Laboratory
     and MRI 721
     Warwick Ames, Kevin Hill, and Edmund H. Jooste

41 Anesthetic Considerations for Children with Congenital
     Heart Disease Undergoing Non-cardiac Surgery 743
     Lawrence I. Schwartz, Richard J. Ing, and Mark D. Twite

42 Databases and Outcomes in Congenital Cardiac
     Anesthesia Patients 759
     David F. Vener

Section VI   Cardio-Pulmonary Bypass 769
Ross M. Ungerleider

43 Mechanical Aspects of Pediatric Cardio
     Pulmonary Bypass 771
     Scott Lawson, Cory Ellis, Craig McRobb, and Brian Mejak

44 Systemic Inflammatory Response to Cardiopulmonary
     Bypass in Pediatric Patients and Related Strategies
     for Prevention 791
     Tara Karamlou and Ross M. Ungerleider

45 Neuroprotection Strategies During
     Cardiopulmonary Bypass 801
     Yoshio Ootaki and Ross M. Ungerleider

Section VII   Monitoring of the Cardiac Patient 819
George Hoffman and Stuart Berger

46 Standard Monitoring Techniques in the Pediatric
     Cardiac Intensive Care Unit 821
     Ryan J. Butts, Thomas Bao Do, and Andrew M. Atz

47 Non-invasive Monitoring of Oxygen Delivery 835
     George M. Hoffman, Nancy S. Ghanayem, and
     James S. Tweddell

48 Biomarkers in Pediatric Cardiology and Cardiac Surgery 857
Angela Lorts, David Hehir, and Catherine Krawczeski

49 Echocardiography in the ICU 879
Edward Kirkpatrick, Amanda J. Shillingford, and Meryl S. Cohen

50 Developing Techniques: The Future of Monitoring 901
Kyle Lieppman, Alejandro A. Floh, and Steven M. Schwartz

Section VIII Cardiopulmonary and Intracardiac Interactions **915**
Lara Shekerdemian

51 Intracardiac Interactions 917
Andrew Redington and Michael Mendelson

52 Cardiopulmonary Interactions 933
Ronald A. Bronicki and Daniel J. Penny

53 Airway Management in Congenital Heart Disease 955
Dean B. Andropoulos

Section IX Cardiovascular Pharmacology **971**
Ricardo Muñoz, Carol G. Vetterly, and Donald Berry

54 Pharmacokinetics and Application to Pediatric Practice 973
Denise L. Howrie and Carol G. Vetterly

55 Pharmacogenomics: A Pathway to Individualized Medicine 981
Denise L. Howrie and Raman Venkataramanan

56 Ionotropic, Lusitropics, Vasodilators and Vasoconstrictors 989
Ryan Flanagan, Carol G. Vetterly, and Ricardo Muñoz

57 Diuretics 1003
Donald Berry

58 Beta-Blockers 1009
Emily Polischuk and Donald Berry

59 Other Drugs: Fenoldopam, Levosemendan, Nesiritide 1015
Kelli L. Crowley and Ricardo Muñoz

60 Antiarrhythmic Drugs 1023
Alejandro J. López-Magallón, Nils Welchering, Juliana Torres Pacheco, Donald Berry, and Ricardo Muñoz

Section X General Principles of Interventional Cardiac Catheterization **1049**
Shakeel Qureshi

61 Catheter-Based Interventions on Right Ventricular
    Outflow Tract 1051
    Gianfranco Butera, Alessandra Frigiola, and
    Philipp Bonhoeffer

62 Catheter-Based Interventions on Pulmonary Arteries 1069
    Frank F. Ing

63 Catheter-Based Interventions on Left Ventricular
    Outflow Tract 1083
    Otto Rahkonen and Lee Benson

64 Catheter-Based Interventions of the Aorta 1101
    Marc Gewillig, Derize Boshoff, and Werner Budts

65 Catheter-Based Interventions on Intracardiac Shunts 1127
    Mazeni Alwi and Ming Chern Leong

66 Catheter-Based Interventions on Extracardiac Arterial
    and Venous Shunts 1153
    Jeffrey R. Darst and Thomas E. Fagan

67 Catheter-Based Interventions for
    Univentricular Hearts 1183
    Ralf J. Holzer, Mark Galantowicz, and John P. Cheatham

Volume 3

Section XI Innovative Interventional Techniques **1217**
Lee Benson

68 Biodegradable Implants 1219
    Daniel S. Levi and Andrew L. Cheng

69 Robotic Surgery 1237
    Nikolay V. Vasilyev, Pedro J. del Nido, and
    Pierre E. Dupont

70 Hybrid Strategies (Non-HLHS) 1251
    Darren P. Berman and Evan M. Zahn

Section XII Cardiopulmonary Resuscitation **1273**
Robert Berg

71 Epidemiology of Pediatric Cardiac Arrest 1275
    Joseph W. Rossano, Maryam Y. Naim, Vinay M. Nadkarni,
    and Robert A. Berg

72 Current CPR Recommendations 1289
    Maryam Y. Naim, Joseph W. Rossano, Vinay M. Nadkarni,
    and Robert A. Berg

Section XIII   Nursing Issues Related to the Cardiac Patient **1305**
Patricia Lincoln and Sandra Staveski

73   Introduction to Nursing Issues 1307
Sandra Staveski and Patricia Lincoln

74   Congential Cardiac Patients – Fetus to Adult: Nursing
Considerations 1309
Patricia Lincoln, Megan Cusick, John Fantegrossi,
Lindsey Katzmark, Terra Lafranchi, Christine Peyton,
and Mary Rummell

75   Pediatric Cardiac Intensive Care – Cardiovascular
Management: Nursing Considerations 1329
Patricia Lincoln, Dorothy Beke, Nancy Braudis,
Elizabeth Leonard, Sherry Pye, and Elisabeth Smith

76   Pediatric Cardiac Intensive Care – Postoperative
Management: Nursing Considerations 1349
Patricia Lincoln, Jeanne Ahern, Nancy Braudis,
Loren D. Brown, Kevin Bullock, Janine Evans,
Yong Mein Guan, Wenyi Luo, Nanping Sheng,
and Margaret Schroeder

77   Chronically Critically Ill Pediatric Cardiac Patient:
Nursing Considerations 1371
Sandra Staveski, Elizabeth Price, Esther Liu, Aileen Lin,
Elisabeth Smith, and Michelle Ogawa

78   Acquired Heart Disease, Arrhythmias and
Transplantation: Nursing Considerations 1383
Cecila St. George-Hyslop, Kelly Kirby, Deborah Gilbert,
and Bethany Diamond

79   Pediatric Cardiac Intensive Care: Nursing Education
and Leadership 1403
Sandra Staveski, Patricia Lincoln, Heather Freeman,
Debra Morrow, and Christine Peyton

**Section XIV   Congenital Cardiovascular Diseases
in Pediatrics** **1417**
*Eduardo M. da Cruz, Dunbar Ivy, James Jaggers, and
Viktor Hraska*

80   Spectrum of Congenital Cardiac Defects 1419
Michael S. Schaffer

81   Persistent Arterial Duct 1425
Enrique García, Miguel A. Granados, Mario Fittipaldi, and
Juan V. Comas

82 Atrial Septal Defect 1439
Shellie Kendall, John Karamichalis, Tara Karamlou,
David Teitel, and Gordon Cohen

83 Ventricular Septal Defects 1455
Beatrice Bonello, Virginie Fouilloux, Stephane Le Bel,
Alain Fraisse, Bernard Kreitmann, and Dominique Metras

84 Atrioventricular Septal Defects 1479
Aditya K. Kaza, L. LuAnn Minich, and Lloyd Y. Tani

85 Aortopulmonary Window 1493
Moritz C. Wyler von Ballmoos, Michael Barnes,
Stuart Berger, Michael E. Mitchell, and James S. Tweddell

86 Tetralogy of Fallot 1505
Jennifer S. Nelson, Edward L. Bove, and
Jennifer C. Hirsch-Romano

87 Pulmonary Atresia with Ventricular Septal Defect 1527
Asad A. Shah, John F. Rhodes, Jr., and Robert D. B. Jaquiss

88 Pulmonary Atresia with Intact Ventricular Septum 1543
Mark G. Hazekamp, Adriaan W. Schneider, and
Nico A. Blom

89 Pulmonary Stenosis and Insufficiency 1557
James Jaggers, Cindy Barrett, and Bruce Landeck

90 Congenital Aortic Valve Stenosis and Regurgitation 1577
Viktor Hraška, Joachim Photiadis, Peter Zartner, and
Christoph Haun

91 Sub-aortic Stenosis 1599
Johann Brink and Christian Brizard

92 Supravalvar Aortic Stenosis 1615
Max B. Mitchell and Eduardo M. da Cruz

93 Coarctation of the Aorta 1631
Melissa Lee, Yves d'Udekem, and Christian Brizard

94 Interrupted Aortic Arch 1647
Melissa Lee, Yves d'Udekem, and Christian Brizard

95 Supramitral Stenosis 1659
David Kalfa and Emile Bacha

96 Acquired Mitral Valve Stenosis and Regurgitation 1669
Cécile Tissot, Sanjay Cherian, Shannon Buckvold, and
Afksendyos Kalangos

97 Acquired Tricuspid Stenosis and Regurgitation 1701
Sanjay Cherian, Anuradha Sridhar, Raghavan Subramanyan,
and Afksendyos Kalangos

98 Ebstein Malformation of the Tricuspid Valve: Early Presentation 1717
Christopher J. Knott-Craig and Steven P. Goldberg

Volume 4

99 Ebstein Malformation of the Tricuspid Valve in Children, Adolescents and Young Adults 1729
Joseph A. Dearani, Jose Pedro da Silva,
Luciana Fonseca da Silva, and Sameh M. Said

100 Prosthetic Valves 1751
Peter D. Wearden

101 Biventricular Repair in Patients with a Borderline Left Heart 1765
Christopher W. Baird, Patrick O. Myers, Gerald Marx,
Meena Nathan, Brian T. Kalish, Wayne Tworetzky,
Puja Banka, Sitaram M. Emani, John E. Mayer,
and Pedro J. del Nido

102 Surgical Approaches to the Hypoplastic Left Heart Syndrome 1787
Peter J. Gruber and Thomas L. Spray

103 Peri-operative and Interstage Considerations for the Hybrid Approach for Hypoplastic Left Heart Syndrome 1809
Mark Galantowicz, Andrew Yates, Clifford Cua,
Aymen Naguib, Janet Simsic, and John P. Cheatham

104 Orthotopic Heart Transplantation as an Alternative Treatment Strategy for Hypoplastic Left Heart Syndrome 1825
Scott R. Auerbach, David N. Campbell, and
Shelley D. Miyamoto

105 Cardiac Malpositions and Anomalies of Situs 1843
Shinya Ugaki, Prashant Bobhate, Charissa Pockett, and
Ian Adatia

106 Single Ventricle (Non HLHS) 1861
Puja Banka, Diego Porras, John E. Mayer, and
Sitaram M. Emani

107 Partial and Total Anomalous Pulmonary Venous Connections and Associated Defects 1885
Parth M. Patel, Alexandre T. Rotta, and John W. Brown

108 Pulmonary Vein Stenosis 1905
François Lacour-Gayet, Leo Lopez, Jesse Davidson, and
Eduardo M. da Cruz

109 Simple Transposition of the Great Arteries 1919
Shriprasad Deshpande, Michael J. Wolf, Dennis W. Kim,
and Paul M. Kirshbom

**110 Congenitally Corrected Transposition of the
Great Arteries** 1941
Alain Serraf and James Jaggers

111 Complex Transposition of the Great Arteries 1965
Victor Morell, Alejandro J. López-Magallón,
Nils Welchering, Juliana Torres Pacheco, and
Ricardo Muñoz

112 Truncus Arteriosus 1983
Steve Bibevski, Joshua Friedland-Little, Richard G. Ohye,
Thorsson Thor, and Michael G. Gaies

113 Double Outlet Right Ventricle 2003
François Lacour-Gayet, Leo Lopez, and Eduardo M. da Cruz

**114 Congenital and Acquired Coronary Artery Anomalies
in Newborns, Infants, Children, and Young Adults** 2019
Ali Dodge-Khatami, Constantine Mavroudis, and
Carl L. Backer

Section XV Cardiac Failure and Cardiomyopathies **2043**
Eduardo M. da Cruz and Dunbar Ivy

115 Congestive Heart Failure 2045
Cécile Tissot, Eduardo M. da Cruz, and
Shelley D. Miyamoto

116 Cardiomyopathies and Acute Myocarditis 2063
Brian Feingold and Steven A. Webber

Section XVI Pulmonary Hypertension **2079**
Rolf Berger

**117 Pathology, Pathobiology and Pathophysiology of
Pulmonary Arterial Hypertension** 2081
Marlene Rabinovitch

**118 Animal Models for PAH and Increased Pulmonary
Blood Flow** 2103
Michael G. Dickinson, Beatrijs Bartelds, and
Rolf M. F. Berger

119 Epidemiology of Pediatric Pulmonary Hypertension 2123
Johannes M. Douwes and Rolf M. F. Berger

120 Idiopathic Pulmonary Arterial Hypertension in the Pediatric Age Group 2139
Usha Krishnan and Erika Berman Rosenzweig

121 Pulmonary Hypertension in Congenital Heart Disease 2159
Prashant Bobhate and Ian Adatia

122 Postoperative Pulmonary Hypertension in Children with Congenital Heart Disease 2201
Dunbar Ivy and Eduardo M. da Cruz

Section XVII Systemic Vasculopathies **2217**
Carl L. Backer

123 Vascular Rings and Slings 2219
Carl L. Backer, Andrada R. Popescu, Jeffrey C. Rastatter, and Hyde M. Russell

124 Takayasu Arteritis 2239
Eduardo M. da Cruz, Lorna Browne, Jeffrey R. Darst, Brian Fonseca, and James Jaggers

125 Extracardiac Arteriovenous and Venovenous Malformations 2253
Philippe Durand, Virginie Lambert, Augustin Ozanne, and Stéphanie Franchi-Abella

Section XVIII Acquired Cardiac Diseases **2273**
Philippe Acar

126 Primary and Secondary Cardiac Tumors 2275
Rebecca S. Beroukhim and Tal Geva

127 Prevention of Infective Endocarditis in Patients with Congenital Heart Disease 2297
Sylvie Di Filippo

128 Diagnosis and Management of Infective Endocarditis 2307
Michael G. W. Camitta, Joseph W. St. Geme, III, and Jennifer S. Li

129 Acute Rheumatic Fever and Chronic Rheumatic Disease 2329
Bo Remenyi and Jonathan Carapetis

130 Kawasaki's Disease 2351
Shinichi Takatsuki, Marsha S. Anderson, and Tsutomu Saji

131 Pericardial Diseases 2369
Cécile Tissot

132   **Cardiac Traumatic Lesions in Children**   2395
      Alexandre Cazavet, Hanane Ouald Ali, and
      Bertrand Leobon

133   **Trypanosomiasis and Cardiac Disease**   2407
      Lísia Esper, Fatima Brant, Louis M. Weiss,
      Herbert Bernard Tanowitz, and Fabiana Simão Machado

134   **Endomyocardial Fibrosis**   2421
      Ana Olga H. Mocumbi

135   **Hypereosinophilic Heart Disease**   2439
      Pierre-Emmanuel Séguéla and Philippe Acar

Volume 5

**Section XIX   The Adult With Congenital Cardiac
Defects**   2453
Gary Webb

136   **Controversies in Our Current Decade Surrounding
      the Management of the Adult with Congenital
      Heart Disease**   2455
      Scott Cohen, Peter Bartz, Tejas Shah, and
      Michael G. Earing

137   **Congenital Heart Disease: A Life-Cycle Condition –
      Understanding Demographic Trends and Estimating
      Disease Burden**   2469
      Ariane Marelli

138   **Eisenmenger Syndrome and Other Types of
      Pulmonary Arterial Hypertension Related to
      Congenital Heart Disease**   2481
      Konstantinos Dimopoulos, Matina Prapa, and
      Michael A. Gatzoulis

139   **Arrhythmias, Conduction Disorders and
      Electrophysiological Anomalies in the Adult with
      Congenital Cardiac Disease**   2495
      Jeremy P. Moore, Ravi Mandapati, Kevin Shannon,
      Anjan S. Batra, and Seshadri Balaji

140   **Aortic Coarctation in the Adult**   2521
      Barry A. Love, Gregory W. Fischer, Paul Stelzer, and
      Valentin Fuster

141   **Tetralogy of Fallot in the Adult**   2551
      Massimo Chessa, Alessandro Giamberti, Sara Foresti, and
      Marco Ranucci

142 **Univentricular Heart Physiology and Associated Anomalies in the Adult** 2569
Jamil Aboulhosn, Leigh Reardon, Reshma Biniwale, and Johanna Schwarzenberger

143 **Principles of the Fontan Conversion Operation** 2589
Constantine Mavroudis, Barbara J. Deal, and Carl L. Backer

144 **Late Sequelae in the Adult Patient with Congenital Heart Disease** 2609
Joseph D. Kay and Amber Khanna

145 **Transfer and Transition in Congenital Heart Disease** 2633
Eva Goossens, Adrienne H. Kovacs, Andrew S. Mackie, and Philip Moons

146 **Aortopathy in Adults with Congenital Heart Disease** 2651
Ali N. Zaidi, W. Aaron Kay, and Curt J. Daniels

147 **Pregnancy and Contraception in ACHD Patients** 2669
Rachel M. Wald, Jack M. Colman, Mathew Sermer, Jose C. A. Carvalho, Eric M. Horlick, Nadine Shehata, and Candice K. Silversides

148 **Heart Failure in Adult Congenital Heart Disease** 2695
Joel McLarry and Craig S. Broberg

Section XX   Extracorporeal Life Support (ECLS) of the Cardiac Patient 2713
Heidi Dalton and Paul Bakerman

149 **New and Developing Technologies for Ventricular Assistance** 2715
David Michael McMullan and Jeffrey M. Pearl

150 **Extra-Corporeal Membrane Oxygenation** 2723
Warwick Butt and Shannon Buckvold

151 **Uni and Biventricular Assistance (LVAD-RVAD)** 2755
Brigitte Stiller and Holger Buchholz

152 **Drugs and ECMO** 2767
Julia Stegger, Anne Susen, Christoph Haun, and Hans-Joerg Hertfelder

Section XXI   Heart and Lung Transplant **2781**
Steven Webber

153 **Basic Principles of Transplant Immunology** 2783
     Biagio A. Pietra

154 **Immunosuppressive Medications** 2809
     Donald Berry and Brian Feingold

155 **Heart Transplantation** 2827
     Shelley D. Miyamoto, David N. Campbell, and
     Scott R. Auerbach

156 **Lung and Heart Lung Transplantation** 2851
     Stuart C. Sweet and Charles B. Huddleston

Section XXII   Arrhythmias and Conductive Disorders **2881**
Kathy Collins

157 **Diagnosis of Arrhythmias and Conductive
     Disorders** 2883
     Salim F. Idriss and Ronald J. Kanter

158 **Supraventricular Tachycardias** 2937
     Carolina Escudero, Nico A. Blom, and
     Shubhayan Sanatani

159 **Ventricular Tachycardiac and Sudden
     Arrhythmic Death** 2971
     Georgia Sarquella-Brugada, Oscar Campuzano,
     Antonio Berruezo, and Josep Brugada

160 **Medical Management of Arrhythmias and Conduction
     Disorders** 2999
     Anthony C. McCanta and Kathryn K. Collins

161 **Temporary and Permanent Pacemakers and
     Automated Internal Defibrillators** 3019
     Elizabeth A. Stephenson and Charles I. Berul

162 **Electrophysiology of Heart Failure and Cardiac
     Re-synchronization Therapy** 3049
     Jan Janoušek

163 **Ablation Therapy for Arrhythmias and Conductive
     Disorders** 3063
     Jennifer Silva and George Van Hare

164 Surgical Therapy of Arrhythmias and Conductive
     Disorders 3089
     Constantine Mavroudis, Barbara J. Deal, and
     Carl L. Backer

Volume 6

Section XXIII Upper Airway and Tracheal Pathology 3107
Michael J. Rutter

165 Upper Airway Anomalies 3109
     Alessandro de Alarcón, Aliza P. Cohen, and
     Michael J. Rutter

166 Tracheal Anomalies and Reconstruction 3129
     Michael J. Rutter, Alessandro de Alarcón, and
     Peter B. Manning

Section XXIV Extra-Cardiac Issues and
Complications 3145
Jonathan Kaufman and Steven Choi

167 Mechanical Ventilation, Cardiopulmonary
     Interactions, and Pulmonary Issues in Children
     with Critical Cardiac Disease 3147
     William L. Stigall and Brigham C. Willis

168 Gastrointestinal Complications in the
     Perioperative Period 3183
     James Pierce, Sylvia del Castillo, and Rula Harb

169 Nutrition in Congenital Heart Disease: Challenges,
     Guidelines and Nutritional Support 3201
     Piyagarnt E. Vichayavilas, Heather E. Skillman, and
     Nancy F. Krebs

170 Endocrinological Issues 3213
     Rambod Amirnovin and Grant L. Burton

171 Venous Thromboembolism 3235
     Courtney Lyle and Neil Goldenberg

172 Acute Kidney Injury 3257
     Scott Aydin, Samriti Dogra, and Marcela Del Rio

173 Stroke 3279
     Maryam Y. Naim and Daniel J. Licht

174 Intracranial Hemorrhage 3289
     Dusty M. Richardson and Todd C. Hankinson

175   Neurologic Complications and Neuromonitoring in
      Pediatric Congenital Heart Disease 3299
      Philip Overby

176   Therapeutic Hypothermia After Cardiac Arrest 3309
      Emily L. Dobyns

177   Sepsis and the Cardiac Patient: Diagnosis
      and Management 3321
      Jennifer Exo

178   End of Life: Ethical and Legal Considerations 3337
      Denis Devictor, Mostafa Mokhtari, and Pierre Tissières

179   Quality and Performance Improvement: Challenges
      for the Congenital Heart Center 3351
      Steven Choi and Jonathan Kaufman

Section XXV   Leadership Issues of a Pediatric
Heart Center 3367
David Moromisato and Niurka Rivero

180   Complexity of Caring for Complex Pediatric
      Congenital Heart Disease 3369
      Samuel D. Yanofsky, Randall M. Schell, and Roberta Williams

181   Leadership in a High-Stakes Service Line 3383
      Lara P. Nelson, Barry P. Markovitz, and
      Cynthia Herrington

182   Intersection of Leadership, Organizational Culture,
      and Clinical Performance 3391
      Niurka Rivero, Beth Zemetra, and Cynde Herman

183   Performance Management in a Multidisciplinary
      Service Line 3409
      Jeannine Acantilado, Jacqueline N. Hood, and
      David Moromisato

184   Seven Practices of Highly Resonant Teams 3423
      Jamie Dickey Ungerleider and Ross M. Ungerleider

Section XXVI   Miscellanous 3451
Matthias Siepe

185   Animal Research in Pediatric Cardiology and
      Cardiac Surgery 3453
      Suzanne Osorio-da Cruz, Paul Flecknell, and
      Claire Richardson

186   Patient-Specific Imaging-Based Techniques for
      Optimization of Pediatric Cardiovascular Surgery 3471
      Kiran Dyamenahalli and Robin Shandas

**187 Clinical and Translational Research in Pediatric
      Cardiology and Cardiac Surgery** 3491
      Michael G. Gaies, Sara K. Pasquali, Mark Russell, and
      Richard G. Ohye

**188 Training, Continuous Education and Simulation in
      Pediatric Cardiac Surgery** 3507
      Patrick O. Myers

**189 Soft Skills in Pediatric Cardiology, Cardiac Surgery
      and Cardiac Intensive Care** 3519
      Brigitte Stiller

**190 Psycho-emotional Stress in Pediatric
      Cardiac Units** 3527
      Jeannie Zuk and Ayelet Talmi

**191 Surgical Site Infection in Pediatric Cardiac
      Surgery: Classification, Risk Factors, Prevention
      and Management** 3541
      Faith A. Fisher and James Jaggers

Index 3551

Contributors

Jamil Aboulhosn Ahmanson/UCLA Adult Congenital Heart Disease Center, Division of Cardiology, David Geffen School of Medicine at UCLA, Los Angeles, CA, USA

Jeannine Acantilado Élan Consulting Services, Albany, GA, USA

Philippe Acar Paediatric Cardiology Unit, Children's Hospital – Toulouse University Hospital, Toulouse, France

Ian Adatia Pediatric Cardiac Intensive Care, Pediatric Cardiology, Stollery Children's Hospital, University of Alberta, Mazankowski Alberta Heart Institute, Edmonton, AB, Canada

Jeanne Ahern Staff Nurse III, Cardiac Operating Room, Boston Children's Hospital, Boston, MA, USA

Alessandro de Alarcón Division of Pediatric Otolaryngology–Head and Neck Surgery, Cincinnati Children's Hospital Medical Center, Cincinnati, OH, USA

Department of Otolaryngology–Head and Neck Surgery, University of Cincinnati College of Medicine, Cincinnati, OH, USA

Mazeni Alwi Paediatric Cardiology, Institut Jantung Negara, Kuala Lumpur, Malaysia

Warwick Ames Department of Anesthesiology, Duke University Medical Center, Duke Children's Hospital, Durham, NC, USA

Rambod Amirnovin Department of Anesthesiology Critical Care Medicine, Children's Hospital Los Angeles, Department of Pediatrics, University of Southern California Keck School of Medicine, Los Angeles, CA, USA

Marsha S. Anderson Department of Pediatrics, School of Medicine, University of Colorado, Children's Hospital Colorado, Aurora, CO, USA

Robert H. Anderson Institute of Genetic Medicine, Newcastle University, London, UK

Institute of Child Health, University College Cardiac Unit, London, UK

Dean B. Andropoulos Division of Pediatric Cardiovascular Anesthesiology, Texas Children's Hospital, Houston, TX, USA

Department of Anesthesiology and Pediatrics, Baylor College of Medicine, Houston, TX, USA

Philip Arnold Jackson Rees Department of Paediatric Anaesthesia, Alder Hey Children's Hospital, Liverpool, UK

Andrew M. Atz Department of Pediatrics, Medical University of South Carolina, Charleston, SC, USA

Scott R. Auerbach Division of Pediatric Cardiology, University of Colorado Health Science Center, The Heart Institute, Children's Hospital Colorado, Aurora, CO, USA

Scott Aydin Division of Pediatric Cardiology, Children's Hospital at Montefiore, Albert Einstein College of Medicine, Bronx, NY, USA

Emile Bacha Congenital and Pediatric Cardiac Surgery, Columbia-University, Morgan Stanley Children's Hospital of New York-Presbyterian, New York, NY, USA

Carl L. Backer Pediatric Cardiovascular-Thoracic Surgery, Department of Surgery, Division of Cardiovascular-Surgery, Children's Memorial Hospital, Northwestern University Feinberg School of Medicine, Chicago, IL, USA

Christopher W. Baird Department of Cardiac Surgery, Boston Children's Hospital, Boston, MA, USA

Seshadri Balaji Department of Pediatrics, Division of Cardiology, Oregon Health and Science University, Portland, OR, USA

Simon D. Bamforth Institute of Genetic Medicine, Newcastle University, London, UK

Puja Banka Department of Cardiology, Boston Children's Hospital, Boston, MA, USA

Michael Barnes Cardiothoracic Surgery Department, Children's Hospital of Wisconsin, Milwaukee, WI, USA

Cindy Barrett Division of Pediatric Cardiology, Department of Pediatrics, Childrens Hospital of Colorado, University of Colorado School of Medicine, Aurora, CO, USA

Beatrijs Bartelds Center for Congenital Heart Diseases, devision Pediatric Cardiology, Beatrix Children's Hospital, University Medical Center Groningen, Groningen, The Netherlands

Peter Bartz Wisconsin Adult Congenital Heart Disease Program (WAtCH), Medical College of Wisconsin, Milwaukee, WI, USA

Anjan S. Batra Department of Pediatrics, Division of Cardiology, UC Irvine, Children's Hospital of Orange County, Orange, CA, USA

Dorothy Beke Clinical Nurse Specialist, Cardiac Intensive Care Unit, Boston Children's Hospital, Boston, MA, USA

Stephane Le Bel Pediatric Intensive Care, Children's Hospital La Timone Aix-Marseille University (France), Marseille, France

Lee Benson The Department of Pediatrics, Division of Cardiology, The University of Toronto School of Medicine, The Labatt Family Heart Center, The Hospital for Sick Children, Toronto, ON, Canada

Robert A. Berg Department of Anesthesia and Critical Care, Perelman School of Medicine at the University of Pennsylvania, Philadelphia, PA, USA

Department of Anesthesiology and Critical Care Medicine, The Children's Hospital of Philadelphia, Philadelphia, PA, USA

Rolf M. F. Berger Center for Congenital Heart Diseases, Department of Pediatric Cardiology, Beatrix Children's Hospital, University Medical Center Groningen, University of Groningen, Groningen, The Netherlands

Stuart Berger Department of Pediatrics, Division of Pediatric Cardiology, The Herma Heart Center The Medical College of Wisconsin, Children's Hospital of Wisconsin, Milwaukee, WI, USA

Lisa Bergersen Department of Cardiology, Farley – 2, Boston Children's Hospital, Boston, MA, USA

Darren P. Berman Cardiology, Miami Children's Hospital, Miami, FL, USA

Rebecca S. Beroukhim Pediatric Cardiology, Boston Children's Hospital, Boston, MA, USA

Antonio Berruezo Unit of Arrhythmias, Hospital Clinic de Barcelona, University of Barcelona, Barcelona, Spain

Donald Berry Clinical Pharmacy Specialist, Cardiac Intensive Care, Department of Pharmacy, Children's Hospital of Pittsburgh of UPMC, Pittsburgh, PA, USA

Charles I. Berul Division of Cardiology, Children's National Medical Center, George Washington University School of Medicine, Washington, DC, USA

Steve Bibevski Section of Pediatric Cardiovascular Surgery, Department of Cardiac Surgery, University of Michigan Medical School, Ann Arbor, MI, USA

Reshma Biniwale Division of Cardiothoracic Surgery, David Geffen School of Medicine at UCLA, Los Angeles, CA, USA

Nico A. Blom Department of Cardiothoracic Surgery, Leiden University Medical Center, Leiden and Academic Medical Center, Amsterdam, The Netherlands

Prashant Bobhate Pulmonary Hypertension Clinic, Pediatric Cardiology, and Cardiac Critical Care, Stollery Children's Hospital Mazankowski Alberta Heart Institute, University of Alberta, Edmonton, AB, Canada

Beatrice Bonello Pediatric Cardiology, Children's Hospital La Timone Aix-Marseille University (France), Marseille, France

Philipp Bonhoeffer Fondazione G. Monasterio, Pisa, Italy

Derize Boshoff Pediatric Cardiology, University Hospital Leuven, Leuven, Belgium

Edward L. Bove Department of Cardiac Surgery, University of Michigan Medical School, Ann Arbor, MI, USA

Fatima Brant Department of Biochemistry and Immunology, Institute of Biological Science, Federal University of Minas Gerais, Belo Horizonte, MG, Brazil

Program in Health Sciences: Infectious Diseases and Tropical Medicine, Medical School, Federal University of Minas Gerais, Belo Horizonte, MG, Brazil

Nancy Braudis Clinical Nurse Specialist, Cardiac Intensive Care Unit, Boston Children's Hospital, Boston, MA, USA

Johann Brink Cardiac Surgery, The Royal Children's Hospital, Melbourne, VIC, Australia

Christian Brizard Cardiac Surgery, The Royal Children's Hospital, Melbourne, VIC, Australia

Craig S. Broberg Oregon Health and Sciences University, Portland, OR, USA

Ronald A. Bronicki Cardiac Intensive Care, Texas Children's Hospital, Houston, TX, USA

Baylor College of Medicine, Houston, TX, USA

John W. Brown Riley Hospital for Children at Indiana University Health; Harris B. Shumacker Professor Emeritus of Surgery, Section of Cardiothoracic Surgery, Indiana University School of Medicine, Indianapolis, IN, USA

Loren D. Brown Clinical Educator, Cardiac Catheterization Laboratory, Boston Children's Hospital, Boston, MA, USA

Nigel A. Brown Division of Biomedical Sciences, St. George's University of London, London, UK

Lorna Browne Pediatric Radiology Department, Children's Hospital Colorado, University of Colorado Denver, School of Medicine, Aurora, CO, USA

Josep Brugada Unit of Arrhythmias, Hospital Clinic de Barcelona, University of Barcelona, Barcelona, Spain

Holger Buchholz University of Alberta Hospital, Stollery Children's Hospital, Mazankowski Alberta Heart Institute, Edmonton, AB, Canada

Shannon Buckvold The Heart Institute, Department of Pediatrics, Children's Hospital Colorado, School of Medicine, University of Colorado, Denver, CO, USA

Werner Budts Congenital & Structural Cardiology, University Hospital Leuven, Leuven, Belgium

Kevin Bullock Supervisor, Respiratory Therapy Department, Boston Children's Hospital, Boston, MA, USA

Grant L. Burton Departments of Pediatrics and Critical Care Medicine, Section of Pediatric Cardiac Intensive Care, Medical City Children's Hospital, Dallas, TX, USA

Gianfranco Butera IRCCS, Policlinico San Donato Milanese, Milan, Italy

Warwick Butt Paediatric Intensive Care Unit, Roayl Children's Hospital, The University of Melbourne, Melbourne, VIC, Australia

Ryan J. Butts Medical University of South Carolina, Charleston, SC, USA

Antonio G. Cabrera Baylor College of Medicine/Texas Children's Hospital, Houston, TX, USA

Michael G. W. Camitta Division of Cardiology, Department of Pediatrics, Duke University Medical Center, Durham, NC, USA

David N. Campbell Pediatric Cardiac Surgery, Department of Surgery, University of Colorado Denver Health Science Center, Aurora, CO, USA

Oscar Campuzano Cardiovascular Genetics Center, University of Girona – IdIBGi, Girona, Spain

Jonathan Carapetis Menzies School of Health Research, Charles Darwin University, Darwin, Australia

Pediatric infectious Disease, Telethon Institute for Child Health Research, West Perth, Australia

Michelle Carr Children's Hospital Colorado Anschutz Medical Campus, Aurora, CO, USA

Jose C. A. Carvalho University of Toronto, Mount Sinai Hospital and University Health Network, Toronto, ON, Canada

Sylvia del Castillo Critical Care, USC Keck School of Medicine, Children's Hospital Los Angeles, Los Angeles, CA, USA

Alexandre Cazavet Department of Pediatric Cardiac Surgery, University Children Hospital of Purpan, Toulouse, France

David S. Celermajer Department of Medicine, Sydney Medical School, The University of Sydney, Sydney, Australia

Scott R. Ceresnak Pediatric Electrophysiology, Division of Pediatric Cardiology, Department of Pediatrics, The Children's Hospital at Montefiore and the Albert Einstein College of Medicine, New York, USA

Sarah Chambers Children's Hospital at Montefiore and Albert Einstein College of Medicine, Bronx, NY, USA

John R. Charpie Department of Pediatrics, Congenital Heart Center, University of Michigan, C.S. Mott Children's Hospital, Ann Arbor, MI, USA

Kathryn C. Chatfield Children's Hospital Colorado Anschutz Medical Campus, Aurora, CO, USA

Bill Chaudhry Institute of Genetic Medicine, Newcastle University, London, UK

John P. Cheatham Paediatric Cardiology, The Heart Center, Nationwide Children's Hospital The Ohio State University College of Medicine, Columbus, OH, USA

Andrew L. Cheng Department of Pediatrics, Mattel Children's Hospital University of California, Los Angeles, Los Angeles, CA, USA

Sanjay Cherian Cardiovascular Surgery Service, The University Hospital of Geneva, Geneva, Switzerland

Frontier Lifeline & Dr. K. M. Cherian Heart Foundation, Chennai, India

Massimo Chessa Pediatric and Adult Congenital Heart Center, IRCCS-Policlinico San Donato, San Donato Milanese, Milan, Italy

Steven Choi Division of Cardiology, Children's Hospital at Montefiore, Albert Einstein College of Medicine, Bronx, NY, USA

Nadine Choueiter Department of Pediatrics, Albert Einstein College of Medicine, New York, NY, USA

Devyani Chowdhury LGH Pediatric Specialists, Lancaster, PA, USA

Aliza P. Cohen Division of Pediatric Otolaryngology–Head and Neck Surgery, Cincinnati Children's Hospital Medical Center, Cincinnati, OH, USA

Gordon Cohen Division of Pediatric Cardiac Surgery, UCSF School of Medicine, Benioff Children's Hospital, San Francisco, CA, USA

Meryl S. Cohen Department of Pediatrics, Children's Hospital of Philadelphia, The Cardiac Center, Philadelphia, PA, USA

Scott Cohen Wisconsin Adult Congenital Heart Disease Program (WAtCH), Medical College of Wisconsin, Milwaukee, WI, USA

Kathryn K. Collins Section of Pediatric Cardiology, Electrophysiology, The Heart Institute, Children's Hospital Colorado, University of Colorado Denver, School of Medicine, Aurora, CO, USA

Jack M. Colman Toronto Congenital Cardiac Centre for Adults, Peter Munk Cardiac Centre, University of Toronto, University Health Network, Mount Sinai Hospital, Toronto, ON, Canada

Juan V. Comas Pediatric Heart Institute, Hospital Universitario "12 de Octubre", Madrid, Spain

Andrew C. Cook Institute of Cardiovascular Science, University College, London, UK

Kelli L. Crowley Pediatric Critical Care, School of Pharmacy, University of Pittsburgh, Children's Hospital of Pittsburgh of UPMC, Pittsburgh, PA, USA

Eduardo M. da Cruz The Heart Institute, Department of Pediatrics, Children's Hospital Colorado, University of Colorado School of Medicine, Aurora, CO, USA

Clifford Cua Department of Pediatrics, The Heart Center, Nationwide Children's Hospital The Ohio State University College of Medicine, Columbus, OH, USA

Bettina Cuneo Heart Institute for Children, Advocate Medical Group, Hope Children's Hospital, Oak Lawn, IL, USA

Megan Cusick Nurse Practitioner, Cardiology Pre Procedure Suite, Boston Children's Hospital, Boston, MA, USA

Curt J. Daniels Adult Congenital Heart Disease Program, Nationwide Children's Hospital, The Ohio State University, Columbus, OH, USA

Stephen R. Daniels Department of Pediatrics, University of Colorado School of Medicine and Children's Hospital Colorado, Aurora, CO, USA

Jeffrey R. Darst The Heart Institute, Department of Pediatrics, Children's Hospital Colorado, University of Colorado Denver, School of Medicine, Denver, Aurora, CO, USA

Jesse Davidson The Heart Institute, Department of Pediatrics, Children's Hospital Colorado, University of Colorado Denver, School of Medicine, Aurora, USA

Barbara J. Deal Cardiology, Ann & Robert H Lurie Children's Hospital of Chicago, Northwestern University Feinberg School of Medicine, Chicago, IL, USA

Joseph A. Dearani Section of Cardiovascular Surgery, Mayo Clinic, Rochester, MN, USA

Matthew A. Deardorff The Children's Hospital of Philadelphia, Philadelphia, PA, USA

Marcela Del Rio Division of Pediatric Nephrology, Children's Hospital at Montefiore, Albert Einstein College of Medicine, Bronx, NY, USA

Shriprasad Deshpande Department of Pediatrics, Emory University School of Medicine, Atlanta, GA, USA

Denis Devictor Pediatric Intensive care Unit, Department of research in ethics, Paris Sud-11 University, Assistance Publique-Hôpitaux de Paris, Bicêtre, France

Aaron G. DeWitt Department of Pediatrics, Congenital Heart Center, University of Michigan, C.S. Mott Children's Hospital, Ann Arbor, MI, USA

Bethany Diamond Children's Hospital of Colorado, Aurora, CO, USA

Heather A. Dickerson Baylor College of Medicine/Texas Children's Hospital, Houston, TX, USA

Michael G. Dickinson Center for Congenital Heart Diseases, devision Pediatric Cardiology, Beatrix Children's Hospital, University Medical Center Groningen, Groningen, The Netherlands

Konstantinos Dimopoulos Adult Congenital Heart Centre and Centre for Pulmonary Hypertension, Royal Brompton Hospital and the National Heart & Lung Institute, Imperial College, London, UK

Thomas Bao Do Medical University of South Carolina, Charleston, SC, USA

Emily L. Dobyns Critical Care, Children's Hospital Colorado and University of Colorado at Denver, School of Medicine, Aurora, CO, USA

Ali Dodge-Khatami Division of Pediatric and Congenital Heart Surgery, Batson Children's Hospital, Department of Surgery, University of Mississippi Medical Center, Jackson, MS, USA

Samriti Dogra Division of Pediatric Nephrology, Children's Hospital at Montefiore, Bronx, NY, USA

Johannes M. Douwes Center for Congenital Heart Diseases, Department of Pediatric Cardiology, Beatrix Children's Hospital, University Medical Center Groningen, University of Groningen, Groningen, The Netherlands

Yves d'Udekem Cardiac Surgery, The Royal Children's Hospital, Melbourne, VIC, Australia

Pierre E. Dupont Pediatric Cardiac Bioengineering, Boston Children's Hospital, Boston, MA, USA

Department of Surgery, Harvard Medical School, Boston, MA, USA

Philippe Durand Pediatric Intensive Care Unit, Department of Pediatrics, Hôpitaux Universitaires Paris Sud, site Bicêtre, Assistance Publique Hôpitaux de Paris, Le Kremlin Bicêtre, France

Kiran Dyamenahalli Department of Bioengineering, Anschutz Medical Campus, University of Colorado Denver, Aurora, CO, USA

School of Medicine, Anschutz Medical Campus, University of Colorado Denver, Aurora, CO, USA

Michael G. Earing Wisconsin Adult Congenital Heart Disease Program (WAtCH), Medical College of Wisconsin, Milwaukee, WI, USA

Robert Eckel Department of Medicine, Division of Endocrinology, Diabetes and Metabolism, Division of Cardiology, University of Colorado School of Medicine, Aurora, CO, USA

Cory Ellis The Heart Institute, Children's Hospital Colorado, Aurora, CO, USA

Sitaram M. Emani Department of Cardiology, Boston Children's Hospital, Boston, MA, USA

Carolina Escudero The Division of Pediatric Cardiology, British Columbia Children's Hospital, University of British Columbia, Vancouver, BC, Canada

Lísia Esper Department of Biochemistry and Immunology, Institute of Biological Science, Federal University of Minas Gerais, Belo Horizonte, MG, Brazil

Program in Health Sciences: Infectious Diseases and Tropical Medicine, Medical School, Federal University of Minas Gerais, Belo Horizonte, MG, Brazil

Janine Evans Clinical Nurse Consultant, Royal Children's Hospital, Melbourne Parkville/Victoria, Australia

Jennifer Exo Section of Pediatric Critical Care, Children's Hospital Colorado, Aurora, CO, USA

Thomas E. Fagan Paediatric Cardiology, Children's Hospital, Denver, CO, USA

John Fantegrossi Nurse Practitioner, Cardiology Pre Procedure Suite, Boston Children's Hospital, Boston, MA, USA

Brian Feingold Heart Failure and Cardiac Transplantation, Children's Hospital of Pittsburgh of UPMC, School of Medicine, University of Pittsburgh, Pittsburgh, PA, USA

Sylvie Di Filippo Department of Pediatric and Congenital Heart Disease, Cardiovascular Hospital Louis Pradel, Lyon, France

Gregory W. Fischer Department of Anesthesia, Mount Sinai Medical Center, New York, NY, USA

Faith A. Fisher School of Medicine, Children's Hospital of Colorado, University of Colorado, Aurora, CO, USA

Mario Fittipaldi Pediatric Heart Institute, Hospital Universitario "12 de Octubre", Madrid, Spain

Ryan Flanagan CHP Department of Pediatric Cardiology, Medical Corps US Army, Washington, DC, USA

Paul Flecknell Comparative Biology Centre, The Medical School, University of Newcastle, Newcastle upon Tyne, UK

Alejandro A. Floh Department of Critical Care Medicine, Labatt Family Heart Centre, The Hospital for Sick Children, Toronto, ON, Canada

Joseph T. Flynn Division of Nephrology, Seattle Children's Hospital, Seattle, WA, USA

Pediatrics, University of Washington School of Medicine, Seattle, WA, USA

Brian Fonseca The Heart Institute, Department of Pediatrics, Children's Hospital Colorado, University of Colorado Denver, School of Medicine, Denver, Aurora, CO, USA

Pediatric Radiology Department, Children's Hospital Colorado, University of Colorado Denver, School of Medicine, Aurora, CO, USA

Sara Foresti Arrhythmia and Electrophysiology Center, IRCCS- Policlinico San Donato, San Donato Milanese, Milan, Italy

Virginie Fouilloux Cardiothoracic Surgery, Children's Hospital La Timone Aix-Marseille University (France), Marseille, France

Alain Fraisse Pediatric Cardiology, Children's Hospital La Timone Aix-Marseille University (France), Marseille, France

Stéphanie Franchi-Abella Pediatric Radiology, Hôpitaux Universitaires Paris Sud, site Bicêtre, Assistance Publique Hôpitaux de Paris, Le Kremlin Bicêtre, France

Heather Freeman Lucile Packard Children's Hospital at Stanford, Palo Alto, CA, USA

Joshua Friedland-Little Division of Pediatric Cardiology, Department of Pediatrics and Communicable Disease, University of Michigan Medical School, Ann Arbor, MI, USA

Alessandra Frigiola UCLH, The Heart Hospital, London, UK

Valentin Fuster Division of Cardiology, Mount Sinai Medical Center, New York, NY, USA

Michael G. Gaies Division of Pediatric Cardiology, Department of Pediatrics and Communicable Diseases, University of Michigan Medical School, Ann Arbor, MI, USA

Mark Galantowicz Paediatric Cardiology, Heart Center, Nationwide Children's Hospital, Columbus, OH, USA

Department of Cardiothoracic Surgery, The Heart Center, Nationwide Children's Hospital The Ohio State University College of Medicine, Columbus, OH, USA

Enrique García Pediatric Heart Institute, Hospital Universitario "12 de Octubre", Madrid, Spain

Michael A. Gatzoulis Adult Congenital Heart Centre and Centre for Pulmonary Hypertension, Royal Brompton Hospital and the National Heart & Lung Institute, Imperial College, London, UK

Kimberlee Gauvreau Department of Cardiology, Farley – 2, Boston Children's Hospital, Boston, MA, USA

Joseph W. St. Geme, III Division of Infectious Diseases, Department of Pediatrics, Duke University Medical Center, Durham, NC, USA

Cecila St. George-Hyslop Advanced Nursing Practice Educator, Hospital for Sick Children, Canada, Toronto, ON, Canada

Welton M. Gersony Division of Pediatric Cardiology, Columbia University and the Morgan Stanley Children's Hospital of New York Presbyterian, New York, NY, USA

Tal Geva Department of Cardiology, Boston Children's Hospital, Boston, MA, USA

Marc Gewillig UZ Leuven, Leuven, Belgium

Nancy S. Ghanayem Departments of Pediatrics (Critical Care Medicine), Medical College of Wisconsin and Herma Heart Center at Children's Hospital of Wisconsin, Milwaukee, WI, USA

Alessandro Giamberti Cardio-Thoracic Surgery–Pediatric and Adult Congenital Heart Center, IRCCS- Policlinico San Donato, San Donato Milanese, Milan, Italy

Deborah Gilbert Nurse Practioner Cardiac Surgery, Children's Hospital of Colorado, Aurora, CO, USA

Steven P. Goldberg Pediatric Cardiothoracic Surgery, University of Tennessee Health Science Center, Le Bonheur Children's Hospital, Memphis, TN, USA

Neil Goldenberg Departments of Pediatrics and Medicine, Divisions of Hematology, Johns Hopkins University School of Medicine, Baltimore, MD, USA

Eva Goossens Centre for Health Services and Nursing Research, KU Leuven, Leuven, Belgium

Miguel A. Granados Pediatric Heart Institute, Hospital Universitario "12 de Octubre", Madrid, Spain

Peter J. Gruber Primary Children's Medical Center, Salt Lake City, UT, USA

Division of Cardiothoracic Surgery, University of Utah, Salt Lake City, UT, USA

Yong Mein Guan Head Nurse, Cardiac Intensive Care Unit, Shanghai Children's Medical Center, Pudong, Shanghai, China

Todd C. Hankinson Neurosurgery, Children's Hospital Colorado B330, Aurora, CO, USA

Rula Harb USC Keck School of Medicine, Children's Hospital Los Angeles, Los Angeles, CA, USA

George Van Hare Division of Pediatric Cardiology, St. Louis Children's Hospital, Washington University School of Medicine, Saint Louis, MO, USA

Christoph Haun Neonatal and Pediatric Cardiac Intensive Care, German Pediatric Heart Center, Sankt Augustin, Germany

Mark G. Hazekamp Leiden University Medical Center, Leiden, The Netherlands

Departments of Cardiothoracic Surgery, Leiden University Medical Center, Leiden and Academic Medical Center, Amsterdam, The Netherlands

David Hehir Department of Pediatics, Division of Critical Care, Children's Hospital of Wisconsin, Medical College of Wisconsin, Milwaukee, WI, USA

Deborah J. Henderson Institute of Genetic Medicine, Newcastle University, London, UK

Cynde Herman Leadership and Organizational Effectiveness, Children's Hospital Los Angeles, Los Angeles, CA, USA

Cynthia Herrington Department of Surgery, Keck USC School of Medicine, Los Angeles, USA

Hans-Joerg Hertfelder Clinical Haemostasis Unit, Institute of Exp. Haematology and Transfusion Medicine, University Hospital Bonn, Bonn, Germany

Kevin Hill Division of Pediatric Cardiology, Duke University Medical Center, Duke Clinical Research Institute, Durham, NC, USA

Jennifer C. Hirsch-Romano Department of Cardiac Surgery, University of Michigan Medical School, Ann Arbor, MI, USA

Anthony J. Hlavacek Division of Pediatric Cardiology, Medical University of South Carolina, Charleston, SC, USA

George M. Hoffman Departments of Anesthesiology and Pediatrics (Critical Care Medicine), Medical College of Wisconsin and Herma Heart Center at Children's Hospital of Wisconsin, Milwaukee, WI, USA

Ralf J. Holzer Paediatric Cardiology, Heart Center, Nationwide Children's Hospital, Columbus, OH, USA

Department of Paediatric Cardiology, The Heart Center, Nationwide Children's Hospital The Ohio State University College of Medicine, Columbus, OH, USA

Jacqueline N. Hood The University of New Mexico, The Robert O. Anderson School and Graduate School of Management, Albuquerque, NM, USA

Eric M. Horlick Toronto Congenital Cardiac Centre for Adults, Peter Munk Cardiac Centre, University of Toronto, University Health Network, Toronto, ON, Canada

Lisa K. Hornberger Fetal & Neonatal Cardiology Program, Pediatric Cardiology, Stollery Children's Hospital, Edmonton, AB, Canada

Women's & Children's Health Research Institute, University of Alberta Mazankowski Alberta Heart Institute, Edmonton, Canada

Richard F. Howard Department of Anesthesia and Pain Medicine, Great Ormond Street Hospital for Children, London, UK

Lisa Howley School of Medicine, The Heart Institute, Department of Pediatrics, Children's Hospital Colorado, University of Colorado at Denver, Aurora, CO, USA

Denise L. Howrie Department of Pharmacy Services, Children's Hospital of Pittsburgh, University of Pittsburgh School of Pharmacy & Medicine, Pittsburgh, PA, USA

Viktor Hraška German Pediatric Heart Center, Asklepios Clinic Sankt Augustin, Sankt Augustin, Germany

Daphne T. Hsu Division of Pediatric Cardiology, Children's Hospital at Montefiore and the Albert Einstein College of Medicine, Bronx, NY, USA

Charles B. Huddleston Department of Surgery, St. Louis University School of Medicine, St. Louis, MO, USA

S. Adil Husain Department of Cardiothoracic Surgery, Division of Pediatric Cardiothoracic Surgery, Cardiothoracic Fellowship Training Program, University of Texas Health Sciences Center, San Antonio, TX, USA

Salim F. Idriss Pediatric Cardiology and Electrophysiology, Duke University School of Medicine, Durham, NC, USA

Frank F. Ing Paediatric Cardiology, Children's Hospital Los Angeles, University of Southern California, Los Angeles, TX, USA

Richard J. Ing Department of Anesthesiology, Children's Hospital Colorado & University of Colorado Anschutz Medical Campus, Aurora, CO, USA

Dunbar Ivy Children's Hospital Colorado, Aurora, CO, USA

Jeffrey P. Jacobs All Children's Hospital, The Congenital Heart Institute of Florida (CHIF), Saint Petersburg, FL, USA

Department of Surgery, University of South Florida (USF), Saint Petersburg, FL, USA

James Jaggers The Heart Institute, Department of Pediatrics, Children's Hospital Colorado, University of Colorado School of Medicine, Denver, Aurora, CO, USA

Cardiothoracic Surgery, University of Colorado School of Medicine The Children's Hospital Pediatrics, Aurora, CO, USA

Jan Janoušek Children's Heart Center, University Hospital Motol, Prague, Czech Republic

Robert D. B. Jaquiss Section of Pediatric Cardiac Surgery, Duke Children's Hospital & Duke University School of Medicine, Durham, NC, USA

John L. Jefferies Pediatric Cardiology and Adult Cardiovascular Diseases, The Heart Institute, Cincinnati Children's Hospital Medical Center, Cincinnati, OH, USA

Kathy Jenkins Department of Cardiology, Farley – 2, Boston Children's Hospital, Boston, MA, USA

Caroline B. Jones Fetal Cardiology Unit, Department of Congenital Heart Disease, Evelina Children's Hospital, Guy's and St. Thomas' NHS Trust, London, UK

Edmund H. Jooste Department of Anesthesiology, Duke University Medical Center, Duke Children's Hospital, Durham, NC, USA

Afksendyos Kalangos Cardiovascular Surgery Service, The University Hospital of Geneva, Geneva, Switzerland

David Kalfa Congenital and Pediatric Cardiac Surgery, Columbia University, Morgan Stanley Children's Hospital of New York-Presbyterian, New York, NY, USA

Brian T. Kalish Harvard Medical School, Boston, MA, USA

Ronald J. Kanter Pediatric Cardiology and Electrophysiology, Duke University School of Medicine, Durham, NC, USA

John Karamichalis Division of Pediatric Cardiac Surgery, UCSF School of Medicine, Benioff Children's Hospital, San Francisco, CA, USA

Tara Karamlou Division of Pediatric Cardiac Surgery, UCSF School of Medicine, Benioff Children's Hospital, San Francisco, CA, USA

Lindsey Katzmark Nurse Practitioner, Adult Congenital Heart Disease Progam, Children's Hospital of Wisconsin, Medical College of Wisconsin, Wauwatosa, WI, USA

Jonathan Kaufman The Heart Institute, Department of Pediatrics, Children's Hospital Colorado, University of Colorado Denver, School of Medicine, Aurora, CO, USA

W. Aaron Kay Adult Congenital Heart Disease Program, Nationwide Children's Hospital, The Ohio State University, Columbus, OH, USA

Joseph D. Kay University of Colorado School of Medicine, Aurora, CO, USA

Aditya K. Kaza Section of Pediatric Cardiothoracic Surgery, Department of Surgery, University of Utah School of Medicine, Salt Lake City, UT, USA

Aaron S. Kelly Department of Pediatrics, University of Minnesota, Minneapolis, MN, USA

Shellie Kendall Division of Pediatric Cardiology, UCSF School of Medicine, Benioff Children's Hospital, San Francisco, CA, USA

Amber Khanna University of Colorado School of Medicine, Aurora, CO, USA

Dennis W. Kim Department of Pediatrics, Emory University School of Medicine, Atlanta, GA, USA

Thomas R. Kimball Cincinnati Children's Hospital Medical Center, Cincinnati, OH, USA

Kelly Kirby Heart Rhythm Service, Lucile Packard Children's Hospital at Stanford, Palo Alto, CA, USA

Edward Kirkpatrick Department of Pediatics, Children's Hospital of Wisconsin Medical College of Wisconsin, Milwaukee, WI, USA

Paul M. Kirshbom Department of Surgery, Yale School of Medicine and Connecticut Children's Medical Center, New Haven, CT, USA

Christopher J. Knott-Craig Pediatric Cardiothoracic Surgery, University of Tennessee Health Science Center, Le Bonheur Children's Hospital, Memphis, TN, USA

Joshua Kovach Department of Pediatrics, Children's Hospital of Wisconsin, The Medical College of Wisconsin, Milwaukee, WI, USA

Adrienne H. Kovacs Toronto Congenital Cardiac Center for Adults, Peter Munk Cardiac Centre, University Health Network, University of Toronto, Toronto, ON, Canada

Catherine Krawczeski Department of Pediatics, The Heart Institute, Cincinnati Children's Hospital Medical Center, University of Cincinnati, Cincinnati, OH, USA

Nancy F. Krebs Department of Clinical Nutrition, Children's Hospital Colorado B270, Aurora, CO, USA

Section of Nutrition, Department of Pediatrics, University of Colorado School of Medicine, Aurora, USA

Bernard Kreitmann Cardiothoracic Surgery, Children's Hospital La Timone Aix-Marseille University (France), Marseille, France

Usha Krishnan Department of Pediatrics, Columbia University College of Physicians and Surgeons, New York, NY, USA

François Lacour-Gayet Children's Hospital at Montefiore, Albert Einstein College of Medicine, New York, USA

Cardiovascular and Thoracic Surgery, Montefiore Medical Center, Bronx, New York, USA

Terra Lafranchi Fetal Cardiology Coordinator, Nurse Practitioner, Advanced Fetal Care Center, Boston Children's Hospital, Boston, MA, USA

Virginie Lambert Department of Pediatric Cardiac Surgery, Centre Chirurgical Marie Lannelongue, Le Plessis Robinson, France

Bruce Landeck Division of Pediatric Cardiology, Department of Pediatrics, Childrens Hospital of Colorado, University of Colorado School of Medicine, Aurora, CO, USA

Scott Lawson Department of Circulatory Support, The Heart Institute, Children's Hospital Colorado, Aurora, CO, USA

Melissa Lee Cardiac Surgery, The Royal Children's Hospital, Melbourne, VIC, Australia

Bertrand Leobon Cardiac Surgery, Hôpital des enfants, Toulouse, France

Elizabeth Leonard Critical and Cardiorespiratory Unit, Great Ormond Street Hospital for Children NHS Foundation Trust, London, England, UK

Ming Chern Leong Paediatric Cardiology, Institut Jantung Negara, Kuala Lumpur, Malaysia

Daniel S. Levi Division of Pediatric Cardiology, Mattel Children's Hospital University of California, Los Angeles, Los Angeles, CA, USA

Jennifer S. Li Division of Cardiology, Department of Pediatrics, Duke University Medical Center, Durham, NC, USA

Daniel J. Licht Department of Neurology, Department of Pediatrics, The University of Pennsylvania Perelman School of Medicine, and The Children's Hospital of Philadelphia, Philadelphia, PA, USA

Kyle Lieppman Department of Critical Care Medicine, Labatt Family Heart Centre, The Hospital for Sick Children, Toronto, ON, Canada

Aileen Lin Heart Failure Program, Lucile Packard Children's Hospital at Stanford, Palo Alto, CA, USA

Patricia Lincoln Clinical Nurse Specialist, Cardiac Intensive Care Unit, Boston Children's Hospital, Boston, MA, USA

Esther Liu Heart Failure Program, Lucile Packard Children's Hospital at Stanford, Palo Alto, CA, USA

Leo Lopez Children's Hospital at Montefiore, Albert Einstein College of Medicine, New York, USA

Cardiovascular and Thoracic Surgery, Medical Center, Bronx, NY, USA

Alejandro J. López-Magallón Pediatric Critical Care Division, Cardiac Intensive Care unit, University of Pittsburgh, Children's Hospital of Pittsburgh of UPMC, Pittsburgh, PA, USA

Angela Lorts Department of Pediatics, The Heart Institute, Cincinnati Children's Hospital Medical Center, University of Cincinnati, Cincinnati, OH, USA

Barry A. Love From the Division of Pediatric Cardiology, Mount Sinai Medical Center, New York, NY, USA

George Lui Medical Director, Adult Congential Heart Program at Stanford, Medicine/Cardiology, Clinial Assistant Professor of Medicine, Stanford University School of Medicine, Stanford, CA, USA

Wenyi Luo Clinical Staff Nurse, Cardiac Intensive Care Unit, Shanghai Children's Medical Center, Pudong, Shanghai, China

Courtney Lyle Department of Pediatrics, Division of Hematology/Oncology, Billings Clinic, Billings, MT, USA

Fabiana Simão Machado Department of Biochemistry and Immunology, Institute of Biological Science, Federal University of Minas Gerais, Belo Horizonte, MG, Brazil

Program in Health Sciences: Infectious Diseases and Tropical Medicine, Medical School, Federal University of Minas Gerais, Belo Horizonte, MG, Brazil

Andrew S. Mackie Division of Cardiology, Stollery Children's Hospital and Department of Pediatrics, University of Alberta, Edmonton, Alberta, Canada

William Mahle Emory University and Children's Hospital of Atlanta, Atlanta, GA, USA

Ravi Mandapati UCLA Cardiac Arrhythmia Center, UCLA Health System, University of California at Los Angeles, UCLA, Los Angeles, CA, USA

Peter B. Manning Division of Pediatric Cardiothoracic Surgery, Saint Louis Children's Hospital, Washington University School of Medicine, St. Louis, MO, USA

Ariane Marelli McGill Adult Unit for Congenital Heart Disease (MAUDE Unit), McGill University, McGill University Health Center, Montreal, QC, Canada

Barry P. Markovitz Division of Critical Care Medicine, Keck USC School of Medicine, Los Angeles, USA

Hugo R. Martinez Department of Pediatrics, University of Texas Medical Branch, Galveston, TX, USA

Gerald Marx Department of Cardiology, Boston Children's Hospital, Boston, MA, USA

Constantine Mavroudis Congenital Heart Institute, Walt Disney Pavilion, Florida Hospital for Children, Orlando, FL, USA

John E. Mayer Department of Cardiac Surgery, Boston Children's Hospital, Boston, MA, USA

Anthony C. McCanta Section of Pediatric Cardiology, Electrophysiology, The Heart Institute, Children's Hospital Colorado, University of Colorado Denver, School of Medicine, Aurora, CO, USA

Joel McLarry Oregon Health and Sciences University, Portland, OR, USA

David Michael McMullan University of Washington School of Medicine, Seattle Children's Hospital, Seattle, WA, USA

Craig McRobb The Heart Institute, Children's Hospital Colorado, Aurora, CO, USA

Jeff Meadows Department of Cardiology, Boston Children's Hospital, Boston, MA, USA

Brian Mejak Department of Perfusion, Heart Institute, Children's Hospital Colorado, Aurora, CO, USA

Michael Mendelson Department of Cardiology, Hospital for Sick Children, Toronto, ON, Canada

Dominique Metras Cardiothoracic Surgery, Children's Hospital La Timone Aix-Marseille University (France), Marseille, France

L. LuAnn Minich Division of Pediatric Cardiology, Department of Pediatrics, University of Utah School of Medicine, Salt Lake City, UT, USA

Michael E. Mitchell Department of Cardiothoracic Surgery, Children's Hospital of Wisconsin, Milwaukee, WI, USA

Max B. Mitchell Department of Surgery, Heart Institute, The Children's Hospital Colorado, University of Colorado at Denver, School of Medicine, Aurora, CO, USA

Alexander Mittnacht Anesthesiology, Icahn School of Medicine at Mount Sinai, New York, NY, USA

Shelley D. Miyamoto The Heart Institute, Department of Pediatrics, University of Colorado Denver, Children's Hospital Colorado, School of Medicine, Aurora, CO, USA

Ana Olga H. Mocumbi Instituto Nacional de Saúde and Universidade Eduardo Mondlane, Maputo, Moçambique

Timothy J. Mohun National Institute for Medical Research, London, UK

Mostafa Mokhtari Pediatric Intensive care Unit, Department of research in ethics, Paris Sud-11 University, Assistance Publique-Hôpitaux de Paris, Bicêtre, France

Anita J. Moon-Grady Fetal Cardiovascular Program, Department of Pediatrics, Division of Cardiology, University of California, San Francisco, CA, USA

Philip Moons Centre for Health Services and Nursing Research, KU Leuven, Leuven, Belgium

Division of Congenital and Structural Cardiology, University Hospitals Leuven, Leuven, Belgium

The Heart Centre, Rigshospitalet, Copenhagen University Hospital, Copenhagen, Denmark

Jeremy P. Moore Department of Pediatrics, Division of Pediatric Cardiology, UCLA, Los Angeles, CA, USA

Antoon F. M. Moorman Department of Anatomy and Embryology, Academic Medical Center, University of Amsterdam, Amsterdam, The Netherlands

Victor Morell Division of Pediatric Cardiothoracic, University of Pittsburgh School of Medicine, Pittsburgh, PA, USA

David Moromisato Children's Hospital Los Angeles University of Southern California Keek School of Medicine, Los Angeles, CA, USA

Debra Morrow Cardiac Intensive Care Unit, Boston Children's Hospital, Boston, MA, USA

Ricardo Muñoz Division of Pediatric Cardiology, Children's Hospital of Pittsburgh of UPMC, Pittsburgh, PA, USA

Horia Muresian Cardiovascular Surgery Department, The University Hospital of Bucharest, Bucharest, Romania

Patrick O. Myers Division of Cardiovascular Surgery, Geneva University Hospitals & School of Medicine, Geneva, Switzerland

Department of Cardiac Surgery, Boston Children's Hospital and Harvard Medical School, Boston, MA, USA

Vinay M. Nadkarni Department of Anesthesia and Critical Care, Perelman School of Medicine at the University of Pennsylvania, Philadelphia, PA, USA

Center for Simulation, Advanced Education and Innovation, The Children's Hospital of Philadelphia, Philadelphia, PA, USA

Aymen Naguib Department of Anesthesia, The Heart Center, Nationwide Children's Hospital The Ohio State University College of Medicine, 43207, Columbus, OH, USA

Maryam Y. Naim Department of Anesthesia and Critical Care, Perelman School of Medicine at the University of Pennsylvania, Philadelphia, PA, USA

Department of Anesthesiology and Critical Care Medicine, The Children's Hospital of Philadelphia, Philadelphia, PA, USA

Meena Nathan Department of Cardiology, Farley – 2, Boston Children's Hospital, Boston, MA, USA

Jennifer S. Nelson Department of Cardiac Surgery, University of Michigan Medical School, Ann Arbor, MI, USA

Lara P. Nelson Division of Critical Care Medicine, Keck USC School of Medicine, Los Angeles, USA

Pedro J. del Nido Department of Cardiac Surgery, Boston Children's Hospital, Boston, MA, USA

Michelle Ogawa Pulmonary Hypertension Program, Lucile Packard Children's Hospital at Stanford, Palo Alto, CA, USA

Richard G. Ohye Division of Cardiology, Department of Pediatrics, and Duke Clinical Research Institute, Duke University School of Medicine, Duke University Medical Center, Ann Arbor, MI, USA

Yoshio Ootaki Pediatric Cardiothoracic Surgery, Wake Forest Baptist Health/Brenner Children's Hospital, Winston-Salem, NC, USA

Suzanne Osorio-da Cruz Department of Pediatrics, Children's Hospital Colorado University of Colorado Denver & Health Sciences Center Denver, Aurora, CO, USA

Hanane Ouald Ali Department of Pediatric Cardiac Surgery, University Children Hospital of Purpan, Toulouse, France

Philip Overby Neurology, Children's Hospital at Montefiore and Albert Einstein College of Medicine, Bronx, NY, USA

Augustin Ozanne Interventional Neuroradiology and Centre de Référence des Maladies Neurovasculaires Malformatives de l'Enfant, Hôpitaux Universitaires Paris Sud, site Bicêtre, Assistance Publique Hôpitaux de Paris, Le Kremlin Bicêtre, France

Juliana Torres Pacheco Pediatric Cardiology, Pediatric Critical Care Medicine, Beneficência Portuguesa Hospital, São Paulo, SP, Brazil

Sara K. Pasquali Division of Cardiology, Department of Pediatrics, and Duke Clinical Research Institute, Duke University School of Medicine, Duke University Medical Center, Durham, NC, USA

Robert H. Pass Pediatric Electrophysiology, Division of Pediatric Cardiology, Department of Pediatrics, The Children's Hospital at Montefiore and the Albert Einstein College of Medicine, New York, USA

Parth M. Patel Indiana University School of Medicine, Indianapolis, IN, USA

Jeffrey M. Pearl University of Arizona College of Medicine–Phoenix, Phoenix, AZ, USA

Cardiothoracic Surgery, Phoenix Children's Hospital, Phoenix, AZ, USA

Mayo Clinic Hospital, Scottsdale, AZ, USA

Daniel J. Penny Cardiac Intensive Care, Texas Children's Hospital, Houston, TX, USA

Department of Cardiology, Texas Children's Hospital, Houston, TX, USA

Baylor College of Medicine, Houston, TX, USA

Christine Peyton Cardiac Intensive Care Unit, Clinical Nurse Specialist, Children's Hospital Colorado, Aurora, CO, USA

Joachim Photiadis German Pediatric Heart Center, Asklepios Clinic Sankt Augustin, Sankt Augustin, Germany

James Pierce Pediatric General Surgery, USC Keck School of Medicine, Children's Hospital Los Angeles, Los Angeles, CA, USA

Biagio A. Pietra The Heart Institute, Department of Pediatrics, Children's Hospital Colorado, Aurora, CO, USA

Department of Pediatrics, Division of Cardiology, University of Colorado Health Sciences Center, Aurora, CO, USA

Charissa Pockett Pediatric Cardiology, Stollery Children's Hospital, University of Alberta, Mazankowski Alberta Heart Institute, Edmonton, AB, Canada

Emily Polischuk Department of Pharmacy, Children's Hospital of Pittsburgh of UPMC, Pittsburgh, PA, USA

Andrada R. Popescu Division of Medical Imaging, Ann & Robert H. Lurie Children's Hospital of Chicago, Chicago, IL, USA

Diego Porras Department of Cardiology, Boston Children's Hospital, Boston, MA, USA

Matina Prapa Adult Congenital Heart Centre and Centre for Pulmonary Hypertension, Royal Brompton Hospital and the National Heart & Lung Institute, Imperial College, London, UK

Elizabeth Price Pediatric Cardiovascular Intensive Care Unit, Lucile Packard Children's Hospital at Stanford, Palo Alto, CA, USA

Sherry Pye Pediatric heart Transplant Coordinator, Department of Pediatric Cardiology, University of Arkansas for Medical Sciences, Arkansas Children's Hospital, Little Rock, AR, USA

Marlene Rabinovitch Department of Pediatrics, Stanford University School of Medicine, Stanford, CA, USA

Otto Rahkonen The Department of Pediatrics, Division of Cardiology, The University of Toronto School of Medicine, The Labatt Family Heart Center, The Hospital for Sick Children, Toronto, ON, Canada

Marco Ranucci Cardio-Thoracic Anesthesia and ICU, IRCCS- Policlinico San Donato, San Donato Milanese, Milan, Italy

Jeffrey C. Rastatter Division of Otolaryngology, Ann & Robert H. Lurie Children's Hospital of Chicago, Chicago, IL, USA

Ellen Rawlinson Department of Anesthesia and Pain Medicine, Great Ormond Street Hospital for Children, London, UK

Leigh Reardon Ahmanson/UCLA Adult Congenital Heart Disease Center, Division of Cardiology, David Geffen School of Medicine at UCLA, Los Angeles, CA, USA

Andrew Redington Department of Cardiology, Hospital for Sick Children, Toronto, ON, Canada

Bo Remenyi Menzies School of Health Research, Charles Darwin University, Darwin, Australia

Jonathan Rhodes Harvard Medical School, Children's Hospital Boston, Boston, MA, USA

John F. Rhodes, Jr. The Heart Program at Miami Children's Hospital, Miami, FL, USA

Claire Richardson Medical School, Framlington Place, Institute for Neuroscience Henry Wellcome Building, Newcastle upon Tyne, UK

Dusty M. Richardson Neurosurgery, Children's Hospital Colorado B330, Aurora, CO, USA

Niurka Rivero Division of Critical Care Medicine, Children's Hospital Los Angeles, USC Keck School of Medicine, Los Angeles, CA, USA

Cesar Rodriguez-Diaz Icahn School of Medicine at Mount Sinai, New York, NY, USA

Erika Berman Rosenzweig Department of Pediatrics, Columbia University College of Physicians and Surgeons, New York, NY, USA

Joseph W. Rossano Department of Pediatrics, Perelman School of Medicine at the University of Pennsylvania, Philadelphia, PA, USA

The Cardiac Center, The Children's Hospital of Philadelphia, Philadelphia, PA, USA

Alexandre T. Rotta Riley Hospital for Children at Indiana University Health; Indiana University School of Medicine, Indianapolis, IN, USA

Mary Rummell Clinical Nurse Specialist, Pediatric Cardiology, Doernbecher Children's Hospital, Oregon Health & Science University, Portland, OR, USA

Hyde M. Russell Division of Cardiovascular–Thoracic Surgery, Ann & Robert H. Lurie Children's Hospital of Chicago, Chicago, IL, USA

Northwestern University Feinberg School of Medicine, Chicago, IL, USA

Mark Russell Division of Pediatric Cardiology, Department of Pediatrics and Communicable Diseases, University of Michigan Medical School, Ann Arbor, MI, USA

Michael J. Rutter Division of Pediatric Otolaryngology–Head and Neck Surgery, Cincinnati Children's Hospital Medical Center, Cincinnati, OH, USA

Department of Otolaryngology–Head and Neck Surgery, University of Cincinnati College of Medicine, Cincinnati, OH, USA

Jack Rychik Pediatrics, Fetal Heart Program, The Cardiac Center, The Children's Hospital of Philadelphia Cardiology, Philadelphia, PA, USA

Pereleman School of Medicine, The University of Pennsylvania, Philadelphia, PA, USA

Sameh M. Said Division of Cardiovascular Surgery, Mayo Clinic, Rochester, MN, USA

Tsutomu Saji Department of Pediatrics, Toho University Omori Medical Center, Tokyo, Japan

Shubhayan Sanatani The Division of Pediatric Cardiology, British Columbia Children's Hospital, University of British Columbia, Vancouver, BC, Canada

Georgia Sarquella-Brugada Unit of Arrhythmias, Hospital Sant Joan de Déu, University of Barcelona, Barcelona, Spain

Michael S. Schaffer Cardiology, Heart Institute, University of Colorado School of Medicine, Children's Hospital Colorado, Aurora, CO, USA

Randall M. Schell Department of Anesthesiology, University of Kentucky Chandler Medical Center, Lexington, KY, USA

Myles S. Schiller Children's Hospital at Montefiore, Albert Einstein College of Medicine, Bronx, NY, USA

Adriaan W. Schneider Departments of Cardiothoracic Surgery, Leiden University Medical Center, Leiden and Academic Medical Center, Amsterdam, The Netherlands

Margaret Schroeder Nurse Practitioner Inpatient Cardiology, Boston Children's Hospital, Boston, MA, USA

Lawrence I. Schwartz Department of Anesthesiology, Children's Hospital Colorado & University of Colorado Anschutz Medical Campus, Aurora, CO, USA

Steven M. Schwartz Department of Critical Care Medicine, Labatt Family Heart Centre, The Hospital for Sick Children, Toronto, ON, Canada

Johanna Schwarzenberger Department of Anesthesiology, David Geffen School of Medicine at UCLA, Los Angeles, CA, USA

Mathew Sermer University of Toronto, Mount Sinai Hospital and University Health Network, Toronto, ON, Canada

Alain Serraf Department of Congenital Heart Surgery, Marie Lannelongue Hospital, University Paris-Sud, Le Plessis-Robinson, France

Pierre-Emmanuel Séguéla Service de Cardiologie Pédiatrique et Congénitale, Hôpital Haut Lévèque – CHU de Bordeaux, Pessac, France

Asad A. Shah Duke University Medical Center, Durham, NC, USA

Tejas Shah Wisconsin Adult Congenital Heart Disease Program (WAtCH), Medical College of Wisconsin, Milwaukee, WI, USA

Robin Shandas Department of Bioengineering, Anschutz Medical Campus, University of Colorado Denver, Aurora, CO, USA

Department of Pediatrics, Division of Cardiology, Children's Hospital Colorado, Aurora, CO, USA

Kevin Shannon Department of Pediatrics, Division of Pediatric Cardiology, UCLA, Los Angeles, CA, USA

Nadine Shehata University of Toronto, Mount Sinai Hospital and University Health Network, Toronto, ON, Canada

Nanping Sheng Vice Director of the Nursing Department, Nursing Department, Shanghai Children's Medical Center, Pudong, Shanghai, China

Amanda J. Shillingford Department of Pediatics, Children's Hospital of Wisconsin Medical College of Wisconsin, Milwaukee, WI, USA

Luciana Fonseca da Silva Cardiovascular Surgeon, Hospital Sao Paulo Federal University of São Paulo, São Paulo, SP, Brazil

Jennifer Silva Division of Pediatric Cardiology, St. Louis Children's Hospital, Washington University School of Medicine, Saint Louis, MO, USA

Jose Pedro da Silva Clinica Cardiocirúrgica J.P.DaSilva 1984-2010, São Paulo, SP, Brazil

Candice K. Silversides Toronto Congenital Cardiac Centre for Adults, Peter Munk Cardiac Centre, University of Toronto, University Health Network, Mount Sinai Hospital, Toronto, ON, Canada

John M. Simpson Department of Congenital Heart Disease, London, UK

Fetal Cardiology Unit, Department of Congenital Heart Disease, Evelina Children's Hospital, Guy's and St. Thomas' NHS Trust, London, UK

Janet Simsic Department of Pediatrics, The Heart Center, Nationwide Children's Hospital The Ohio State University College of Medicine, Columbus, OH, USA

Heather E. Skillman Department of Clinical Nutrition, Children's Hospital Colorado B270, Aurora, CO, USA

Michael R. Skilton Boden Institute of Obesity, Nutrition, Exercise and Eating Disorders, Sydney Medical School, The University of Sydney, Sydney, Australia

Elisabeth Smith Great Ormond Street Hospital for Children NHS Foundation Trust, London, England, UK

Diane E. Spicer Division of Pediatric Cardiology, University of Florida, Gainesville, USA

Congenital Heart Institute of Florida, St. Petersburg, FL, USA

Thomas L. Spray Division of Cardiothoracic Surgery, The Children's Hospital of Philadelphia, Philadelphia, PA, USA

Anuradha Sridhar Frontier Lifeline & Dr. K. M. Cherian Heart Foundation, Chennai, India

Sandra Staveski Pediatric Cardiovascular Intensive Care Unit, Lucile Packard Children's Hospital at Stanford, Palo Alto, CA, USA

Julia Stegger Neonatal and Pediatric Cardiac Intensive Care, German Pediatric Heart Center, Sankt Augustin, Germany

Julia Steinberger Division of Cardiology/Department of Pediatrics, University of Minnesota, Amplatz Children's Hospital, Minneapolis, MN, USA

Paul Stelzer Department of Cardiothoracic Surgery, Mount Sinai Medical Center, New York, NY, USA

Elizabeth A. Stephenson Department of Pediatrics, Division of Cardiology, The Hospital for Sick Children, University of Toronto, Toronto, ON, Canada

William L. Stigall Critical Care, Medical City Children's Hospital, Dallas, Irving, TX, USA

Philosophy Department, University of Dallas, Irving, TX, USA

Brigitte Stiller Department of Congenital Heart Defects and Pediatric Cardiology, University Heart Center Freiburg/Bad Krozingen, Freiburg, Germany

Raghavan Subramanyan Frontier Lifeline & Dr. K. M. Cherian Heart Foundation, Chennai, India

Anne Susen Neonatal and Pediatric Cardiac Intensive Care, German Pediatric Heart Center, Sankt Augustin, Germany

Stuart C. Sweet Department of Pediatrics, Division of Pediatric Allergy, Immunology and Pulmonary Medicine, Washington University School of Medicine, St. Louis, MO, USA

Anita Szwast Pediatrics, Fetal Heart Program, The Cardiac Center, The Children's Hospital of Philadelphia Cardiology, Philadelphia, PA, USA

Pereleman School of Medicine, The University of Pennsylvania, Philadelphia, PA, USA

Shinichi Takatsuki Department of Pediatrics, Toho University Omori Medical Center, Tokyo, Japan

Ayelet Talmi Departments of Psychiatry and Pediatrics, University of Colorado School of Medicine, Aurora, CO, USA

Lloyd Y. Tani Division of Pediatric Cardiology, Department of Pediatrics, University of Utah School of Medicine, Salt Lake City, UT, USA

Herbert Bernard Tanowitz Department of Medicine and Pathology, Albert Einstein College of Medicine, Jack and Pearl Resnick Campus, Bronx, NY, USA

David Teitel Division of Pediatric Cardiology, UCSF School of Medicine, Benioff Children's Hospital, San Francisco, CA, USA

Ravi Thiagarajan Department of Cardiology, Farley – 2, Boston Children's Hospital, Boston, MA, USA

Thorsson Thor Division of Pediatric Cardiology, Department of Pediatrics and Communicable Disease, University of Michigan Medical School, Ann Arbor, MI, USA

Pierre Tissières Pediatric Intensive care Unit, Department of research in ethics, Paris Sud-11 University, Assistance Publique-Hôpitaux de Paris, Bicêtre, France

Cécile Tissot Pediatric Cardiology Unit, Department of Pediatrics, University Children's Hospital of Geneva, Geneva, Switzerland

Jeffrey A. Towbin The Heart Institute, Division of Pediatric Cardiology, Cincinnati Children's Hospital Medical Center, Cincinnati, OH, USA

James S. Tweddell Department of Pediatrics and Surgery (Cardiothoracic), Medical College of Wisconsin and Herma Heart Center at Children's Hospital of Wisconsin, Milwaukee, WI, USA

Mark D. Twite Department of Anesthesiology, Children's Hospital Colorado & University of Colorado Anschutz Medical Campus, Aurora, CO, USA

Wayne Tworetzky Pediatrics, Boston Children's Hospital Harvard Medical School, Boston, MA, USA

Shinya Ugaki Cardiac Surgery, Stollery Children's Hospital, University of Alberta, Mazankowski Alberta Heart Institute, Edmonton, AB, Canada

Sana Ullah Department of Anesthesiology, UT Southwestern Medical Center, Children's Medical Center, Dallas, Dallas, TX, USA

Jamie Dickey Ungerleider Family and Community Medicine, Wake Forest University School of Medicine, Winston Salem, NC, USA

Ross M. Ungerleider Pediatric Cardiac Surgery, Wake Forest University, Winston-Salem, NC, USA

Nikolay V. Vasilyev Department of Cardiac Surgery, Boston Children's Hospital, Boston, MA, USA

Department of Surgery, Harvard Medical School, Boston, MA, USA

David F. Vener Departments of Pediatrics and Anesthesia, Baylor College of Medicine Texas Childrens Hospital, Houston, TX, USA

Raman Venkataramanan University of Pittsburgh School of Pharmacy, Pittsburgh, PA, USA

Thomas Starzl Transplantation Institute, Magee Womens Research Institute, Pittsburgh, PA, USA

Prem Venugopal Department of Cardiac Surgery, Alder Hey Children's Hospital, Liverpool, UK

Carol G. Vetterly Department of Pharmacy Services, Children's Hospital of Pittsburgh, University of Pittsburgh School of Pharmacy, Pittsburgh, PA, USA

Piyagarnt E. Vichayavilas Department of Clinical Nutrition, Children's Hospital Colorado B270, Aurora, CO, USA

Rachel M. Wald Toronto Congenital Cardiac Centre for Adults, Peter Munk Cardiac Centre, University of Toronto, University Health Network, Hospital for Sick Children and Mount Sinai Hospital, Toronto, ON, Canada

Christine A. Walsh Children's Hospital at Montefiore, Albert Einstein College of Medicine, Bronx, NY, USA

Peter D. Wearden Department of Cardiothoracic Surgery, University of Pittsburgh School of Medicine Children's Hospital of Pittsburgh of UPMC, Pittsburgh, PA, USA

Steven A. Webber Department of Pediatrics, School of Medicine, Monroe Carell Jr. Children's Hospital at Vanderbilt, Vanderbilt University, Nashville, TN, USA

Louis M. Weiss Departments of Medicine and Pathology, Albert Einstein College of Medicine, Jack and Pearl Resnick Campus, Bronx, NY, USA

Nils Welchering Department of Critical Care Medicine, School of Medicine, University of Pittsburgh, Children's Hospital of Pittsburgh of UPMC, Pittsburgh, PA, USA

Roberta Williams Department of Pediatrics, Keck School of Medicine Children's Hospital Los Angeles, Los Angeles, CA, USA

Brigham C. Willis Department of Child Health, University of Arizona College of Medicine, Phoenix, Phoenix, AZ, USA

Division of Cardiovascular Critical Care Medicine, Phoenix Children's Hospital, University of Arizona COM – PHX, Phoenix, AZ, USA

Michael J. Wolf Department of Pediatrics, Emory University School of Medicine, Atlanta, GA, USA

Moritz C. Wyler von Ballmoos Division of Cardiothoracic Surgery, Department of Surgery, Medical College of Wisconsin, Wauwatosa, WI, USA

Samuel D. Yanofsky Department of Anesthesiology Critical Care Medicine, Children's Hospital Los Angeles Keck USC School of Medicine, Los Angeles, CA, USA

Andrew Yates Department of Pediatrics, The Heart Center, Nationwide Children's Hospital The Ohio State University College of Medicine, Columbus, OH, USA

Elizabeth Yeung Department of Pediatrics, University of Colorado School of Medicine, Children's Hospital Colorado, Aurora, CO, USA

Luis M. Zabala Department of Anesthesiology, UT Southwestern Medical Center, Children's Medical Center, Dallas, Dallas, TX, USA

Evan M. Zahn Cardiology, Cedars-Sinai Medical Center, Los Angeles, CA, USA

Ali N. Zaidi Adult Congenital Heart Disease Program, Nationwide Children's Hospital, The Ohio State University, Columbus, OH, USA

Peter Zartner German Pediatric Heart Center, Asklepios Clinic Sankt Augustin, Sankt Augustin, Germany

Beth Zemetra Cardiothoracic Intensive Care Unit, Children's Hospital Los Angeles, Los Angeles, CA, USA

Jeannie Zuk Department of Anesthesiology and Pediatrics, Children's Hospital Colorado, University of Colorado School of Medicine, Aurora, CO, USA

Division of Cardiothoracic Surgery, The Children's Hospital of Philadelphia, Philadelphia, PA, USA

Section XI

Innovative Interventional Techniques

Lee Benson

Biodegradable Implants

68

Daniel S. Levi and Andrew L. Cheng

Abstract

Most devices used to repair congenital heart lesions only need to serve as temporary scaffoldings. Because the ideal devices would ultimately vanish after serving its purpose, biodegradable materials are now being utilized for pediatric transcatheter and surgical vascular and cardiac devices. Because pediatric patients have growing cardiovascular structures, there is great interest in use of bioresorbable stents for the treatment of coarctation of the aorta and pulmonary artery stenosis. Eventual complete resorption of these stents and other devices will avoid the complications associated with traditional devices and may eliminate the possible need to remove the device in the future. Biodegradable devices for congenital heart patients can also facilitate other interventions at the same site and will allow for improved radiographic imaging of lesions. Having a basic understanding of the types of materials available for use in biodegradable devices is important for pediatric interventional cardiologists and cardiothoracic surgeons. This chapter includes a discussion of biodegradable polymers, biocorrodible metals, and biodegradable surgical materials. An overview of currently investigated biodegradable materials and cardiovascular devices, including their applications to pediatric cardiology, is also presented.

D.S. Levi (✉)
Division of Pediatric Cardiology, Mattel Children's
Hospital University of California, Los Angeles,
Los Angeles, CA, USA
e-mail: dlevi@ucla.edu; dlevi@mednet.ucla.edu

A.L. Cheng
Department of Pediatrics, Mattel Children's Hospital
University of California, Los Angeles, Los Angeles,
CA, USA
e-mail: acheng@mednet.ucla.edu

E.M. da Cruz et al. (eds.), *Pediatric and Congenital Cardiology, Cardiac Surgery and Intensive Care*,
DOI 10.1007/978-1-4471-4619-3_128, © Springer-Verlag London 2014

Keywords

Antiproliferative drug • ASD • Biocorrodible material • Biodegradable material • Closure device • Coarctation • Congenital heart disease • Coronary artery disease • Percutaneous intervention • Polymer • Prosthetic valve • Recoil • Small intestinal submucosa • Stenosis • Stent • Thrombosis • Tissue scaffold

Introduction

Although biodegradable materials have been used in medicine for several decades, these materials only recently have been utilized for pediatric transcatheter and surgical vascular and cardiac devices. Most devices used to repair congenital heart lesions only need to serve as temporary scaffoldings – ideally they would ultimately disappear. For example, a stent provides support to a stenotic vessel while it heals from angioplasty, but also can lead to complications such as thrombosis and late restenosis. Furthermore, the ability to stent the vessel of a small infant is limited, as the infant can eventually grow beyond any stent's capacity to expand. A bioresorbable stent can potentially solve these problems.

Biodegradable implants have many potential advantages over conventional devices such as bare metal stents (BMS) and nitinol closure devices. The interest in these materials for pediatric applications is primarily to accommodate growth. Lesions such as coarctation of the aorta and pulmonary artery stenosis could be temporarily augmented with a bioresorbable stent, allowing time for remodeling. As the patient grows and the vessel regains adequate functionality, the stent is slowly resorbed. Eventual complete resorption of the stent avoids the complications associated with traditional stents and eliminates the possible need to remove the device in the future. Recent studies of such devices have been promising – the ABSORB trial of the bioresorbable vascular scaffold (BVS) everolimus-eluting stent showed restoration of a functionally normal endothelium at the stented site in some patients [1], suggesting that these vessels may also gain the ability to grow after being stented. Similar benefits are also likely to be seen with surgically placed materials and closure devices.

Biodegradable devices for congenital heart patients can also facilitate other interventions at the same site. For example, traditional ASD closure devices significantly impede future transseptal left heart catheterization and metallic stents limit future dilations. Biodegradable stents and devices will completely avoid these "full metal jacket" situations and may even preserve side branches near the site of intervention. These devices also will allow for improved radiographic imaging of lesions with MRI or CT. Many bioresorbable stents range from being completely radiolucent to having isolated radioopaque markers, resulting in minimal or absent artifact [2].

Reduction or avoidance of late stent restenosis has been ascribed at least to some degree to inflammation around metallic struts after coronary stenting [3]. Replacement of the conventional metallic scaffold with an absorbable biopolymer, therefore, theoretically should decrease the rate of restenosis. This has been the impetus for the maturation of biodegradable stent technology, and currently a variety of biodegradable coronary stents are now being tested in the adult population. As many bioresorbable stents are embedded with drug-eluting agents, they may even provide an opportunity to improve results in stenting difficult lesions such as pulmonary vein stenoses.

Having a basic understanding of the types of materials available for use in biodegradable devices is important for pediatric interventional cardiologists and cardiothoracic surgeons. This chapter includes a discussion of biodegradable polymers, biocorrodible metals, and biodegradable surgical materials. An overview of currently investigated biodegradable materials and cardiovascular devices, including their applications to pediatric cardiology, is also presented.

Main Text

Definitions

A biodegradable material is one that is primarily degraded by a biological agent like an enzyme or microbe. Bioresorption and bioabsorption refer to removal of degradation products by cellular activity, such as phagocytosis, in a biological environment. A bio-erodible or biocorrodible material is a water-insoluble substance that is converted under physiologic conditions into a water-soluble material [4]. A tissue scaffold is a material that promotes the growth of surrounding tissue into a device [5]. Although they are not technically biodegradable, tissue scaffolds are an important related technology that also likely will have a significant impact on the future of pediatric cardiology.

Biodegradable Materials

Biodegradable materials have been used in medicine for several decades, but only more recently have they been investigated for use in cardiovascular interventions. The first bioabsorbable suture was created from polyglycolic acid in the 1960s, and subsequent use in the surgical arena has been widespread [6]. In the 1990s resorbable plates and screws were introduced for use in orthopedic surgery, eliminating the need for secondary device-related procedures while maintaining safety and efficacy [7].

Most biodegradable devices to date have been made from biodegradable polymers. These are a heterogeneous family of molecules created by linkage of a variety of simple monomeric units. These molecules degrade in the body into normal metabolites or into products that can be completely eliminated from the body with or without further metabolic transformation.

Aliphatic polyesters, the most commonly used synthetic biodegradable polymers, are synthesized by polycondensation of diacids and diols, self-polycondensation of hydroxyacids, or by ring-opening polymerization of cyclic diesters, lactones, glycolides, and lactides. The most commonly used monomers (lactide, glycolide, and caprolactone) have been combined to create several different polymers with a wide spectrum of physical properties (Fig. 68.1) [6].

Both the mechanical and biological properties of the polymers can be chemically programmed during their synthesis. The radial strength and degradation time can be "engineered" by manipulation of the monomers used to synthesize the polymer, by utilization of enantiomer monomers, by blending polymers, or by inclusion of side chains. Both the mechanical and biological properties of devices made from polyester polymers are already well known, and many processes can be used to manufacture devices from a wide range of polymers. The extensive knowledge of the material science of these molecules should help doctors and engineers to produce devices with very specific desired properties.

Other major bioresorbable polymer families include polyanhydrides, polyhydroxyalkanoates (PHA), tyrosine-derived polycarbonates, and polyether-esters. While all of these are currently being investigated for a variety of clinical applications, tyrosine-derived polycarbonates are notable since they have been used successfully to create a bioabsorbable stent that has undergone clinical trials [5]. Tyrosine-derived polycarbonates are a subgroup of synthetic poly (amino acids). In contrast to early synthetic poly (amino acids), which had unfavorable physical properties, recently developed pseudo poly (amino acid) polymers like tyrosine-derived polycarbonates have been more promising. These polymers are made by linking amino acid monomers with non-amide bonds, and their physiochemical properties can be altered by varying the pendant alkyl ester chain. Degradation results in tyrosine and the diols used to esterify the side chain [6]. Overall these polymers have a slow degradation rate, high strength, and good biocompatibility [5].

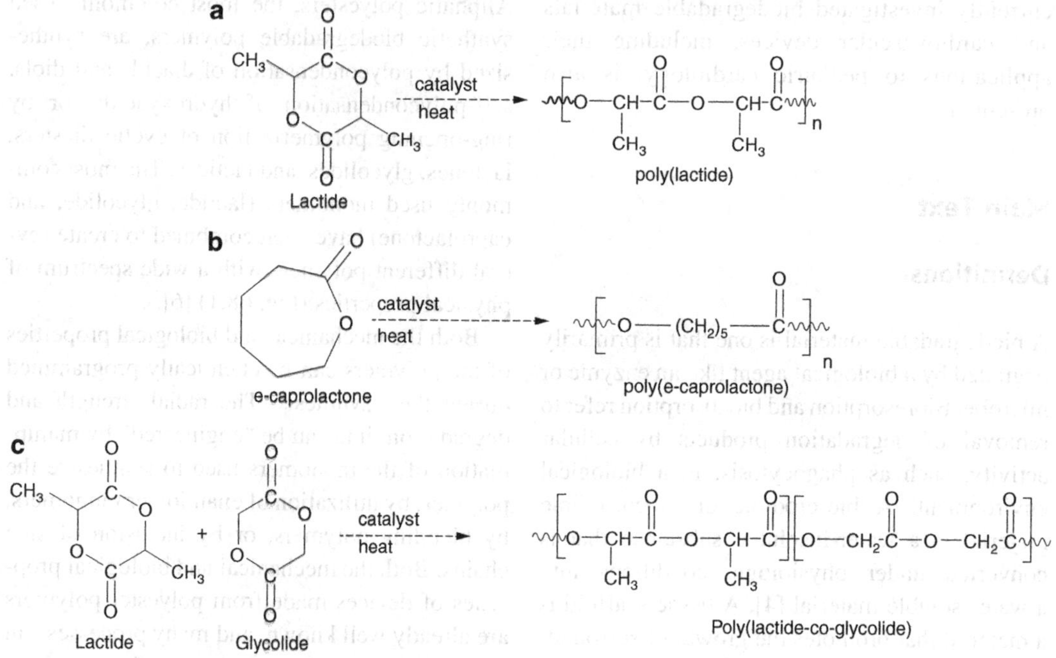

Fig. 68.1 Synthesis of commonly used synthetic biodegradable polymers: (**a**) poly(lactide), (**b**) poly(caprolactone), (**c**) poly(lactide-co-glycolide) [6]

Several criteria are important to consider when developing polymers for biomedical applications including mechanical properties (e.g., strength, radial force, elasticity), degradation time, toxicity, route of metabolism, shelf life, and ability to sterilize. Due to improved control of these properties and minimal immunogenicity, synthetic polymers have been utilized to a much greater degree than natural polymers for these applications. For biodegradable polymers, these variables can be manipulated by altering the type of monomers and the ratio of enantiomers used to make the polymer. For example, poly(L-lactic acid) (PLLA) is a semicrystalline material with high modulus and degradation time of 3–5 years, whereas poly(D,L-lactic acid) (PDLLA) is an amorphous material with lower modulus and shorter degradation time of 12–16 months [8]. Due to its favorable mechanical properties, PLLA has been approved for many clinical uses including absorbable sutures and orthopedic plates. Physical properties can be altered by copolymerizing individual monomers and by varying the copolymer ratio. Copolymers of

poly(lactic acid) and poly(glycolic acid) (PLAGA) have been studied for a variety of medical applications such as stents, drug delivery devices, and scaffolds for tissue engineering [6]. Similarly, the rate of degradation and stress transfer can be tailored by blending or layering different polymers.

After implantation in the body, a biodegradable device should maintain structural integrity for a desired amount of time and then be degraded, absorbed, and excreted by the body. Degradation of the polymer occurs by hydrolysis of the unstable backbone. This process occurs in two phases for semicrystalline polymers. First, water preferentially penetrates the bulk of the device, and primarily hydrolyzes the covalent bonds in the amorphous regions of the polymer matrix, converting long polymer chains into shorter water-soluble fragments. This initially results in a loss of molecular weight but not radial strength, as strength primarily comes from the crystalline domains that exist in between the long polymer chains (Fig. 68.2). As the crystalline domains are hydrolyzed, there is

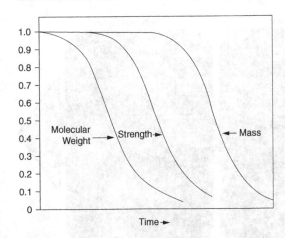

Fig. 68.2 Sequence of polymer-molecular weight, strength, and mass reduction over time [6]

subsequent loss of strength. Second, the water-soluble fragments are degraded, resulting in loss of polymer mass [8]. Thus, the rate of degradation depends on water accessibility to the matrix, which in turn depends on hydrophilicity/hydrophobicity of the polymer, crystallinity of the polymer, and overall structure of the device [9]. Due to this mechanism of degradation, factors that contribute to higher polymer degradation include more hydrophilic monomers, more hydrophilic and acidic end groups, more reactive hydrolytic groups in the polymer backbone, less crystallinity, and smaller device size [8].

After hydrolysis of the polymer, the body metabolizes the monomeric components. For example, PLLA hydrolyzes to lactic acid, which is metabolized through the Krebs cycle to be excreted as carbon dioxide and water. The location where a device is implanted must be carefully considered, as these metabolites can accumulate and become harmful, such as might be the case with a large implant placed in an area of poor vascularization [8]. An acidic environment will catalyze further degradation and exacerbate acidosis, which may also lead to adverse tissue reactions [10, 11].

As biodegradable polymers are hydrolytically unstable, exposure to moisture must be minimized throughout the processing, packaging, and sterilization processes. Therefore, the polymers are packaged quickly and double-bagged in an inert atmosphere or vacuum soon after manufacturing. They are then frozen to minimize the effect of the remaining moisture. Final device packaging is comprised of an airtight moisture-proof container and often a desiccant to reduce moisture. Sterilization typically occurs by gamma radiation, ethylene oxide, or other less common techniques such as plasma etching to avoid structural compromise [8].

The ideal biodegradable device should transition through three distinct stages (Fig. 68.3). Initially, the stent should perform similarly to a conventional device with smooth deliverability and minimum acute recoil upon insertion. For the first 3 months, postimplantation the stent should maintain high radial strength, allowing for revascularization of the diseased vessel (as discussed further below). From 3 to about 6 months postimplantation, the stent should transition from scaffolding to a discontinuous structure. Gradually the stent will lose radial strength and the struts will be incorporated into the vessel wall, allowing for vessel growth and response to physiologic stimuli. Finally around 9 months postimplantation, after the vessel has had sufficient time to heal and grow, the stent should be discontinuous and inert and resorb in a benign fashion.

Biodegradable Stents

Biodegradable stents have been the most heavily investigated biodegradable cardiovascular devices to date. Completely biodegradable stents represent the third generation of drug-eluting stents (DES). First-generation DES improved on the conventional bare metal stent (BMS) by releasing antithrombotic or antiproliferative medications such as paclitaxel or sirolimus. Compared to BMS, first-generation DES significantly decreased both angiographic and clinical measures of restenosis in randomized clinical trials [12]. More widespread use of first-generation DES, however, revealed an increased risk of late (6 month to 1 year) and very late (beyond 1 year) stent thrombosis, a well-described complication of percutaneous coronary

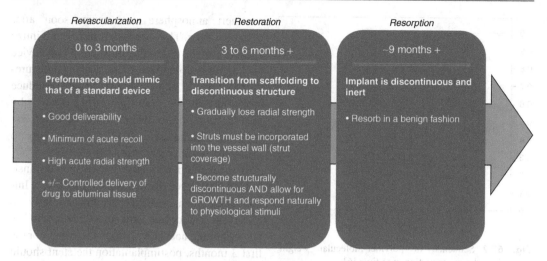

Fig. 68.3 Behavior of an ideal biodegradable device over time

intervention (PCI) with BMS that can lead to myocardial infarction or death [13, 14]. In addition to patient comorbidities, lesion complexity, and procedural difficulty, device-related factors were also implicated in this increased risk. First-generation DES were typically coated with permanent polymers that facilitated release of medication; these polymers could cause inflammation, delayed endothelialization, positive remodeling, and hypersensitivity reactions, all of which could result in thrombosis. Second-generation DES, such as the Endeavor zotarolimus-eluting stent (Medtronic, Minneapolis, MN) and the Xience V everolimus-eluting stent (Advanced Cardiovascular Systems, Santa Clara, CA), reduced the risk of thrombosis by utilizing innovative polymeric coatings, anti-restenotic agents, and thinner stent platforms [12]. Biodegradable stents have been hypothesized to cause an even further decreased incidence of late thrombosis, since the devices are eventually completely resorbed [2]. The new generation of fully absorbable stents will hopefully minimize or completely eliminate late thrombosis.

Like other DES, biodegradable stents have the ability to deliver antiproliferative medications, such as sirolimus, directly to the site of disease [2]. The FUTURE trials of an everolimus-eluting metallic stent showed promising results in reducing in-stent restenosis [15, 16]. Studies of the bioresorbable vascular scaffold (BVS) everolimus-eluting stent have shown similar clinical outcomes at 2 years to metallic DES [1]. In the pediatric population, such devices may be particularly valuable for systemic or pulmonary vein stenting, as restenosis in this setting is extremely common [17]. A bioresorbable antiproliferative-releasing stent could potentially combat this complication by decreasing neointimal proliferation.

Several biodegradable stents that have undergone clinical trials will now be discussed (Table 68.1).

Igaki-Tamai Stent

The Igaki-Tamai stent (Igaki Medical Planning Company, Kyoto, Japan) was the first absorbable stent to be implanted in a human. It is made from PLLA and configured in a zigzag helical coil with straight bridges. Strut thickness is 170 μm and vessel coverage by the struts is 24 %, both of which are larger than conventional metal stents (Fig. 68.4a). The device is delivered via a balloon-mounted self-expanding sheath system, whose expansion is quickened by dilatation with warmed contrast medium. Gold markers at each end of the stent allow for radiographic localization. Absorption is by bulk erosion and results in release of lactic acid, which is metabolized through the Krebs cycle [2].

Table 68.1 Comparison of biodegradable stents that have undergone clinical trials in humans. BTI Bioabsorbable Therapeutics Inc., BVS bioresorbable vascular scaffold, AMS Biotronik absorbable magnesium stent, PLLA poly(L-lactic acid), PDLLA poly(D,L-lactic acid)

Stent	Material	Coating	Design	By-products	Drug elution	Radioopacity	Strut thickness, μm	Crossing profile, mm	Stent-to-artery coverage, %	Radial support duration	Absorption time
Igaki-Tamai	PLLA	None	Zigzag helical coils with straight bridges	Lactic acid, CO_2, H_2O	None	Gold markers	170	?	24	6 months	2 years
REVA	Poly (12DTE-12DT carbonate)	None	Slide and lock	L-tyrosine, ethanol, CO_2	None	Iodine impregnated	200	1.7	55	3–6 months	2 years
BTI	Salicylate + linker polymer	Salicylate + adipic acid	Tube with laser-cut voids	Salicylate, CO_2, H_2O	Sirolimus, salicylate	None	200	2.0	65	3 months	6 months
BVS	PLLA	PDLLA	1.0: out-of-phase sinusoidal hoops with straight and direct links. 1.1: in-phase hoops with straight links	Lactic acid, CO_2, H_2O	Everolimus	Platinum markers	156	1.4	25	1.0: weeks. 1.1: 3 months	2 years
AMS	Magnesium alloy	None	Sinusoidal in-phase hoops linked by straight bridges	N/A	None	None	165	1.2	10	Days–weeks	<4 months

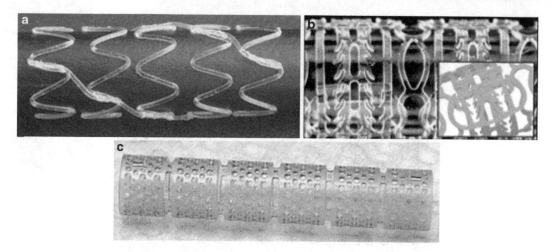

Fig. 68.4 Biodegradable stents: (**a**) the Igaki-Tamai stent, (**b**) the REVA stent, (**c**) the BTI stent [2]

A first-in-man prospective nonrandomized clinical trial of the stent was performed in 50 patients with a low complication rate including 18 % repeat PCI, one Q-wave myocardial infarction, and one noncardiac death. Although no further human coronary implants have been performed with this stent, it is being explored for peripheral applications and is clearly the predecessor to the current generation of coronary and peripheral biodegradable stents [2].

REVA Stent

The REVA stent (Reva Medical Inc., San Diego, CA) is made from an absorbable tyrosine-derived polycarbonate polymer, poly(12DTE-12DT carbonate) [5], configured in a slide and lock (ratchet) structure that allows for expansion without deformation. Strut thickness is significant at 200 μm and crossing profile is 1.7 mm when balloon mounted, requiring a 7 F guide catheter (Fig. 68.4b). The stent-to-artery ratio is 55 % after expansion [2]. Polyethylene glycol (PEG) is added for increased blood compatibility and the tyrosine backbone is iodinated to provide radio-opacity. Degradation results in L-tyrosine, ethanol, carbon dioxide, and PEG [5]. The main interest in this stent form a pediatric standpoint is its slide and lock design. This design may allow for increased radial force in stents designed for pulmonary artery and coarctation stenting.

The RESORB first-in-man trial was a prospective nonrandomized single-arm safety study of 27 patients with a nondrug-eluting version of the REVA stent. At 30 days 2 patients experienced a Q-wave myocardial infarction and 1 had target lesion revascularization. Poor outcomes were noted at 4–6 months postimplantation with higher-than-anticipated target lesion revascularization due mainly to reduced stent diameter [2]. A susbsequent iteration of this stent, the ReZolve stent, includes an antiproliferative agent and soon will be undergoing clinical testing in the RESTORE trial.

BTI Stent

The BTI stent (Bioabsorbable Therapeutics Inc., Menlo Park, CA) is a bioabsorbable sirolimus-eluting stent. Because this device incorporates a polymer backbone made from repeating salicylate molecules joined by a linker molecule, it is worth a brief discussion. It is also coated with a polymer composed of repeating salicylic acid molecules linked by adipic acid. The device dimensions are similar to the REVA stent; strut thickness is 200 μm, crossing profile is 2.0 mm, and artery coverage is 65 % (Fig. 68.4c). Resorption of the device releases salicylic acid, which is anticipated to decrease the inflammation associated with PCI. Sirolimus is also released at a dose and rate similar to that of the Cypher stent [2].

Fig. 68.5 The BVS
everolimus-eluting stent:
(**a**) BVS 1.0, (**b**) BVS 1.1

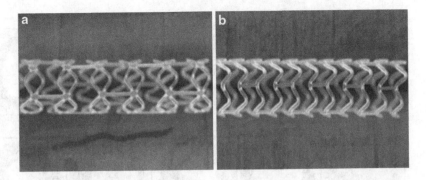

The Whisper first-in-man trial studied 8 patients implanted with the BTI stent. Higher-than-expected neointimal hyperplasia was observed. Thus the design is currently being revised to include thinner struts, decreased wall coverage, and a higher dose of sirolimus [2].

BVS Everolimus-Eluting Stent

The bioresorbable vascular scaffold (BVS) everolimus-eluting stent (Abbott Vascular, Santa Clara, CA) is the first biodegradable stent to have comparable clinical and imaging outcomes to metallic DES 2 years after implantation (Fig. 68.5a) [2]. This stent deserves the most attention as it has the most extensive record in human use. A larger version of this stent – possibly one designed for peripheral interventions – could be the first stent widely used for palliation of congenital heart disease.

The BVS stent is composed of a PLLA backbone with a coating of a 1:1 mixture of PDLLA and the antiproliferative drug everolimus. PDLLA regulates controlled release of everolimus [18]. The rate of everolimus delivery (80 % by 30 days) is similar to that from the permanent polymer on the metallic Xience V stent. The ABSORB trials studied two different revisions of the stent. BVS stent revision 1.0 is configured in circumferential out-of-phase zigzag hoops linked either directly or by straight bridges; strut thickness is 150 μm and crossing profile is 1.4 mm. Revision 1.1 is configured in circumferential in-phase zigzag hoops linked by straight bridges; strut thickness is the same (Fig. 68.5b). Both models have vessel coverage of 25 % and a total absorption time of about 2 years. Compared to the original device, revision 1.1 has increased duration of radial support due to different polymer processing methods [2]. It also provides more uniform vessel wall support and drug delivery and has improved device retention [19]. Platinum radio-opaque markers are present on the ends of both models, allowing for clear identification on fluoroscopy. Absorption of the both is by bulk erosion and the resulting lactic acid is metabolized by the Krebs cycle [2].

The ABSORB cohort A first-in-man trial was a prospective nonrandomized study of BVS stent revision 1.0. Stents were placed in 30 patients with simple de novo native coronary artery stenoses. At 3 years postimplantation the ischemia-driven major adverse cardiac event rate was very favorable and there were no stent thromboses. Intravascular ultrasound (IVUS) showed no vessel shrinkage at 6 months; however, stent area was reduced 11–12 %. Moreover intimal hyperplastic tissue caused the luminal area to be reduced by a total of almost 17 %. This angiographic late loss was similar to some metallic DES (Fig. 68.6). Despite this shrinkage, the stent resisted negative remodeling well. In fact, between 6 months and 2 years, both IVUS and optical coherence tomography (OCT) detected lumen enlargement. Vasoactivity in the stented segment was also noted in the small number of patients who were tested. These vessels showed vasoconstriction induced by methylergonovine maleate and vasodilatation induced by nitroglycerin. This observation suggests that the return of a physiologic response to vasoactive stimuli and the potential for arterial dilation in response to local ischemia is possible with bioresorbable stents [18].

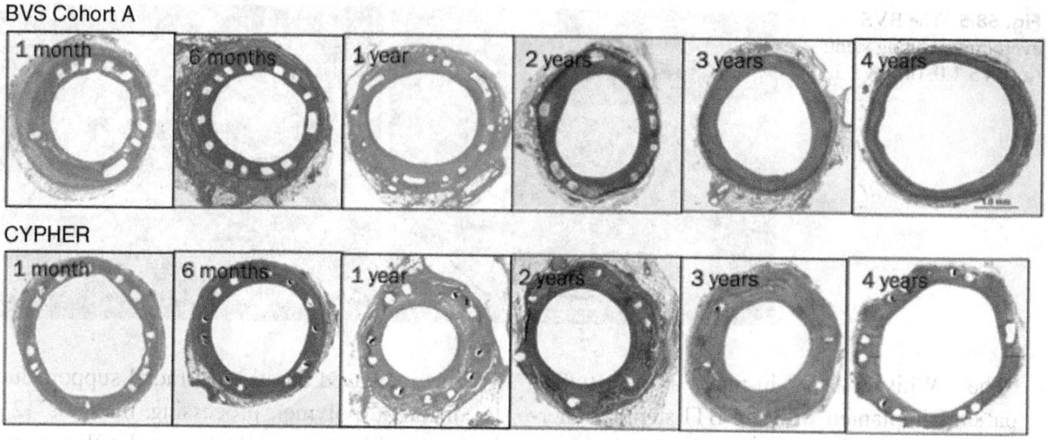

BVS Cohort A

CYPHER

Fig. 68.6 Histologic comparison of BVS 1.0 and Cypher stents in porcine model. The neointimal response was comparable between the two implants at 28 and 90 days in terms of neointimal composition and coverage. At later time points, however, the neointimal response to BVS stents was milder

The ABSORB cohort B trial is a prospective nonrandomized study of BVS stent revision 1.1. As previously mentioned, the scaffold design and manufacturing process of its polymer were modified for BVS 1.1. Based on results seen with BVS 1.0, these modifications were made to maintain the mechanical integrity of the stent up to 6 months with the goal of reducing scaffold shrinkage and eventual late luminal loss, and to reduce acute and late recoil. BVS 1.1 was placed in 101 patients with a maximum of two de novo native coronary artery lesions. This cohort was divided into two subgroups based on timing of follow-up imaging. By IVUS, OCT, and angiography, the overall performance of BVS 1.1 at 6 months was significantly improved over BVS 1.0 [19]. Absolute acute recoil was not statistically different from BVS 1.0 or the metallic everolimus-eluting stent Xience V [20, 21]. Late luminal loss was in the same range seen with current metallic DES. Evaluation of the stent by IVUS-VH and OCT showed little change over the trial period, suggesting increased mechanical integrity over BVS 1.0 [19]. A substudy of BVS 1.1 implanted in small coronary vessels <2.5 mm showed similar clinical and angiographic outcomes compared to those with larger vessels [22].

The ABSORB EXTEND trial is a single-arm study currently aiming to enroll about 1,000 patients at 100 sites throughout Europe, Asia, Canada, and Latin America. The trial will include patients with more complex coronary artery disease than those in the previous ABSORB cohorts. Stent size will limit the treatable lesion length to <28 mm; however, a subgroup of patients at selected investigational sites are planned to receive overlapping stents to treat longer lesions. Clinical outcomes will include ischemia-driven major adverse cardiac events, ischemia-driven target vessel failure, ischemia-driven target vessel revascularization, ischemia-driven target lesion revascularization, and stent thrombosis. Follow-up will be similar to the prior ABSORB trials, including evaluation with angiography, IVUS, and OCT.

Biocorrodible Materials

Corrosion is a design consideration that must be taken into account for any metallic implant. It can lead to premature device failure and can affect biocompatibility by releasing metal ions/particles [5]. While typically a hindrance that must be carefully combated, this property is now being investigated for positive uses. Biocorrodible metallic implants have the mechanical advantages of stainless steel, while also incorporating the benefits of a temporary scaffold like the previously described biodegradable devices.

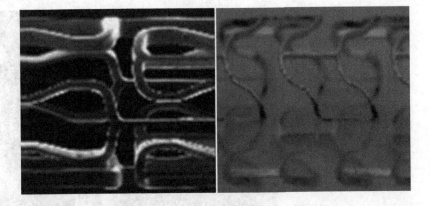

Fig. 68.7 The Biotronik absorbable magnesium stent [2]

Toxicity may be a concern, however, and is related to the rate of biocorrosion. Recent research demonstrated the safety of a corrodible pure iron stent placed in the descending aorta of a pig for 12 months. No evidence of local or systemic toxicity from corrosion by-products was observed [23]. Magnesium was also recently successfully used to develop an absorbable stent that performed well in animal studies and a first-in-man trial for peripheral vascular interventions. Animal studies showed complete and rapid endothelialization, minimal inflammatory changes, and complete absorption within 2 months with residual deposition of calcium and phosphorus [24].

Absorbable Magnesium Stent

The absorbable magnesium stent (AMS) (Biotronik, Berlin, Germany) was the first metallic bioabsorbable stent to be implanted in a human. The device is laser cut from tubular magnesium WE-43 and is configured in sinusoidal in-phase hoops linked by straight bridges. It has strut thickness of 165 μm and crossing profile of 1.2 mm, which is compatible with a 6 F guide catheter (Fig. 68.7). Arterial wall coverage is 10 %, which is comparable to that of conventional BMS. The device is balloon expandable. Initial radial strength is similar to stainless steel stents. It is radiolucent and lacks radio-opaque markers. Absorption is by surface erosion, so strut thickness decreases as the stent is absorbed [2].

The PROGRESS-AMS trial was a prospective nonrandomized study of 63 patients with simple de novo native coronary artery lesions in whom 71 magnesium stents (10–15 mm in length) were implanted. Angiographic results immediately after implantation were similar to those seen with conventional BMS. Radial support, however, was lost very early, perhaps within days. Accordingly there was a high restenosis rate of almost 50 % at 4 months. No stent thromboses, myocardial infarctions, or deaths were observed [24].

While the AMS stent is clearly not ideal for use in coronary applications, it may be well suited for pediatric applications. The AMS was successfully implanted in two newborns for emergency off-label uses. Its first use was in a 6-week-old female baby who had been born prematurely at 26 weeks gestation. During an attempt to ligate a patent ductus arteriosus, her left pulmonary artery was accidentally ligated. After surgical removal of the ligature, both echocardiography and angiography showed persistent occlusion. Selective angiography suggested possible reperfusion of the vessel; however, passage with a catheter was not possible because of the vessel anatomy. Due to the small size of the patient and partial atrophy of the vessel wall caused by ligation, surgical patch angioplasty was not considered to be a viable option. Implantation of a conventional coronary stent would have limited the artery size and required future surgical intervention. Instead an AMS was implanted via a catheter through a surgical cutdown of the pulmonary bifurcation. Good perfusion of the left lung was demonstrated by angiography at 1 month postimplantation. At 5 months, after

Fig. 68.8 Angiograms of
the descending aortic arch.
(**a**) Postoperative long-
segment recoarctation.
(**b**) Angiography after
placement of the
3.5×15 mm^2 AMS.
(**c**) Recoarctation during
degradation of the previous
stent. (**d**) Immediate
angiographic result after
placement of the
4×15 mm^2 AMS [26]

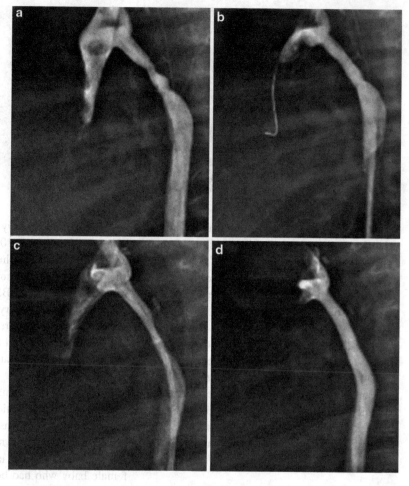

the stent had been completely degraded, left lung perfusion remained adequate with only a slight difference in size between the right and left pulmonary arteries [25].

The second pediatric application the AMS was in a 3-week-old male baby with a postsurgical long-segment recoarctation. He was born with critical aortic coarctation, which was repaired by resection of the narrowed isthmus and end-to-end anastamosis; recoarctation seen intraoperatively prompted an additional subclavian-flap repair. Unfortunately, the second surgery was also unsatisfactory. Residual long-segment stenosis of the descending aortic arch as well as a VSD resulted in pulmonary hypertension and subsequent ventilator dependence. As with the prior patient, alternative

treatment modalities had significant disadvantages. Angioplasty seemed contraindicated so soon after surgery, and a conventional metal stent was limited by the size of the patient and need for future surgical removal. An AMS was placed instead. Initially a 3.5 mm diameter AMS was implanted: however, at 3 weeks postimplantation recatheterization showed a reduced diameter of the stented area and a comparable vessel shape to that preimplantation. Subsequently an additional 4 mm diameter AMS was placed (Fig. 68.8). The patient did well with this second stent and was discharged home. At 3 months he underwent VSD closure because of excess left-to-right shunting and previously stented segment was patch augmented because of the systolic pressure gradient [26].

Tissue Scaffolds

Making the distinction between biodegradable materials and tissue scaffolds is important. While biodegradable materials are actually metabolized, tissue scaffolds are meant to promote tissue growth into a device. Although biodegradable materials in some forms serve as tissue scaffolds, scaffolds also include synthetic materials such as Dacron, xenografts, and allografts. A discussion of porcine small intestinal submucosa (SIS) and intestinal collagen layer (ICL) is relevant to this chapter. Although SIS is not completely biodegradable, it is essentially bioreplaceable. SIS is marketed as CorMatrix and has become very popular for use among congenital heart surgeons. ICL is used in the BioSTAR ASD closure device.

Biologic sources of extracellular matrix (ECM) include xenografts, autografts, and allografts. Xenografts have been used in a variety of medical applications, including porcine valve replacements and catgut suture. Both xenografts and allografts have the potential for disease transmission from donor to recipient. Conversely, autologous tissue has minimal risk for disease transmission but is much more scarce. In general, the ECM provides a collagen network that serves as a scaffold for cellular growth and healing. In addition to collagen, an ECM scaffold can include growth factors, fibronectin, laminin, and other bioactive molecules to help regulate the healing response [5].

Different harvesting and processing techniques can result in altered strength, growth factor concentration, immune response, degradation time, sterility, and bioburden of a tissue scaffold. After harvesting, tissues are chemically and mechanically cleaned, cross-linked, and sterilized. Cleaning reduces host response to a tissue but may remove growth factors and other components that promote cellular proliferation. Cross-linking increases resorption time, but can also reduce cellular infiltration. Sterilization, most often through gamma radiation, can affect cross-linking and result in reduced mechanical strength [5].

Scaffold architecture plays a critical role in how the material behaves. Mesh scaffolds can be made by weaving, while nonwoven scaffolds can be made by mechanical entanglement, melt blown, dry spun, wet spun, or electrospun processes. Cellular interaction with a scaffold can be greatly influenced by this microarchitecture. For example, the BioTREK septal occluder when made with a nonwoven tissue scaffold is almost completely covered with neoendothelium at 1 month postimplantation, while when made with a film tissue scaffold remains significantly covered with unorganized plasma protein after the same time period. Like DES, tissue scaffolds can also incorporate drugs or other biological response modifiers to regulate thromboresistance and endothelialization. These can be directly integrated into absorbable devices to provide controlled release during the lifespan of the device [5].

ICL is made from the tunica submucosa of porcine small intestine, which is purified to create a sheet of acellular type 1 collagen. ICL is reproducible with undetectable amounts of porcine DNA. Materials like ICL have been shown to remodel into functional native-like tissue, which promotes site-specific tissue regeneration instead of scar formation. During remodeling, the matrix is infiltrated by cells, undergoes phagocytosis, and degrades into peptides [5].

SIS is usually derived from porcine small intestine as well and consists of collagen, proteoglycan glycosaminoglycan, glycoprotein, and growth factors. Like ICL it signals surrounding host cells to grow and initiates site-specific tissue remodeling. It has very low immunogenicity but has the potential to cause a significant inflammatory response if not adequately decellularized. SIS has been widely used for a variety of tissue-engineering applications as a scaffold for the artery, bladder, intestine, and tendon. It is also FDA-approved for urogenital procedures such as hernia repairs and ureteral reconstructions [27]. In the cardiovascular realm, research has shown promising results for using SIS as a vascular graft in animal models. For pediatric cardiologists, it is of particular interest because of its growth potential [28]. Currently it is being investigated for a variety of novel applications including three-dimensional myocardial patches and injectable biomaterial for myocardial infarct repair [29–31].

Nanotechnology can be used to produce novel nanocomposite polymers. These man-made polymers can be made to encourage cell growth or to deliver stem cells. Interest in these materials to date has been for uses as an arterial surgical graft to reduce risk of rupture or rejection after implantation. These materials have also been used to engineer grafts for tracheal replacement. Potentially they also could be used in transcatheter and surgically placed devices.

Tissue Scaffold Devices

BioSTAR Closure Device

The BioSTAR biodegradable implant (NMT Medical, Boston, MA) consists of a metallic frame covered by a type I collagen matrix or porcine submucosa (ICL). This material is coated with heparin and cross-linked. The framework is a double umbrella of stainless steel (MP35N) arms with interposed spring hinges along each arm and a nitinol wire at the end of each arm. Two discs of ICL are attached over the metal frame. The ICL discs are completely resorbed within 6 months, leaving only the metallic framework. Histology in animals showed breakdown of the collagen ICL by inflammatory cells and then gradual replacement with host tissue. The device is available in 22, 28, and 33 mm diameters (Fig. 68.9) [32].

A study of the BioSTAR biodegradable implant for closure of small to moderate ASD showed similar closure rates to the AMPLATZER Septal Occluder (ASO). Ten children with isolated ASD (<16 mm diameter) and evidence of right ventricular volume overload on echocardiography underwent ASD closure with the BioSTAR device. They were matched with children at the same institution undergoing closure with the ASO. Follow-up at 24 h and 6 months showed similar occlusion rates between the two groups. One child in the BioSTAR group had a trivial leak related to prolapse of one of the device arms, which decreased on serial exams. There were no vascular complications in either group [32].

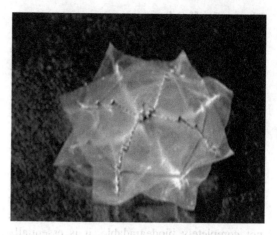

Fig. 68.9 The BioSTAR closure device [32]

Another study of the BioSTAR showed similar success in closure of atrial-level shunts in patients with more complicated anatomy, including multiple defects and Fontan circulation. Two devices were implanted in one patient for closure of a multifenestrated aneurismal ASD. Complete and early closure was seen in all nine patients and follow-up echocardiography did not detect any residual shunts. No significant complications were observed [33]. It is hoped that there will be overall comparable efficacy and safety between the BioSTAR device and the current commercially available devices, but with the potential additional benefits of decreased inflammatory response, reduced arrythmogenicity and erosion, improved transseptal access, and decreased thrombogenicity.

A fully absorbable version of the implant, the BioTREK (NMT Medical, Boston, MA), has undergone preclinical trials [32]. This next generation device is designed to be completely bioabsorbable and to incorporate drugs to reduce thrombosis and encourage endothelialization. It is made from poly-4-hydroxybutyrate (P4HB), a biosynthetic polymer made using recombinant DNA technology. P4HB is less inflammatory than some of the more commonly used bioabsorbable polymers such as PLA and PGA. It is broken down by hydrolysis and surface erosion. The decreased inflammatory response in combination with complete absorbability could improve upon BioSTAR's side effect profile [34].

Biodisk Closure Device

The Biodisk closure device (Cook Medical, Bloomington, IN) is composed of two nitinol wire components covered with platinum coil, a flexible ring with a cross bar covered with SIS, and an anchor with a delivery bar. Its low profile allows delivery through an 8 F catheter. A study in pigs demonstrated simple device implantation for correction of PFO. No shunting of contrast medium was observed after initial device deployment nor at serial assessments up to 4 months. The device was easily retrievable after intentional embolization into the right and left atria. In the subset of animals in which the device was left in place, progressive increase in neointima was seen with near complete remodeling and revascularization at 4 months. The Biodisk induced minimal inflammatory response and foreign body reactions. No significant adverse events, including thrombosis, embolization, or arrhythmia were noted [35].

SIS Pulmonary Valve

A prosthetic pulmonary valve, constructed from a square stent with four barbs (Cook Inc., Bloomington, IN) and a sheet of SIS (Cook Biotech, Lafayette, IN), was also recently tested in animals. A stent was placed in the native pulmonary valve of 12 pigs to induce pulmonary insufficiency. The animals were monitored for several weeks until significant right ventricular dilatation was seen on echocardiography, after which a prosthetic pulmonary valve was placed by PCI in each. Placement of the prosthetic valve resulted in effective reversal of pulmonary insufficiency and follow-up by echocardiography at 1 year showed minimal regurgitation and no stenosis. Histologic examination demonstrated endothelialization of the surface of the device by 1 month and progressive significant remodeling over the next several months. No evidence of immunologic rejection was observed. At 1 year, progressive valve thickening led to a moderate reduction in valve motility. Adaptation of the valve to the growing pulmonary artery appeared to be limited by the metallic stent and not by the SIS leaflets [36]. While a prosthetic SIS valve is far from being ready for human trials, this study suggests

that SIS has significant potential. An SIS valve could potentially be placed percutaneously with a low-profile delivery system and be remodeled to resemble native tissue. Such a valve could provide graft longevity without the need for anticoagulation or immunosuppression.

Summary

Because of their use in coronary stents, biodegradable polymers have been developed for use in medical devices. The use of these materials for devices also now has been developed, and biodegradable stents and closure devices are in clinical trials. The chemistry and mechanical properties of these materials are well known. It is possible to engineer devices with very predictable degradation times, biology and radial force. Biodegradable materials are likely to replace many of the conventional metals in the current surgical and transcatheter pediatric devices. In general, the ideal material will always need to be nontoxic and non-thrombogenic and will need to have appropriate strength, elasticity, and degradation rate. Because the ideal biodegradable material will need to be tailored from device to device, there is unlikely to ever be one "ideal" biodegradable material. Nonetheless, many challenges remain for the development of devices in the pediatric community. A wide range of potential biodegradable devices possible can be realized in the pediatric community if the significant biological, regulatory and financial issues in bringing new pediatric biodegradable devices to market can be overcome.

References

1. Serruys PW, Ormiston J, Onuma Y et al (2009) A bioabsorbable everolimus-eluting coronary stent system (absorb): two-year outcomes and results from multiple imaging methods. Lancet 373:897–910
2. Ormiston JA, Serruys PWS (2009) Bioabsorbable coronary stents. Circ Cardiovasc Interv 2:255–260
3. Kimura T, Abe K, Shizuta S et al (2002) Long-term clinical and angiographic follow-up after coronary stent placement in native coronary arteries. Circulation 105:2986–2991

4. Ratner BD, Hoffman AS, Schoen FJ et al (1996) Bio-materials science: an introduction to materials in medicine. Academic, San Diego

5. Devellian SA, Kladakis SM, Opolski SW, Wright JA (2010) Engineering aspects of metallic and bioabsorbable devices. In: Hijazi ZM, Feldman T, Abdullah Al-Qbandi MH, Sievert H (eds) Transcatheter closure of ASDs and PFOs: a comprehensive assessment. Cardiotext, Minneapolis

6. Nair LS, Laurencin CT (2006) Polymers as biomaterials for tissue engineering and controlled drug delivery. Adv Biochem Eng Biotechnol 102:47–90

7. Eppley BL, Morales L, Wood R et al (2003) Resorbable PLLA-PGA plate and screw fixation in pediatric craniofacial surgery: clinical experience in 1883 patients. Pediatr Cranio-fac Surg 114(4):850–856

8. Middleton JC, Tipton AJ (2000) Synthetic biodegradable polymers as orthopedic devices. Biomaterials 21:2335–2346

9. Griffith LG (2000) Polymeric biomaterials. Acta Mater 48(1):263–277

10. Athanasiou KA, Agrawal CE, Barber FA, Burkhart SS (1998) Orthopaedic applications for PLA-PGA biodegradable polymers. Arthrosc J Arthrosc Relat Surg 14(7):726–737

11. Suganuma J, Alexandar H (1993) Biological response of intramedullary bone to poly(L-lactic acid). J Appl Biomater 4:13–27

12. Akin I, Schneider H, Ince H et al (2011) Second- and third-generation drug eluting coronary stents: progress and safety. Herz 36:190–197

13. Stone G, Ellis S, Colombo A et al (2007) Offsetting impact of thrombosis and restenosis on occurrence of death and myocardial infarction after paclitaxel-eluting and bare metal stent implantation. Circulation 115:2842–2847

14. Serruys PW, Daemen J (2007) Late stent thrombosis: a nuisance in both bare metal and drug-eluting stents. Circulation 115:1433–1439

15. Costa RA, Lansky AJ, Mintz GS et al (2005) Angiographic results of the first human experience with everolimus-eluting stents of the treatment of coronary lesions (the FUTURE I trial). Am J Cardiol 95(1):113–116

16. Grube E, Sonoda S, Ikeno F et al (2004) Six- and twelve-month results from first human experience using everolimus-eluting stents with bioabsorbable polymer. Circulation 109;2168–2171

17. Tomita H, Watanabe K, Yazaki S et al (2003) Stent implantation and subsequent dilatation for pulmonary vein stenosis in pediatric patients: maximizing effectiveness. Circ J 67:187–190

18. Onuma Y, Serruys PW, Ormiston JA et al (2010) Three-year results of clinical follow-up after a bioresorbable everolimus-eluting scaffold in patients with de novo coronary artery disease: the ABSORB trial. EuroIntervention 6(4):447–453

19. Serruys PW, Onuma Y, Ormiston JA et al (2010) Evaluation of the second generation of a bioresorbable everolimus drug-eluting vascular scaffold for treatment of de novo coronary artery stenosis. Circulation 122:2301–2312

20. Onuma Y, Serruys PW, Gomez J et al (2011) Comparison of in vivo acute stent recoil between the bioresorbable everolimus-eluting coronary scaffolds (revision 1.0 and 1.1) and the metallic everolimus-eluting stent. Catheter Cardiovasc Interv 78:3–12

21. Tanimoto S, Serruys PW, Thuesen L et al (2007) Comparison of in vivo acute stent recoil between the bioabsorbable everolimus-eluting coronary stent and the everolimus-eluting cobalt chromium coronary stent. Catheter Cardiovasc Interv 70:515–523

22. Diletti R, Onuma Y, Farooq V et al (2011) 6-month clinical outcomes following implantation of the bioresorbable everolimus-eluting vascular scaffold in vessels smaller or larger than 2.5 mm. J Am Coll Cardiol 58(3):258–264

23. Peuster M, Hesse C, Schloo T et al (2006) Long-term biocompatibility of a corrodible peripheral iron stent in the porcine descending aorta. Biomaterials 27(28):4955–4962

24. Erbel R, Di Mario C, Bartunek J et al (2007) - Temporary scaffolding of coronary arteries with bioabsorbable magnesium stents: a prospective non-randomized multicentre trial. Lancet 369: 1869–1875

25. Zartner P, Cesnjevar R, Singer H, Weyand M (2005) First successful implantation of a biodegradable metal stent into the left pulmonary artery of a preterm baby. Catheter Cardiovasc Interv 66: 590–594

26. Schranz D, Zartner P, Michel-Behnke I, Akinturk H (2006) Bioabsorbable metal stents for percutaneous treatment of critical recoarctation of the aorta in a newborn. Catheter Cardiovasc Interv 67:671–673

27. Luo JC, Chen W, Chen XH et al (2011) A multi-step method for preparation of porcine small intestinal submucosa (SIS). Biomaterials 32:706–713

28. Robotin-Johnson MC, Swanson PE, Johnson DC et al (1998) An experimental model of small intestinal submucosa as a growing vascular graft. J Thorac Cardiovasc Surg 116(5):805–811

29. Hata H, Bar A, Dorfman S et al (2010) Engineering a novel three-dimensional contractile myocardial patch with cell sheets and decellularised matrix. Eur J Cardiothorac Surg 38(4):450–455

30. Crapo PM, Wang Y (2010) Small intestinal submucosa gel as a potential scaffolding material for cardiac tissue engineering. Acta Biomater 6(6): 2091–2096

31. Okada M, Payne TR, Oshima H et al (2010) Differential efficacy of gels derived from small intestinal submucosa as an injectable biomaterial for myocardial infarct repair. Biomaterials 31(30): 7678–7683

32. Morgan G, Lee KJ, Chaturvedi R, Benson L (2010) A biodegradable device (BioSTAR) for atrial septal defect closure in children. Catheter Cardiovasc Interv 76(2):241–245

33. Hoehn R, Hesse C, Ince H, Peuster M (2010) First experience with the Biostar-device for various applications in pediatric patients with congenital heart disease. Catheter Cardiovasc Interv 75:72–77

34. Majunke N, Sievert H (2007) ASD/PFO devices: what is in the pipeline? J Interv Cardiol 20:517–523

35. Pavcnik D, Takulve K, Uchida BT et al (2010) Biodisk: a new device for closure of patent foramen ovale: a feasibility study in swine. Catheter Cardiovasc Interv 75:861–867

36. Ruiz CE, Iemura M, Medie S et al (2005) Transcatheter placement of a low-profile biodegradable pulmonary valve made of small intestinal submucosa: a long-term study in a swine model. J Thorac Cardiovasc Surg 130(2): 477–484

Robotic Surgery

Nikolay V. Vasilyev, Pedro J. del Nido, and Pierre E. Dupont

Abstract

Currently available robotic surgical and catheter-based systems have limited application in pediatric cardiac procedures. For surgical systems, the main obstacles include extended setup time and complexity of the procedures, as well as the large size of the instruments with respect to the size of the child. For intracardiac surgery, while the main advantage of robotic systems is the ability to minimize incision size, use of cardiopulmonary bypass is still required. Catheter-based robotic systems, on the other hand, have been expanding rapidly in both application and complexity of procedures and lesions treated. However, despite the development of sophisticated devices, robotic systems to aid catheter procedures have not been commonly applied in children. There are a few transcardiac and percutaneous robotic delivery platforms currently under development. These systems aim to facilitate safe navigation through confined spaces and, combined with novel instruments and devices, enable complex repairs, such as tissue approximation and fixation, and tissue removal, inside the beating heart under image guidance. Promising solutions for image-compatible and multifunctional robotic tools are also described.

N.V. Vasilyev (✉)
Department of Cardiac Surgery, Boston Children's
Hospital, Boston, MA, USA

Department of Surgery, Harvard Medical School, Boston,
MA, USA
e-mail: Nikolay.Vasilyev@childrens.harvard.edu

P.J. del Nido
Department of Cardiac Surgery, Boston Children's
Hospital, Boston, MA, USA
e-mail: Pedro.DelNido@childrens.harvard.edu

P.E. Dupont
Pediatric Cardiac Bioengineering, Boston Children's
Hospital, Boston, MA, USA

Department of Surgery, Harvard Medical School, Boston,
MA, USA
e-mail: Pierre.Dupont@childrens.harvard.edu

E.M. da Cruz et al. (eds.), *Pediatric and Congenital Cardiology, Cardiac Surgery and Intensive Care*,
DOI 10.1007/978-1-4471-4619-3_129, © Springer-Verlag London 2014

Keywords

Atrial septal defects • Beating heart • Cardiac surgery • Cardiovascular diseases • Catheters • Echocardiography • Endovascular • Heart defects congenital • Heart septal defects • Image-guided • Imaging • Interventions • Minimally invasive • Mitral valve • Navigation • Patent foramen ovale • Pediatrics • Percutaneous • Robotics • Robotically assisted • Transcatheter • Transcardiac • Ultrasonics • Ventricular septal defects

Introduction

In the last two decades, minimally invasive image-guided techniques have been gradually adapted to cardiac surgical specialties, from the initial attempts of video-assisted procedures through small incisions, toward fully endoscopic complex reconstructive procedures using telemanipulation systems and specialized instruments and devices. Among the advantages over conventional open-heart surgery, robotically assisted techniques offer less trauma to neighboring structures, which leads to less patient discomfort postoperatively and faster recovery. In addition, newly available specialized surgical tools and imaging aids provide the surgeon the ability to operate precisely in confined spaces and then assess the results of repair in physiologic conditions, which results in safe and effective repairs.

Robotic Surgical Systems

Currently, the da Vinci® Surgical System (Intuitive Surgical, Inc., Sunnyvale, CA) is the only FDA-approved system for intracardiac procedures. It consists of several components that include a surgical console, a patient-side cart, four interactive robotic arms, a 3D vision system, and proprietary EndoWrist® instruments. The surgeon operates from a console that is located remotely from the patient while using the 3D high-definition high-magnification endoscopic vision system for imaging. The patient-side cart is where the patient is positioned during surgery. It includes four robotic arms that accept the EndoWrist® instruments

and a dual-camera endoscope. These 7-degree-of-freedom instruments essentially represent mechanical wrists and are designed to function as the surgeon's forearm and wrist but with dexterity provided at the operative site through the entry ports. While the surgeon operates using the master control clutches at the console, a computer system causes the robot arms to transmit the surgeon's hand motions to the instruments while also enabling the features of tremor elimination, motion scaling, and motion indexing.

Robotically Assisted Pediatric Cardiac Surgery

The first report of robotically assisted cardiac surgical procedure was published in 1998 by Carpentier and colleagues [1]. The authors used a prototype of the current da Vinci® Surgical system and performed successful closure of an atrial septal defect (ASD) in a 52-year-old woman. Shortly thereafter, Mohr and colleagues performed the first coronary artery bypass in five patients, which was reported in 1999 [2]. Initially, the procedures were performed through small thoracotomy incisions. In the following years, the da Vinci® Surgical system has gained acceptance among adult cardiac surgeons and, with the improved instruments and visualization system, has been used in patients undergoing totally endoscopic coronary artery bypass or mitral valve repair [3, 4]. Despite increasing reports in adults, there is limited experience with robotically assisted procedures in children.

Pediatric Extracardiac Procedures

Le Bret and colleagues first reported robotically assisted patent ductus arteriosus (PDA) ligation in 2002 [5] using the discontinued ZEUS® Surgical System (Computer Motion, Inc., Goleta, CA, USA). The authors compared a robotically assisted technique for PDA closure with the standard video-assisted thoracoscopic surgery technique in 56 patients weighing 2.3–57 kg (mean = 12 kg), 28 patients per group. The robotic group ranged from 2 months to 5.5 years in age and from 3.2 to 22.5 kg in weight. The investigators found that the operation time was significantly longer in the robotically assisted group because of the incremental complexity, but no complications were noted. Suematsu and colleagues reported the successful use of the da Vinci® Surgical System for PDA closure in nine patients and vascular ring division in six patients weighing 14.1–77.0 kg (mean = 35.5 kg) [6]. It was found that, despite the long operative times, the robotic procedures were feasible and safe, largely due to advantage of 3D visualization and dexterous manipulation afforded by the surgical robotic system. The conclusions of these reports and others [7, 8], however, are that due to the large instrument size and need for entry port sites that are relatively far apart to avoid interference between the robotic arms, use of this system in children less than about 30 kg is quite difficult. For these reasons, most surgeons who have utilized the da Vinci® Surgical system in children believe that a robotic approach is comparable but has no major advantages over non-robotic thoracoscopic instruments using video-assisted techniques.

Pediatric Intracardiac Procedures

The reports of robotically assisted intracardiac procedures have been limited to a small series of adult size patients undergoing ASD closure. Torracca and colleagues used da Vinci® Surgical System for the repair of ASD in seven patients [9]. In their report, five patients had ASD, whereas the other two patients had a patent foramen ovale (PFO) with atrial septal aneurysm. The authors established cardiopulmonary bypass (CPB) via peripheral cannulation and used an endoaortic balloon occlusion of the ascending aorta. All procedures were completed endoscopically; no conversion was needed. Argenziano and colleagues and Wimmer-Greinecker and colleagues reported a totally endoscopic ASD repair procedure using the da Vinci® Surgical system in 17 and ten patients, respectively [10, 11]. In the report by Argenziano et al., one patient required reoperation due to a recurrent shunt. In the study by Wimmer-Greinecker et al., no complications occurred, although conversion to a minithoracotomy was required in two patients due to endoaortic balloon failure. Bacha and colleagues reported closure of sinus venosus defect in 40-year-old patient via a 3-cm right anterolateral minithoracotomy [12]. Baird and colleagues reported closure of ASD using the da Vinci® system and hypothermic fibrillatory arrest in a 14-year-old female weighting 35 kg [13]. In all these reports, the operative times and CPB times still exceed those needed for a conventional procedure due to extended setup time and complexity of the procedure. In addition, in most of the series, 8 mm instruments were used, which have a larger working area and therefore limited the use of the robotic system in younger patients. Recently, Intuitive Surgical introduced a new 5 mm instrument set; however, there is limited experience with these instruments.

Despite the fact that the robotically assisted approach contributes to reduced invasiveness of the procedure, there is still a need for the use of CPB, which may potentially lead to neurologic among other complications [14]. Furthermore, since in most of these procedures bypass is achieved by peripheral vessel cannulation, the small size of children's vessels with respect to cannula size introduces the added risk of permanent vessel damage and its impact on limb growth [15].

Catheter-Based Robotic Interventions

Catheter-based percutaneous interventions have evolved significantly over the past decades and have become routine procedures in most centers [16]. Robotically assisted catheter-based interventions, however, are still early in development and have not been widely used in pediatric practice. Currently, there are two robotic catheter technologies available, an electromechanically based system and a magnetically controlled system. Hansen Medical (Mountain View, CA) offers the Sensei X robotic navigation system designed for electrophysiology interventions, while their novel Magellan system is a platform for peripheral vascular interventions. The Niobe magnetic navigation system (Stereotaxis, St. Louis, MO) is operated by a magnetic field created by two computer-controlled 0.08 T permanent magnets. The magnets are mounted on articulating arms that are enclosed within a stationary housing, with one magnet on either side of the patient table. By changing the positions of these magnets with respect to the patient, deflection of the magnetic tip of the catheter can be precisely controlled. Recently, a magnetically controlled system that utilizes a technology of dynamically shaped magnetic fields was introduced (Catheter Guidance Control and Imaging, CGCI, Magnetecs, Los Angeles, CA). Currently, robotic catheter applications in adults include electrophysiological procedures for arrhythmia ablation, peripheral vascular interventions and coronary interventions, and more frequently transcatheter valve interventions [17–25].

Despite recent development of novel technologies, most of the robotically assisted catheter interventions are still fundamentally device deployment or tissue ablation rather than tissue reconstructive procedures. The limitations of current robotic catheter design include inadequate ability for significant force application, especially in a lateral direction from the axis of the catheter, and, at the same time, stable tip position control that is sufficient for tissue manipulation. These limitations impair the surgeon's ability to grasp, plicate, approximate, and remove tissue as it is done during complex repairs in open-heart surgery.

Beating-Heart Intracardiac Image-Guided Surgery

In light of the deleterious effects of CPB and with growing availability of new imaging techniques and device development, there has been an ongoing interest in developing techniques to perform the same types of repairs currently done as open procedures but with the heart beating to avoid use of CPB. Initial attempts have been reported, mostly methods of septal defect closure and mitral valve repair. Warinsirikul and colleagues reported ASD patch closure in 76 patients, whereas the patch was attached with blind suture fixation followed by intra-atrial stapling under transesophageal echocardiography (TEE) guidance [26]. Beating-heart repair of mitral valve prolapse in an animal model has been reported by Seeburger and colleagues. The authors used a novel system developed by NeoChord (NeoChord, Inc. Minnetonka, MN) and were able to insert artificial chords via a transapical approach under echocardiography guidance [27].

Initial laboratory efforts have included direct image-guided approaches such as optical imaging with an endocardioscope in eight dogs for septal defect repair [28] and TEE-guided mitral valve suturing in a porcine model. Vasilyev and colleagues reported beating-heart ASD and ventricular septal defect (VSD) closure under image guidance in swine models [29, 30]. A patch delivery device and handheld anchor delivery system were utilized for atrial and ventricular septal defect closure under real-time 3D echocardiography. Video-assisted cardioscopy was used for intraoperative imaging and instrument navigation.

In order to bring these initial attempts to wide clinical practice, some major developments are required. New robotic delivery platforms need to be developed that provide steerability, precise repeatable motion control, and safe navigation and manipulation of rapidly moving intracardaic structures. In addition, new instruments and devices need to be developed that enable complex tissue manipulations inside the beating heart, limit interference with imaging techniques, and ideally can be integrated with a delivery platform.

Experimental Systems Under Development

Robotic Platforms for Beating-Heart Intracardiac Procedures

Concentric Tube Robots

Recently, a new class of robots for minimally invasive surgery has been developed called concentric tube robots [31–39]. While potentially appropriate for many types of minimally invasive surgery, their size and steerability make them particularly appropriate for intracardiac beating-heart surgery [37, 39–41]. These robots are similar in size to catheters but differ in construction since they are formed from the concentric, telescoping, curved superelastic metal tubes. The shape of the robots is a smooth three-dimensional curve that is controlled by rotating and translating the individual tubes within each other. While their construction makes these robots significantly stiffer than conventional catheters, the ability to precisely control robot shape enables safe navigation inside vessels and

the heart. Tools and devices are deployed through the central lumen of the robot that serves as a working channel.

The family of shapes that a concentric tube robot can assume is determined by the shape and length of the individual tubes that comprise it. Sets of tubes for specific procedures can be designed that provide the robot shapes necessary to enable navigation to the surgical site as well as to perform the procedure [32, 39]. These tube sets can be made either for single use or for repeated use with sterilization. A motorized drive system, compatible with all tube sets, is used to control the motion of the individual tubes while the surgeon controls commands the overall motion of the robot using a joystick. Robot design algorithms are available to develop tube sets for new intracardiac procedures. These algorithms use image-based models of the anatomy together with geometric descriptions of the procedure to compute the appropriate lengths, shapes, and stiffness of individual tubes [39].

Robots similar to the design shown in Fig. 69.1 have been employed in percutaneous beating-heart tissue-to-tissue approximation for PFO closure in the right atrium [37]. Entry to the heart was gained via the internal jugular vein. For imaging, a combination of 3D ultrasound and fluoroscopy was employed. The stiffness and steerability of the robot enabled precise positioning on the septum and also the ability to "park" the robot in a particular shape and position so that imaging studies could be performed.

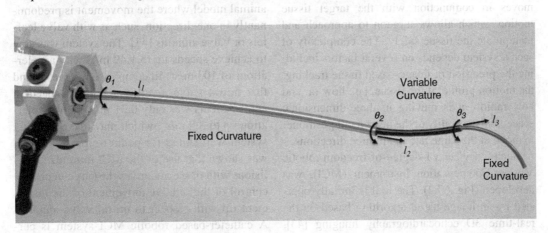

Fig. 69.1 Robot used for PFO closure. Design consists of three telescoping sections

Fig. 69.2 Handheld
1-degree-of-freedom
Motion Compensation
Instrument

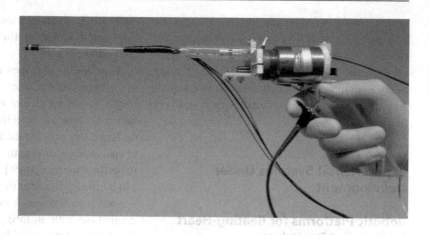

Robotically Assisted Motion Compensation Tools

While atrial septal motion over the cardiac cycle is modest, this is not true for other structures inside the beating heart. Interacting with valvar structures may not be achieved solely with robotically assisted tool tip stabilization, and a different method is required to avoid collision with such delicate structures. One option is to capture and immobilize a valve leaflet first, which then allows performing necessary manipulations with it. This approach is used in several tools for beating-heart mitral valve repair including MitraClip (Abbott Laboratories, Abbott Park, IL) and NeoChord (NeoChord, Inc. Minnetonka, MN), and others [27, 42]. An alternative approach is called robotically assisted motion cancellation, where the instrument moves in conjunction with the target tissue motion, which allows surgeon to approach and manipulate the tissue safely. The complexity of such a system depends on several factors including the precision of image-based tissue tracking; the motion profile of the tissue, i.e., how far and how rapidly it is moving in three-dimensional space; and the ability of the instrument positioner to move at the same rate in all three directions.

Such a device, a 1-degree-of-freedom robotic Motion Compensation Instrument (MCI), was developed (Fig. 69.2). The tool is initially operated by an image-based algorithm based on the real-time 3D echocardiography imaging [43]. The system identifies and tracks the position of

the tissue target directly in front of the tool, and a linear motor moves the instrument shaft according to the target motion.

One of the limitations of image-based tracking is that once the surgical instrument tip comes into contact with the tissue target, the algorithm can no longer separate tissue movement from the instrument tip and therefore cannot control the instrument accurately. To address this limitation, a force control tracking algorithm is utilized in addition to the image-based tracking [44]. A force sensor, which is placed on the tip of the MCI, reads the force that the surgeon applies to the target tissue in real time. The force control algorithm thus enables maintenance of constant force against the tissue, which significantly increases the safety of the procedure. The MCI system was tested in an animal model where the movement is predominantly in one direction, such as with valve leaflets or valve annulus [43]. The system was able to achieve speeds up to 1.49 m/s, with accelerations of 103 m/s^2. In comparison, it was found that mitral valve annulus maximum speed in adult patients was only 0.21 m/s, with acceleration up to 3.8 m/s^2, which may make the MCI system well suited for pediatric procedures. It was shown that use of the MCI minimizes collisions with tissue and gives the surgeon precise control of the relative movement of the instrument tip with respect to mitral valve annulus. A catheter-based robotic MCI system is currently under development (Fig. 69.3).

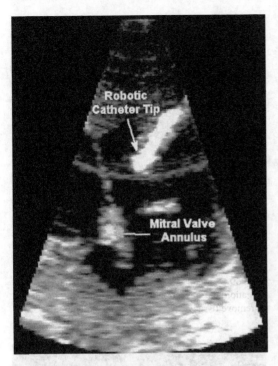

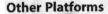

Fig. 69.3 3D-echocardiography image of the catheter-based Motion Compensation Instrument

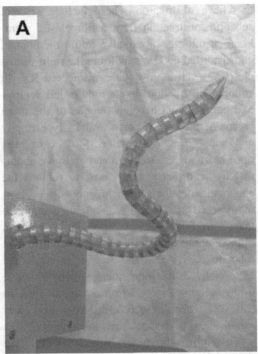

Fig. 69.4 CardioARM robotic surgical

Other Platforms

Robotic platforms for extracardiac procedures have also been under development. The articulated robotic surgical system CardioARM (Cardiorobotics Inc., Middletown, RI) is a snake-type robot composed of series of rigid cylindrical links serially connected by three cables (Fig. 69.4).

The distal apparatus is 10 mm in diameter and 300 mm in length, with 105° of freedom, and is operated by a 2-degree-of-freedom joystick to control the most distal link together with a button to control forward/backward motions. All of the links are not individually controlled, as the robot employs the so-called "follow-the-leader" motion strategy. It possesses significant strength in the longitudinal direction but less so in the lateral direction. Catheter-based tools can be passed through the robot, and a fiber scope can be used for visible light pericardioscopy imaging. The robot was successfully tested in large swine animal model, where epicardial navigation and left atrial ablation trials were performed [45].

There are no reports, however, on possible use of such a system for pediatric extracardiac or intracardiac applications.

Instruments and Devices

In open-heart procedures, fundamental surgical maneuvers, such as tissue removal and approximation, are usually performed with standard surgical instruments. In cases of endoscopically guided minimally invasive procedures, long shaft endoscopic tools are used. However, both of these designs are not applicable inside the beating heart on rapidly moving structures in the presence of blood. The instruments also need to be compatible with the imaging modality used for procedure guidance and should be integrated with the robotic platforms.

Tissue Removal Tools

There are several clinical applications where precise tissue removal in confined spaces is required to relieve obstruction. These include discrete subaortic obstruction from a fibroelastic membrane or muscle, supra-valve mitral membrane, and abnormal muscle bundles in the right ventricle (RV) such as in double-chambered RV. In children, obstructions in the right or left ventricular outflow tract account for one of the more common causes of myocardial hypertrophy and subsequent dysfunction [46]. Currently, open-heart surgery to completely remove abnormal tissue or, in severe cases, to replace the abnormal structure is often the only option. Beating-heart tissue removal is an alternate approach that is currently being developed. Tissue removal in these applications utilizes the concentric tube robot to navigate to the area of interest, and a specialized microdebrider, which is made using metal micro electromechanical systems (MEMS) technology, is used to sculpt away excess tissue from the desired location [41].

To remove abnormal obstructions from the right ventricular outflow tract (RVOT), the concentric tube robotic system, similar to Fig. 69.1, is delivered percutaneously via a trans-jugular approach. The tool, containing rotating cutting blades, performs the combined functions of tissue cutting, morselizing, and particle entrainment as well as disposal (Fig. 69.5). The latter are implemented by including irrigation and aspiration channels inside the robot lumen. The results of ex vivo tests are shown in Fig. 69.6. As shown, this tool can be used to remove millimeter-thick surface layers of endocardium. It can also be used to create deeper cavities in the tissue. While aspiration removes the bulk of the tissue debris, a downstream embolization filter may need to be deployed into the main pulmonary artery to collect any particulate emboli that may be dislodged by the process of tissue removal.

Tissue Approximation Tools

Tissue approximation is a fundamental maneuver in surgical reconstruction and involves grasping one part of tissue and attaching it to another or to an artificial material. Novel devices have been under development that may enable these precise maneuvers during beating-heart procedures.

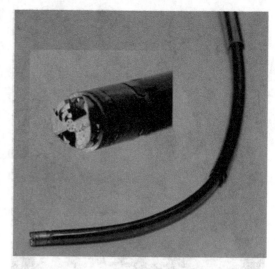

Fig. 69.5 Metal MEMS tissue removal device. Both irrigation and aspiration are incorporated into the design to remove tissue debris through the robot lumen

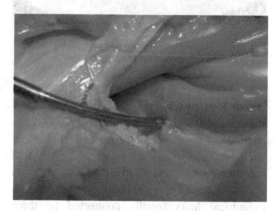

Fig. 69.6 Ex vivo example of tissue removal in the right ventricular outflow tract

One specific example of tissue approximation is PFO closure. Current approaches to closure include open-heart surgery and catheter-based deployment of an occluder device. Experience with device closure, however, shows that serious complications such as hemorrhage, cardiac tamponade, the need for surgery, pulmonary embolism, and death occur in 1.5 % of patients and minor complications (arrhythmia, device fracture or embolization, air embolism, femoral hematoma, and fistula) in another 7.9 % [47]. Results with open-heart surgery indicate significantly lower risk of complications and no

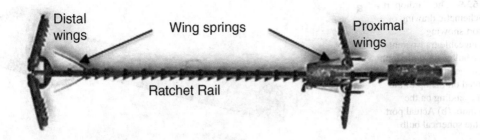

Fig. 69.7 Metal MEMS tissue approximation device

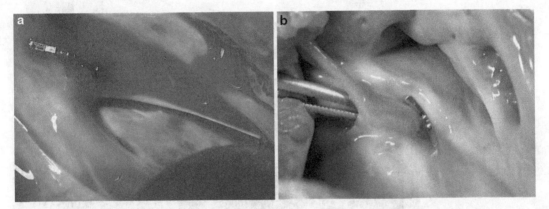

Fig. 69.8 Implanted tissue approximation device. (**a**) Right atrial view, (**b**) left atrial view

recurrence at 23 months of follow-up [48]. A device and technique of PFO closure that mimics surgical closure was developed (Fig. 69.7). The device is manufactured fully assembled using a metal MEMS fabrication process. It is comprised of two pairs of expanding spring-loaded wings that are used to pull the tissue layers together. The wing pairs are attached by a ratcheting mechanism that enables the tissue layer approximation distance to be adjusted with submillimeter accuracy. During device deployment, the robotic delivery platform enables accurate approximation of the septum secundum and primum by first piercing the secundum and then dragging it laterally to achieve the desired overlap with the septum primum (Fig. 69.8).

Successful PFO closure using the device has been demonstrated in porcine in vivo trials [37]. With further development, this device concept may serve as a platform for other procedures such as valve repair.

Imaging-Compatible Tools

For intracardiac robotically assisted beating-heart surgery, imaging plays a critical role. Real-time high-resolution imaging is necessary for the surgeon to navigate to the target, perform the required task, and then confirm adequate and accurate completion of the repair. In addition, imaging data often serves as an input for image-based robotic control algorithms. Therefore, its spatial and temporal resolution must meet the highest performance standards.

Recently, real-time 3D echocardiography has been gaining acceptance as often the sole imaging modality for guiding beating-heart intracardiac interventions given its relatively large field of view and its ability to image the surgical tool and the tissue structures simultaneously [49–53]. Most traditional surgical instruments, however, are made of hard materials with smooth surfaces, which produce a variety of image artifacts when ultrasound waves interact with their surfaces, and

Fig. 69.9 The Cardioport. (a) Schematic drawing of the port showing exchangeable transparent plastic bulbs; the bulbs with various geometries can be mounted on the tip of the port depending on the procedure. (b) Actual port with the spherical bulb

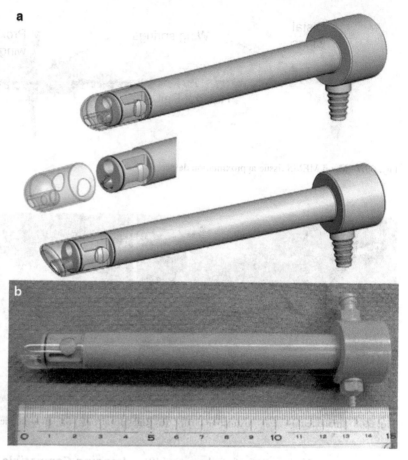

can make it difficult to clearly visualize the instrument as well as nearby tissue [54, 55]. A variety of solutions to the artifact problem have been introduced. These include instrument modification, image processing techniques, active tracking sensors, and fiduciary markers. Instrument modification involves the application of coatings or surface modifications to reduce the specular reflectivity or to increase absorption [54–58]. Image processing methods apply search techniques to locate an instrument in an image [59–63]. Tracking sensors can also be placed on the surgical tool to detect instrument position and by registering the position relative to the ultrasound image provide real-time information as to the position of the tool within the image [64]. Fiduciary markers on the instruments that are strongly echogenic can also be used to enable the instrument position and orientation to be detected using image-based algorithms from the marker image [65, 66].

Multifunctional Tools

Most of the currently available instruments for minimally invasive surgery and catheter-based procedures are designed as single-function tools and have to be continually exchanged during the procedure. Although tool multifunctionality has the advantage of having a single tool for various tasks performed inside the heart, the design concept increases device complexity, particularly at the instrument tip and handle mechanisms. An intermediate step toward a fully multifunctional tool may be a single access multi-tool approach, where various tools are introduced via a single entry point into the patient's body significantly minimizing trauma and eliminating the need for instrument exchanges at the same time. There are new designs of such dexterous multifunctional robotic tools offered for endoscopic "single-port" surgical procedures. Intuitive Surgical has announced a single-port instrument set, which is not yet available on the market for cardiac procedures, and is undergoing feasibility studies in adult laparoscopic procedures [67]. It is yet to be seen, if such an approach is feasible for pediatric beating-heart interventions.

An additional feature to increase the functionality of the instrument is to incorporate an imaging modality. With recent technological developments for gastroenterologic natural orifice translumenal endoscopic surgical procedures, there have been a few commercially available systems that combine endoscopic imaging and dexterous instrumentation [68]. For cardiac applications, there is no commercially available multifunctional instrument. Vasilyev and colleagues reported development of a Cardioport that combines video-assisted optical cardioscopy and an instrument channel to access structures inside the beating heart [69] (Fig. 69.9).

The optical channel contained in the instrument is used to image the cardiac structure by pressing the scope against the tissue, displacing the blood, and permitting optical imaging of the heart surface. A fluid purging and valve system is utilized in the instrument channel, in order to prevent blood loss and air entry during instrument introduction and exchanges. In animal experiments, the Cardioport was successfully used for beating-heart atrial and septal defect closure and tricuspid valve annular dilation model creation [70].

Conclusion

Despite the fact that robotic systems have evolved significantly over the past decades, there is still limited application of these technologies in extracardiac and intracardiac pediatric procedures. Current clinically available systems have been designed primarily for adult surgical applications. Pediatric intracardiac interventions present an additional challenge, since the complex maneuvers required have to be performed in an even smaller space while operating on delicate tissue. In the research and development pipeline, there are promising

platforms for robotically assisted beating-heart intracardiac procedures, which meet the challenges of accessing rapidly moving intracardiac structures. These nonrigid systems can be delivered either transcardiac or percutaneously, much like catheter-based interventions, but with the added functionality of providing a stable platform with the ability to manipulate tissue in a precise and controlled manner. Newly developed instruments combined with smaller, more steerable robotic delivery platforms and enhanced imaging form a single multifunctional tool platform technology, which may enable development of pediatric beating-heart reconstructive interventions currently not feasible with available robotic systems or by conventional catheter-based techniques.

References

1. Carpentier A, Loulmet D, Aupècle B et al (1998) Computer assisted open-heart surgery. First case operated on with success. C R Acad Sci III 321(5):437–442
2. Mohr FW, Falk V, Diegeler A, Autschback R (1999) Computer-enhanced coronary artery bypass surgery. J Thorac Cardiovasc Surg 117(6):1212–1214
3. Anderson CA, Chitwood WR (2009) Advances in mitral valve repair. Future Cardiol 5(5):511–516
4. Bonatti J, Schachner T, Bonaros N, Lehr EJ, Zimrin D, Griffith B (2011) Robotically assisted totally endoscopic coronary bypass surgery. Circulation 124(2):236–244
5. Le Bret E, Papadatos S, Folliguet T et al (2002) Interruption of patent ductus arteriosus in children: robotically assisted versus videothoracoscopic surgery. J Thorac Cardiovasc Surg 123(5):973–976
6. Suematsu Y, Mora BN, Mihaljevic T, del Nido PJ (2005) Totally endoscopic robotic-assisted repair of patent ductus arteriosus and vascular ring in children. Ann Thorac Surg 80(6):2309–2313
7. Mihaljevic T, Cannon JW, del Nido PJ (2003) Robotically assisted division of a vascular ring in children. J Thorac Cardiovasc Surg 125(5):1163–1164
8. Meehan JJ, Sandler AD (2008) Robotic resection of mediastinal masses in children. J Laparoendosc Adv Surg Tech A 18(1):114–119
9. Torracca L, Ismeno G, Quarti A, Alfieri O (2002) Totally endoscopic atrial septal defect closure with a robotic system: experience with seven cases. Heart Surg Forum 5(2):125–127
10. Argenziano M, Oz MC, Kohmoto T et al (2003) Totally endoscopic atrial septal defect repair with robotic assistance. Circulation 108(Suppl 1): II191–II194

11. Wimmer-Greinecker G, Dogan S, Aybek T et al (2003) Totally endoscopic atrial septal repair in adults with computer-enhanced telemanipulation. J Thorac Cardiovasc Surg 126(2):465–468

12. Bacha EA, Bolotin G, Consilio K, Raman J, Ruschhaupt DG (2005) Robotically assisted repair of sinus venosus defect. J Thorac Cardiovasc Surg 129(2):442–443

13. Baird CW, Stamou SC, Skipper E, Watts L (2007) Total endoscopic repair of a pediatric atrial septal defect using the da Vinci robot and hypothermic fibrillation. Interact Cardiovasc Thorac Surg 6(6):828–829

14. Menache CC, du Plessis AJ, Wessel DL, Jonas RA, Newburger JW (2002) Current incidence of acute neurologic complications after open-heart operations in children. Ann Thorac Surg 73(6):1752–1758

15. Gander JW, Fisher JC, Reichstein AR et al (2010) Limb ischemia after common femoral artery cannulation for venoarterial extracorporeal membrane oxygenation: an unresolved problem. J Pediatr Surg 45(11):2136–2140

16. Hijazi ZM, Awad SM (2008) Pediatric cardiac interventions. JACC Cardiovasc Interv 1(6):603–611

17. Antoniou GA, Riga CV, Mayer EK, Cheshire NJ, Bicknell CD (2011) Clinical applications of robotic technology in vascular and endovascular surgery. J Vasc Surg 53(2):493–499

18. Bismuth J, Kashef E, Cheshire N, Lumsden A (2011) Feasibility and safety of remote endovascular catheter navigation in a porcine model. J Endovasc Ther 18:243–249

19. Wood MA, Orlov M, Ramaswamy K, Haffajee C, Ellenbogen K, Stereotaxis Heart Study Investigators (2008) Remote magnetic versus manual catheter navigation for ablation of supraventricular tachycardias: a randomized, multicenter trial. Pacing Clin Electrophysiol 31(10):1313–1321

20. Di Biase L, Fahmy TS, Patel D et al (2007) Remote magnetic navigation: human experience in pulmonary vein ablation. J Am Coll Cardiol 50(9):868–874

21. Miyazaki S, Shah AJ, Xhaët O et al (2010) Remote magnetic navigation with irrigated tip catheter for ablation of paroxysmal atrial fibrillation. Circ Arrhythm Electrophysiol 3(6):585–589

22. Gang ES, Nguyen BL, Shachar Y et al (2011) Dynamically shaped magnetic fields: initial animal validation of a new remote electrophysiology catheter guidance and control system. Circ Arrhythm Electrophysiol 4(5):770–777

23. Lüthje L, Vollmann D, Seegers J et al (2011) Remote magnetic versus manual catheter navigation for circumferential pulmonary vein ablation in patients with atrial fibrillation. Clin Res Cardiol 100(11):1003–1011

24. Lumsden AB, Anaya-Ayala JE, Birnbaum I et al (2010) Robot-assisted stenting of a high-grade anastomotic pulmonary artery stenosis following single lung transplantation. J Endovasc Ther 17(5):612–616

25. Riga CV, Bicknell CD, Hamady MS, Cheshire NJ (2011) Evaluation of robotic endovascular catheters for arch vessel cannulation. J Vasc Surg 54(3):799–809

26. Warinsirikul W, Sangchote S, Mokarapong P, Chaiyodsilp S, Tanamai S (2001) Closure of atrial septal defects without cardiopulmonary bypass: the sandwich operation. J Thorac Cardiovasc Surg 121(6):1122–1129

27. Seeburger J, Leontjev S, Neumuth M et al (2011) Trans-apical beating-heart implantation of neo-chordae to mitral valve leaflets: results of an acute animal study. Eur J Cardiothorac Surg May 17

28. Sogawa M, Moro H, Tsuchida M, Shinonaga M, Ohzeki H, Hayashi J (1999) Development of an endocardioscope for repair of an atrial septal defect in the beating heart. ASAIO J 45(1):90–93

29. Vasilyev NV, Martinez JF, Freudenthal FP, Suematsu Y, Marx GR, del Nido PJ (2006) Three-dimensional echo and videocardioscopy-guided atrial septal defect closure. Ann Thorac Surg 82(4):1322–1326

30. Vasilyev NV, Melnychenko I, Kitahori K et al (2008) Beating-heart patch closure of muscular ventricular septal defects under real-time 3D echo guidance: a pre-clinical study. J Thorac Cardiovasc Surg 135(3):603–609

31. Sears P, Dupont P (2006) A steerable needle technology using curved concentric tubes. ConfProc IEEE/RSJ Intelligent Robots and Systems (IROS), pp 2850–2856

32. Dupont P, Lock J, Itkowitz B, Butler E (2010) Design and control of concentric tube robots. IEEE Trans Robot 26(2):209–225

33. Rucker D, Webster R III, Chirikjian G, Cowan N (2010) Equilibrium conformations of concentric-tube continuum robots. Int J Robotics Research 29(10):1263–1280

34. Lock J, Laing G, Mahvash M, Dupont P (2010) Quasistatic modeling of concentric tube robots with external loads. Conf Proc IEEE/RSJ Intelligent Robots and Systems (IROS), pp 2325–2332

35. Rucker DC, Jones BA, Webster RJ III (2010) A geometrically exact model for externally loaded concentric-tube continuum robots. IEEE Trans Robotics 26(5):769–780

36. Mahvash M, Dupont P (2011) Stiffness control of surgical continuum manipulators. IEEE Trans Robot 27(2):334–345

37. Butler E, Folk C, Cohen A et al (2011) Metal MEMS tools for beating-heart tissue approximation. Conf Proc IEEE International Conference on Robotics and Automation, pp 411–416

38. Lock J, Dupont P (2011) Friction modeling in concentric tube robots. Conf Proc IEEE International Conference on Robotics and Automation, pp 1139–1146

39. Bedell C, Lock J, Gosline A, Dupont P (2011) Design optimization of concentric tube robots based on task and anatomical constraints. Conf Proc IEEE International Conference on Robotics and Automation, pp 398–403

40. Gosline A, Vasilyev N, Veeramani A et al (2012) Metal MEMS tools for beating-heart tissue removal. Conf Proc IEEE International Conference on Robotics and Automation, pp 1921–1936

41. Gosline A, Vasilyev NV, Butler E et al (2012) Percutaneous intracardiac beating-heart surgery using metal MEMS tissue approximation tools. Int J Robotics Research 31:1081–1093

42. Goldberg SL, Feldman T (2010) Percutaneous mitral valve interventions: overview of new approaches. Curr Cardiol Rep 12(5):404–412

43. Yuen SG, Kesner SB, Vasilyev NV, Del Nido PJ, Howe RD (2008) 3D ultrasound-guided motion compensation system for beating heart mitral valve repair. Med Image Comput Comput Assist Interv 11(Pt 1):711–719

44. Yuen SG, Yip MC, Vasilyev NV, Perrin DP, Del Nido PJ, Howe RD (2009) Robotic force stabilization for beating heart intracardiac surgery. Med Image Comput Comput Assist Interv 5761(2009):26–33

45. Ota T, Degani A, Schwartzman D, Zubiate B, McGarvey J, Choset H, Zenati MA (2009) A highly articulated robotic surgical system for minimally invasive surgery. Ann Thorac Surg 87(4):1253–1256

46. Margossian R (2008) Contemporary management of pediatric heart failure. Expert Rev Cardiovasc Ther 6(2):187–197

47. Khairy P, O'Donnell CP, Landzberg MJ (2003) Transcatheter closure versus medical therapy of patent foramen ovale and presumed paradoxical thromboemboli: a systematic review. Ann Intern Med 139:753–760

48. Devuyst G, Bogousslavsky J, Ruchat P et al (1996) Prognosis after stroke followed by surgical closure of patent foramen ovale: a prospective follow-up study with brain MRI and simultaneous transesophageal and transcranial Doppler ultrasound. Neurology 47.1162–1166

49. Suematsu Y, Marx GR, Stoll JA et al (2004) Three-dimensional echocardiography-guided beating-heart surgery without cardiopulmonary bypass: a feasibility study. J Thorac Cardiovasc Surg 128(4):579–587

50. Suematsu Y, Martinez JF, Wolf BK et al (2005) Three-dimensional echo-guided beating heart surgery without cardiopulmonary bypass: atrial septal defect closure in a swine model. J ThoracCardiovasc Surg 130(5):1348–1357

51. Cannon J, Stoll J, Salgo I et al (2003) Real-time three-dimensional ultrasound for guiding surgical tasks. Computer Aid Surg 8(2):82–90

52. Balzer J, Kuhl H, Rassaf T et al (2008) Real-time transesophageal three-dimensional echocardiography for guidance of percutaneous cardiac interventions: first experience. Clin Res Cardiol 97:565–574

53. Deng J, Rodeck C (2006) Current applications of fetal cardiac imaging technology. Curr Opin Obst Gynec 18(2):177

54. Huang J, Dupont P, Undurti A, Triedman J, Cleveland R (2006) Producing diffuse ultrasound reflections from medical instruments using the quadratic residue diffuser. Ultrasound Med Biol 32(5):721–727

55. Huang J, Triedman JK, Vasilyev NV, Suematsu Y, Cleveland RO, Dupont PE (2007) Imaging artifacts of medical instruments in ultrasound-guided interventions. J Ultrasound Med 26(10):1303–1322

56. Nichols K, Wright L, Spencer T, Culp W (2003) Changes in ultrasonographic echogenicity and visibility of needles with changes in angles of insonation. J VascInterv Radiol 14(12):1553–1557

57. Reading C, Charboneau J, James E, Hurt M (1988) Sonographically guided percutaneous biopsy of small (3 cm or less) masses. AJR Am J Roentgenol 151(1):189

58. Culp W, McCowan T, Goertzen T et al (2000) Relative ultrasonographic echogenicity of standard, dimpled, and polymeric-coated needles. J Vasc Interv Radiol 11(3):351–358

59. Ding M, Fenster A (2003) A real-time biopsy needle segmentation technique using hough transform. Medical Physics 30(8):2222–2233

60. Draper KJ, Blake CC, Gowman L, Downey DB, Fenster A (2000) An algorithm for automatic needle localization in ultrasound-guided breast biopsies. Medical Physics 27(8):1971–1979

61. Novotny P, Cannon J, Howe R (2003) Tool localization in 3d ultrasound images. Medical Image Computing and Computer-Assisted Intervention-MICCAI, pp 969–970

62. Ren H, Vasilyev N, Dupont P (2011) Detection of curved robots using 3D ultrasound. Conf Proc IEEE/RSJ Intelligent Robots and Systems (IROS), pp 2083–2089

63. Ren H, Dupont P (2011) Tubular structure enhancement for surgical instrument detection in 3D ultrasound. Conf Proc IEEE Engineering in Medicine and Biology Conference (EMBC) pp 7203–7206

64. Leotta D (2004) An efficient calibration method for freehand 3-d ultrasound imaging systems. Ultrasound Med Bio 30(7):999–1008

65. Stoll J, Dupont P (2005) Passive markers for ultrasound tracking of surgical instruments. ConfProc Medical Image Processing and Computer-Assisted Intervention (MICCAI), pp II41–II48

66. Stoll J, Ren H, Dupont P (2012) Passive markers for tracking surgical instruments in real-time 3D ultrasound imaging. IEEE Transactions on Medical Imaging 31(3):563–575

67. Kroh M, El-Hayek K, Rosenblatt S et al (2011) First human surgery with a novel single-port robotic system: cholecystectomy using the da Vinci Single-Site platform. Surg Endosc 25(11):3566–3573

68. Swanstrom LL (2011) NOTES: Platform development for a paradigm shift in flexible endoscopy. Gastroenterology 140(4):1150–1154

69. Vasilyev NV, Kawata M, DiBiasio CM et al (2011) A novel cardioport for beating-heart, image-guided intracardiac surgery. J Thorac Cardiovasc Surg 142(6):1545–1551

70. Walter EM, Vasilyev NV, Sill B, Padala M et al (2011) Creation of a tricuspid valve regurgitation model from tricuspid annular dilatation using the cardioport video-assisted imaging system. J Heart Valve Dis 20(2):184–188

Hybrid Strategies (Non-HLHS)

70

Darren P. Berman and Evan M. Zahn

Abstract

Over the past 20 years, survival for patients with congenital heart disease has improved dramatically. With this, has come a fundamental shift in the field from simply maintaining survival to developing better ways to both minimize the cumulative therapeutic trauma that congenital heart disease patients must endure while improving functional outcomes. A variety of hybrid procedures that utilize a combination of surgical and interventional catheterization techniques have been developed to advance this strategy.

Keywords

Aorta • Coarctation • Hybrid procedures • Intravascular stent • Pediatric interventions • Pulmonary arteries

Introduction

Survival for patients with congenital heart disease (CHD) has improved dramatically over the past 20 years. Emphasis within the field has thus begun to shift from simply maintaining survival to finding new and better ways to improve functional outcomes while at the same time minimizing the cumulative therapeutic trauma that patients must endure throughout their lifetime. The advent of procedures which utilize a combination of surgical

D.P. Berman (✉)
Cardiology, Miami Children's Hospital, Miami, FL, USA
e-mail: darren.berman@mch.com

E.M. Zahn
Cardiology, Cedars-Sinai Medical Center, Los Angeles, CA, USA
e-mail: Evan.Zahn@cshs.org

and interventional catheterization techniques, so-called hybrid procedures, has the potential to play a prominent role in this strategy.

Houde et al. published the first description of a hybrid procedure used for the treatment of CHD nearly 20 years ago with a combined approach to stent placement in a child with pulmonary atresia [1]. Currently, hybrid procedures are defined as any technique that utilizes both surgery and interventional catheterization in a single procedure. An important goal of any hybrid strategy should be to maximize patient outcomes while minimizing morbidity through a combination of decreasing the total number of procedures a patient must undergo as well as reduction of operative or interventional trauma caused by each procedure performed. In this chapter a number of hybrid procedures exclusive of the treatment of hypoplastic left heart syndrome (HLHS) will be

E.M. da Cruz et al. (eds.), *Pediatric and Congenital Cardiology, Cardiac Surgery and Intensive Care*,
DOI 10.1007/978-1-4471-4619-3_130, © Springer-Verlag London 2014

discussed. Elsewhere in this textbook, a specific chapter dedicated to hybrid procedures in HLHS can be found.

Restoration or Maintenance of Pulmonary Blood Flow

Pulmonary Artery Stent Implantation

Placement of intravascular stents into central and branch pulmonary arteries is a well-accepted therapeutic option for the treatment of pulmonary artery (PA) stenoses [2, 3]. In general, the goal is to deliver a stent that provides not only complete and immediate stenosis relief but also has the ability to be re-dilated at a future date to keep pace with a child's somatic growth. Due to improvements in delivery techniques and balloons, stents, and sheath technologies, the majority of PA stents can be delivered percutaneously [4, 5]; however, there are several important scenarios where hybrid delivery of a PA stent may be advantageous [6]. These include small patient size (e.g., infants and neonates), limited vascular access, the need for concomitant surgical procedures, and as rescue therapy for either a failed percutaneous stent attempt or for a patient unable to separate from cardiopulmonary bypass due to PA stenosis. Advantages to hybrid PA stent implantation include:

1. The ability to implant a stent with the capability of achieving an adult diameter regardless of patient size at the time of implant (including young infants)
2. Avoidance of intracardiac catheter manipulation, which may be important for critically ill patients, particularly in the early postoperative period [7]
3. Minimization or avoidance of ionizing radiation
4. Reduction of total number of invasive procedures by combining several procedures (e.g., conduit replacement and bilateral PA stent placement) into one
5. Improved accuracy of stent placement including the ability to redo the implant if desired and/or flair proximal stents against the PA wall to facilitate future vessel reentry

Technique: Two different techniques have evolved for the hybrid delivery of PA stents. The first, stent implantation under direct or endoscopic visualization, is typically a planned procedure performed in the operating room or a hybrid suite. The second, stent implantation via surgically provided vascular access supported with fluoroscopic imaging, can be used to treat not only PA stenoses but several other lesions that will be discussed in later sections. This approach can be performed in a standard catheterization suite, surgical operating room (with portable fluoroscopic imaging), or hybrid suite.

Direct or videoscopic-guided stent implantation: This procedure is typically performed at the time of other required surgical procedures such as right ventricular outflow tract reconstruction, conduit replacement, delayed ventricular septal defect (VSD) closure (in the setting of pulmonary atresia and VSD), bidirectional Glenn, or Fontan palliation. A critical component to success is a thorough quantitative assessment of all pertinent anatomy *prior to* the procedure. Until recently, this has typically been done with preoperative biplane angiography, although preoperative 3-dimensional rotational angiography may supplant this [8]. Since these implants are done without fluoroscopy or angiography, decisions regarding implant location, stent type, length, and the diameter of the implantation balloon are made prior to the procedure based upon pre-procedural imaging (Fig. 70.1). Typically, stents with adult size potential are chosen and stent length is determined based on pre-procedural imaging combined with known foreshortened length-diameter relationships, paying special attention to the takeoff of side branches. The diameter of the implant balloon is chosen to approximate normal vessel diameter adjacent to the stenosis [9].

The surgeon decides upon the timing of stent implantation in relation to other parts of the planned operation. This varies based on the location of the lesion(s) to be treated and the operation being performed. When ready, the interventional cardiologist and assistant join the case, temporarily replacing the surgeon's first assistant. Since in most institutions the

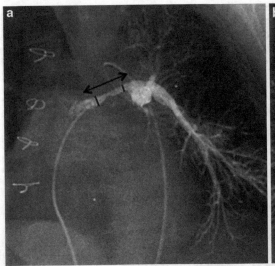
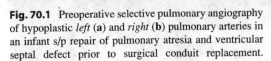
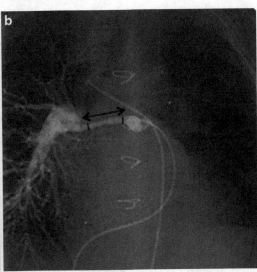

Fig. 70.1 Preoperative selective pulmonary angiography of hypoplastic *left* (**a**) and *right* (**b**) pulmonary arteries in an infant s/p repair of pulmonary atresia and ventricular septal defect prior to surgical conduit replacement. Measurements of vessel length (*arrow*) as well as vessel diameter are used to determine the stent and balloon size for hybrid videoscopic stent implantation

catheterization suite and operating room are in separate physical locations, the interventional equipment that will be needed are brought to the operating room, and a "runner" is designated to obtain any unexpected items. A separate sterile "cath table" holding the needed equipment is set up and includes a heparinized bowl of saline, mosquito clamp, a 0.035″ hi-torque floppy guidewire (e.g., Wholey wire, Mallinckrodt, St. Louis, MO), a pressure manometer, and the anticipated stent and balloon.

Prior to implantation, the target stenosis and surrounding vessel is examined internally and externally using direct visual and/or digital videoscopic examination. A videoscope limits the amount of dissection required to visualize the target lesion, thereby shortening operative and cardiopulmonary bypass times, minimizing trauma to surrounding structures, and preserving supporting tissue as the target stenosis and surrounding vessel are forced to expand with balloon inflation. Landmarks that have been identified on pre-procedural imaging such as side branches are reidentified with the videoscope as final plans for implant are made. Preparation of the stent and balloon differ slightly from normal in several respects. The balloon catheter lumen is flushed,

and the balloon itself is inflated and deflated with saline (contrast not needed) prior to mounting the stent to improve stent adherence since no sheath is utilized and low-profile balloons are preferred for this application (see below). After crimping the stent onto the balloon, stent slippage is assessed by applying gentle traction on the stent. If the stent is loose despite vigorous crimping, the balloon may be inflated slightly to form a "dumbbell" shape which helps to minimize stent slippage (Fig. 70.2). A slight "hockey stick" curve is placed on the guidewire, which is "preloaded" within the balloon catheter lumen such that a few centimeters extend beyond the catheter tip. Typically balloons with moderate burst pressure with low deflation profiles are used to minimize the chance of pulling back the stent after it has been deployed.

The prepared balloon-stent-wire complex is brought to the operating table, and access to the target vessel is provided by the surgeon – typically through a partially completed suture line. While the surgeon manages the videoscope, the cardiologist places the balloon tip at the orifice of the vessel and advances the tip of the guidewire down the target vessel, directing the wire so as to align the tip with the

Fig. 70.2 (a) As
a protective delivery sheath
is not used for videoscopic-
guided operative stent
implantation, and vascular
access is not an issue, the
delivery balloon may be
slightly inflated to form
a "dumbbell" shape
(*arrows*) to prevent stent
slippage. (**b**) A "hockey
stick" curve on the end of
a high-torque floppy
guidewire helps to facilitate
atraumatic passage of the
stent-balloon complex
down a branch pulmonary
artery without the use of
fluoroscopy

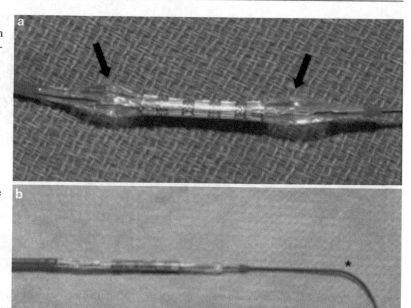

course of the target vessel. With the wire now advanced several centimeters into a distal branch, the back of the wire is stabilized as the balloon-stent complex is advanced over the wire and across the target lesion. Care should be taken to not damage the balloon or stent if a forceps is being used to advance the complex forward. The videoscope is then advanced down the vessel to confirm and fine tune positioning prior to inflation (Fig. 70.3). Inflation is typically performed to the manufacturers' specified burst pressure, followed by balloon deflation. The balloon catheter is removed over the guidewire in the usual fashion as the surgeon holds gentle pressure on the proximal stent struts to prevent proximal dislodgement. The videoscope is then advanced down the newly stented vessel to assess the end result prior to removal of the wire. Particular attention is paid to presence or absence of vascular tears, apposition of the entire stent to the vessel wall, patency of any side branches thought to be at risk, and the integrity of any suture lines that were crossed by the stent. If need be, the stent can be re-dilated with a larger balloon (+/- higher pressure) if it does not appear fully expanded or apposed to the vessel wall.

When satisfied with the end result, the wire is removed and the surgeon may flare any proximal struts that may be protruding into the main PA, particularly when treating ostial stenoses.

While this is a fairly simple technique, several words of caution are worth mentioning. If being performed in the operating room and not in a hybrid suite, this procedure puts the interventional team in an unfamiliar environment without the aid of fluoroscopy or angiography. This requires excellent communication and cooperation with the surgical team and careful preprocedural planning. A thorough review of the pre-procedural angiography and careful calibration to ensure accurate measurements is essential. Use of floppy-tipped guidewires and avoiding rigid high-pressure balloons are important safety measures to prevent vessel damage, particularly from the distal balloon catheter tip which is not seen during inflation with this technique.

Institutional experience: Between 1998 and 2008, this approach was utilized to implant 41 stents into the PAs of 34 patients. Median age and weight at time of implant was 36 months (5 days–31 years) and 13.8 kg (2.9–67 kg), respectively. There was one procedural failure

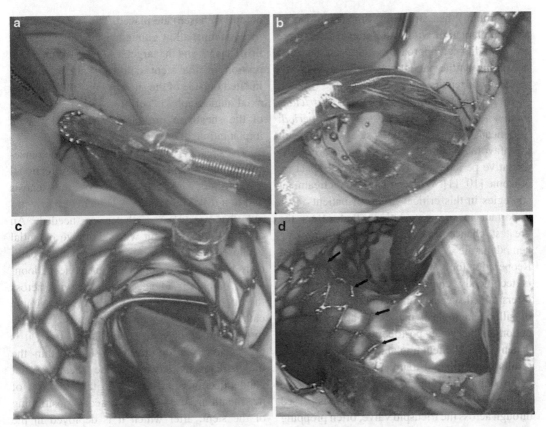

Fig. 70.3 Videoscopic stent implantation procedure to treat central pulmonary artery (PA) stenosis. Pre-implant image used to position stent-balloon complex in the right PA (**a**). Note how the proximal stent is brought to the ostium of the vessel. The appearance of the balloon during implantation (**b**). Videoscopic examination of the vessel following stent implantation shows good apposition of the stent to the vessel wall, absence of any side-branch crossing, and no obvious vessel tear (**c**). Following bilateral stent placement, the surgeon has flared the proximal stent struts (*arrows*) to facilitate future catheter reentry (**d**)

in a child with previously implanted stents that were incompletely removed at a prior operation, which resulted in rupture of the implantation balloon and prevented hybrid stent placement. Technical success rate 97 %. During a median follow-up of 94 months (22 months–11.5 years), 19 patients (22 stents) underwent follow-up catheterization. Angiographic assessment of vessel size showed a statistically significant improvement in mean minimal luminal diameter and the consistent ability to further expand these stents to keep up with patient growth. There were four cases of side-branch crossing resulting in stenosis of that branch; however, only one resulted in complete occlusion. Late distal stent migration occurred in one case without clinical sequelae,

and that stent has remained in place with good flow around and through it. Four patients have undergone unremarkable surgical enlargement (longitudinal splitting) of their hybrid placed stents during a subsequent operation.

Stent implantation via *surgically provided vascular access*: A second, more common hybrid approach to PA stent implantation involves provision of surgical access to deliver stents to otherwise difficult or impossible to reach areas. In general, this technique has evolved to treat two distinct patient populations: (1) infants and neonates who are critically ill in the early postoperative period or (2) more stable patients presenting with unusual lesions or limited vascular access making more percutaneous stent implantation impossible. When applying this technique to stent implantation within the branch PAs, there are two distinct approaches that can be used depending on the patient's underlying diagnosis and stage of repair:

PA stent implantation via *the right ventricular outflow tract in the early postoperative period*: Significant residual branch PA stenosis can result in unfavorable hemodynamics in the early post-operative period and have a negative impact on outcome [10, 11]. When embarking on treatment strategies in this critical group of patients, it is important to use a technique that offers the greatest chance for success while minimizing hemodynamic instability and morbidity. Reoperation for branch PA stenosis in this setting is technically challenging and traumatic and offers mixed success. Likewise, the unreliability of balloon angioplasty makes this an unattractive option in the acute postoperative, critically ill patient [12, 13]. Stent implantation offers reliable results with minimal trauma; however, percutaneous delivery of these rigid devices may be poorly tolerated as the delivery system is passed through across the tricuspid valve, often propping it open and causing hypotension, arrhythmia, and low cardiac output [4]. These problems are amplified in the young infant where the additional issue of limited vascular access may preclude placement of stents with adult-sized potential. Use of a direct right ventricular outflow approach for stent implantation in this population minimizes hemodynamic stability, eliminates sheath size constraints, and improves accuracy of implantation.

Technique: Most experience with this procedure is in patients in the early postoperative period who arrive in the catheterization suite with their sternum open, with or without mechanical cardiopulmonary support. Typically, a diagnostic catheterization is performed from a conventional access route (e.g., femoral vein) to delineate both the hemodynamics and postsurgical anatomy. The surgical team then places a purse-string suture into the proximal right ventricular outflow tract through which a standard vascular sheath and dilator (larger enough to accommodate the predicted balloon stent complex chosen) are placed. The location of this incision must allow enough distance between the tip of sheath and the target lesion, so the proximal portion of the stent delivery balloon can be inflated outside of the sheath (Fig. 70.4). Biplane axial angiography is performed via the side arm of the sheath to provide a roadmap for stent implantation.

The sheath is secured by tightening the purse-string suture, and a floppy-tipped directional 0.035" guidewire is directed across the stenosis and to a distal posterior PA branch with or without the use of a catheter as needed. An appropriate-sized stent with adult size potential is chosen and hand-crimped onto a balloon catheter. Under fluoroscopic guidance the balloon-stent complex is advanced over the wire, across the target lesion. Owing to the short and simple catheter course provided by access directly through the right ventricular outflow tract, it is not necessary to protect the stent within the bloodstream by advancing the sheath. Serial hand injections performed via the side arm of the sheath are used to aid in precise positioning of the stent, after which it is deployed in the typical fashion. As with a standard stent deployment, follow-up angiography and hemodynamics are performed; after which the surgical team reenters the field to remove the sheath and repair the incision in the right ventricular outflow tract.

Institutional experience: Between 1999 and 2011, 10 patients underwent placement of 12 PA stents using this technique. Median weight was 6 kg and all were critically ill. Several were on mechanical cardiopulmonary support. There were no procedural complications or deaths. All stents were successfully placed (as judged by standard criteria and by clinical improvement). In follow-up, all stents placed using this technique have been further expanded via percutaneous routes with no cases of late complications. One patient, who did not have "adult-sized" stents placed at the time of the procedure, has undergone successful surgical enlargement (longitudinal splitting) of the stents during a subsequent operation.

PA stent implantation through an aortopulmonary shunt via *carotid arterial access*: Institutional experience with this

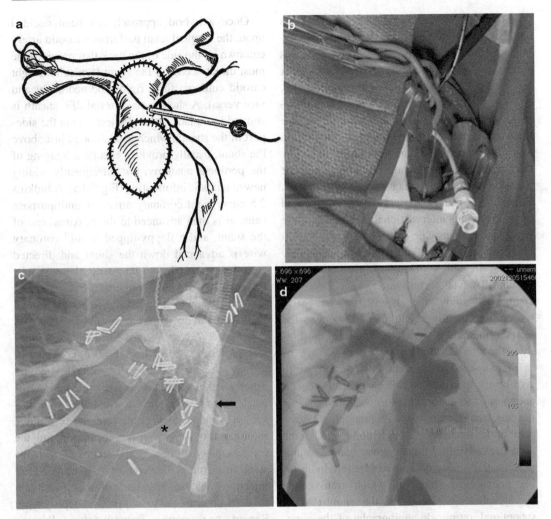

Fig. 70.4 Hybrid pulmonary artery (PA) stent implantation via the right ventricular outflow in a critically ill infant after repair of pulmonary atresia and ventricular septal defect in association of hypoplastic PAs. A schematic diagram demonstrating the desired location of a vascular sheath for placement of hybrid PA stents using this technique (**a**). An intraoperative photograph showing the delivery sheath within the outflow tract (**b**). An angiogram performed through the side arm of the sheath demonstrates severe bilateral branch PA stenosis. Note the venous cannula (*), which needed to maintain the infant on mechanical cardiopulmonary support (**c**). Following placement of bilateral PA stents, there is a marked improvement in bilateral branch PA caliber allowing the infant to be successfully separated from mechanical circulatory support (**d**)

procedure is restricted to neonates and infants who were either (1) critically ill in the immediate postoperative period following placement of an aortopulmonary shunt (central shunt or modified Blalock-Taussig shunt) or (2) infants that presented in early follow-up after surgical shunt placement with a change in their clinical status suspicious of decreased pulmonary blood flow. Severe PA and/or shunt stenoses following shunt placement typically present in a dramatic fashion with profound systemic oxygen desaturation, increased ventilator and inotropic requirements, and circulatory collapse. PA-shunt stenosis can be more difficult to diagnose. These infants may have nothing more than prolonged intubation and ventilator reliance and/or the need to maintain slightly higher systemic blood pressures to achieve acceptable saturations in the postoperative period. After discharge, symptoms may be even subtler such as poor feeding, irritability, and pallor. Noninvasive imaging of this area may be difficult and important shunt or PA stenoses can be under diagnosed. Additionally, shunt or PA stenosis may have long-term negative effects on PA growth in this setting. For these reasons, maintaining a high index of suspicion in this patient population and advocating for a low threshold for cardiac catheterization may be warranted when this diagnosis is entertained. While many shunt-PA stenoses can be treated by percutaneous interventional techniques, there are certain patients who due to issues with vascular access, shunt position, or clinical instability are best treated with stent implantation into a shunt-PA via carotid arterial access. This approach avoids the need for an early reoperation, greatly simplifies and shortens the intervention, and may reduce long-term morbidity to the arterial vascular system.

Technique: This procedure is performed in a catheterization (or hybrid) suite using general anesthesia and endotracheal intubation. In stable patients, hemodynamic and angiographic assessment of the shunt-PA via the femoral vein (as the aorta in nearly all of these patients can be cannulated via the venous system) is preferred. In unstable patients or those in which transvenous angiographic assessment of the shunt-PAs is suboptimal, retrograde angiography of the aorta, shunt, and pulmonary arteries should be performed from a femoral arterial approach. Once an area of stenosis has been identified, consultation with cardiac surgery is prudent to finalize a treatment plan. The decision as to whether to attempt the planned intervention from a conventional access route or hybrid carotid approach is predicated upon several factors:

1. Sheath size required for the intervention (particularly important in small neonates, e.g., <3.0 kg).
2. Hemodynamic status of the patient. The faster and more direct hybrid approach may be preferable in unstable patients.
3. Catheter course. Patients with an acute angle of the shunt from the systemic artery may benefit from the hybrid approach.

Once a hybrid approach has been decided upon, the surgical team performs a carotid artery cutdown on the side of the neck that provides the most direct access to the shunt (typically a right carotid cutdown for a right modified shunt and vice versa). A short radial arterial 4Fr. sheath is sutured into place. A hand injection via the side-port of the sheath, which is positioned just above the shunt, usually provides excellent imaging of the pertinent anatomy, not infrequently adding new diagnostic information (Fig. 70.5). A Judkins 2.5 curve right coronary artery or multipurpose catheter is then advanced to the proximal end of the shunt, and a floppy-tipped 0.014″ coronary wire is advanced down the shunt and directed across the target lesion into a distal lower lobe PA branch. After measurements are taken, a premounted coronary stent with a balloon diameter that approximates adjacent normal PA diameter is selected. Advantages of these stents include low profile, excellent tractability, avoidance of a long sheath, and excellent radial strength. Since all these patients will require future surgery, a team commitment (including the surgeons) is made to surgically enlarge or remove these stents at a later date thereby eliminating the concern of creating a "fixed stenosis" with the stent (maximum diameter of 5–6 mm). Hand injections via the side-port of the sheath are used to confirm position prior to deployment. Repeat angiography immediately following stent deployment prior to removing the guidewire is routinely performed. Addressing the most distal lesion first and then working proximally (e.g., stent the branch PA first followed by a shunt stent that may be needed) minimizes the risk of dislodging or disrupting a newly placed stent. Following successful stent deployment, the surgeon removes the sheath from the carotid artery and repairs the vessel and incision.

Institutional experience: Between 1999 and 2011, 24 patients underwent catheterization to treat 36 PA or aorta-pulmonary shunt stenoses. All were treated with initial angioplasty. Fifteen patients required definitive treatment with stent implantation. Twelve of these 15 patients were treated via a surgically accessed carotid artery.

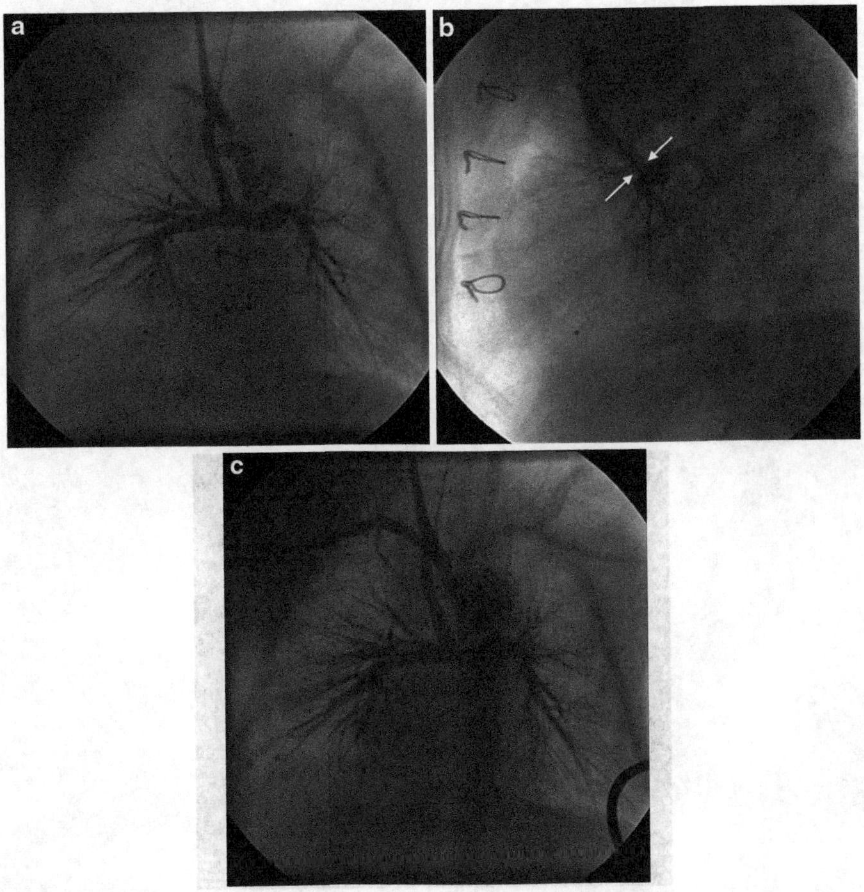

Fig. 70.5 A 2-week-old neonate after Norwood I palliation for hypoplastic left heart syndrome developed slowly worsening cyanosis. A frontal angiogram failed to demonstrate any obvious shunt or pulmonary artery stenosis (**a**); however, a lateral projection with caudal angulation demonstrated a subtle but significant shunt stenosis at the insertion into the pulmonary artery (*arrow*) (**b**). Following stent implantation from a carotid approach, there was obvious enlargement of the distal shunt (**c**), which correlated to improved systemic oxygen saturations

Stent implantation was successful in all cases (as judged by standard criteria as well as by clinical improvement). There were no instances of shunt thrombosis or procedural deaths.

Hybrid Arterial Duct Stent Implantation for Ductal-Dependent Pulmonary Blood Flow

Initial attempts at arterial duct stent implantation as an alternative to surgical shunt placement were discouraging due to a combination of technical constraints of the time as well as the initial strategic goal of having this palliation provide reliable pulmonary blood flow for a prolonged period of time (>6 months) [14, 15]. Advancements in stent technology coupled with a trend towards earlier surgical repair have revived an interest in arterial duct stent implantation [16, 17]. While the majority of these cases can be performed via a percutaneous approach, there is a subset of patients that may benefit from a hybrid carotid arterial approach [18]. These include neonates with tortuous ducts, ducts which arise in a proximal location from the under surface of the transverse aortic arch, and small infants where concerns for vascular access exist.

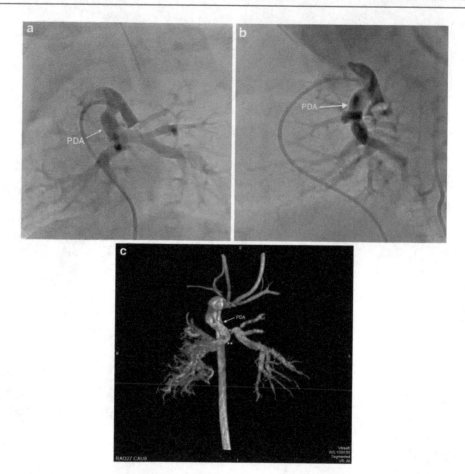

Fig. 70.6 Imaging of neonatal duct to evaluate for suitability stent. Initially a transvenous standard 2-dimensional balloon occlusion descending aortogram was performed in multiple views (**a, b**) to assess the ductal and pulmonary artery (PA) morphology. While these images demonstrated a large and somewhat tortuous duct arising from the undersurface of the aorta, it was not possible to completely assess the details of the ductal anatomy at its insertion point into the branch PAs. Volume-rendered 3-dimensional rotational aortography (**c**) clearly showed a complex ductus with an early and stenotic take off of the left PA(*) with continuation of a ductal stenosis onto the origin of the right PA(**). This patient was sent for a surgical shunt

Technique: Prostaglandin is discontinued 3–6 h prior to the beginning of the case so that the duct (which is typically quite large) may partially constrict and allow for stent implantation. As time to ductal closure is unpredictable, careful patient monitoring is needed during this time, and PGE_1 is kept at the bedside ready to be reinstituted immediately if patients deteriorate. Aortic angiography is typically performed from a femoral venous approach. It can be quite challenging to profile a tortuous duct despite the use of multiple axial projections and injections. Three-dimensional rotational angiography may be useful in these cases (Fig. 70.6). This is a critical decision point in the case as not only the suitability of the duct for stenting is determined but also the decision to approach the intervention from either a percutaneous or hybrid approach.

When a hybrid approach is chosen, the surgical team accesses the right or left carotid artery (whichever is felt to give more direct access to the arterial duct) and secures a 4Fr. radial short sheath in place. The interventional team then approaches this intervention in a similar fashion as described above for shunt-PA stenting with

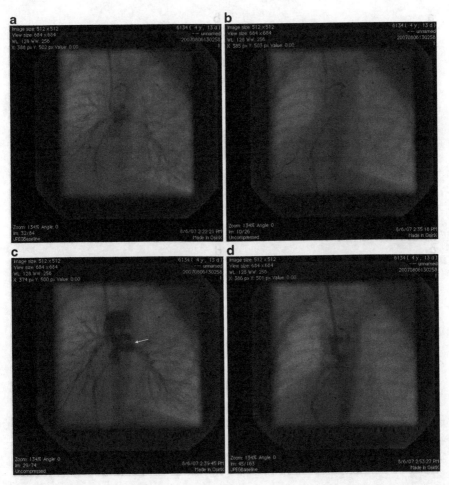

Fig. 70.7 Premature ductal closure induced by attempted ductal stent. A frontal injection via a right carotid arterial approach demonstrates a tortuous duct with a nearly circular course (**a**), confirmed by positioning a coronary guidewire into the right pulmonary artery (**b**). Angiography shortly after positioning the guidewire (**c**) demonstrates the development of an important ductal stenosis (*) followed shortly thereafter with abrupt ductal closure (**d**). After removal of the guidewire and bolus dosing of prostaglandin, the duct was reopened and the child sent for a surgical shunt

some important differences owing to the friable, tortuous, and reactive nature of the neonatal duct, which can close abruptly and unexpectedly with disastrous results (Fig. 70.7). Attempts are made to minimize catheter and wire manipulation across these reactive vessels. After passing a medium-stiff 0.014″ coronary guidewire across the duct, angiography is repeated via the side arm of the hybrid sheath. These wires serve to partially straighten the duct and provide more precise sizing used to determine stent length. Pre-mounted, non-drug-eluting, coronary artery stents (Driver stents, Medtronic, Minneapolis, MN) are again preferred

for this procedure and implanted at 3.5–4.0 mm based on body weight and ductal length (larger infants and/or longer duct = larger implant diameter). It is important that the entire length of the arterial duct is covered by stent while attempting to leave as little stent material in the PA and aortic lumen as possible (Fig. 70.8). While the goal is to use one single stent of optimal length, if the aortic end of the arterial duct appears uncovered after deployment of the initial stent, then a second stent is telescoped within. Angiography both before and after removing the guidewire position is performed to ensure that the

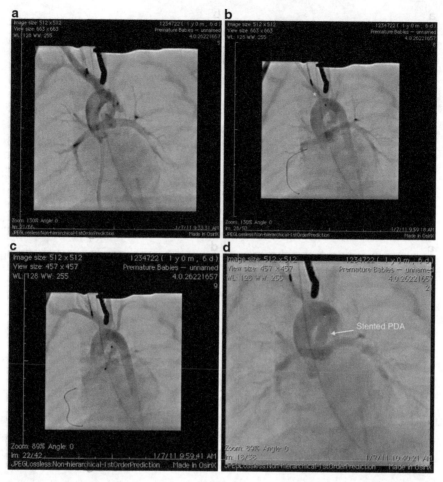

Fig. 70.8 Successful hybrid stenting of a tortuous duct. A frontal angiogram performed via the right carotid artery demonstrates a tortuous arterial duct with at least two acute turns (**a**). With the direct access provided by the hybrid approach, a guidewire was easily passed into the right pulmonary artery (**b**) followed by a coronary stent (*). Once the stent is positioned within the duct, follow-up angiography through the side arm of the sheath (**c**) is used to fine tune the position, followed by deployment of the stent (**d**). Note the straightening of the ductus with stent deployment

entire arterial duct is in fact stented and that both PAs fill well.

Institutional experience: Between 2007 and 2011, eight patients underwent attempted arterial duct stent implantation via a hybrid approach for the treatment of ductal-dependent cyanotic CHD. Median weight was 2.8 kg (1.8–3.5 kg). Stent implantation was successful in seven patients. One patient developed profound cyanosis upon catheter manipulation across the arterial duct that required emergent surgical aortopulmonary shunt placement. There were no procedural deaths. Several have had ultrasound evaluation for patency of the accessed carotid artery, and there have been no instances of clinically significant carotid artery stenosis.

Pulmonary Valve Perforation in Pulmonary Atresia with Intact Ventricular Septum

Many algorithms have been developed for treatment of this complex lesion reflecting the wide variation in anatomic subtypes [19]. This customized approach based upon an individual patient's anatomy has been shown to improve outcomes [20, 21]. The subset of patients with an adequate-sized tricuspid valve, right ventricle, and absence of right ventricular dependent coronary blood flow may be candidates for right ventricular decompression and biventricular repair. Numerous catheter-based methods to perforate and then dilate the atretic pulmonary valve membrane have been described as an alternative to surgical valvotomy or reconstruction of the right ventricular outflow tract [22–24]. In the current era, the preferred method for perforating the atretic valve is through the use of radiofrequency (RF) energy delivered via a wire or catheter. In certain patients it can be difficult to achieve a stable position in a central location beneath the atretic valve prior to perforation. This is particularly true in smaller infants and those with some hypoplasia of the inlet or outlet portion of the right ventricle. Perforation anywhere but in a central location may result in cardiac perforation, tamponade, and death [25]. A hybrid approach via a direct right ventricular puncture through a limited subxiphoid incision offers a safe and simple alternative in high-risk situations [26].

Technique: As these patients are arterial duct dependent, intravenous prostaglandins are continued throughout the case. Via the femoral vein, a right and left (via a patent foramen ovale or atrial septal defect) heart catheterization is performed. Angiography in the right ventricle and aorta is performed to rule out right ventricular dependent coronary circulation and assess right ventricular morphology, suitability of the valve for perforation, and ductal and PA anatomy. If a hybrid approach is chosen, the chest is sterilely prepared and draped and a 1–2 cm lower sternal incision is made. The xiphoid process is removed and the pericardium is opened, exposing the diaphragmatic surface of the right ventricle. A purse-string suture is placed into the right ventricle, through which an 18 ga needle is passed into the RV cavity through which a 0.035″ guidewire is advanced. Importantly, the right ventricular access point must be chosen far enough from the imperforate valve to ensure enough distance between the sheath tip and

valve for complete balloon expansion later in the case. The needle is then exchanged for a 4 Fr. sheath, which is secured by tightening the purse-string suture (Fig. 70.9). A contrast injection via the side arm of the sheath confirms its position and is used to direct a Judkins right or multipurpose catheter a short distance to the center of the imperforate valve membrane in a central location. The anterior to posterior orientation of the sheath greatly facilitates central and stable positioning of the catheter in the center of the imperforate membrane. After confirmatory angiography through the tip of this catheter, an RF wire and accompanying coaxial microcatheter are advanced in a coaxial fashion to the undersurface of the valve and RF energy applied until perforation is confirmed visually. The floppy RF wire is advanced down the arterial duct followed by the microcatheter which can be used to exchange the soft RF wire for a stiffer 0.014″ or 0.018″ guidewire. Serial balloon dilations of the valve can then be performed. Since the hybrid approach provides such direct access to the valve, anchoring the guidewire with a snare from the systemic circulation, as has been previously described, is not necessary.

Following valvuloplasty, hemodynamic assessment and angiography can be performed easily using this approach after which the sheath is removed from the right ventricle, the purse-string suture closed, and a small pericardial drain left in place.

Published experience: The largest series [27] reported using this technique involves 30 newborns over a 5-year period. Technical success was achieved in all patients. Follow-up ranged from 1.5 months to 5 years with 83 % survival. The majority of patients have gone on to achieve biventricular circulation.

Shunt Lesions

Ventricular Septal Defect Closure

Over the past decade, defects of the muscular and perimembranous septum have been treated with increasing frequency using catheter-delivered

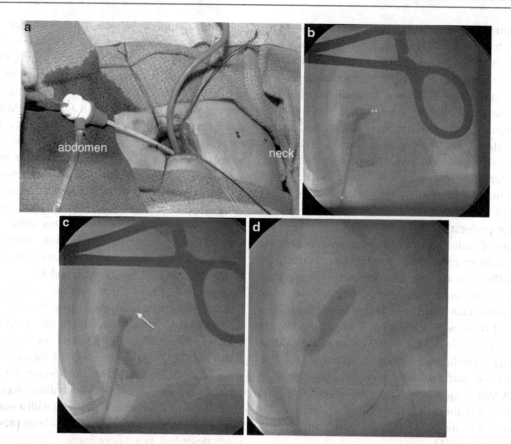

Fig. 70.9 Hybrid approach to pulmonary atresia with intact ventricular septum. After removing the xiphoid process and exposing the anterior free wall of the right ventricle (RV), a 4Fr. radial arterial sheath is placed directly into the right ventricular cavity (**a**). A Judkins right coronary artery catheter (**b**) is positioned centrally under the atretic valve membrane which is typically identified by its beak-like appearance (**). Using the Judkins catheter to stabilize position, after the application of radiofrequency energy, the wire (*arrow*) is passed into the pulmonary artery (**c**), exchanged for a stiffer guidewire, after which balloon pulmonary valvotomy can be performed (**d**)

devices [28, 29]. While the majority of these procedures can be performed from either a transfemoral or transjugular venous percutaneous approach, there are certain clinical scenarios in which a hybrid approach should be considered. Clinical scenarios in which a hybrid approach should be considered include (1) infants (weight <5 kg), (2) failed percutaneous approach (i.e., inability to position device correctly), and (3) requirement of a concomitant surgical procedure (i.e., PA band removal). The discussion below applies only to the closure of muscular ventricular septal defect (VSD).

Technique: While fluoroscopy may be useful in selected cases, the majority of these procedures can be guided with echocardiography alone (either transesophageal (TEE) in older patients or epicardial echocardiography in infants). Prior to the procedure an expert in congenital heart imaging must perform a complete cardiac transthoracic echocardiographic assessment. During this examination, the VSD should be assessed in multiple planes and measurements of VSD diameter (made in diastole when the VSD is at its largest), distance from the superior rim of the defect to the aortic and atrioventricular valves, and a thorough search for any associated defects performed. These values are used for device selection. Via a lower mini sternotomy, the pericardium is opened and the right ventricular free

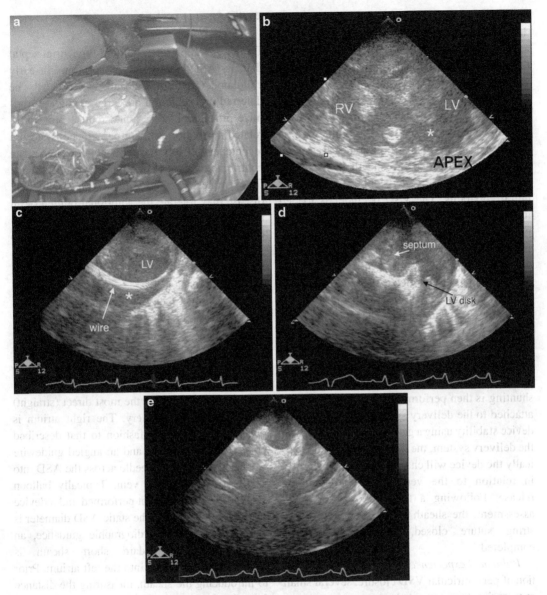

Fig. 70.10 Hybrid approach to apical muscular ventricular septal defect (VSD) closure in a 4-week-old, 2.1 kg neonate. Positioning the echocardiography transducer on the surface of the right ventricle (**a**) can be a challenge in small infants but will provide accurate images (**b**) of the VSD (*) and guide device placement: from identifying wire position (**c**), through opening the left ventricular disk (**d**), to assessing the final result (**e**)

wall is exposed. Under echocardiographic guidance, gentle pressure is placed on various areas of the free wall (usually with a finger tip or forceps) to ascertain the best place to insert the needle as it relates to crossing the VSD (Fig. 70.10). This is an important part of the procedure as the angle at which the needle approaches the VSD is critical for successful crossing of the defect with the guidewire. Once this area has been identified, a purse-string suture is placed in the right ventricular free wall, and an 18 ga needle is advanced into the right ventricle and held in position as the tip is carefully angled towards the defect. Under echocardiographic guidance, an angled hydrophilic guidewire is advanced across the defect, into the left ventricle.

Care must be taken to ensure that the guidewire does not become ensnared with mitral valve apparatus. With stable wire position achieved, the needle is exchanged for a standard short vascular sheath, which is advanced across the VSD into the left ventricle. When it has been confirmed that the tip of the sheath is free within the left ventricular cavity, the guidewire is removed. Careful echocardiographic assessment is used to ensure that the sheath tip is not in contact with the left ventricular free wall or mitral apparatus. The VSD occluder is loaded into the sheath and under echocardiographic guidance, advanced to the tip of the sheath. Gentle retraction of the sheath while holding the device in place results in expansion of the left ventricular disk, which is then pulled against the left side of the septum. With the left disk anchored against the septum, the sheath is again slowly retracted, deploying the remainder of the device across the defect and in the right ventricle. A complete echocardiographic assessment of device position and residual ventricular level shunting is then performed with the device still attached to the delivery system. After assessing device stability using a gentle "push and pull" on the delivery system, the device is released. Typically the device will change orientation slightly in relation to the ventricular septum upon release. Following a final echocardiographic assessment, the sheath is removed, the purse-string suture closed, and the procedure completed.

Published experience: Since the first description of perventricular VSD closure, several small case series have reported encouraging results using this hybrid technique [30–32]. Collectively, they report 100 % technical success with the majority of patients demonstrating immediate complete closure of the VSD. Hemodynamically insignificant residual shunts were present in a minority of patients immediately following device deployment; however, most of these spontaneously resolve by 1 year. Complications were rare but included wire perforation of the left ventricle associated with hemopericardium, device migration, and transient electromechanical dissociation.

Atrial Septal Defects

Clinically important secundum-type atrial septal defects (ASD) rarely cause symptoms in early childhood. Therefore, closure can typically be deferred until children are large enough to optimize procedural success and reduce procedure-related morbidity utilizing percutaneous closure techniques [33, 34]. Rarely, secundum ASDs can contribute to clinical morbidity in small infants; for example, premature infants with chronic lung disease may tolerate the additional burden of an atrial level left-to-right shunt poorly. In selected circumstances such as this, a hybrid approach to ASD closure may be considered as an alternative to traditional surgical repair or a high-risk percutaneous approach [35].

Technique: Either transesophageal or epicardial echocardiography is required for full assessment of the ASD and device selection and guidance. Single-plane fluoroscopy may be helpful but is not mandatory. Via a median sternotomy a purse-string suture is placed in a part of the right atrium that will provide the most direct (straight) course for device delivery. The right atrium is punctured in a similar fashion to that described above for VSD closure and an angled guidewire advanced through the needle across the ASD into a left-sided pulmonary vein. Typically balloon sizing of the defect is not performed and a device ~20–25 % larger than the static ASD diameter is chosen. Under echocardiographic guidance, an appropriate-sized standard short sheath is advanced over the wire into the left atrium. Prior to introducing the sheath, measuring the distance from the right atrial puncture site to the posterior wall of the left atrium (by transesophageal echocardiography) provides a guide for how far the sheath should be advanced, thereby minimizing the chance of perforating the left atrium. This distance can be marked on the sheath providing the operator with a visual indicator. After removing the guidewire and dilator, the sheath is de-aired and the device loaded into the short sheath and advanced into the left atrium. Standard transcatheter deployment methods, as described above for hybrid VSD closure, are then used to deploy the device. Of note is that in small infants the close proximity of the TEE probe to the left atrium can complicate left atrial disk deployment and positioning. Following completion of device deployment, a final echocardiographic assessment is performed and the device released from the delivery cable.

Published experience: Several reports from China provide data on the largest cohorts of hybrid per-atrial ASD closures. Li et al. reported technical success in 95 % of cases (n = 39) and Yin et al. technical success in 99 % of cases (n = 115) [36, 37]. This technique avoided cardiopulmonary bypass, shortened hospital stay, and exhibited excellent immediate and short-term results. Long-term follow-up is pending.

Left Heart Obstructive Lesions

Valvar Aortic Stenosis

Transcatheter treatment of congenital aortic valve stenosis was first described over 25 years ago [38] and in many centers is accepted as first-line treatment for this lesion. Neonates with critical aortic valve stenosis pose several unique challenges to the interventional cardiologist including hemodynamic instability, ventilator and/or inotropic dependence, and limited vascular access. While femoral arterial-venous and umbilical arterial-venous access routes have all been utilized to perform this intervention, all have been associated with significant complications including peripheral vascular and aortic wall damage, resultant aortic insufficiency, circulatory collapse, and death [39, 40]. As these infants can be quite unstable during the procedure, minimizing the time it takes to cross the aortic valve (often the most time consuming part of the intervention) is beneficial. Using a hybrid approach from the carotid artery provides the operator with a direct approach to the valve (facilitating valve crossing), minimizes the risks of vascular damage, and brings the surgical team into the procedure, should they be needed emergently [7, 40].

Technique: In those patients with a left aortic arch and normal vessel branching, the right carotid artery is surgically accessed as described above. The technical procedure from this point is quite similar as to what has been previously described for standard valvar aortic stenosis, i.e., crossing the valve with a soft-tipped coronary guidewire followed by serial balloon dilation up no greater than 90 to −100 % of the valve diameter. Approaching the valve from the right carotid artery not only facilitates valve crossing but also provides for a more stable position of the balloon during inflation and deflation, which may be important in minimizing the development of aortic insufficiency. Following balloon valvuloplasty and assessment of the result, the surgeon reenters the field, removes the carotid sheath, and repairs the carotid arteriotomy.

Aortic Recoarctation After Stage 1 Palliation for Hypoplastic Left Heart Syndrome

Survival after stage 1 palliative surgery for hypoplastic left heart syndrome has improved remarkably over the past decade; however, recurrent or residual aortic arch obstruction continues to be a serious problem [41–46]. Typically, obstruction occurs in the area of the distal anastomosis of the aortic gusset [45]. In addition to upper body hypertension, aortic obstruction in this setting has a number of other undesirable physiologic effects including pulmonary over-circulation resulting in ventricular volume overload, systemic atrioventricular valve regurgitation, and diminished cardiac output from an already burdened systemic right ventricle [41, 47]. Surgical revision of this area is difficult and may not completely relieve the obstruction. Balloon angioplasty, while often successful, may not provide adequate relief if the stenosis is long segment and may carry an increased risk compared with simple recurrent coarctation angioplasty [41, 48–52]. While stent implantation has become accepted therapy for older children and adults with native and/or recurrent coarctation of the aorta, it is not typically considered an option in this setting secondary to technical considerations and concerns regarding future stent enlargement as an infant grows.

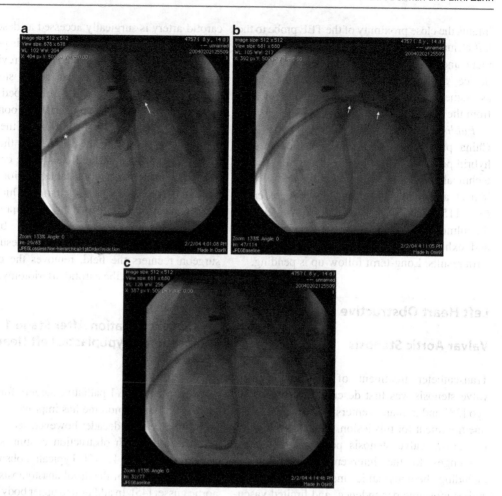

Fig. 70.11 Hybrid aortic stent placement in a 14-day-old, 2.90 kg neonate. Following stage 1 Norwood reconstruction, a contrast injection via a hybrid placed sheath within the neo-ascending aorta (*) demonstrates severe aortic arch obstruction (*arrow*). Repeat injection through the side arm of the sheath shows the relationship of the stent (*arrows*) to the area of obstruction to guide placement (**b**). Final contrast injection prior to removal of the sheath demonstrates good stent positioning and an improved diameter of the aortic arch (**c**)

Recently, a hybrid approach to this difficult problem has been described [53].

Technique: To date this procedure has been performed at the time of cavopulmonary anastomosis in infants who have had unsuccessful balloon angioplasty for recurrent coarctation after Stage 1 palliation (Fig. 70.11). Via a median sternotomy a 6–10 Fr. introducer sheath is advanced to the proximal transverse aortic arch via a purse-string incision in the neo-ascending aorta. The side arm of the sheath is utilized for serial angiography and aortic pressure measurements throughout the procedure. Typically a 0.035″ guidewire is advanced under fluoroscopic guidance across the obstructed segment into the descending aorta. A stent with adult-sized potential diameter is manually crimped onto an angioplasty balloon and passed over the guidewire to the narrowed area of the distal arch without the use of a long sheath as the distance is short and the catheter course quiet simple. After confirming position with angiography, the stent is deployed in typical fashion. Angiography and hemodynamic measurements are repeated after stent deployment. The guidewire and sheath are removed and the arteriotomy repaired.

Institutional experience: From 2002 to 2011, this procedure was performed in 11 children. Median weight and age were 6.1 kg (2.9–18 kg) and 4.5 months (0.5 months–3.5 years), respectively. Nearly all had at least moderately depressed ventricular function at the time of the procedure. Successful stent implantation was achieved in all patients without immediate or late procedure-related complications. In follow-up, all stents have been successfully re-dilated when needed. One stent (Double Strut LD; ev3, Plymouth, MN) became significantly distorted with re-dilation and was surgically removed at the time of the Fontan operation. This stent is no longer used for this application. While ventricular function has improved in several patients, several others continue to show persistent poor ventricular function despite an unobstructed aortic arch.

Miscellaneous Hybrid Procedures

A number of additional rarely performed hybrid procedures have been described including pulmonary valve placement, bailout of malpositioned devices, treatment of a variety of venous obstructions (pulmonary veins, superior vena cava), and the occlusion of aortopulmonary collaterals. Literature describing these novel techniques is referenced at the end of the chapter [36, 54–58].

Conclusions

Most lesions encountered in CHD can be treated with either conventional transcatheter or surgical techniques. In a select group of patients including neonates and infants, patients in the early postoperative period, hemodynamically unstable patients, and those with limited vascular access hybrid techniques to treat a variety of lesions appear to be beneficial. These procedures may serve to reduce the cumulative trauma CHD patients must endure throughout their lifetimes by minimizing individual procedure morbidity as well as the total number of procedures that

a patient must experience. The success of these approaches requires careful long-term planning and a well-coordinated multidisciplinary team approach.

References

1. Houde C, Zahn EM, Benson LN et al (1992) Intraoperative placement of endovascular stents. J Thorac Cardiovasc Surg 104(2):530–532
2. O'Laughlin MP, Perry SB, Lock J et al (1991) Use of endovascular stents in congenital heart disease. Circulation 83(6):1923–1939
3. O'Laughlin MP, Slack MC, Grifka RG et al (1993) Implantation and intermediate-term follow-up of stents in congenital heart disease. Circulation 88(2):605–614
4. Pass RH, Hsu DT, Garabedian CP et al (2002) Endovascular stent implantation in the pulmonary arteries of infants and children without the use of a long vascular sheath. Catheter Cardiovasc Interv 55(4):505–509
5. McMahon CJ, El Said HG, Vincent JA et al (2002) Refinements in the implantation of pulmonary arterial stents: impact on morbidity and mortality of the procedure over the last two decades. Cardiol Young 12(5):445–452
6. Ungerleider RM, Johnston TA, O'Laughlin MP et al (2001) Intraoperative stents to rehabilitate severely stenotic pulmonary vessels. Ann Thorac Surg 71(2): 476–481
7. Davenport JJ, Lam L, Whalen-Glass R et al (2008) The successful use of alternative routes of vascular access for performing pediatric interventional cardiac catheterization. Catheter Cardiovasc Interv 72(3): 392–398
8. Berman DP, Khan D, Zahn EM (2012) The use of three-dimensional rotational angiography to assess the pulmonary circulation following cavo-pulmonary connection in patients with single ventricle. Catheter Cardiovasc Interv. 80(6):922–30
9. Fogelman R, Nykanen D, Smallhorn JF et al (1995) Stents in the pulmonary circulation. Clinical impact on management and medium-term follow-up. Circulation 92(4):881–885
10. Chau AK, Leung MP (1997) Management of branch pulmonary artery stenosis: balloon angioplasty or endovascular stenting. Clin Exp Pharmacol Physiol 24(12):960–962
11. Hosking MC, Thomaidis C, Hamilton R et al (1992) Clinical impact of balloon angioplasty for branch pulmonary arterial stenosis. Am J Cardiol 69(17): 1467–1470
12. Rothman A, Perry SB, Keane JF et al (1990) Early results and follow-up of balloon angioplasty for branch pulmonary artery stenosis. J Am Coll Cardiol 15:1109–1117

13. Gentles T, Lock J, Perry S (1993) High pressure balloon angioplasty for branch pulmonary artery stenosis: early experience. J Am Coll Cardiol 22:867–872

14. Gibbs JL, Uzun O, Blackburn ME et al (1999) Fate of the stented arterial duct. Circulation 99(20): 2621–2625

15. Gibbs JL, Rothman MT, Rees MR et al (1992) Stenting of the arterial duct: a new approach to palliation for pulmonary atresia. Br Heart J 67(3):240–245

16. Schranz D, Michel-Behnke I, Heyer R et al (2010) Stent implantation of the arterial duct in newborns with a truly duct-dependent pulmonary circulation: a single-center experience with emphasis on aspects of the interventional technique. J Interv Cardiol 23(6):581–588

17. Alwi M, Choo KK, Latiff HA et al (2004) Initial results and medium-term follow-up of stent implantation of patent ductus arteriosus in duct-dependent pulmonary circulation. J Am Coll Cardiol 44(2): 438–445

18. Kenny D, Berman D, Zahn E et al (2012) Variable approaches to arterial ductal stenting in infants with complex congenital heart disease. Catheter Cardiovasc Interv 79(1):125–130

19. Freedom RM, Mawson JB, Yoo S, Benson LN (1997) Congenital heart disease. Textbook of angiocardiography. Futura, New York

20. Hannan RL, Zabinsky JA, Stanfill RM et al (2009) Midterm results for collaborative treatment of pulmonary atresia with intact ventricular septum. Ann Thorac Surg 87(4):1227–1233

21. Rychik J, Levy H, Gaynor JW et al (1998) Outcome after operations for pulmonary atresia with intact ventricular septum. J Thorac Cardiovasc Surg 116(6): 924–931

22. Piéchaud JF, Ladeia AM, Da Cruz E et al (1993) Perforation-dilatation of pulmonary atresia with intact interventricular septum in neonates and infants. Arch Mal Coeur Vaiss 86(5):581–586

23. Giusti S, Spadoni I, De Simone L et al (1996) Radiofrequency perforation in pulmonary valve atresia and intact ventricular septum. G Ital Cardiol 26(4):391–397

24. Justo RN, Nykanen DG, Williams WG et al (1997) Transcatheter perforation of the right ventricular outflow tract as initial therapy for pulmonary valve atresia and intact ventricular septum in the newborn. Cathet Cardiovasc Diagn 40(4):408–413

25. Agnoletti G, Piechaud JF, Bonhoeffer P et al (2003) Perforation of the atretic pulmonary valve. Long-term follow-up. J Am Coll Cardiol 41(8): 1399–1403

26. Burke RP, Hannan RL, Zabinsky JA et al (2009) Hybrid ventricular decompression in pulmonary atresia with intact septum. Ann Thorac Surg 88(2):688–689

27. Li S, Chen W, Zhang Y et al (2011) Hybrid therapy for pulmonary atresia with intact ventricular septum. Ann Thorac Surg 91(5):1467–1471

28. Carminati M, Butera G, Chessa M et al (2007) Investigators of the European VSD Registry. Transcatheter closure of congenital ventricular septal defects: results of the European Registry. Eur Heart J 28(19): 2361–2368

29. Holzer R, Balzer D, Cao QL, Amplatzer Muscular Ventricular Septal Defect Investigators et al (2004) Device closure of muscular ventricular septal defects using the Amplatzer muscular ventricular septal defect occluder: immediate and mid-term results of a U.S. registry. J Am Coll Cardiol 43(7):1257–1263

30. Bacha EA, Cao QL, Galantowicz ME et al (2005) Multicenter experience with periventricular device closure of muscular ventricular septal defects. Pediatr Cardiol 26(2):169–175

31. Crossland DS, Wilkinson JL, Cochrane AD et al (2008) Initial results of primary device closure of large muscular ventricular septal defects in early infancy using periventricular access. Catheter Cardiovasc Interv 72(3):386–391

32. Diab KA, Cao QL, Mora BN et al (2007) Device closure of muscular ventricular septal defects in infants less than one year of age using the Amplatzer devices: feasibility and outcome. Catheter Cardiovasc Interv 70(1):90–97

33. Masura J, Gavora P, Podnar T (2005) Long-term outcome of transcatheter secundum-type atrial septal defect closure using Amplatzer septal occluders. J Am Coll Cardiol 45(4):505–507

34. Butera G, De Rosa G, Chessa M et al (2003) Transcatheter closure of atrial septal defect in young children: results and follow-up. J Am Coll Cardiol 42(2):241–245

35. Pedra SF, Jatene M, Pedra CA (2010) Hybrid management of a large atrial septal defect and a patent ductus arteriosus in an infant with chronic lung disease. Ann Pediatr Cardiol 3(1):68–73

36. Li SJ, Zhang H, Sheng XD et al (2010) Intraoperative hybrid cardiac surgery for neonates and young children with congenital heart disease: 5 years of experience. Ann Thorac Cardiovasc Surg 16(6): 406–409

37. Yin N, Zhao T, Yang Y et al (2011) Evaluation of minimally invasive peratrial device closure of secundum atrial septal defects in children. Zhong Nan Da Xue Xue Bao Yi Xue Ban 36(6): 576–580

38. Lababidi Z, Wu JR, Walls JT (1984) Percutaneous balloon aortic valvuloplasty: results in 23 patients. Am J Cardiol 53(1):194–197

39. Brown DW, Chong EC, Gauvreau K et al (2008) Aortic wall injury as a complication of neonatal aortic valvuloplasty: incidence and risk factors. Circ Cardiovasc Interv 1(1):53–59

40. Rossi RI, Manica JL, Petraco R et al (2011) Balloon aortic valvuloplasty for congenital aortic stenosis using the femoral and the carotid artery approach: a 16-year experience from a single center. Catheter Cardiovasc Interv 78(1):84–90

41. Tworetzky W, McElhinney DB, Burch GH et al (2000) Balloon arterioplasty of recurrent coarctation after the modified Norwood procedure in infants. Catheter Cardiovasc Interv 50:54–58

42. Meliones JN, Snider AR, Bove EL et al (1990) Longitudinal results after first-stage palliation for hypoplastic left heart syndrome. Circulation 82:151–156

43. Murdison KA, Baffa JM, Farrell PE Jr et al (1990) Hypoplastic left heart syndrome. Outcome after initial reconstruction and before modified Fontan procedure. Circulation 82:199–207

44. Ishino K, Stumper O, De Giovanni JJ et al (1999) The modified Norwood procedure for hypoplastic left heart syndrome: early to intermediate results of 120 patients with particular reference to aortic arch repair. J Thorac Cardiovasc Surg 117:920–930

45. Bartram U, Grunenfelder J, Van Praagh R (1997) Causes of death after the modified Norwood procedure: a study of 122 postmortem cases. Ann Thorac Surg 64:1795–1802

46. Zellers TM (1999) Balloon angioplasty for recurrent coarctation of the aorta in patients following staged palliation for hypoplastic left heart syndrome. Am J Cardiol 84:231–233

47. Pearl JM, Nelson DP, Schwartz SM et al (2002) First-stage palliation for hypoplastic left heart syndrome in the twenty-first century. Ann Thorac Surg 73:331–339

48. Anderson JB, Beekman RH 3rd, Border WL et al (2009) Lower weight-for-age z score adversely affects hospital length of stay after the bidirectional Glenn procedure in 100 infants with a single ventricle. J Thorac Cardiovasc Surg 138:397–404

49. Saul JP, Keane JF, Fellows KE et al (1987) Balloon dilation angioplasty of postoperative aortic obstructions. Am J Cardiol 59:943–948

50. Moore JW, Spicer RL, Mathewson JW et al (1993) High-risk angioplasty. Coarctation of the aorta after Norwood stage 1. Tex Heart Inst J 20:48–50

51. Yetman AT, Nykanen D, McCrindle BW et al (1997) Balloon angioplasty of recurrent coarctation: a 12-year review. J Am Coll Cardiol 30:811–816

52. Chessa M, Dindar A, Vettukattil JJ et al (2000) Balloon angioplasty in infants with aortic obstruction after the modified stage I Norwood procedure. Am Heart J 140:227–231

53. Kutty S, Burke RP, Hannan RL et al (2011) Hybrid aortic reconstruction for treatment of recurrent aortic obstruction after stage 1 single ventricle palliation: medium term outcomes and results of redilation. Catheter Cardiovasc Interv 78(1):93–100

54. Berman DP, Burke R, Zahn EM (2012) Use of a novel hybrid approach to salvage an attempted transcatheter pulmonary valve implant. Pediatr Cardiol 33(5): 839–842

55. Amanullah MM, Siddiqui MT, Khan MZ et al (2011) Surgical rescue of embolized amplatzer devices. J Card Surg 26(3):254–258

56. Cubeddu RJ, Hijazi ZM (2011) Bailout perventricular pulmonary valve implantation following failed percutaneous attempt using the Edwards Sapien transcatheter heart valve. Catheter Cardiovasc Interv 77(2):276–280

57. Sareyyupoglu B, Burkhart HM, Hagler DJ et al (2009) Hybrid approach to repair of pulmonary venous baffle obstruction after atrial switch operation. Ann Thorac Surg 88(5):1710–1711

58. Hannan RL, Zabinsky JA, Hernandez A et al (2009) Hybrid treatment of superior vena cava syndrome in a child. Ann Thorac Surg 88(1):277–278

Section XII

Cardiopulmonary Resuscitation

Robert Berg

Epidemiology of Pediatric Cardiac Arrest

71

Joseph W. Rossano, Maryam Y. Naim, Vinay M. Nadkarni, and Robert A. Berg

Abstract

Cardiac arrest is not rare in children, accounting for up to one quarter of the total pediatric mortalities. Infants represent the largest group at risk for a cardiac arrest, in and out of the hospital. While outcomes remain suboptimal, especially for out-of-hospital cardiac arrests, survival from in-hospital cardiac arrests has approached 50 % in some studies. A number of risk factors for cardiac arrest in children have been identified and potential therapeutic interventions to improve outcomes are discussed.

J.W. Rossano (✉)
Department of Pediatrics, Perelman School of Medicine at the University of Pennsylvania, Philadelphia, PA, USA

The Cardiac Center, The Children's Hospital of Philadelphia, Philadelphia, PA, USA
e-mail: RossanoJ@email.chop.edu

M.Y. Naim • R.A. Berg
Department of Anesthesia and Critical Care, Perelman School of Medicine at the University of Pennsylvania, Philadelphia, PA, USA

Department of Anesthesiology and Critical Care Medicine, The Children's Hospital of Philadelphia, Philadelphia, PA, USA
e-mail: naim@email.chop.edu; bergra@email.chop.edu

V.M. Nadkarni
Department of Anesthesia and Critical Care, Perelman School of Medicine at the University of Pennsylvania, Philadelphia, PA, USA

Center for Simulation, Advanced Education and Innovation, The Children's Hospital of Philadelphia, Philadelphia, PA, USA
e-mail: nadkarni@email.chop.edu

Keywords

Arrhythmia • Asystole • Automated external defibrillator • Bradycardia • Cardiac arrest etiology • Cardiac arrest incidence • Cardiac arrest outcomes • Cardiac arrest prevalence • Cardiac arrest risk factors • Cardiopulmonary resuscitation • Defibrillation • Epidemiology • In-hospital cardiac arrest • Neurological outcome • Out-of-hospital cardiac arrest • Pulseless electrical activity • Sudden cardiac death • Survival • Ventricular fibrillation • Ventricular tachycardia

Introduction

Heart disease remains the largest cause of death among people in the United States, accounting for greater 860,000 deaths per year which is over 35 % of all deaths [1]. Sudden cardiac death represents over 50 % of these deaths [2] and is greater than the annual deaths from breast cancer, colon cancer, and prostate cancer combined [3]. While many adults who suffer sudden cardiac death will have no previously recognized risk factors for cardiac arrest, adults with underlying coronary artery disease, risk factors for coronary artery disease, and heart failure [4] are among those at greatest risk for a cardiac arrest. Interestingly, there are some data to suggest that the overall risk of sudden cardiac death may be decreasing among adults [5]. This may in part be secondary to prevention strategies including the use of implantable defibrillators [6].

Compared with adults, children differ in terms of the overall risk for a cardiac arrest, etiologies, outcomes, and potential for prevention. This chapter will focus on these issues regarding cardiac arrests in children.

Incidence of Cardiac Arrest: Out-of-Hospital Cardiac Arrest

It is difficult to know precisely how many children suffer an out-of-hospital cardiac arrest, but the contribution to pediatric mortality is substantial, possibly accounting for up to one quarter of all mortalities [7]. There have been several population-based studies that have attempted to define the incidence (Table 71.1). A meta-analysis of published studies on pediatric out-of-hospital cardiac arrests from 1983 to 2004 found eight studies where the incidence of cardiac arrests was determined or could be calculated [8]. The incidence ranged from 2.6 to 19.7 per 100,000 person-years. The greatest incidence reported was from a population-based study from Houston, Texas, reporting on 300 children presenting to emergency medical services with a cardiac arrest [9]. The incidence was 19.7 per 100,000 person-years. Unlike most of the other studies, cardiac arrests from injuries were included and accounted for 29 % of the total arrests.

The largest and most comprehensive prospective population-based study was reported from the NHLBI-funded Resuscitation Outcome Consortium, a ten-center emergency medical systems consortium covering >21 million people in North America (December 2005–March 2007). The overall incidence of nontraumatic cardiac arrests was 8.04 per 100,000 person-years in the pediatric population and 126 per 100,000 person-years in adults [10]. The rate was significantly increased in infants (72.71 per 100,000 person-years) compared to children (3.73 per 100,000 person-years) and adolescents (6.37 per 100,000 person-years). Similar to adults, there was a gender predisposition to cardiac arrests, with males accounting for 62 % of the cases.

The reported incidences of cardiac arrests in children from different populations around the world are similar to what has been reported from the United States, though there are no published reports from many parts of the world.

Table 71.1 Incidence and outcome of out-of-hospital cardiac arrest

Author (year)	Population	Incidence per 100,000 person-years	Survival
Kuisma et al. (1995)	Cardiac arrests in Helsinki, Finland; age <16 years	Overall – 9.8	9.6 % – 1-year survival
		"Natural" – 7.5	14.7 % – 1-year survival for attempted resuscitation
		"Nonnatural" – 2.3	7.7 % – 1-year neurologically favorable survival
Sirbaugh et al. (1999)	Cardiac arrest in Houston, Texas; age <18 years	Overall – 19.7	2.3 % – overall survival to hospital discharge
		Nontraumatic – 14.0	2.9 % – nontraumatic survival to hospital discharge
		Traumatic – 5.7	1.1 % – traumatic survival to hospital discharge
			0.4 % – neurologically favorable survival
Gerein et al. (2006)	Cardiac arrest in Ontario, Canada; age <18 years	Overall – 9.1	2 % – overall survival to hospital discharge
		Nontraumatic – 5.7	
		Traumatic – 3.4	
Atkins et al. (2009)	Nontraumatic cardiac arrests in United States and Canada (11 geographic areas), age <20 years	8.04	6.4 % – survival to hospital discharge
Park et al. (2009)	Nontraumatic cardiac arrests in Korea, age <20 years	4.2	4.7 % – survival to hospital discharge
			5.0 % – survival to hospital discharge for attempted resuscitation
Kitamura et al. (2010)	Cardiac arrests in Japan, age <18 years	8.0	9.2 % – 1-month survival
			3.2 % – 1-month neurologically favorable survival
Nitta et al. (2011)	Cardiac arrests in Osaka, Japan; age <18 years	Overall – 8.6	Nontraumatic:
		Nontraumatic – 7.3	8 % – 1-month survival
		Traumatic – 1.3	3 % – 1-month neurologically favorable survival
Bardai et al. (2011)	Cardiac arrest in North Holland province of the Netherlands, age <21	Overall – 9.0	24 % – survival to hospital discharge for attempted resuscitation
		"Natural" – 4.5	
		"Nonnatural" – 4.5	20 % – neurologically favorable survival at hospital discharge for attempted resuscitation

A recent study from Korea found the incidence of nontraumatic cardiac arrests to be 4.2 per 100,000 person-years, with infants having a risk of 67.1 per 100,000 person-years [11]. A retrospective study from Helsinki documented 79 cardiac arrests in children (<16 years) during a 10-year time period that corresponded to an incidence of 9.8 per 100,000 person-years, and sudden infant death syndrome was the most common etiology

[12]. A similar incidence of 9.0 per 100,000 person-years was found from the North Holland province of the Netherlands [7]. Kitamura et al. recently reported 5,578 out-of-hospital arrests among children (≤17 years) during a 3-year prospective population-based observational study, including the entire Japanese population. This corresponded to a incidence of 8.0 per 100,000 person-years [13]. The incidence

among infants, 65.9 per 100,000 person-years, was similar to the incidence from the Resuscitation Outcome Consortium study. Given the potential life expectancy for infants and children, the potential number of persons-years saved is great.

Prevalence of Cardiac Arrest: In-Hospital Cardiac Arrest

Inpatient cardiac arrests are also not rare occurrences in pediatric patients (Table 71.2). A recent population-based study from a nationwide administrative database in the United States reported that 5,807 patients received in-hospital cardiopulmonary resuscitation (95 %CI 5,259–6,355) in 2006 or 0.77 patients receiving cardiopulmonary resuscitation per 1,000 hospital admissions, among all types of hospitals [14]. An increased rate was observed from a 5-year review of all cardiac arrests at the Hospital for Children and Adolescents in Helsinki, Finland, at 0.7 per 100 admissions [15]. These overall rates are lower than has been reported from a large children's hospital in Brazil, which reported 176 patients with a cardiac arrest out of over 6,000 hospital admissions (3 %) [16]. Patients with cardiovascular disease, not surprisingly, have an increased risk for a cardiac arrest while hospitalized, with a rate of one event per 135 admissions compared to one event per 1,850 admissions in children without cardiovascular disease [17].

Children admitted to an intensive care unit also have a higher likelihood of a cardiac arrest with rates ranging from as low as 1 % of admissions in a multidisciplinary intensive care units [18, 19] to as high as 4 % in a cardiac intensive care unit [20, 21]. One study from the University of Minnesota reported that almost 6 % of their medical-surgical pediatric intensive care unit patients underwent at least one episode of cardiopulmonary resuscitation and that an event occurred on average every 62 patient-days [22]. Because of the long life expectancy of infants and children, the potential for life-years added by providing successful in-hospital resuscitations is great.

Etiology of Cardiac Arrest: Out-of-Hospital Cardiac Arrest

Sudden infant death syndrome is the most common etiology of cardiac arrest reported in many studies [12, 23, 24]. In contrast to adult out-of-hospital cardiac arrests, pediatric out-of-hospital cardiac arrests are mostly the result of progressive hypoxemia from a respiratory disease, including drowning [9, 12, 23, 24]. This has important implications regarding the need for rescue breathing during resuscitation of children with out-of-hospital cardiac arrest. A prospective observational study from Japan demonstrated lower rates of survival with neurologically favorable outcome among children with noncardiac etiology for the arrest who received bystander cardiopulmonary resuscitation without assisted ventilations versus conventional cardiopulmonary resuscitation with rescue breaths [13]. Other etiologies, including trauma, are also frequently reported [10, 23–25]. If an underlying chronic medical condition is known prior to the arrest, it is frequently a cardiac condition [7, 11, 12, 23, 24, 26, 27]. As noted above, a male predominance is evident for pediatric cardiac arrests among all age groups, including infants [7, 10, 23, 28].

A sudden cardiac event during exercise in young people is of special interest. This disease often strikes those in peak physical condition with no prior warning signs or symptoms. These events can have a profound impact on the communities where these events occur. While the true incidence of sudden cardiac death in young athletes is difficult to ascertain in the United States because of the lack of a mandatory centralized reporting system, it has been estimated at 0.6 per 100,000 person-years [29]. A recent study from the United States suggested that the incidence may be even higher among elite college athletes [30]. In certain regions, such as the Veneto region of Italy, the application of intense screening programs has been associated with a decrease in the incidence from 3.6 to 0.4 per 100,000 person-years [31]. The etiology of sudden cardiac death in athletes

Table 71.2 Prevalence and outcome of in-hospital cardiac arrest

Author (year)	Population	Prevalence	Survival
Slonim et al. (1997)	32 PICUs in the United States	1.8 % – PICU admissions	14 % – survival to hospital discharge
Souminen et al. (2000)	Tertiary care children's hospital in Helsinki, Finland (NICU excluded); age <16 years	0.7 % – all admissions	19 % – survival to hospital discharge
		5.5 % – PICU admissions	18 % – survival at 1 year
			13 % – survival with favorable neurological outcome at hospital discharge
Parra et al. (2000)	Tertiary care children's hospital CICU in Miami, Florida; age ≤21 years	4.1 % – CICU admissions	42 % – survival to hospital discharge
Reis et al. (2002)	Tertiary care children's hospital in Sao Paulo, Brazil (no NICU or cardiac surgery in hospital); age <21 years	3 % – all admissions	16 % – survival to hospital discharge
		14 % – PICU admissions	15 % – survival at 1 year
			12 % – neurologically favorable 1-year survival
de Mos et al. (2006)	Tertiary care children's hospital PICU in Toronto, Canada; age <18 years	0.9 % – PICU admissions	25 % – survival to hospital discharge
			23 % – survival at 1 year
			16 % – survival with favorable neurological outcome at discharge
Peddy et al. (2007)	Tertiary care children's hospital in Philadelphia, Pennsylvania	3.1 % – CICU admissions	46 % – survival to hospital discharge
Knudson et al. (2010)	Pediatric admissions throughout the United States, age <21 years	0.07 % – all admissions	48 % – survival to hospital discharge

is usually cardiac, with hypertrophic cardiomyopathy, and congenital cardiac anomalies being the most common diseases identified [32]. Primary arrhythmias such as long QT syndrome and other ion channel disorders account for approximately 3 % of cases [29]. Certain regions, such as the Veneto region of Italy, have a high incidence of arrhythmogenic right ventricular dysplasia [31]. In order to prevent sudden cardiac death in this population, some have advocated more intensive screening studies with the addition of electrocardiography and echocardiography to the standard pre-participation sports history and physical examination. Many organizations in the United States such as the American Academy of Pediatrics, American Heart Association, and American Red Cross have also advocated for the availability of automated external defibrillators at schools [33].

Etiology of Cardiac Arrests: In-Hospital Cardiac Arrests

The reported etiologies of in-hospital cardiac arrests in children have varied depending on the population, but respiratory illness, cardiac disease, sepsis/shock, and central nervous system disorders are among the most commonly reported [16, 22, 34]. According to data from the large American Heart Association Get With The Guidelines-Resuscitation Registry, formerly known as the National Registry of CPR or NRCPR, the immediate cause of 880 pediatric in-hospital cardiac arrests was most commonly hypotension (61 %) or acute respiratory insufficiency (57 %) [35]. Notably many patients had both. In addition, ventricular fibrillation was the presenting rhythm in 10 % of arrests, but occurred in 27 % of in-hospital arrests at some

Precipitating Cause of Cardiac Arrest

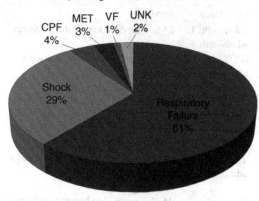

Fig. 71.1 Precipitating causes of cardiac arrests and bradycardic events treated with CPR. *CPF* cardiopulmonary failure, *MET* metabolic, *VF* ventricular fibrillation, *UNK* unknown (Adapted from Reis et al. [16])

time during resuscitation [36]. A more recent Get With The Guidelines-Resuscitation report by Ortmann and colleagues also revealed that most pediatric cardiac surgical and cardiac medical patients had their cardiac arrests precipitated by hypotension and/or acute respiratory insufficiency [37]. Arrhythmias were also present in 46–61 % of patients. Reis et al. performed a prospective observation study from a large children's hospital in Brazil that does not perform cardiac surgery, and found respiratory failure or circulatory shock was the precipitating cause in 90 % of patients (Fig. 71.1) [16]. Other centers have reported cardiovascular disease as the most common underlying diagnosis reported from arrests on the ward and in the intensive care unit [18, 22, 38–40].

Outcome of Cardiac Arrests: Out-of-Hospital Cardiac Arrests

Recent large-scale studies from North America, the Netherlands, and Japan have reported the overall survival of out-of-hospital cardiac arrests in children ranging from 6 % to 24 % [7, 10, 41]. The Resuscitation Outcomes Consortium reported on 624 pediatric cardiac arrests from geographically diverse areas in the United States

and Canada covering over 23 million people [10]. The overall pediatric survival of nontraumatic out-of-hospital cardiac arrest was 6.4 %, with survival to hospital discharge of 3.3 % among infants, 9.1 % among children, and 8.9 % among adolescents. This was significantly higher than the overall survival among adults (4.5 %). A prospective, population-based, observational study from Osaka, Japan reported on 740 pediatric nontraumatic cardiac arrests that underwent resuscitation attempt [41]. The overall 1-month survival was similar to the Resuscitation Outcomes Consortium at 8 %, which ranged from 5 % in infants to 14 % in adolescents. Neurologically favorable outcome, defined as a Cerebral Performance Category scale score of 1 or 2 or no change in the Cerebral Performance Category scale score from the pre-arrest baseline, was 3 % overall. Neurologically favorable outcome was highest in adolescents (11 %) and lowest in infants (1 %). The proportion of children with overall survival and neurologically favorable survival was higher than reported from adults. The largest percentage of survivors for out-of-hospital arrests was recently reported from the prospective, population-based study from the North Holland province of the Netherlands. In this study, of the 51 pediatric-aged victims of out-of-hospital cardiac arrest that underwent an attempt at resuscitation, the overall survival to hospital discharge was 24 % [7].

A review of the published literature from 1970 to 1997 by Young and Seidel found that 8.4 % of children with an arrest survived to hospital discharge [28]. Another review by Donoghue et al. of 41 studies of pediatric out-of-hospital arrests found an overall survival to hospital discharge of 12 % and 4 % survival with favorable neurological outcomes, though most of the articles reviewed did not use a validated scale of neurological outcomes [8]. In special populations, such as submersion victims, survival rates are much higher, with up to one third surviving after a cardiac arrest [42].

The presenting arrest rhythm also greatly affects the likelihood of survival. Children found asystolic or with pulseless electrical activity have overall low survival, with the majority of the studies reporting 0–8 % survival to hospital discharge [9–11, 13, 25, 43, 44], though one study reported a survival rate for asystole of 18.5 % [12]. The Resuscitation Outcomes Consortium reported an overall survival of 5 % for children found in pulseless electrical activity or asystole [10]. Nitta et al. separated those with a first documented rhythm of pulseless electrical activity (91 children) from those with asystole (591 children) and found increased survival with pulseless electrical activity (21 %) versus asystole (5 %) [41]. The low overall survival from asystole and pulseless electrical activity is likely a manifestation of prolonged hypoxemia leading to bradycardia and eventual pulselessness. Those in asystole were less likely to have a witnessed arrest, less likely to have bystander cardiopulmonary resuscitation, and more likely to require prolonged resuscitations, all of which likely contributed to the observed outcomes of this group [23, 43, 45–47].

Conversely, patients presenting with ventricular fibrillation or pulseless ventricular tachycardia have fared significantly better in many [10, 13, 27, 41, 43], but not all studies of out-of-hospital cardiac arrests [7, 9, 12]. Nitta et al. from Osaka, Japan, reported a 26 % 1-month survival after ventricular fibrillation or ventricular tachycardia, with a neurologically favorable outcome in 19 % [41]. A study from King County, Washington, over a 6-year time period reported a survival to hospital discharge rate in patients with ventricular fibrillation of 37 % with 17 % neurologically intact survivors [43]. A similar percentage of survivors was reported form a more recent study in the same geographic area [27]. Large population-based observational studies from North America [10], Korea [11], and Japan [13] have also found a survival advantage for children found in ventricular tachycardia or ventricular fibrillation with survival rates ranging from 20 % to 32 %. The increased survival seen in patients that present with ventricular fibrillation or ventricular tachycardia is likely multifactorial and related to the increased incidence of witnessed arrest, increased incidence

of bystander cardiopulmonary resuscitation, decreased likelihood of severe hypoxemia preceding the arrest, and shorter duration of onset of symptoms to appropriate therapy (defibrillation). Of interest, a recent population-based study from the Netherlands reported a relatively high overall survival to hospital discharge rate of 24 %; however, the presenting rhythm was not associated with survival [7]. Sirbaugh et al., however, reported a low rate of survival after ventricular tachycardia or ventricular fibrillation from the Houston, Texas, area in the 1990s with a survival of only 8 % [9].

Age is an important factor in terms of the etiology, presenting rhythm, and likelihood of survival to discharge. As noted above, infants represent the largest group of children that suffer out-of-hospital cardiac arrests and also have the poorest outcomes [10, 11, 13, 28, 48]. This group most commonly has an etiology of sudden infant death syndrome and a presenting rhythm of asystole/pulseless electrical activity, which are associated with very poor outcome. In the large review by Young et al., sudden infant death syndrome accounted for 62 % of infant cardiac arrests [28]. In the Resuscitation Outcomes Consortium study, infants accounted for 44 % of the total arrests in children and asystole/pulseless electrical activity as the initial rhythm in 84 % of these, with survival to hospital discharge in only 3 % [10]. Conversely, older children and adolescents are more likely to have ventricular fibrillation or ventricular tachycardia as the initial rhythm during the cardiac arrest with a reported incidence as high as 15–80 % and a survival rate as high as 30–40 % among adolescents [7, 10, 11].

Beyond merely survival, the neurological status of children suffering a cardiac arrest is of great importance. As stated above, the recent population-based observational study from Osaka, Japan, reported an overall neurologically favorable outcome 1 month after an out-of-hospital cardiac arrest of 3 % [41]. However, certain subgroups, such as adolescents with a presenting rhythm of ventricular fibrillation or ventricular tachycardia, had neurologically favorable survival as high as 26 %. Conversely, only 1 % of cardiac arrests in infants had neurologically favorable survival [13, 41]. Factors associated with neurologically favorable outcome included bystander-witnessed arrest and rhythm other than asystole. The population-based study from the Netherlands reported that 10 of the 51 (20 %) children who underwent a resuscitation attempt survived to hospital with a favorable neurological outcome [7]. Several older studies, however, have suggested that most survivors had severe neurologic impairment [9, 25, 33, 49]. There are, however, other studies to suggest that the neurological outcome is not as grim, with over 50 % of survivors having good neurological outcome or a return to their pre-arrest neurological outcome [7, 23, 50]. Standardized reporting and longer-term follow-up of survivors has been advocated to clarify the true neurological morbidity in children suffering out-of-hospital cardiac arrests [8, 28].

Improving the overall outcomes of out-of-hospital cardiac arrests is of paramount importance. Primary and secondary prevention, mainly through activity restrictions and implantable cardioverter defibrillator placement, certainly has a role in patients identified as high risk including certain patients with hypertrophic cardiomyopathy [32], dilated cardiomyopathy [6, 51], and some channelopathies [52]. However, many children have not previously been identified as high risk for a cardiac arrest prior to the arrest. Therefore, this form of prevention may not greatly alter the current incidence of out-of-hospital arrests in children [29].

Data from animal models have established that the quality of cardiopulmonary resuscitation greatly affects the likelihood of return of spontaneous circulation, myocardial and brain perfusion, and survival with favorable neurological outcome. Particularly important factors seem to be prompt resuscitation, performance of adequately deep and fast chest compressions, minimizing interruptions to compressions, and avoidance of hyperventilation [53]. The presence of bystander cardiopulmonary resuscitation has long been noted to be associated with improved outcomes compared to children and adults who do not have cardiopulmonary resuscitation until the arrival of emergency personnel [13, 46]. Encouraging the initiation of cardiopulmonary resuscitation by the public once an arrest is witnessed is one strategy of improving outcomes [53, 54].

Another advocated method of accomplishing these goals is to perform continuous chest compressions without assisted ventilation or protocols that greatly minimize the ventilations given. These strategies have been adopted by several pre-hospital emergency medical systems and are associated with improved survival among adult out-of-hospital cardiac arrests, especially when ventricular fibrillation or ventricular tachycardia is the initial rhythm [53–56]. However, as children have a greater frequency of respiratory arrests, this method may prove detrimental to many children. A prospective observational study from Japan found lower rates of neurologically favorable survival among children provided bystander cardiopulmonary resuscitation without assisted ventilation versus conventional bystander cardiopulmonary resuscitation with rescue breaths when the arrest was presumed to be noncardiac in etiology [13]. However, the same investigators noted that outcomes were similar following bystander CPR with or without rescue breathing for children with presumed cardiac etiology for their cardiac arrest.

Outcomes of Cardiac Arrests: In-Hospital Cardiac Arrests

Overall, children suffering a cardiac arrest while in the hospital appear to have a greater likelihood of survival to hospital discharge than children suffering a cardiac arrest at home, with reported overall survival as high as 27–48 % [14, 21, 34, 35, 57–59]. Recent reports from the American Heart Association Get With The Guidelines-Resuscitation Registry, formerly known as the National Registry of CPR or NRCPR, reported an overall survival to hospital discharge rate of 25–27 % for in-hospital pulseless cardiac arrest, excluding the neonatal intensive care unit [35, 37], and 22 % of cardiac arrests that occurred in the intensive care unit [60]. Recent single-center studies have also demonstrated similar survival to hospital discharge rates [21, 58]. A 4-year study from a large cardiac intensive care unit reported a 46 % survival to hospital discharge [21], and a study of all cardiac arrests at a children's hospital in Australia from over a 3-year time period found a 1-year survival of 26 % for pulseless cardiac arrests [58]. The greater survival reported from in-hospital cardiac arrest in children as opposed to out-of-hospital cardiac arrest is likely secondary to many factors including shorter duration to recognition of cardiopulmonary compromise and initiation of cardiopulmonary resuscitation and possibly quicker access to more expert application of basic and advanced life support [57].

Similar to out-of-hospital cardiac arrests, infants comprise the largest group of pediatric patients undergoing cardiopulmonary resuscitation while hospitalized [14, 16]. However, unlike the experience with out-of-hospital arrests where the survival is dismal, many studies report superior survival among infants compared to older children [14, 40, 60, 61]. While ventricular tachycardia or ventricular fibrillation has been associated with improved survival for out-of-hospital arrests, most studies of in-hospital arrests have not found improved survival with ventricular fibrillation/ventricular tachycardia compared to asystole/pulseless electrical activity [34]. This may, in part, be secondary to the improved survival of asystole/pulseless electrical activity among hospitalized children compared to hospitalized adults or out-of-hospital arrests in children [35]. However, children who have ventricular fibrillation or tachycardia as the initial rhythm present during the cardiac arrest have improved survival compared to those who develop it during the course of the arrest [36].

Whether hospital-based programs aimed at rapid defibrillation through the use of automated external defibrillators will have a role in pediatric patients remains uncertain [62]. Importantly, in-hospital use of automated external defibrillators for adults is associated with worse outcomes, especially for patients without a shockable rhythm [63]. The worse outcomes were presumably partly related to the required "hands-off" time for the application of the automated external defibrillator pads and rhythm analysis. Because most pediatric in-hospital cardiac arrests are not associated with a shockable rhythm, these findings are especially concerning for children.

Factors appearing to influence survival include obesity [59], initiating cardiopulmonary resuscitation for bradycardia with poor perfusion as opposed to asystole/pulseless electrical activity [57], shorter duration of cardiopulmonary resuscitation [15, 16, 34, 38, 40, 64, 65], and respiratory failure as the etiology of the arrest [15, 16, 34]. Survival appears to be particularly low among patients with sepsis, renal failure, and cancer [14, 16, 34, 36, 66]. Some studies, however, have demonstrated increased survival among patients with underlying cardiac disease, especially with the use of extracorporeal membrane oxygenation [18, 66–70]. Similar to out-of-hospital cardiac arrests, the reported neurological outcome of in-hospital arrest is varied [16, 19, 34, 38, 71]. Studies in the 1980s and 1990s have reported overall very few survivors with favorable neurologic outcomes [38, 71]. More recent studies have reported improved outcomes, ranging from >50 % to >80 % of survivors with either favorable neurological outcome or no change in their neurological status from baseline [16, 19, 34, 35]. Interestingly, the use of extracorporeal membrane oxygenation during CPR (E-CPR) has been associated with relatively high rates of survivors with favorable neurologic outcomes, even with quite prolonged resuscitations [18, 66, 70, 72–74].

Several multifaceted strategies have been employed in hope of improving the outcome of in-hospital cardiac arrest in children. Prevention of a cardiac arrest would be an obvious goal. Some centers have reported a decreased incidence of cardiac arrests and cardiac arrests outside of intensive care units with the addition of medical response teams [75, 76]. These teams can help identify patients on the general wards who may be deteriorating and help facilitate the provision of more intensive care prior to circulatory collapse. While these programs have great appeal, they have not been uniformly successful in improving mortality [77]. Other programs such as identifying high-risk patients in the intensive care unit and reviewing with medical team procedures in the event of an arrest likely improve the delivery of care to these patients [78]. If an arrest has occurred, insuring high-quality cardiopulmonary resuscitation may also improve outcomes, and there has been some encouraging data using devices capable of delivering real-time feedback to the rescuer [79]. If cardiopulmonary resuscitation is not successful, some centers have reported good outcomes with the use of rescue extracorporeal membrane oxygenation in select patients [18, 66, 68–70, 72–74, 80]. The eventual role and widespread application of these approaches will await further study.

Conclusion

Cardiac arrest is unfortunately not a rare event in children. The incidence of out-of-hospital cardiac arrests in infants approaches that of adults. Cardiac arrest in hospitalized children is also not rare, occurring in up to 4 % of specialty intensive care units. Many children who suffer a cardiac arrest have an underlying disease, usually a cardiac abnormality, which predisposes them to the event. However, many of these conditions are not diagnosed until after death. Outcomes of cardiac arrest children remain poor; however, survival of in-hospital arrests has approached 50 % in some studies, though the neurological outcome of survivors has not been consistently reported. A renewed focus on the quality of cardiopulmonary resuscitation and the use of aggressive modalities such as extracorporeal membrane oxygenation may have a more important role in the future.

References

1. Lloyd-Jones D, Adams RJ, Brown TM et al (2010) Heart disease and stroke statistics–2010 update: a report from the American Heart Association. Circulation 121:e46–e215
2. Zheng ZJ, Croft JB, Giles WH et al (2001) Sudden cardiac death in the United States, 1989 to 1998. Circulation 104:2158–2163
3. Heron M, Hoyert DL, Murphy SL et al (2009) Deaths: final data for 2006. Natl Vital Stat Rep 57:1–134
4. Herre JM, Sauve MJ, Malone P et al (1989) Long-term results of amiodarone therapy in patients with recurrent sustained ventricular tachycardia or ventricular fibrillation. J Am Coll Cardiol 13:442–449
5. Fox CS, Evans JC, Larson MG et al (2004) Temporal trends in coronary heart disease mortality and sudden cardiac death from 1950 to 1999: the Framingham Heart Study. Circulation 110:522–527
6. Bardy GH, Lee KL, Mark DB et al (2005) Amiodarone or an implantable cardioverter-defibrillator for congestive heart failure. N Engl J Med 352:225–237
7. Bardai A, Berdowski J, van der Werf C et al (2011) Incidence, causes, and outcomes of out-of-hospital cardiac arrest in children. A comprehensive, prospective, population-based study in the Netherlands. J Am Coll Cardiol 57:1822–1828
8. Donoghue AJ, Nadkarni V, Berg RA et al (2005) Out-of-hospital pediatric cardiac arrest: an epidemiologic review and assessment of current knowledge. Ann Emerg Med 46:512–522
9. Sirbaugh PE, Pepe PE, Shook JE et al (1999) A prospective, population-based study of the demographics, epidemiology, management, and outcome of out-of-hospital pediatric cardiopulmonary arrest. Ann Emerg Med 33:174–184
10. Atkins DL, Everson-Stewart S, Sears GK et al (2009) Epidemiology and outcomes from out-of-hospital cardiac arrest in children: the Resuscitation Outcomes Consortium Epistry-Cardiac Arrest. Circulation 119:1484–1491
11. Park CB, Shin SD, Suh GJ et al (2010) Pediatric out-of-hospital cardiac arrest in Korea: a nationwide population-based study. Resuscitation 81:512–517
12. Kuisma M, Suominen P, Korpela R (1995) Paediatric out-of-hospital cardiac arrests–epidemiology and outcome. Resuscitation 30:141–150
13. Kitamura T, Iwami T, Kawamura T et al (2010) Conventional and chest-compression-only cardiopulmonary resuscitation by bystanders for children who have out-of-hospital cardiac arrests: a prospective, nationwide, population-based cohort study. Lancet 375:1347–1354
14. Knudson JD, Neish SR, Cabrera AG et al (2012) Prevalence and outcomes of pediatric in-hospital cardiopulmonary resuscitation in the United States: an analysis of the Kids' Inpatient Database. Crit Car Med 40:2940–2944
15. Suominen P, Olkkola KT, Voipio V et al (2000) Utstein style reporting of in-hospital paediatric cardiopulmonary resuscitation. Resuscitation 45:17–25
16. Reis AG, Nadkarni V, Perondi MB et al (2002) A prospective investigation into the epidemiology of

in-hospital pediatric cardiopulmonary resuscitation using the international Utstein reporting style. Pediatrics 109:200–209

17. Lowry AW, Cabrera AG, Morales DL et al (2011) Frequency of cardiopulmonary resuscitation among children with cardiovascular disease hospitalized in the United States: an analysis of 22 million hospitalizations (abstract). Congenit Heart Dis 6:528

18. de Mos N, van Litsenburg RR, McCrindle B et al (2006) Pediatric in-intensive-care-unit cardiac arrest: incidence, survival, and predictive factors. Crit Care Med 34:1209–1215

19. Horisberger T, Fischer E, Fanconi S (2002) One-year survival and neurological outcome after pediatric cardiopulmonary resuscitation. Intensive Care Med 28:365–368

20. Parra DA, Totapally BR, Zahn E et al (2000) Outcome of cardiopulmonary resuscitation in a pediatric cardiac intensive care unit. Crit Care Med 28:3296–3300

21. Peddy SB, Hazinski MF, Laussen PC et al (2007) Cardiopulmonary resuscitation: special considerations for infants and children with cardiac disease. Cardiol Young 17(Suppl 2):116–126

22. Von Seggern K, Egar M, Fuhrman BP (1986) Cardiopulmonary resuscitation in a pediatric ICU. Crit Care Med 14:275–277

23. Young KD, Gausche-Hill M, McClung CD et al (2004) A prospective, population-based study of the epidemiology and outcome of out-of-hospital pediatric cardiopulmonary arrest. Pediatrics 114:157–164

24. Gerein RB, Osmond MH, Stiell IG et al (2006) What are the etiology and epidemiology of out-of-hospital pediatric cardiopulmonary arrest in Ontario, Canada? Acad Emerg Med 13:653–658

25. Schindler MB, Bohn D, Cox PN et al (1996) Outcome of out-of-hospital cardiac or respiratory arrest in children. N Engl J Med 335:1473–1479

26. Friesen RM, Duncan P, Tweed WA et al (1982) Appraisal of pediatric cardiopulmonary resuscitation. Can Med Assoc J 126:1055–1058

27. Rossano JW, Quan L, Kenney MA et al (2006) Energy doses for treatment of out-of-hospital pediatric ventricular fibrillation. Resuscitation 70:80–89

28. Young KD, Seidel JS (1999) Pediatric cardiopulmonary resuscitation: a collective review. Ann Emerg Med 33:195–205

29. Maron BJ, Doerer JJ, Haas TS et al (2009) Sudden deaths in young competitive athletes: analysis of 1866 deaths in the United States, 1980–2006. Circulation 119:1085–1092

30. Harmon KG, Asif IM, Klossner D et al (2011) Incidence of sudden cardiac death in national collegiate athletic association athletes. Circulation 123:1594–1600

31. Corrado D, Basso C, Pavei A et al (2006) Trends in sudden cardiovascular death in young competitive athletes after implementation of a preparticipation screening program. JAMA 296:1593–1601

32. Maron BJ (2010) Risk stratification and role of implantable defibrillators for prevention of sudden death in patients with hypertrophic cardiomyopathy. Circ J 74:2271–2282

33. Hazinski MF, Chahine AA, Holcomb GW 3rd et al (1994) Outcome of cardiovascular collapse in pediatric blunt trauma. Ann Emerg Med 23:1229–1235

34. Rodriguez-Nunez A, Lopez-Herce J, Garcia C et al (2006) Effectiveness and long-term outcome of cardiopulmonary resuscitation in paediatric intensive care units in Spain. Resuscitation 71:301–309

35. Nadkarni VM, Larkin GL, Peberdy MA et al (2006) First documented rhythm and clinical outcome from in-hospital cardiac arrest among children and adults. JAMA 295:50–57

36. Samson RA, Nadkarni VM, Meaney PA et al (2006) Outcomes of in-hospital ventricular fibrillation in children. N Engl J Med 354:2328–2339

37. Ortmann L, Prodhan P, Gossett J et al (2011) Outcomes after in-hospital cardiac arrest in children with cardiac disease: a report from Get With the Guidelines-Resuscitation. Circulation 124:2329–2337

38. Gillis J, Dickson D, Rieder M et al (1986) Results of inpatient pediatric resuscitation. Crit Care Med 14:469–471

39. Nichols DG, Kettrick RG, Swedlow DB et al (1986) Factors influencing outcome of cardiopulmonary resuscitation in children. Pediatr Emerg Care 2:1–5

40. Slonim AD, Patel KM, Ruttimann UE et al (1997) Cardiopulmonary resuscitation in pediatric intensive care units. Crit Care Med 25:1951–1955

41. Nitta M, Iwami T, Kitamura T et al (2011) Age-specific differences in outcomes after out-of-hospital cardiac arrests. Pediatrics 128:e812–e820

42. Quan L, Wentz KR, Gore EJ et al (1990) Outcome and predictors of outcome in pediatric submersion victims receiving prehospital care in King County, Washington. Pediatrics 86:586–593

43. Mogayzel C, Quan L, Graves JR et al (1995) Out-of-hospital ventricular fibrillation in children and adolescents: causes and outcomes. Ann Emerg Med 25:484–491

44. Safranek DJ, Eisenberg MS, Larsen MP (1992) The epidemiology of cardiac arrest in young adults. Ann Emerg Med 21:1102–1106

45. Ong ME, Ng FS, Anushia P et al (2008) Comparison of chest compression only and standard cardiopulmonary resuscitation for out-of-hospital cardiac arrest in Singapore. Resuscitation 78:119–126

46. SOS-KANTO study group (2007) Cardiopulmonary resuscitation by bystanders with chest compression only (SOS-KANTO): an observational study. Lancet 369:920–926

47. Petrie DA, De Maio V, Stiell IG et al (2001) Factors affecting survival after prehospital asystolic cardiac arrest in a Basic Life Support-Defibrillation system. CJEM 3:186–192

48. Suominen P, Korpela R, Kuisma M et al (1997) Paediatric cardiac arrest and resuscitation provided by physician-staffed emergency care units. Acta Anaesthesiol Scand 41:260–265

49. Torphy DE, Minter MG, Thompson BM (1984) Cardiorespiratory arrest and resuscitation of children. Am J Dis Child 138:1099–1102

50. Teach SJ, Moore PE, Fleisher GR (1995) Death and resuscitation in the pediatric emergency department. Ann Emerg Med 25:799–803

51. Dimas VV, Denfield SW, Friedman RA et al (2009) Frequency of cardiac death in children with idiopathic dilated cardiomyopathy. Am J Cardiol 104:1574–1577

52. Goldenberg I, Moss AJ (2008) Long QT syndrome. J Am Coll Cardiol 51:2291–2300

53. Berg RA, Hemphill R, Abella BS et al (2010) Part 5: adult basic life support: 2010 American Heart Association Guidelines for Cardiopulmonary Resuscitation and Emergency Cardiovascular Care. Circulation 122: S685–S705

54. Bobrow BJ, Spaite DW, Berg RA et al (2010) Chest compression-only CPR by lay rescuers and survival from out-of-hospital cardiac arrest. JAMA 304:1447–1454

55. Bobrow BJ, Clark LL, Ewy GA et al (2008) Minimally interrupted cardiac resuscitation by emergency medical services for out-of-hospital cardiac arrest. JAMA 299:1158–1165

56. Kellum MJ, Kennedy KW, Barney R et al (2008) Cardiocerebral resuscitation improves neurologically intact survival of patients with out-of-hospital cardiac arrest. Ann Emerg Med 52:244–252

57. Donoghue A, Berg RA, Hazinski MF et al (2009) Cardiopulmonary resuscitation for bradycardia with poor perfusion versus pulseless cardiac arrest. Pediatrics 124:1541–1548

58. Tibballs J, Kinney S (2006) A prospective study of outcome of in-patient paediatric cardiopulmonary arrest. Resuscitation 71:310–318

59. Srinivasan V, Nadkarni VM, Helfaer MA et al (2010) Childhood obesity and survival after in-hospital pediatric cardiopulmonary resuscitation. Pediatrics 125:e481–e488

60. Meaney PA, Nadkarni VM, Cook EF et al (2006) Higher survival rates among younger patients after pediatric intensive care unit cardiac arrests. Pediatrics 118:2424–2433

61. del Castillo J, Lopez-Herce J (2010) Age related differences in in-hospital pediatric cardiac arrest in European and Latin-American hospitals (abstract). Resuscitation 81:S27

62. Rossano JW, Jefferson LS, Smith EO et al (2009) Automated external defibrillators and simulated in-hospital cardiac arrests. J Pediatr 154:672–676

63. Chan PS, Krumholz HM, Spertus JA et al (2010) Automated external defibrillators and survival after in-hospital cardiac arrest. JAMA 304:2129–2136

64. Innes PA, Summers CA, Boyd IM et al (1993) Audit of paediatric cardiopulmonary resuscitation. Arch Dis Child 68:487–491

65. Torres A Jr, Pickert CB, Firestone J et al (1997) Long-term functional outcome of inpatient pediatric cardiopulmonary resuscitation. Pediatr Emerg Care 13:369–373

66. Raymond TT, Cunnyngham CB, Thompson MT et al (2010) Outcomes among neonates, infants, and children after extracorporeal cardiopulmonary resuscitation for refractory in hospital pediatric cardiac arrest: a report from the National Registry of Cardiopulmonary Resuscitation. Pediatr Crit Care Med 11:362–371

67. Kane DA, Thiagarajan RR, Wypij D et al (2010) Rapid-response extracorporeal membrane oxygenation to support cardiopulmonary resuscitation in children with cardiac disease. Circulation 122:S241–S248

68. Chan T, Thiagarajan RR, Frank D et al (2008) Survival after extracorporeal cardiopulmonary resuscitation in infants and children with heart disease. J Thorac Cardiovasc Surg 136:984–992

69. Morris MC, Wernovsky G, Nadkarni VM (2004) Survival outcomes after extracorporeal cardiopulmonary resuscitation instituted during active chest compressions following refractory in-hospital pediatric cardiac arrest. Pediatr Crit Care Med 5: 440–446

70. Alsoufi B, Al-Radi OO, Nazer RI et al (2007) Survival outcomes after rescue extracorporeal cardiopulmonary resuscitation in pediatric patients with refractory cardiac arrest. J Thorac Cardiovasc Surg 134: 952e2–959e2

71. Bos AP, Polman A, van der Voort E et al (1992) Cardiopulmonary resuscitation in paediatric intensive care patients. Intensive Care Med 18:109–111

72. Sivarajan VB, Best D, Brizard CP et al (2011) Duration of resuscitation prior to rescue extracorporeal membrane oxygenation impacts outcome in children with heart disease. Intensive Care Med 37:853–860

73. Chen YS, Yu HY, Huang SC et al (2008) Extracorporeal membrane oxygenation support can extend the duration of cardiopulmonary resuscitation. Crit Care Med 36:2529–2535

74. Huang SC, Wu ET, Chen YS et al (2008) Extracorporeal membrane oxygenation rescue for cardiopulmonary resuscitation in pediatric patients. Crit Care Med 36:1607–1613

75. Anwar UH, Saleem AF, Zaidi S et al (2010) Experience of pediatric rapid response team in a tertiary care hospital in Pakistan. Indian J Pediatr 77:273–276

76. Sharek PJ, Parast LM, Leong K et al (2007) Effect of a rapid response team on hospital-wide mortality and code rates outside the ICU in a Children's Hospital. JAMA 298:2267–2274

77. Joffe AR, Anton NR, Burkholder SC (2011) Reduction in hospital mortality over time in a hospital without a pediatric medical emergency team: limitations of before-and-after study designs. Arch Pediatr Adolesc Med 165:419–423

78. Niles D, Sutton RM, Donoghue A et al (2009) "Rolling Refreshers": a novel approach to maintain CPR psychomotor skill competence. Resuscitation 80:909–912

79. Niles D, Nysaether J, Sutton R et al (2009) Leaning is common during in-hospital pediatric CPR, and decreased with automated corrective feedback. Resuscitation 80:553–557

80. Alsoufi B, Al-Radi OO, Gruenwald C et al (2009) Extra-corporeal life support following cardiac surgery in children: analysis of risk factors and survival in a single institution. Eur J Cardiothorac Surg 35:1004–1011, discussion 11

Maryam Y. Naim, Joseph W. Rossano,
Vinay M. Nadkarni, and Robert A. Berg

Abstract

The year 2010 marked the 50th anniversary of modern resuscitation. In October 2010, the American Heart Association released updated guidelines for cardiopulmonary resuscitation (CPR) and emergency cardiovascular care. This chapter will outline current CPR recommendations and review the evidence for major changes in pediatric basic and advanced life support with a special emphasis on children with cardiac disease.

Keywords

Cardiopulmonary resuscitation • Cardiac arrest • Extracorporeal circulatory support • Extracorporeal membrane oxygenation (ECMO) • Pediatric bradycardia • Pediatric ventricular fibrillation • Pediatric ventricular tachycardia

M.Y. Naim (✉) • R.A. Berg
Department of Anesthesia and Critical Care, Perelman
School of Medicine at the University of Pennsylvania,
Philadelphia, PA, USA

Department of Anesthesiology and Critical Care
Medicine, The Children's Hospital of Philadelphia,
Philadelphia, PA, USA
e-mail: naim@email.chop.edu; bergra@email.chop.edu

J.W. Rossano
Department of Pediatrics, Perelman School of Medicine
at the University of Pennsylvania, Philadelphia, PA, USA

The Cardiac Center, The Children's Hospital of
Philadelphia, Philadelphia, PA, USA
e-mail: RossanoJ@email.chop.edu

V.M. Nadkarni
Department of Anesthesia and Critical Care, Perelman
School of Medicine at the University of Pennsylvania,
Philadelphia, PA, USA

Center for Simulation, Advanced Education and
Innovation, The Children's Hospital of Philadelphia,
Philadelphia, PA, USA
e-mail: nadkarni@email.chop.edu

E.M. da Cruz et al. (eds.), *Pediatric and Congenital Cardiology, Cardiac Surgery and Intensive Care*,
DOI 10.1007/978-1-4471-4619-3_59, © Springer-Verlag London 2014

Introduction

In 1947, Claude Beck reported the first use of electrical shock for prolonged ventricular fibrillation in a human. The following decade saw the birth of modern resuscitation with the description of mouth-to-mouth ventilation by James Elam; "closed-chest cardiac massage" by William Kouwenhoven, Guy Knickerbocker, and James Jude; and the use of the external defibrillator in humans by Paul Zoll. In 1960, Kouwenhoven, Knickerbocker, and Jude published their landmark article on 20 patients with in-hospital cardiac arrest treated with closed-chest massage, with an astonishing 70 % rate of survival to hospital discharge [1].

The year 2010 marked the 50th anniversary of modern resuscitation. In October 2010, the American Heart Association (AHA) released updated guidelines for cardiopulmonary resuscitation (CPR) and emergency cardiovascular care. Based on the best available evidence, the updated guidelines for pediatric basic [2] and advanced [3] life support reinforce the emphasis on high-quality basic CPR and recommend a few major changes compared to the 2005 guidelines.

Special resuscitation situations that have been addressed in the updated guidelines include pediatric cardiac patients, specifically the single ventricle patient and the child with pulmonary hypertension. Although the management of these special patients before a cardiac arrest may differ from children without these cardiac challenges, there is no evidence for alteration of good quality standard CPR (push hard, push fast, minimize interruptions, allow full chest recoil, don't overventilate) for these children during cardiac arrest. This chapter will focus on the current CPR recommendations, reviewing the evidence for major changes in pediatric basic and advanced life support.

Physiology and Pathophysiology

Physiology of Cardiac Arrest

The three common pathways to cardiac arrest are asphyxial, ischemic, and arrhythmogenic. Asphyxial cardiac arrests are precipitated by acute hypoxia and/or hypercarbia and are the most common pathway in children [4–6]. Ischemic arrests in children are precipitated by inadequate myocardial blood flow. In adults, the primary cause of ischemic cardiac arrests is atherosclerotic coronary artery disease, whereas in children they are most commonly due to shock from hypovolemia, sepsis, or myocardial dysfunction. In children with congenital heart disease, this type of arrest may result from a coronary artery abnormality, or following an arterial switch operation for transposition of the great arteries. Finally, arrhythmogenic arrests are precipitated by ventricular fibrillation (VF) or ventricular tachycardia (VT). The immediate cause of arrest in two recent pediatric in-hospital studies was arrhythmogenic for 10 %, asphyxial for 67 %, and ischemic for 61 % (many had both asphyxia and ischemia) [5, 6]. The vast majority of out-of-hospital arrests are also either asphyxial or ischemic, and 5–20 % are arrhythmogenic [7].

Clinical Features

The triad of pulselessness, apnea, and unresponsiveness define the clinical state of cardiac arrest. For decades, published guidelines on the assessment of patients suspected to be in cardiac arrest used the mnemonic A-B-C (airway-breathing-circulation) for the stepwise assessment and intervention sequence. This sequence included the opening of the airway, assessing respirations using the "look-listen-feel" technique for up to 10 seconds (s), providing two rescue breaths, and checking for a central pulse (brachial or femoral in children, carotid in adults). For the first time in 2005, Consensus on Science and Treatment Recommendations published by International Liaison Committee on Resuscitation (ILCOR) removed the pulse check as a necessary step for lay rescuers and limited the duration and reliance on pulse check for healthcare providers based on data demonstrating poor specificity and sensitivity of a 10-s carotid pulse check by healthcare providers [8, 9]. The implication for rescuers is that any patient who is unresponsive and apneic and appears "lifeless" by gross appearance (i.e., "appears dead") should have chest compressions initiated immediately without delay to check for a pulse. This recommendation may have particular pertinence for children because of the high prevalence of bradycardia and hypoperfusion in the pre-arrest phase and the potential improvement in outcomes when CPR is provided for bradycardia and poor pulses [10].

Studies on the pulse check in pediatrics have predominantly focused on healthy children, where the data on the accuracy of brachial and femoral pulse checks is varied [11, 12]. A recent pediatric study examined the accuracy of the pulse check by healthcare providers on children receiving extracorporeal circulatory support, where native pulsatile cardiac activity was variably diminished or absent. A 10-s femoral or brachial pulse check had a sensitivity of 86 % and a specificity of 64 % for presence of pulse [13]. In other words, making a decision to provide CPR based on the pulse check alone in this patient set would have resulted in chest compressions provided to 36 % of patients when they were not indicated and compressions withheld from 14 % of patients who were either pulseless or critically hypoperfused enough to require them. Based largely on this study, the 2010 ILCOR guidelines for pediatric resuscitation have removed the pulse check for lay rescuers. Healthcare providers should spend no more than 10 s assessing a central pulse. They should either provide chest compressions without a pulse check or provide chest compressions within 10 s.

The 2010 AHA recommendation is to change the algorithmic sequence of rescue interventions for the arrested patient from A-B-C to C-A-B (compressions-airway-breathing). The main rationale for this change is to prevent a delay in initiation of chest compressions because blood flow during cardiac arrest depends on chest compressions and efforts to address A and B first delay the time to reestablishment of blood flow [14]. The value of this approach is most dramatically demonstrated by the success of compression-only CPR (i.e., without rescue breathing) [15]. Therefore, C-A-B is the adult recommendation, and it is reasonable to use the same approach in children to simplify training for the lay rescuer. Additionally, starting resuscitation for an arrested child with compressions instead of ventilations will result in only a brief delay prior to the first rescue breath (18 s for the lone rescuer, 9 s for multiple rescuers). Finally, in a healthcare setting where a team of providers responds to an arrest, multiple tasks are undertaken simultaneously by task-specific personnel. Because chest compressions can be applied instantaneously and positive-pressure ventilation requires several seconds of equipment preparation and application to the patient's face, C-A-B is typically the best approach for providing circulation, oxygenation, and ventilation as promptly as possible.

Phases of Cardiac Arrest

The cardiac arrest process can be divided into four distinct phases: (1) pre-arrest, (2) no flow (untreated cardiac arrest), (3) low flow (cardiopulmonary resuscitation), and (4) post-resuscitation.

Pre-arrest

The pre-arrest phase focuses on preventing the arrest (i.e., recognizing precipitating events/changes in physiologic status and intervening). In this phase, attention is directed to early recognition and treatment of the most common causes of pediatric cardiac arrest: respiratory failure and shock. Rapid response teams or medical emergency teams (METs) are in-hospital teams designed for this purpose [16–18]. Early warning scores can help screen potential victims. Classically, these teams are comprised of critical care trained care providers who are available to lower acuity care areas to identify children at risk so that they can be transferred to a higher level of care before the event. While METs cannot identify all children at risk, transferring critically ill children to an ICU early in their disease process for better monitoring and more aggressive interventions improves resuscitative care and clinical outcome [16–18].

Patients with cardiac disease may manifest potential pre-arrest signs and symptoms because of low cardiac output states following intra-operative myocardial ischemia, myocarditis or dilated cardiomyopathy, arrhythmias following cardiac surgery, or single ventricle physiology with a high ratio of pulmonary blood flow to systemic blood flow. Pulmonary hypertensive crisis with right ventricular failure, or inadequate flow to the lungs during occlusion of a systemic to pulmonary artery shunt, cyanotic spells, or ductal closure, are other common pathways to cardiac arrest [19]. Early recognition with targeted interventions including inotropic or mechanical support for low cardiac output states, antiarrhythmic therapy for arrhythmias, pulmonary vasodilator therapy for patients with pulmonary hypertension, and reestablishment of blood flow to the lungs in patients with shunt occlusion or ductal closure can prevent a patient in this phase from progressing to cardiac arrest.

Specific recommendations from the 2010 AHA guidelines on single ventricle patients in a pre-arrest state include consideration of increasing partial pressure of CO_2 with controlled hypoventilation, or supplemental inspired CO_2 [20] prior to stage 1 in infants with a pre-arrest low cardiac output condition secondary to a high ratio of pulmonary blood flow to systemic blood flow. In children with a Fontan or hemi-Fontan/bidirectional Glenn physiology in a pre-arrest low cardiac output condition, hypoventilation may improve oxygen delivery [21], and negative pressure ventilation may improve cardiac output [22]. Children with post-operative low cardiac output syndrome may benefit from afterload reduction with phenoxybenzamine [23, 24], milrinone [25], or nitroprusside [24]. Monitoring with near infra-red spectroscopy [26] and systemic venous saturations [27] may detect changes in hemodynamics that may be helpful in detecting impending cardiac arrest. Extracorporeal membrane oxygenation (ECMO) should be considered before or early during cardiac arrest for children following a stage I operation [28], and with Fontan physiology [29].

No Flow

Once a child suffers a cardiac arrest, the focus should shift towards shortening the no-flow phase of untreated cardiac arrest. Early recognition is imperative. When the heart arrests and no blood flows to the aorta, coronary and cerebral blood flow stops [30]. Organs, including the brain, are deprived of life-sustaining perfusion. At that point, provision of CPR is necessary to reestablish flow. Therefore, it is important to triage children at high risk of cardiac arrest to a monitored ICU where cardiac arrest can be promptly recognized and treated.

Low Flow (Cardiopulmonary resuscitation)

Chest Compressions

The goal during CPR is to maximize the myocardial perfusion pressure (MPP). The MPP (aortic diastolic blood pressure [AoDP] minus right atrial pressure [RAP]) improves as the gradient between AoDP and RAP increases. During the downward compression phase, aortic pressure rises at the same time as right atrial pressure with little change in the MPP. However, a pressure gradient is generated during the decompression phase of chest compression as the right atrial pressure falls faster and lower than the aortic pressure. This pressure gradient delivers oxygenated blood during the decompression phase ("diastole") when the blood flows through the coronary arteries. Therefore, full elastic recoil (release) of the chest is important to create a pressure difference between the aortic root and the right atrium. Failure to generate a MPP of at least 15 mm Hg during CPR is a poor prognostic factor for ROSC in both animal and human studies [31–34]. During the low-flow state of CPR, cardiac output and pulmonary blood flow are approximately 25–50 % of that during normal sinus rhythm; therefore, much less ventilation is necessary for adequate gas exchange from the blood traversing the pulmonary circulation [35]. In fact, animal and adult data indicate that a rapid rate of assisted ventilation ("overventilation" from exuberant rescue breathing) during CPR is not only common [36–38] but can substantially compromise venous return and cardiac output by increasing intrathoracic pressure.

The 2010 guidelines continue to emphasize high-quality CPR. Inadequate chest compression depth is common during CPR [39, 40]. In a recent quantitative analysis of CPR quality in children and adolescents with IHCA, AHA targets for depth and rate were not achieved 36.1 % and 48 % of the time, respectively [39]. The updated guidelines reemphasize to "push hard" to a depth of approximately 1½ in. (4 cm) in infants, and approximately 2 in. (5 cm) in children, or *at least* one-third of the anterior-posterior dimension of the chest. New evidence with measurement of optimal depth of compressions with analysis of infant and children's chest tomography scans shows that the previous recommendation to push to one half was probably too deep [41] and may not be achievable. In addition, 2010 guidelines increase emphasis on avoiding "leaning" on the chest that prevents full recoil of the chest and refilling of the heart and avoiding interruptions of CPR (e.g., charge the defibrillator *during* chest compressions).

Neonatal resuscitation guidelines recommend newborns with cardiac arrest receive chest compressions at a ratio of 3:1 (chest compressions: breaths) in the newborn nursery or neonatal intensive care unit [42]. However, if the cardiac arrest is of primary cardiac origin, the new pediatric guidelines recommend a ratio of 15:2 in newborns regardless of location.

Circumferential Versus Focal Sternal Compressions

In adults and animal models of cardiac arrest, circumferential CPR (e.g., "vest CPR") provides better CPR hemodynamics than two-finger compressions. In smaller infants, the recommended CPR technique is to encircle the chest with both hands and depress the sternum with the thumbs, while compressing the thorax circumferentially (when the resuscitator's hands are large enough to do so) [43]. This "two-thumb" circumferential compression technique results in higher systolic and diastolic blood pressures and a higher pulse pressure than traditional two-finger compression of the sternum [44].

Open-Chest Cardiopulmonary Resuscitation

Open-chest CPR is often provided to children after open-heart cardiac surgery and sternotomy. In animal models, high-quality standard, closed-chest CPR generates myocardial blood flow that is >50 % of normal, cerebral blood flow that is approximately 50 % of normal, and cardiac output ~10–25 % of normal [30, 33, 45, 46]. By contrast, open-chest CPR can generate myocardial and cerebral blood flow that approaches *normal*. Although open-chest massage improves coronary perfusion pressure and increases the chance of successful defibrillation in animals and humans [47–49], performing a thoracotomy to allow open-chest CPR is impractical in many situations. Earlier institution of open-chest CPR may warrant consideration in selected special resuscitation circumstances (e.g., children with an open sternum post-cardiac surgery).

Compression-Only CPR

In adults with witnessed cardiac arrest of presumed cardiac etiology, chest-compression-only CPR by lay rescuers has been shown to be associated with increased survival compared with no CPR and equivalent to conventional CPR with rescue breathing [15]. The updated 2010 *adult* basic life support guidelines recommend chest-compression-only CPR by untrained lay rescuers of adults with cardiac arrest [50]. A study done in children in Japan comparing bystander chest-compression-only CPR to bystander conventional

CPR showed that survivors of arrest from noncardiac causes (71 %) had better neurological outcomes following conventional CPR with rescue breathing, compared to chest-compression-only CPR. For children who had arrests from cardiac causes (29 %), there was no difference in neurologic outcome between children who received bystander conventional CPR compared to compression-only CPR [51]. Importantly both bystander CPR groups had better survival than those who did not receive bystander CPR at all. As asphyxial arrests are common in children, the 2010 *pediatric* guidelines recommend conventional CPR for the lay rescuer, unless the rescuer is not trained, not willing or not confident in providing the rescue breaths.

Monitoring During CPR

End-tidal carbon dioxide (ETCO2) monitoring is recommended to confirm tracheal intubation. In addition, quantitative capnography during CPR is recommended to monitor and guide the quality of CPR. ETCO2 during CPR is primarily determined by pulmonary blood flow. Therefore, ETCO2 increases with interventions that increase cardiac output and pulmonary blood flow during CPR. ETCO2 increases abruptly with return of spontaneous circulation (ROSC) [52, 53]. Resuscitation teams can follow ETCO2 to determine ROSC rather than interrupt chest compressions while feeling for pulses to determine ROSC. Echocardiography may also be useful as a monitoring tool during CPR, especially to identify a reversible cause (e.g., pericardial tamponade).

Special Considerations in Cardiac Patients

For a child with cardiac disease important additional considerations include management of a systemic to pulmonary artery shunt occlusion, drainage of pericardial tamponade, potential initiation of epicardial or transcutaneous pacing, and early activation of the ECMO team [19]. In children with shunted single ventricle physiology in cardiac arrest, consideration of bolus heparin therapy is recommended because of the risk of shunt occlusion [3]. A standard PALS approach with conventional CPR should be administered to children with pulmonary hypertension, with special consideration to correcting hypercarbia, assuring adequacy of preload (fluid bolus administration), and reinstituting pulmonary hypertensive therapies (if they were discontinued prior to the event), such as inhaled nitric oxide, inhaled prostacyclin, or intravenous prostacyclin. ECMO may have benefit for reversible conditions, if it is initiated early in the resuscitation [54] and in conjunction with high-quality basic life support.

Advanced Life Support Medications During the Low-Flow Phase of Cardiopulmonary Resuscitation

Although animal studies indicate that epinephrine can improve initial resuscitation success after both asphyxial and VF cardiac arrests, no single medication has been shown to improve survival to hospital discharge outcome from pediatric cardiac arrests. Medications commonly used for CPR in children are vasopressors (epinephrine or vasopressin), calcium salts, sodium bicarbonate, and antiarrhythmics (amiodarone or lidocaine). During CPR, epinephrine's alpha-adrenergic effect increases systemic vascular resistance, increasing diastolic blood pressure, which in turn increases coronary perfusion pressure and myocardial blood flow and increases the likelihood of the return of spontaneous circulation. Epinephrine also increases cerebral blood flow during CPR because peripheral vasoconstriction directs a greater proportion of flow to the cerebral circulation. The beta-adrenergic effect increases myocardial contractility and heart rate and relaxes smooth muscle in the skeletal muscle vascular bed and bronchi, although this effect is of less importance. Epinephrine also changes the character of VF (i.e., higher amplitude, more "coarse"), increasing the likelihood of successful defibrillation (Fig. 72.1 and Table 72.1).

Prospective and retrospective studies indicate that use of high-dose epinephrine in adults or children (0.05–0.2 mg/kg) does not improve survival and may be associated with a worse neurologic outcome. A randomized, blinded, controlled trial of rescue high-dose epinephrine versus standard-dose epinephrine following failed

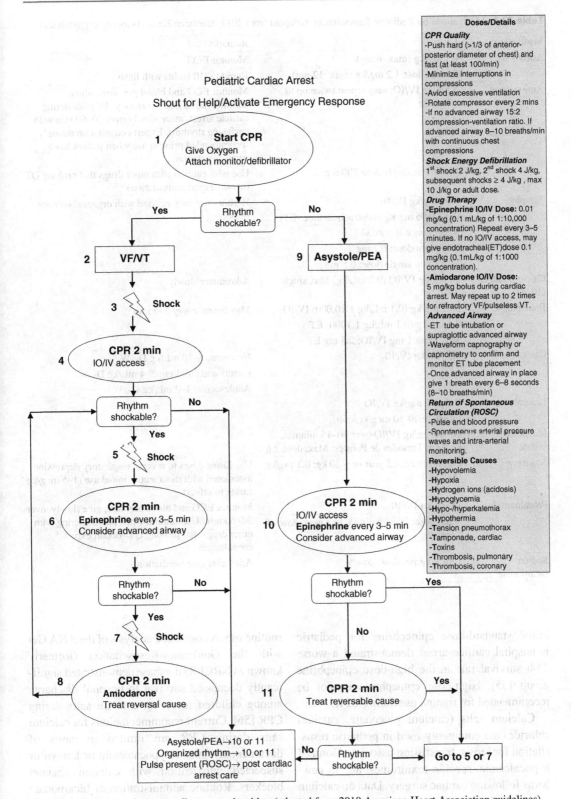

Fig. 72.1 Pediatric pulseless cardiac arrest algorithm (adapted from 2010 American Heart Association guidelines)

Table 72.1 Medications for Pediatric Resuscitation (adapted from 2012 American Heart Association guidelines)

Medication	Dose	Remarks
Adenosine	0.1 mg/kg (max. 6 mg)	Monitor ECG
	Second dose 1.2 mg/kg (max. 12 mg)	Rapid IV/10 Bolus with flush
Amiodarone	5 mg/kg IV/IO; may repeat twice up to 15 mg/kg	Monitor ECG and blood pressure; adjust administration rate to urgency (IV push during cardiac arrest, more slowly over 20–60 min with perfusing rhythm). Expert consultation strongly recommended prior to use when patient has a perfusing rhythm
	Maximum single dose 300 mg	Use with caution with other drugs that prolong QT (obtain expert consultation)
Atropine	0.02 mg/kg IV/10	Higher dose may be used with organophosphate poisoning
	0.04–0.06 mg/kg endotracheal tube (ET)	
	Repeat once if needed	
	Minimum dose: 0.1 mg	
	Maximum single dose: 0.5 mg	
Calcium chloride (10 %)	20 mg/kg IV/IO (0.2 mL/kg) Max single dose 2 g	Administer slowly
Epinephrine	0.01 mg/kg (0.1 mL/kg 1:10,000) IV/IO	May repeat every 3–5 min
	0.1 mg/kg (0.1 mL/kg 1:1000) ET	
	Max. dose 1 mg IV/IO; 2.5 mg ET	
Glucose	0.5–1 g/kg IV/10	Newborn: 5–10 mL/kg $D_{10}W$
		Infants and children: 2–4 mL/kg $D_{25}W$
		Adolescents: 1–2 mL/kg $D_{50}W$
Lidocaine	Bolus: 1 mg/kg IV/IO	
	Infusion: 20-50 mcg/kg/min	
Magnesium sulfate	20–50 mg/kg IV/IO over 10–15 minutes, faster in Torsades de Pointes; Max. dose 2 g	
Naloxone	Full reversal: <5 year or ≤20 kg: 0.1 mg/kg IV/IO/ET	Use lower doses to reverse respiratory depression associated with therapeutic opioid use (1–5 mcg/kg titrate to effect)
Procainamide	15 mg/kg IV/10	Monitor ECG and blood pressure; give slowly–over 30–60 min. Use caution when administering with other drugs that prolong QT (obtain expert consultation)
	Adult dose: 20 mg/min IV to a max. dose of 17 mg/kg	
Sodium bicarbonate	1 mEq/kg per dose slowly	After adequate ventilation

initial standard-dose epinephrine for pediatric in-hospital cardiac arrest demonstrated a worse 24-h survival rate in the high-dose epinephrine group [55]. High-dose epinephrine cannot be recommended for routine use during CPR.

Calcium salts (calcium gluconate, calcium chloride) are commonly used in pediatric resuscitation for sepsis, transfusion-associated ionized hypocalcemia, specific toxidromes, and in newborns following cardiac surgery. Data on calcium salts in cardiac arrest, however, do not support its routine use. A controlled analysis of the AHA Get with the Guidelines-Resuscitation (formerly known as NRCPR) database demonstrated significantly decreased survival to hospital discharge among children receiving calcium salts during CPR [56]. Current recommendations for calcium salts during CPR are limited to cases of documented ionized hypocalcemia or known or suspected intoxication with calcium channel blockers. Routine administration of bicarbonate is also discouraged [3].

Pediatric Ventricular Fibrillation and Ventricular Tachycardia

Although asystole and pulseless electrical activity (PEA) are the most common rhythms seen with in-hospital pediatric cardiac arrest, VF or pulseless VT are not rare [5] and are commonly seen in pediatric cardiac intensive care unit settings. VF/VT may occur as the primary inciting arrest rhythm (i.e., arrhythmogenic arrest) due to a variety of underlying myocardial pathologies (myocarditis, congenital heart disease, long QT syndrome, etc.) or electrolyte derangements. Of 1,005 pediatric in-hospital cardiac arrests in the AHA Get with the Guidelines-Resuscitation database, 27 % had VF/VT at some point during the resuscitation, 10 % as an initial rhythm, and an additional 15 % as subsequent VF/VT (i.e., sometime later during the resuscitation effort) [5].

Traditionally, VF and VT have been considered "good" cardiac arrest rhythms, resulting in much better outcomes than asystole and PEA. However, AHA Get with the Guidelines-Resuscitation data showed that survival to discharge was more common among children with *initial* VF/VT than among children with *subsequent* VF/VT (35 % vs. 11 %) [5]. Surprisingly, the subsequent VF/VT group had worse outcomes than children with asystole/PEA (11 % vs. 27 % survival). These data suggest that outcomes after *initial* VF/VT in children (an arrhythmogenic arrest) are "good," but outcomes after *subsequent* VF/VT (i.e., VF/VT in the setting of an asphyxial or ischemic arrest) are worse, even compared with initial asystole/PEA without subsequent VF/VT.

Defibrillation

Defibrillation is necessary for successful resuscitation from VF cardiac arrest. The goal of defibrillation is return of an organized electrical rhythm with a palpable pulse. When prompt defibrillation is provided soon after the induction of VF in a cardiac catheterization laboratory, the rates of successful defibrillation and survival approach 100 %. In general, the mortality rate increases by 5–10 % per minute of delay to defibrillation [57]. Provision of high-quality CPR can improve outcomes and save lives. Because pediatric cardiac arrests are commonly due to progressive asphyxia or shock (or both), the initial treatment of choice is prompt CPR, not defibrillation. Therefore, rhythm recognition has been deemphasized in the latest PALS guidelines compared with adult cardiac arrests. This historical emphasis must be balanced against the increasing evidence that VF in children is not rare, outcomes from arrhythmogenic VF arrests are superior to those from other types of cardiac arrests, and that early rhythm diagnosis is necessary for optimal care.

Because of the increasing awareness that "shockable" rhythms are not uncommon in children, greater attention has been focused on the dose for pediatric defibrillation. The recommended shock dose is 2–4 J/kg, which is based on animal studies of short-duration VF and a single retrospective study of in-hospital (short duration) VF with 91 % (52/57) defibrillation success [58]. More recent piglet and out-of-hospital pediatric data indicate that 2 J/kg is often ineffective at terminating fibrillation [59, 60]. In-hospital pediatric defibrillation data also suggest that 2 J/kg is often ineffective at terminating fibrillation [61]. Animal and clinical data suggest that a single pediatric dose of 50 J (i.e., the dose in many pediatric AEDs) can be quite effective at terminating fibrillation in children <8 years of age.

The 2010 guidelines address the use of automated external defibrillators (AEDs) for infants with ventricular fibrillation or pulseless ventricular tachycardia. Manual defibrillators are preferred to AEDs in infants; however, if a manual defibrillator is not available, an AED with a dose attenuator can be used. Based on a recent case report, if neither a manual defibrillator or an AED with dose attenuator is available, defibrillation with an AED without a dose attenuator can be safe and effective in infants [62] with cardiac arrest secondary to a shockable rhythm.

CPR in Pediatric Bradycardia

Neonates, infants, and children are primarily dependent on heart rate for maintenance of cardiac output. Their ability to augment stroke volume to increase cardiac output is limited, and physiologic or pathophysiologic states leading to an increase in cardiac output are hallmarked by tachycardia. Conversely, illnesses or injuries resulting in negative chronotropy (e.g., heart block, toxicity of beta-blockers, or calcium channel blockers) tend to result in more profound shock and hypoperfusion in children than in adults with similar processes.

Bradycardia with hypoperfusion (without pulselessness) is a common hemodynamic state for critically ill children during the pre-arrest phase immediately before a pulseless arrest. Early clinical studies of terminally ill children demonstrated almost ubiquitous prevalence of bradycardia prior to onset of cardiac arrest [63]. Animal models of asphyxia have demonstrated a predictable hemodynamic progression from tachycardia to bradycardia with hypotension, followed by pulseless electrical activity and asystole [64], and that CPR earlier in this continuum is associated with more favorable outcomes [65, 66]. Given that the majority of children suffering cardiac arrest are suffering either respiratory and/or circulatory insufficiency prior to the onset of pulselessness, *a bradycardic child in shock should be considered to be in a pre-arrest state*. Multiple reversible causes need to be considered (e.g., hypothermia, increased intracranial pressure) but immediate consideration of the need for support of cardiovascular status is essential.

Neonatal resuscitation algorithms have recommended escalation of respiratory and cardiac support for the neonate, whose heart rate is less than 60 beats per minute, including the provision of chest compressions if bradycardia does not resolve with effective ventilation and oxygenation. Multiple studies of pediatric patients from the Get With The Guidelines-Resuscitation database (formerly known as NRCPR) have shown that nearly half of patients below the age of 18 who receive chest compressions in-hospital are in a state of bradycardia and hypoperfusion, as opposed to pulselessness, when CPR is initiated [5, 10, 67]. Not surprisingly outcomes are superior when CPR is provided for bradycardia and poor perfusion rather than waiting for progression to pulselessness [10]. Current AHA guidelines recommend the consideration of immediate chest compressions for a child with a heart rate of less than 60 with obvious hypoperfusion [3].

Extracorporeal Circulatory Support During Cardiac Arrest (E-CPR)

The use of rescue ECMO in children during cardiac arrest was initially described in two small series. del Nido and colleagues in 1992 reported on ECMO during CPR for 11 children with cardiac arrest following open-heart surgery with 64 % early survival and no apparent long-term cardiac or neurologic sequelae [68]. In 1998, the Children's Hospital of Boston reported their use of rapid deployment ECMO in 11 children with congenital heart disease following cardiac arrest and showed shorter duration of cardiac arrest (55 vs. 90 min) and improved survival (64 % vs. 27 %) compared to historical controls [69].

In a landmark publication, Morris et al. at The Children's Hospital of Philadelphia reported on 66 children placed on ECMO during CPR. The median duration of CPR prior to establishment of ECMO was 50 min, yet 35 % (23/66) of these children survived to hospital discharge. Children with heart disease were more likely to survive compared to children with other medical conditions [71]. Other data from The Children's Hospital of Philadelphia showed that ECMO can be lifesaving after stage 1 operation for single ventricle physiology, especially in infants with reversible conditions like acute shunt thrombosis and transient ventricular dysfunction [28].

Two recent large studies on E-CPR (Extracorporeal-CPR) from the Extracorporeal Life Support Organization (ELSO) database [72] and the American Heart Association's Get With The Guidelines-Resuscitation data [73] have supported the findings above and shown increased use of E-CPR in children. The ELSO study included 110 centers with 14 international centers between 1992 and 2005, 682 pediatric patients had E-CPR, of which 499 were cardiac, with a 38 % survival to hospital discharge. Patients with newborn respiratory disease and cardiac disease had higher survival rates compared to children with sepsis, pediatric respiratory disease and accidental injury. Complications associated with an increased risk of death included central nervous system (CNS) injury, renal injury, a pH <7.2, pulmonary hemorrhage, CPR on ECMO, gastrointestinal hemorrhage, and hyperbilirubinemia. In the AHA Get with the Guidelines-Resuscitation study of 199 E-CPR events over a 7-year period, there was a 43.7 % survival to hospital discharge, with cardiac patients more likely to survive compared to noncardiac patients. Ninety five percent of survivors had favorable neurologic outcomes on pediatric cerebral performance category scores at the time of hospital discharge. Renal insufficiency and metabolic and electrolyte abnormalities with acidosis and administration of sodium bicarbonate or tromethamine were associated with a worse outcome. Interestingly, 5 out of the 7 survivors who had CPR for more than 90 min prior to ECMO cannulation had a good neurologic outcome.

The use of extracorporeal cardiovascular support for cardiac arrest depends on the rapid availability of the resources, equipment, and personnel to establish mechanical circulatory support, most typically extracorporeal membrane oxygenation (ECMO). Current consensus statements from the AHA state that there is insufficient evidence for a time-based threshold within which E-CPR may be beneficial [3]. Centers with resources for E-CPR may consider its use for patients with other epidemiologic features known to be favorable (e.g., witnessed arrests, short CPR times).

4. Post-resuscitation Management

Following return of circulation (spontaneous or ECMO), post-resuscitation management commences. This phase deals with optimizing vital organ perfusion, preventing lethal arrhythmias in the immediate period, initiating potential protective therapies in a timely manner, preventing secondary injury to organs, and ultimately spans a time period lasting months to years with long-term rehabilitation treatment.

Recommendations for post-resuscitation care include close monitoring and support to avoid hyperthermia, hypotension, hypoglycemia, hyperglycemia, hypoxemia or hyperemia, and achieve normocarbia, and avoidance of seizures [74–76]. A goal-directed and meticulous approach is recommended. Increasing evidence is emerging on the deleterious effects of hyperoxia following cardiac arrest [77]; the new guidelines have addressed this by recommending titration of oxygen following return of spontaneous circulation (ROSC) to 94–98 % [3].

In addition, post-resuscitation care includes consideration of therapeutic hypothermia in comatose children following cardiac arrest, [78–81], but cannot be strongly recommended in light of limited data. This issue is being addressed by the ongoing NHLBI multicenter "Therapeutic Hypothermia After Pediatric Cardiac Arrest" (THAPCA) trial.

Outcomes and Long-Term Follow Up

Outcomes from pediatric cardiac arrest have improved significantly over the past 20 years. For example, survival to discharge from pediatric in-hospital cardiac arrest has increased from <10 % in the 1980s [82, 83] to >25 % in the twenty-first century. Survival for children with cardiac disease, cared for in dedicated cardiac intensive care units, is higher than in mixed pediatric intensive care units with survival to hospital discharge >40 % [14, 19, 84]. Specifically, there are higher rates of survival among post-operative cardiac patients compared to preoperative or nonsurgical patients [14, 19]. Of the pediatric patients who survive to hospital discharge, nearly three-quarters will have favorable neurological function defined by specific pediatric cerebral outcome measures and quality of life indicators [5, 14, 85, 86]. Factors that influence outcome from pediatric cardiac arrest include the preexisting condition of the child, the environment in which the arrest occurred, the initial rhythm detected, the duration of no-flow time, the quality of the life-supporting therapies provided during the resuscitation, and the quality of life-supporting therapies administered after resuscitation.

Not surprisingly, outcomes after pediatric out-of-hospital arrests are much worse than those after in-hospital arrests [7, 60, 87–95]. This may be due to the fact that there is a prolonged period of no flow in out-of-hospital arrests, where many of the pediatric cardiac arrests are not witnessed and only 30 % of children are provided with bystander CPR. As a result of these factors, less than 10 % of pediatric out-of-hospital cardiac arrests survive to hospital discharge, and among those who survive, severe neurological injury is common.

Survival outcomes after in-hospital cardiac arrest are higher in the pediatric population compared with adults; 27 % of children survive to hospital discharge compared with only 17 % of adults [5]. For both children and adults, outcomes are better after the arrhythmogenic arrests, ventricular fibrillation/ventricular tachycardia (VF/VT). Importantly, pediatric in-hospital arrests are less commonly caused by arrhythmias (10 % of pediatric arrests vs. 25 % of adult arrests), and approximately one-third of children and adults with these arrhythmogenic arrests survive to hospital discharge. Interestingly, the superior pediatric survival rate following in-hospital cardiac arrest reflects a substantially higher survival rate among children with asystole or pulseless electrical activity (PEA) compared with adults (24 % vs. 11 %). Further investigations have shown that the superior survival rate among children is mostly attributable to a much better survival rate among infants and preschool age children compared with older children [86]. Although speculative, the higher survival rates in children may be due to improved coronary and cerebral blood flow during CPR because of increased chest compliance in these younger arrest victims, with improved aortic diastolic pressure and venous return [67, 96]. In addition, survival of pediatric patients from an in-hospital cardiac arrest is more likely in hospitals staffed with dedicated pediatric physicians [97].

Future Developments

The future of CPR research includes titration of blood flow, oxygen and ventilation to optimize brain and heart function, assessment of long-term neurologic outcomes of survivors with increased attention to validated quality of life assessments, and development of evidence-based neuroprotective strategies. Enhancing the quality of CPR, especially in the neonatal population with development of feedback devices similar to those developed for older children and adults [39, 40], is another area that requires investigation. In the post-resuscitative care phase, further strategies to enhance neuroprotection are being studied including the "therapeutic hypothermia after cardiac arrest" (THAPCA) trial. In addition, with the increasing use of E-CPR, the use of neuroprotective strategies during ECMO is another area ripe for investigation.

References

1. Kouwenhoven WB, Jude JR, Knickerbocker GG (1960) Closed-chest cardiac massage. JAMA 173:1064–1067
2. Berg MD et al (2010) Part 13: pediatric basic life support: 2010 American Heart Association Guidelines for Cardiopulmonary Resuscitation and Emergency Cardiovascular Care. Circulation 122(18 Suppl 3): S862–S875
3. Kleinman ME et al (2010) Part 14: pediatric advanced life support: 2010 American Heart Association Guidelines for Cardiopulmonary Resuscitation and Emergency Cardiovascular Care. Circulation 122(18 Suppl 3):S876–S908
4. Young KD et al (2004) A prospective, population-based study of the epidemiology and outcome of out-of-hospital pediatric cardiopulmonary arrest. Pediatrics 114(1):157–164
5. Nadkarni VM et al (2006) First documented rhythm and clinical outcome from in-hospital cardiac arrest among children and adults. JAMA 295(1):50–57
6. Samson RA et al (2006) Outcomes of in-hospital ventricular fibrillation in children. N Engl J Med 354(22):2328–2339
7. Donoghue AJ et al (2005) Out-of-hospital pediatric cardiac arrest: an epidemiologic review and assessment of current knowledge. Ann Emerg Med 46(6):512–522

8. Dick WF et al (2000) The carotid pulse check revisited: what if there is no pulse? Crit Care Med 28(11 Suppl):N183–N185

9. Eberle B et al (1996) Checking the carotid pulse check: diagnostic accuracy of first responders in patients with and without a pulse. Resuscitation 33(2):107–116

10. Donoghue A et al (2009) Cardiopulmonary resuscitation for bradycardia with poor perfusion versus pulseless cardiac arrest. Pediatrics 124(6):1541–1548

11. Inagawa G et al (2003) A comparison of five techniques for detecting cardiac activity in infants. Paediatr Anaesth 13(2):141–146

12. Sarti A et al (2006) Comparison of three sites to check the pulse and count heart rate in hypotensive infants. Paediatr Anaesth 16(4):394–398

13. Tibballs J, Russell P (2009) Reliability of pulse palpation by healthcare personnel to diagnose paediatric cardiac arrest. Resuscitation 80(1):61–64

14. Parra DA et al (2000) Outcome of cardiopulmonary resuscitation in a pediatric cardiac intensive care unit. Crit Care Med 28(9):3296–3300

15. Bobrow BJ et al (2010) Chest compression-only CPR by lay rescuers and survival from out-of-hospital cardiac arrest. JAMA 304(13):1447–1454

16. Sharek PJ et al (2007) Effect of a rapid response team on hospital-wide mortality and code rates outside the ICU in a Children's Hospital. JAMA 298(19):2267–2274

17. Tibballs J, Kinney S (2009) Reduction of hospital mortality and of preventable cardiac arrest and death on introduction of a pediatric medical emergency team. Pediatr Crit Care Med 10(3):306–312

18. Brilli RJ et al (2007) Implementation of a medical emergency team in a large pediatric teaching hospital prevents respiratory and cardiopulmonary arrests outside the intensive care unit. Pediatr Crit Care Med 8(3):236–246, quiz 247

19. Peddy SB et al (2007) Cardiopulmonary resuscitation: special considerations for infants and children with cardiac disease. Cardiol Young 17(Suppl 2):116–126

20. Tabbutt S et al (2001) Impact of inspired gas mixtures on preoperative infants with hypoplastic left heart syndrome during controlled ventilation. Circulation 104(12 Suppl 1):I159–I164

21. Bradley SM, Simsic JM, Mulvihill DM (2003) Hypoventilation improves oxygenation after bidirectional superior cavopulmonary connection. J Thorac Cardiovasc Surg 126(4):1033–1039

22. Shekerdemian LS et al (1997) Cardiopulmonary interactions after Fontan operations: augmentation of cardiac output using negative pressure ventilation. Circulation 96(11):3934–3942

23. Hoffman GM et al (2004) Alteration of the critical arteriovenous oxygen saturation relationship by sustained afterload reduction after the Norwood procedure. J Thorac Cardiovasc Surg 127(3):738–745

24. Motta P et al (2005) Comparison of phenoxybenzamine to sodium nitroprusside in infants undergoing surgery. J Cardiothorac Vasc Anesth 19(1):54–59

25. Hoffman TM et al (2003) Efficacy and safety of milrinone in preventing low cardiac output syndrome in infants and children after corrective surgery for congenital heart disease. Circulation 107(7):996–1002

26. Johnson BA et al (2009) Near-infrared spectroscopy in neonates before palliation of hypoplastic left heart syndrome. Ann Thorac Surg 87(2):571–577, discussion 577–9

27. Hoffman GM et al (2005) Systemic venous oxygen saturation after the Norwood procedure and childhood neurodevelopmental outcome. J Thorac Cardiovasc Surg 130(4):1094–1100

28. Ravishankar C et al (2006) Extracorporeal membrane oxygenation after stage I reconstruction for hypoplastic left heart syndrome. Pediatr Crit Care Med 7(4):319–323

29. Booth KL et al (2004) Extracorporeal membrane oxygenation support of the Fontan and bidirectional Glenn circulations. Ann Thorac Surg 77(4):1341–1348

30. Berg RA et al (2001) Adverse hemodynamic effects of interrupting chest compressions for rescue breathing during cardiopulmonary resuscitation for ventricular fibrillation cardiac arrest. Circulation 104(20):2465–2470

31. Paradis NA et al (1990) Coronary perfusion pressure and the return of spontaneous circulation in human cardiopulmonary resuscitation. JAMA 263(8):1106–1113

32. Michael JR et al (1984) Mechanisms by which epinephrine augments cerebral and myocardial perfusion during cardiopulmonary resuscitation in dogs. Circulation 69(4):822–835

33. Halperin HR et al (1986) Determinants of blood flow to vital organs during cardiopulmonary resuscitation in dogs. Circulation 73(3):539–550

34. Schleien CL et al (1986) Effect of epinephrine on cerebral and myocardial perfusion in an infant animal preparation of cardiopulmonary resuscitation. Circulation 73(4):809–817

35. Idris AH et al (1994) Effect of ventilation on acid–base balance and oxygenation in low blood-flow states. Crit Care Med 22(11):1827–1834

36. McInnes AD et al (2011) The first quantitative report of ventilation rate during in-hospital resuscitation of older children and adolescents. Resuscitation 82(8):1025–1029

37. Aufderheide TP, Lurie KG (2004) Death by hyperventilation: a common and life-threatening problem during cardiopulmonary resuscitation. Crit Care Med 32(9 Suppl):S345–S351

38. Aufderheide TP et al (2004) Hyperventilation-induced hypotension during cardiopulmonary resuscitation. Circulation 109(16):1960–1965

39. Sutton RM et al (2009) Quantitative analysis of CPR quality during in-hospital resuscitation of older children and adolescents. Pediatrics 124(2):494–499

40. Abella BS et al (2005) Quality of cardiopulmonary resuscitation during in-hospital cardiac arrest. JAMA 293(3):305–310

41. Braga MS et al (2009) Estimation of optimal CPR chest compression depth in children by using computer tomography. Pediatrics 124(1):e69–e74

42. Kattwinkel J et al (2010) Part 15: neonatal resuscitation: 2010 American Heart Association Guidelines for Cardiopulmonary Resuscitation and Emergency Cardiovascular Care. Circulation 122(18 Suppl 3): S909–S919

43. Kleinman ME et al (2010) Part 10: pediatric basic and advanced life support: 2010 International Consensus on Cardiopulmonary Resuscitation and Emergency Cardiovascular Care Science With Treatment Recommendations. Circulation 122(16 Suppl 2): S466–S515

44. Menegazzi JJ et al (1993) Two-thumb versus two-finger chest compression during CRP in a swine infant model of cardiac arrest. Ann Emerg Med 22(2):240–243

45. Berg RA et al (1997) Assisted ventilation does not improve outcome in a porcine model of single-rescuer bystander cardiopulmonary resuscitation. Circulation 95(6):1635–1641

46. Voelckel WG et al (2000) Effects of vasopressin and epinephrine on splanchnic blood flow and renal function during and after cardiopulmonary resuscitation in pigs. Crit Care Med 28(4):1083–1088

47. Fleisher G et al (1985) Open- versus closed-chest cardiac compressions in a canine model of pediatric cardiopulmonary resuscitation. Am J Emerg Med 3(4):305–310

48. Boczar ME et al (1995) A technique revisited: hemodynamic comparison of closed- and open-chest cardiac massage during human cardiopulmonary resuscitation. Crit Care Med 23(3):498–503

49. Sanders AB et al (1984) Improved resuscitation from cardiac arrest with open-chest massage. Ann Emerg Med 13(9 Pt 1):672–675

50. Berg RA et al (2010) Part 5: adult basic life support: 2010 American Heart Association Guidelines for Cardiopulmonary Resuscitation and Emergency Cardiovascular Care. Circulation 122(18 Suppl 3): S685–S705

51. Kitamura T et al (2010) Conventional and chest-compression-only cardiopulmonary resuscitation by bystanders for children who have out-of-hospital cardiac arrests: a prospective, nationwide, population-based cohort study. Lancet 375(9723):1347–1354

52. Pokorna M et al (2010) A sudden increase in partial pressure end-tidal carbon dioxide (P(ET)CO(2)) at the moment of return of spontaneous circulation. J Emerg Med 38(5):614–621

53. Wik L et al (1996) Effects of various degrees of compression and active decompression on haemodynamics, end-tidal CO_2, and ventilation during cardiopulmonary resuscitation of pigs. Resuscitation 31(1):45–57

54. Dhillon R et al (1995) Extracorporeal membrane oxygenation and the treatment of critical pulmonary hypertension in congenital heart disease. Eur J Cardiothorac Surg 9(10):553–556

55. Perondi MBM et al (2004) A comparison of high-dose and standard-dose epinephrine in children with cardiac arrest. N Engl J Med 350(17):1722–1730

56. Srinivasan V et al (2008) Calcium use during in-hospital pediatric cardiopulmonary resuscitation: a report from the National Registry of Cardiopulmonary Resuscitation. Pediatrics 121(5):e1144–e1151

57. Larsen MP et al (1993) Predicting survival from out-of-hospital cardiac arrest: a graphic model. Ann Emerg Med 22(11):1652–1658

58. Gutgesell HP et al (1976) Energy dose for ventricular defibrillation of children. Pediatrics 58(6):898–901

59. Berg RA et al (2005) Better outcome after pediatric defibrillation dosage than adult dosage in a swine model of pediatric ventricular fibrillation. J Am Coll Cardiol 45(5):786–789

60. Berg MD et al (2005) Pediatric defibrillation doses often fail to terminate prolonged out-of-hospital ventricular fibrillation in children. Resuscitation 67(1):63–67

61. Meaney PA et al (2011) Effect of defibrillation energy dose during in-hospital pediatric cardiac arrest. Pediatrics 127(1):e16–e23

62. Bar-Cohen Y et al (2005) First appropriate use of automated external defibrillator in an infant. Resuscitation 67(1):135–137

63. Walsh CK, Krongrad E (1983) Terminal cardiac electrical activity in pediatric patients. Am J Cardiol 51(3):557–561

64. DeBehnke DJ et al (1995) The hemodynamic and arterial blood gas response to asphyxiation: a canine model of pulseless electrical activity. Resuscitation 30(2):169–175

65. Kramer-Johansen J et al (2006) Quality of out-of-hospital cardiopulmonary resuscitation with real time automated feedback: a prospective interventional study. Resuscitation 71(3):283–292

66. Berg RA et al (1996) Ventricular fibrillation in a swine model of acute pediatric asphyxial cardiac arrest. Resuscitation 33(2):147–153

67. Donoghue AJ et al (2006) Effect of hospital characteristics on outcomes from pediatric cardiopulmonary resuscitation: a report from the national registry of cardiopulmonary resuscitation. Pediatrics 118(3):995–1001

68. del Nido PJ et al (1992) Extracorporeal membrane oxygenator rescue in children during cardiac arrest after cardiac surgery. Circulation 86(5 Suppl):II300–II304

69. Duncan BW et al (1998) Use of rapid-deployment extracorporeal membrane oxygenation for the resuscitation of pediatric patients with heart disease after cardiac arrest. J Thorac Cardiovasc Surg 116(2):305–311

70. Alsoufi B et al (2007) Survival outcomes after rescue extracorporeal cardiopulmonary resuscitation in

pediatric patients with refractory cardiac arrest. J Thorac Cardiovasc Surg 134(4):952–959.e2

71. Morris MC, Wernovsky G, Nadkarni VM (2004) Survival outcomes after extracorporeal cardiopulmonary resuscitation instituted during active chest compressions following refractory in-hospital pediatric cardiac arrest. Pediatr Crit Care Med 5(5):440–446

72. Thiagarajan RR et al (2007) Extracorporeal membrane oxygenation to aid cardiopulmonary resuscitation in infants and children. Circulation 116(15):1693–1700

73. Raymond TT et al (2010) Outcomes among neonates, infants, and children after extracorporeal cardiopulmonary resuscitation for refractory inhospital pediatric cardiac arrest: a report from the National Registry of Cardiopulmonary Resuscitation. Pediatr Crit Care Med 11(3):362–371

74. Wright WL, Geocadin RG (2006) Postresuscitative intensive care: neuroprotective strategies after cardiac arrest. Semin Neurol 26(4):396–402

75. Popp E, Bottiger BW (2006) Cerebral resuscitation: state of the art, experimental approaches and clinical perspectives. Neurol Clin 24(1):73–87, vi

76. Sunde K et al (2007) Implementation of a standardised treatment protocol for post resuscitation care after out-of-hospital cardiac arrest. Resuscitation 73(1):29–39

77. Kilgannon JH et al (2010) Association between arterial hyperoxia following resuscitation from cardiac arrest and in-hospital mortality. JAMA 303(21):2165–2171

78. Bernard SA et al (2002) Treatment of comatose survivors of out-of-hospital cardiac arrest with induced hypothermia. N Engl J Med 346(8):557–563

79. Hypothermia after Cardiac Arrest Study Group (2002) Mild therapeutic hypothermia to improve the neurologic outcome after cardiac arrest. N Engl J Med 346(8):549–556

80. Fink EL et al (2010) A tertiary care center's experience with therapeutic hypothermia after pediatric cardiac arrest. Pediatr Crit Care Med 11(1):66–74

81. Doherty DR et al (2009) Hypothermia therapy after pediatric cardiac arrest. Circulation 119(11):1492–1500

82. Zaritsky A et al (1987) CPR in children. Ann Emerg Med 16(10):1107–1111

83. Nichols DG et al (1986) Factors influencing outcome of cardiopulmonary resuscitation in children. Pediatr Emerg Care 2(1):1–5

84. Rhodes JF et al (1999) Cardiac arrest in infants after congenital heart surgery. Circulation 100(19 Suppl): II194–II199

85. Reis AG et al (2002) A prospective investigation into the epidemiology of in-hospital pediatric cardiopulmonary resuscitation using the international Utstein reporting style. Pediatrics 109(2):200–209

86. Meaney PA et al (2006) Higher survival rates among younger patients after pediatric intensive care unit cardiac arrests. Pediatrics 118(6):2424–2433

87. Young KD, Seidel JS (1999) Pediatric cardiopulmonary resuscitation: a collective review. Ann Emerg Med 33(2):195–205

88. Kuisma M, Suominen P, Korpela R (1995) Paediatric out-of-hospital cardiac arrests–epidemiology and outcome. Resuscitation 30(2):141–150

89. Suominen P et al (1997) Paediatric cardiac arrest and resuscitation provided by physician-staffed emergency care units. Acta Anaesthesiol Scand 41(2):260–265

90. Sirbaugh PE et al (1999) A prospective, population-based study of the demographics, epidemiology, management, and outcome of out-of-hospital pediatric cardiopulmonary arrest. Ann Emerg Med 33(2):174–184

91. Schindler MB et al (1996) Outcome of out-of-hospital cardiac or respiratory arrest in children. N Engl J Med 335(20):1473–1479

92. Dieckmann RA, Vardis R (1995) High-dose epinephrine in pediatric out-of-hospital cardiopulmonary arrest. Pediatrics 95(6):901–913

93. Gerein RB et al (2006) What are the etiology and epidemiology of out-of-hospital pediatric cardiopulmonary arrest in Ontario, Canada? Acad Emerg Med 13(6):653–658

94. Tunstall-Pedoe H et al (1992) Survey of 3765 cardiopulmonary resuscitations in British hospitals (the BRESUS Study): methods and overall results. BMJ 304(6838):1347–1351

95. Lopez-Herce J et al (2005) Outcome of out-of-hospital cardiorespiratory arrest in children. Pediatr Emerg Care 21(12):807–815

96. Dean JM et al (1987) Age-related changes in chest geometry during cardiopulmonary resuscitation. J Appl Physiol (Bethesda, Md: 1985) 62(6):2212–22129

97. Chaplik S, Neafsey PJ (1998) Pre-existing variables and outcome of cardiac arrest resuscitation in hospitalized patients. Dimens Crit Care Nurs 17(4):200–207

Section XIII

Nursing Issues Related to the Cardiac Patient

Patricia Lincoln and Sandra Staveski

Introduction to Nursing Issues

73

Sandra Staveski and Patricia Lincoln

Keywords

Acquired heart disease • Admission • Adult • APN role • Cardiac catheterization • Cardiac rehab • Chronically, critically ill • ECLS • Heart transplantation • Newborn • Postoperative care systems

The practice of nursing encompasses various aspects of physiology, psychology, and the caring arts in order to prevent illness and promote healing of patients and their families. Nurses bear witness to their patients' and parents' or caregivers' journey in the healthcare system, by being present with them for extended periods of time. Nursing ill children in the pediatric cardiovascular intensive care unit (PCICU) and cardiology ward is a complex, multifaceted role and an intricate and, at times, intimate social interaction. Throughout hospital stay, nurses stand vigilant to protect their patients from harm and simultaneously create healing environments for them and their families.

Children with heart disease have a lifelong illness and demanding, complex care needs. Nurses provide patients and families a safety net through very challenging times in their lives. Family centered care is a philosophy and a framework adopted by pediatric cardiology nurses as they assume the responsibility and the goal to care for children with heart disease in ways that attend to their physical health while at the same time supporting and promoting healthy emotional and psychological development that occurs in the context of the family [1]. Nurses are the gatekeepers to providing holistic, interdisciplinary care and help children and their families navigate through healthcare systems. The nurse-patient and nurse-parent relationship are best articulated by the concept of mutuality and the percepts of family centered care. Mutuality as defined by Curley (1997) is a "...synchronous, coconstituting relationship that stimulates human becoming" [2].

S. Staveski (✉)
Pediatric Cardiovascular Intensive Care Unit, Lucile Packard Children's Hospital at Stanford, Palo Alto, CA, USA
e-mail: sstaveski@lpch.org

P. Lincoln
Clinical Nurse Specialist, Cardiac Intensive Care Unit, Boston Children's Hospital, Boston, MA, USA
e-mail: Patricia.Lincoln@childrens.harvard.edu

E.M. da Cruz et al. (eds.), *Pediatric and Congenital Cardiology, Cardiac Surgery and Intensive Care*,
DOI 10.1007/978-1-4471-4619-3_198, © Springer-Verlag London 2014

This section has brought together nursing experts from around the globe to assist pediatric cardiac nurses worldwide as they put their patients and families in the best place to heal and to return to their lives outside of the hospital.

References

1. Curley MAQ (1997) Mutuality: an expression of nursing presence. J Pediatr Nurs 12(4):208–213
2. Harrison TM (2010) Family centered pediatric nursing care: state of the science. J Pediatr Nurs 25(5):335–343

Congential Cardiac Patients – Fetus to Adult: Nursing Considerations

74

Patricia Lincoln, Megan Cusick, John Fantegrossi, Lindsey Katzmark, Terra Lafranchi, Christine Peyton, and Mary Rummell

Abstract

Pediatric nursing, involving care of the patient with congenital heart disease, spans the entire age continuum from birth to adults. This chapter will describe preoperative care of the newborn and nursing care of the adult included in this population. Also discussed will be same-day surgery admission practices for all patients with congenital heart disease and the

P. Lincoln (✉)
Clinical Nurse Specialist, Cardiac Intensive Care Unit,
Boston Children's Hospital, Boston, MA, USA
e-mail: patricia.lincoln@childrens.harvard.edu

M. Cusick • J. Fantegrossi
Nurse Practitioner, Cardiology Pre Procedure Suite,
Boston Children's Hospital, Boston, MA, USA
e-mail: meghan.cusick@cardio.chboston.org;
john.fantegrossi@cardio.chboston.org

L. Katzmark
Nurse Practitioner, Adult Congenital Heart Disease
Progam, Children's Hospital of Wisconsin, Medical
College of Wisconsin, Wauwatosa, WI, USA
e-mail: lkatzmark@chw.org

T. Lafranchi
Fetal Cardiology Coordinator, Nurse Practitioner,
Advanced Fetal Care Center, Boston Children's Hospital,
Boston, MA, USA
e-mail: terra.lafranchi@cardio.chboston.org

C. Peyton
Cardiac Intensive Care Unit, Clinical Nurse Specialist,
Children's Hospital Colorado, Aurora, CO, USA
e-mail: christine.peyton@childrenscolorado.org

M. Rummell
Clinical Nurse Specialist, Pediatric Cardiology,
Doernbecher Children's Hospital, Oregon Health &
Science University, Portland, OR, USA
e-mail: rummellm@ohsu.edu

education and counseling involved when caring for the family with a prenatal diagnosis of congenital heart disease.

Keywords

Adult comorbidities • Adult with CHD • Coordination of care • Lifelong care • Newborn with congenital heart disease • Patient/family education • Preductal/postductal oxygen saturations • Prenatal diagnosis • Prostaglandin E_1 infusion • Same-day admission for cardiac surgery

Introduction

Pediatric nursing, involving care of the patient with congenital heart disease (CHD), spans the entire age continuum from birth to adults. This chapter will describe preoperative care of the newborn and nursing care of the adult with congenital heart disease. Also discussed will be same-day surgery admission practices for all patients with CHD and the education and counseling involved when caring for the family with a prenatal diagnosis of CHD.

Preoperative Care of the Newborn with Congenital Heart Disease

CHD accounts for 3 % of all infant deaths regardless of the advances in fetal ultrasound technology and early diagnosis in utero [1]. A review of the literature demonstrates that CHD is 90 % multifactorial with 8 % related to chromosomal/genetic factors and 2 % to environmental teratogens [2]. The preoperative stabilization of the critically ill newborn as well as prompt neonatal resuscitation is essential for improving outcomes and survival rates for this population. Survival and quality of life have improved over the past decade for infants born with complex congenital heart disease due to advances in echocardiography, interventional catheterization, and increased knowledge of newborn physiology [2].

Central cyanosis may be the first clinical presentation for a neonate with parallel circulations, such as complete transposition of the great arteries (complete TGA) or a defect resulting in decreased pulmonary blood flow such as pulmonary atresia (PA) or tricuspid atresia (TA). A bluish discoloration of the tongue and mucous membranes is indicative of central cyanosis. Cyanosis is dependent on anemia, polycythemia, and 2,3 diphosphoglycerate levels; hence, it may take up to a week to present in the newborn. Peripheral cyanosis is a normal finding in the postnatal period due to the result of slow blood flow through the extremities.

Congestive heart failure (CHF), occurring in the first month of life, may present in complete TGA, coarctation of the aorta (CoA), and critical aortic stenosis (AS) or pulmonary stenosis (PS). Three hallmark signs of congestive heart failure include tachycardia, tachypnea at rest, and hepatomegaly. Peripheral pulses are weak and may be accompanied by pale/dusky coloring and decreased urine output. Coarse breath sounds are heard on auscultation due to pulmonary edema. Truncus arteriosus usually presents with CHF, however; a widened pulse pressure and bounding pulses are also present due to increased pulmonary blood flow and decreased pulmonary vascular resistance. Neonates with CHF have difficulty feeding and usually become diaphoretic with feeds due to the energy expenditure.

Neonates with cardiac defects that involve obstruction to systemic blood flow, such as hypoplastic left heart syndrome (HLHS), interrupted aortic arch (IAA), or CoA, may present in cardiogenic shock. These defects are associated with underdevelopment of the left-sided heart structures or a narrowing in the ascending or transverse aortic arch [3]. Signs of shock present once the ductus arteriosus, which in these defects permits blood to flow from the pulmonary to the systemic circulation, has closed. Usually this occurs within the first week of life. Peripheral pulses are decreased or absent, with tachypnea, prolonged capillary refill, and possibly acidosis and rapidly decreasing arterial saturations. The neonate is pale, mottled, and cool to touch. Aggressive medical management and resuscitation is crucial for the stabilization. The newborn should have blood, urine, and respiratory cultures drawn to include septic shock as part of the differential diagnosis. Electrolytes, liver function tests, and the presence of metabolic acidosis require evaluation. Blood glucose and electrolytes are monitored as severe hypoglycemia may present as shock symptoms. Supraventricular tachycardia is also a common cause of shock state presentation in the neonate. An electrocardiogram is done to ensure sinus rhythm.

Weight, length, head circumference, and abdominal girth are measured as part of the admission vital sign parameters. These are important for medication calculations, possible ventilation parameters, and growth patterns. Initial heart rate, respiratory rate, blood pressure, temperature, and oxygen saturations are obtained to establish a patient baseline for stability. Physical exam includes inspection of the skin and mucous membranes for central and peripheral cyanosis. A hyperoxia test is performed to determine if there is a respiratory rather than cardiac cause for the cyanosis. Blood gas determination of partial pressure of oxygen (PaO_2) and partial pressure of carbon dioxide ($PaCO_2$) in the blood are compared on room air and then with the addition of 100 % fractional inspired oxygen (FiO_2). If the infant has a fixed intracardiac right-to-left shunt, the addition of oxygen will result in only a small increase of oxygenation [4]. Palpation and assessment of peripheral and central pulses are done to determine if aortic arch abnormalities are present. Bounding pulses may imply aortic arch runoff, as blood takes the path of least resistance and flows through the ductus arteriosus [4]. Four-extremity blood pressures are also obtained. This is an important parameter to monitor as aortic arch abnormalities are

suspected when systolic blood pressure in the upper extremities is 20 mmHg greater than in the lower extremities [2]. Preductal and postductal arterial saturations are monitored in the critically ill newborn to assure blood flow through the ductus arteriosus. This measurement provides crucial data as PaO_2 directly correlates with oxygen saturation level. Oxygen saturations measured before the level of the ductus arteriosus are considered preductal [4]. The right arm, which is perfused by the right subclavian artery, is the usual preductal site. The postductal saturation is obtained with measurement of the oxygen saturation in the left arm or either lower extremity as the vessels in these extremities are arise at the level of, or distal to, the ductus arteriosus [4]. Auscultation of heart sounds may indicate the presence of a murmur. Murmurs are difficult to differentiate in the newborn period and may not be heard, even when present. Systolic ejection murmurs are heard in aortic stenosis or pulmonary stenosis, tetralogy of Fallot (TOF), and total anomalous pulmonary venous return (TAPVR). Diastolic murmurs are heard with increased pulmonary blood flow over the mitral and tricuspid valves. Panoyotolic murmurs are associated with defects that include a ventricular septal defect (VSD), for example, complete TGA or TOF. A continuous murmur is present with a patent ductus arteriosus (PDA) and is helpful in determining the effectiveness of prostaglandin E_1 (PGE_1) in maintaining an open ductus arteriosus for ductal-dependent lesions. A chest radiograph (CXR) is obtained to evaluate heart size and lung fields. Neonates with complex congenital heart disease are evaluated for arrhythmias with cardiac monitoring and a 12-lead electrocardiogram (ECG). An echocardiogram is done to provide definite imaging and assist with diagnosis. Magnetic resonance imaging (MRI) is utilized for improved viewing of aortic arch abnormalities. A diagnostic cardiac catheterization is useful in assessing pulmonary artery pressures and pulmonary vascular resistance or coronary artery malformations or fistulas. Adequate kidney perfusion is best determined by urine output equal or greater than 1 ml/kg/h. Blood urea nitrogen and creatinine are monitored daily to assess kidney function. Since chromosomal abnormalities may be associated with complex CHD, genetic studies should be considered in infants with dysmorphic features. The most common chromosomal abnormalities associated with CHD are trisomy 21 (Down syndrome), trisomy 13, Turner syndrome, DiGeorge syndrome (22q11 deletion), Williams syndrome, and Noonan syndrome [2, 5]. A baseline head ultrasound and/or computerized tomography (CT) scan may be recommended for neonates at risk to determine the presence of an intraventricular hemorrhage.

Many variables are associated with survival of the newborn with complex congenital heart disease. The following risk factors are related to improved survival and decreased surgical complications: age, weight, the presence of extra cardiac anomalies, the type of congenital heart defect, and length of stay (LOS) in the hospital. Neonates weighing less than 2.0 kg have been found to have increased mortality after surgical repair [6–8]. As age and weight increase in the neonatal period, complications and mortality decrease [9]. The presence of extracardiac anomalies (i.e., tracheoesophageal fistula, diaphragmatic hernia, or asplenia) may increase morbidity and mortality following a cardiac surgical repair. Cardiac defects that involve multiple lesions may also have affected the surgical outcomes. As the number of other diagnoses increase, the probability of complications and death increase [9]. Also, shorter hospital length of stay (LOS) for the neonate, or any patient, results in decreased exposure to and possible development of hospital-acquired infections.

Evaluation of end-organ function is made with arterial blood gas and electrolyte, liver, and renal function tests results that are within normal range. These indicate successful medical management and/or resuscitation of the critically ill newborn in the preoperative period. Infection control practices including hand washing, screening for methicillin-resistant Staphylococcus aureus (MRSA), and proper care and maintenance of central lines are essential in preventing postoperative infection. Prevention of surgical wound infection is optimized with antibiotic prophylaxis intraoperatively and utilization of a chlorhexidine scrub prior to surgery.

Neonates presenting in a collapsed state with shock, cyanosis, or congestive heart failure require urgent pediatric advanced life support [10]. If a ductal-dependent cardiac lesion is suspected, the priority is to establish and maintain an open ductus arteriosus using a PGE_1 infusion. Airway and breathing is supported as needed. Access to circulation is obtained [10], commonly via peripheral or umbilical catheterization, though an intraosseous insertion may be required for an infant in shock. Cardiac output and tissue perfusion are supported with fluids and inotropes. A pediatric cardiologist is consulted for management [11, 12] and a plan for obtaining a definitive diagnosis [10]. Once the infant is resuscitated and stabilized, transfer to the pediatric cardiac intensive care unit (PCICU) within the hospital or transportation to an institution that has expertise in CHD is organized.

The correct amount of oxygen to administer may be difficult to determine in critically ill infants, especially if the diagnosis is not yet known. While excessive oxygen is known to be harmful, critically ill infants with low blood oxygen saturation via pulse oximetry (SpO_2) may require high FiO_2 for adequate tissue oxygenation [13]. If an infant presents in a critical state with an unknown diagnosis, 100 % oxygen is used for resuscitation [13]. Once the infant is resuscitated, FiO_2 is reduced to maintain a SpO_2 in the appropriate target range for the suspected condition. Many infants are diagnosed antenatally, and having that information allows for a more targeted approach to oxygen delivery. For infants with non-cyanotic lesions, a SpO_2 of 94–98 % is adequate. For infants with single ventricle physiology such as TA, PA, or HLHS, the aim is a SpO_2 of 80–85 % [10, 14]. Oxygen is a potent pulmonary vasodilator. Excessive oxygenation will result in pulmonary over circulation at the expense of the systemic circulation. This may result in poor tissue perfusion and symptoms such as metabolic acidosis and poor urine output [14]. Excessive oxygen may cause an elevated PaO_2 which may risk stimulating closure of the needed PDA [15]. Intubation and ventilation may be indicated in some neonates to support cardiac function and relieve severe respiratory distress or apnea [16]. Intubation should be performed by a skilled operator as neonates with CHD have limited reserve and may not tolerate bradycardia or hypoxia induced by unsuccessful intubation attempts [10]. In some CHD, pulmonary vascular resistance (PVR) is elevated. Adequate ventilation and oxygenation may assist in overcoming elevated PVR. However, in neonates with HLHS, ventilation strategies may be used to manipulate PVR and decrease pulmonary blood flow, limiting blood flow to the lungs and increasing blood flow to the systemic circulation, by deliberately increasing PVR [16]. Inhaled nitric oxide (iNO) administration may be used in an effort to reduce pulmonary vascular resistance in some neonates, to increase pulmonary blood flow.

PGE$_1$ is used to maintain a patent ductus arteriosus in infants with ductal-dependent circulation until surgery is performed [14]. PGE$_1$ relaxes the smooth muscle in the ductus arteriosus [17] so blood continues to flow through the vessel. Indications for use include diagnosis of obstruction to pulmonary blood flow lesions, such as PA and TA. In these lesions, bloods flows through the ductus arteriosus from the aorta to the pulmonary arteries providing pulmonary blood flow. With obstruction to systemic blood flow defects, such as HLHS, CoA or IAA, an open ductus arteriosus permits blood flow from the pulmonary artery to the aorta providing systemic blood flow. The use of PGE$_1$ may upset pulmonary/systemic blood flow balance in the neonate with certain defects, such as some forms of TAPVR [1, 6]. PGE$_1$ is most effective if commenced within 96 h of birth, before the ductus begins to close. However, this medication should always be initiated in the setting of low PaO2 (<40 mmHg) [17]. It has a short half-life, 5–10 min, and must be administered as a continuous infusion. The infusion dose may initially be as high as 0.5–1 mcg/kg/min and then reduced to 0.0125–0.2 mcg/kg/min [10, 18]. Side effects of PGE$_1$ infusion include fever, hypotension, and apnea episodes [6]. These are dose related and more likely to occur with higher doses. Some neonates may require respiratory support such as continuous positive airway pressure (CPAP) or mechanical ventilation due to frequent apnea. Nursing considerations for the patients receiving PGE$_1$ infusions include maintaining continuous infusion and observation for effectiveness and side effects [19]. Even brief interruptions to the infusion may result in ductal closure and patient deterioration, due to the short half-life of PGE$_1$. Infants receiving a PGE$_1$ infusion must have their intravenous (IV) access closely observed for signs of extravasation and should have an additional IV access in place when possible. Effectiveness of the PGE$_1$ infusion is observed through close monitoring of heart rate, respiratory rate and pattern, and improvement in pre- and postductal SpO$_2$ [11]. The presence of side effects is also monitored, and since fever may also indicate sepsis, a septic workup should be performed if that occurs. Enteral feeding while receiving PGE$_1$ is controversial due to concerns regarding the possibility of necrotizing enterocolitis [20].

Adequate cardiac output in the preoperative newborn is important to ensure organ perfusion and prevent the development of metabolic acidosis. This involves both effective cardiac output and the balance of sufficient blood flow to both pulmonary and systemic circulations. Perfusion and circulation is assessed by examining heart rate, pulse volume, capillary refill times, peripheral warmth, urine output, and laboratory blood results, including blood gas values, mixed venous saturation, and lactate levels. Inadequate cardiac output is treated initially with a volume administration, followed by reassessment and further fluid boluses if required [12]. If sepsis is present, additional fluid administration may be needed due to capillary leak. Inotropes, such as dopamine or dobutamine [10, 16], are started in response to hypotension. If cardiac output remains inadequate, or if the heart rate is low, starting an adrenaline infusion is considered [10]. It is important to balance flow to both the pulmonary and systemic circulations. Manipulation of vascular resistance using vasodilators may be required to ensure adequate systemic circulation and reduce pulmonary overcirculation [16]. Severe metabolic acidosis is treated with sodium bicarbonate administration [12]. Hypoglycemia and hypocalcaemia are corrected. Calcium is important in the neonatal heart for effective contractility [10]. Fever is avoided as it will increase oxygen consumption and cardiac workload [10]. Diuretics may be needed to treat the development of congestive heart failure. Early surgery is the only effective treatment in a few conditions such as obstructed TAPVR or HLHS with an intact or restrictive atrial septum [19]. If, despite maximal treatment, cardiac output remains inadequate, the infant may require extracorporeal life support (ECLS) or transfer to center where ECLS available.

A balloon atrioseptostomy is a catheter procedure which enlarges the patent foramen ovale (PFO) to allow the mixing of blood to occur between the right and left atria [19]. This procedure is used in conditions such as HLHS with a restrictive atrial septum [14, 16] and complete TGA with restrictive VSD or intact ventricular septum [14]. A deflated balloon is placed into the heart via a catheter inserted through an umbilical or femoral vein. Once in the left atrium, the balloon is inflated and pulled across the PFO thereby enlarging it. Following the procedure there should be improved pre- and postductal SaO_2, as there is now increased mixing of oxygenated and non-oxygenated blood. Post-procedure, the catheter insertion site is observed for signs of bleeding, infection, or pain, and lower limbs are assessed for peripheral perfusion including pulses, warmth, and capillary refill [19]. This procedure may be done in the cardiac catheterization laboratory or in the PCICU at the bedside.

Infants with congenital heart disease have an increased risk of necrotizing enterocolitis (NEC) compared to the general population [21, 22]. NEC is a serious complication and has higher morbidity and mortality in infants with congenital heart disease (CHD) than infants without [21]. Infants with HLHS have the highest incidence of NEC [22]. This may be due to diastolic hypotension and poor end-organ perfusion leading to mesenteric ischemia [16, 21, 22]. PGE_1, particularly in high doses, has been associated with NEC [22], but its true role in this process is unclear. As a result, some institutions may choose to avoid

enteral feedings of newborns receiving PGE_1 until after surgery [20]. These infants may require parenteral nutrition [10]. All preoperative newborns with CHD are observed for signs and symptoms of NEC including abdominal distention, reddened or discolored umbilical area, blood in stool, and bilious aspirate.

Newborns with cardiac conditions are especially fragile. Minimal stimulation is important; however, this may be difficult due to the need for diagnostic echocardiograms, laboratory blood work, ultrasounds, etc. Unnecessary handling should be avoided and neonates observed for tolerance of scheduled procedures. Signs of activity intolerance include hypotension and hypoxia. Also, it is common for infants with CHD to experience growth and feeding issues [23]. Nutritional status and enteral feeding in the preoperative period should be considered for all neonates especially those weighing less than 2.5 kg. Daily caloric and protein needs are calculated and nutrition optimized with enteral and parental nutrition. A dietician may be consulted to assist with nutritional needs for the critically ill newborn along with occupational therapy for the determination of oral feeding readiness.

The nurse will need to recognize the concerns of the family and provide support and encouragement at the time of CHD diagnosis. Nurses guide parents in navigating the healthcare system by providing education on the complex heart defect with the utilization of videos, reputable Internet sites, books, and written information [24]. New mothers need assessment for postpartum depression which may impact their coping mechanisms. Both parents may experience anxiety due to the loss of a healthy newborn. Interdisciplinary members of the healthcare team such as social workers, physicians, surgeons, and psychologists are introduced to parents [24]. A lactation consultant is a valuable resource for the nursing mother who is pumping in preparation for preoperative or postoperative feeding of her newborn. Parental participation is encouraged by including the parents in their baby's daily care and inviting them to participate in medical rounds with the healthcare team. These opportunities will promote bonding and development of parental/newborn attachment. Parents need ample opportunities to ask questions. The nurse answers the questions and validates the concerns of the parents. Anticipatory guidance may be provided by offering a preoperative tour to prepare parents for the postoperative period when their newborn requires more equipment and mechanical support. Many families are overwhelmed with the initial diagnosis of complex CHD as well as the initial stabilization of their critically ill newborn [4]. Nursing must provide emotional support and an ongoing assessment of parental responses.

Care of the Adult with Congenital Heart Disease

With 85 % of infants with congenital heart disease surviving to adulthood are now more adults than children with CHD [25, 26]. Estimates of numbers of adults with congenital heart disease (ACHD) vary but may be as high as 1.8 million adults, three times as many adults as children [27–30]. This increase is the result of improved treatment with surgical survival rate >90 % in most centers. Of these adults, 80,000 are projected to have severe disease [27, 28]. In addition to the survivors of childhood interventions, another 10 % of congenital defects are not discovered until the patient is an adult. Adults may also have defects that were originally diagnosed as not needing intervention or deemed inoperable because of their complexity [31].

The adult patient presents unique and challenging problems for continuing management. Treatment options, both medical and surgical, have evolved since the first intracardiac repair in 1952 [31]. Many historical interventions are no longer performed; however, those adult patients having undergone these procedures present current clinicians with significant problems such as arrhythmias, including sudden death, pulmonary hypertension, altered hemodynamic cardiac function, and complex multiple organ system pathology [32, 33]. In addition to their congenital heart disease symptomatology, the ACHD patient may present with other high-risk comorbidities. These include coronary artery disease, conditions exacerbated by cigarette smoking, obesity, diabetes mellitus, hypercholesterolemia, and hypertension. These comorbidities contribute to chronic lung disease, renal insufficiency, hepatic insufficiency, endocrinopathies, and bleeding/clotting disorders. Other conditions may also exist, such as scoliosis or kyphosis, or genetic syndromes [31, 34].

The ACHD patient requires lifelong surveillance and monitoring. Many who have had childhood interventions experience gaps in their ongoing care [35, 36]. These gaps may result from (1) an understanding that they were "cured" and/or did not need follow-up, (2) lack of transfer to an adult provider, (3) lack of insurance, or (4) fear of hearing bad news [35]. Also there are limits to the number of centers with services for adults with CHD and cardiologists trained in the care of the ACHD patient [37]. Patients who have had a lapse in care seek medical care only when significant symptoms related to advanced heart failure and other comorbidities occur. Management of these problems usually requires hospitalization and urgent intervention [26, 35, 37]. When hospitalized, the ACHD patient presents with complex anatomy, significant multiple organ pathology, and psychosocial issues related to chronic illness [37, 38]. Transition of care from parent to patient in the chronically ill is often difficult. Ideally this transition should start around 12 years of age with the goal that the young adult will assume the responsibility of his/her healthcare management. This is an extended and multifaceted educational process that may be delayed for many reasons [36]. It may be difficult for the parent to relinquish control of care, especially for those who recognize that their attention and dedication to the healthcare of their child is responsible for the positive outcomes. Also the young adult may prefer that their parent continues in the care managing role. These ACHD patients must be supported in making decisions and assuming responsibility for their own care [36, 37, 39]. The complex psychosocial issues with conflict and investment in the role of care manager directly affect the nurse-patient interaction. Additional anxiety may be experienced due to an unfamiliar hospital environment or care providers [40].

Ideally, an interdisciplinary team with expertise in congenital heart disease directs ACHD patient care. Included in the interdisciplinary team is a congenital heart surgeon who is available to perform any necessary surgery. Studies have compared surgical results and have found that mortality in complex lesions, as well as less complicated lesions such as VSD, is significantly less in centers with expertise in CHD [31, 41, 42]. Still, as many as 24 % of ACHD patients experience severe postoperative complications, including arrhythmias, renal failure, stroke, and multisystem failure. The rate of complications, even mortality, is even higher in those with cyanosis and/or very complex disease [27, 43].

The nurse familiar with the pre- and postoperative care of infants and children with CHD will be challenged with the pathophysiology and comorbidities of the ACHD patient. These challenges include understanding the anatomy of the primary defect and previous surgical interventions, the hemodynamic implications of the defect, and chronic problems associated with the pathophysiology of the defect. Additional psychosocial issues of patients are chromosomal abnormalities and chronic disease from childhood.

The ACHD patient with single ventricle physiology has a complex congenital heart disorder. Each variation and surgical approach has altered the patient's hemodynamics and blood flow through the heart and lungs. Intervention includes several operative procedures involving repeated sternotomies. Mortality risk increases to as high as 8 % after four sternotomies [31, 44]. Multiple surgical and catheterization procedures also impact vascular access, especially in the neck and groin. These patients are at significant risk of atrial arrhythmias, compromised lung function, pulmonary and systemic thromboemboli, decreased renal and hepatic function, coagulopathies, progressive cyanosis, residual shunts, conduit failure, peripheral edema, and ascites and chronic diarrhea with protein-losing enteropathy. Cyanotic patients are at risk for the

development of arterio-pulmonary collateral vessels that may compromise cerebral, renal, and mesenteric perfusion [31]. Preoperative assessment of pulmonary, renal, hepatic, and cardiac function is imperative to successful outcomes [31, 32]. Patients must be risk stratified considering the presence of cyanosis, pulmonary vascular disease, cardiac failure, or history of arrhythmia. Patients with hypoxemia have increased blood viscosity and potential iron deficiency and must be adequately hydrated to decrease effects of polycythemia [45]. In patients with decreased pulmonary blood flow, hypoxemia may be avoided with hydration, adequate systemic arterial pressure, avoiding increases in pulmonary vascular resistance and use of measures to reduce oxygen consumption [45].

Adults with infant/childhood repair of TOF usually require either surgical or interventional catheter replacement of their pulmonary valve. With the goal of normal right ventricular size and function, optimal timing for replacement of the pulmonary valve is still under discussion [31]. The Food and Drug Administration (FDA) has approved the use of a Medtronic Melody percutaneous valve for right ventricular outflow tract dysfunction under specific conditions [46]. Midterm results are good with 80–90 % freedom from intervention after 2 years [47]. The patient with TOF may have many surgical interventions throughout their lifetime; pathologies of the right ventricular outflow tract are the most frequent reoperations [48]. The most common long-term complications related to TOF include atrial and ventricular arrhythmias as well as right ventricular dysfunction. Patients may require antiarrhythmic therapy. Some patients undergo a surgical MAZE procedure for treatment of atrial arrhythmias and must be monitored post-procedure for complications, specifically heart block.

Development of right ventricular dysfunction requiring reoperation in patients with TOF is common. Frequently, these patients require inotropic support for several days postoperatively. As inotropic support is weaned, other medications may be utilized for treatment including beta-blockers, Aldactone, ACE inhibitors, and diuretics for several months as the ventricle remodels and function improves. As these medications are initiated, fluid balance and hemodynamics must be followed to maintain adequate preload.

There are two eras of surgical repair for the ACHD patient with complete TGA. Many adults in the first era have undergone an atrial switch procedure, either a Mustard or Senning operation, during which the venous blood returning to the heart was redirected at the atrial level through a baffle to the appropriate ventricle supplying either the lungs or the body. In this repair the right ventricle remains the systemic ventricle.

These patients may experience significant systemic atrioventricular (AV) valve regurgitation related to the tricuspid valve (TV) being the AV valve, arrhythmias, pulmonary hypertension, and both right and left ventricular dysfunction. Patients may also experience problems related to the atrial baffle. An atrial baffle leak may result in the development of a right-to-left shunt and ventricular dysfunction, or baffle placement may obstruct either systemic or pulmonary venous drainage [31, 49, 50].

Many concerns for this population are related to the presence of a systemic right ventricle, leading to ventricular dysfunction and heart failure. Long-term heart failure treatment in this setting may be challenging. Medications, such as diuretics, ACE inhibitors, and beta-blockers, are used for treatment. However, currently there is no data representing the benefit of traditional heart failure medications for a systemic right ventricle. In addition to medical management for heart failure, antiarrhythmic medications may be administered to treat any resulting ventricular arrhythmias. More invasive interventions, such as an automatic implantable defibrillator or pacemaker, may also be required. The benefits of biventricular pacing to manage ventricular dysfunction in the setting of a systemic right ventricle are being discussed and studied [33]. Cardiac transplantation may also be considered for some patients with severe ventricular dysfunction post an atrial switch procedure [31, 51].

The second era of surgical intervention for the complete TGA patient is the arterial switch procedure. This procedure provides a complete anatomical and physiological correction. The first cohort of these patients is now reaching adulthood. The concerns for reintervention for these patients include either right or left outflow tract obstruction, branch pulmonary artery stenosis, coronary artery occlusion, or dilation of the aortic root with aortic regurgitation [31, 49].

Septal defects, primarily a secundum atrial septal defect (ASD), represent about one third of the defects diagnosed in adults. Repair of a secundum ASD a may be accomplished via device closure in the interventional catheterization laboratory [47]. Defects identified as sinus venosus defects, especially those with anomalous pulmonary venous return or primum ASD with involvement of the mitral valve, require surgical repair. Preoperative evaluation includes assessment of pulmonary pressures and possible atrial arrhythmias. Many adults with significant left-to-right shunts will develop irreversible pulmonary vascular disease with right heart failure and arrhythmias [31, 52].

An ASD that is repaired in the operating room carries a good lifetime prognosis [53]. After repair of ostium secundum ASD or sinus venosus ASD, postoperative atrial tachyarrhythmias are the most common complication. The risk of postoperative atrial arrhythmias increases when the arrhythmia was present preoperatively and with increased age at time of repair [53]. When supraventricular atrial tachycardia, atrial fibrillation, or atrial flutter occur following surgical repair, antiarrhythmic medications as well as need for cardioversion are considered, depending on patient hemodynamic tolerance of the arrhythmia.

VSD, as well as atrioventricular septal defects (AVSD), are usually repaired in infancy or early childhood. Many of the ACHD patients with AVSD have chromosomal abnormalities. The most common is trisomy 21, Down syndrome, occurring in 39 % of patients with AVSD [54]. Unrepaired adults present with congestive heart failure, exercise limitations, pulmonary hypertension, cyanosis, and atrial arrhythmias. Repair may not be possible due to pulmonary vascular disease [50]. Patients with AVSD, which was repaired in infancy, may have symptomatic left-sided atrioventricular (AV) valve stenosis or AV valve regurgitation. Additionally these adults may have increase in left ventricle size, decrease in left ventricular function, and experience arrhythmias including heart block. Left AV valve replacement may be necessary, often accompanied by pacemaker placement [49, 54].

Currently, CoA is repaired in the neonatal period with excision of the narrowed segment and extended end-to-end anastomosis or subclavian flap angioplasty. Adults with a historical repair involving use of Dacron or GORE-TEX® are at risk to develop pseudoaneurysm. Those with suture, end-to-end repair may develop re-coarctation at the site of the suture line. Reoperation in these patients comes with significant risk from pleural and mediastinal adhesions, the rare development of an aortobronchial fistula, or pleurodesis. Repair with an ascending-to-descending thoracic aorta bypass and placement of a Dacron tube graft provides a safe repair [31]. Endovascular stenting in the catheterization lab also is an effective, safe alternative procedure. Primary endovascular stenting of a discrete coarctation of the aorta in the young adult patient is advocated [46].

Postoperative monitoring for reperfusion injury, specifically to the pancreas and kidneys, is important. Ventricular dysfunction, if present, may require inotropic support and long-term management. Hypertension must be aggressively treated, as its impact on fresh suture lines is of great concern. Blood pressures should be checked in both upper and lower extremities to monitor for a gradient and the continued presence of an area of narrowing in the aorta.

Discharge considerations of ACHD patients reflect the need lifelong follow-up. Teaching must be individualized. Key considerations include psychosocial factors, including the presence of parents of the ACHD patients in management of the patient's healthcare, any learning disabilities or genetic anomalies, the ability to work preoperatively and postoperatively, and insurance considerations [55].

An understanding of their disease is key to empowering ACHD patients. Upon discharge, patients should receive education on postsurgical management including incision care and activity and diet restrictions, including explanation of the surgical repair and subsequent follow-up appointments and concerns.

Arrhythmias and heart failure are the most common complications that occur following many congenital cardiac surgical procedures. In addition to general postoperative teaching, patients should be instructed to notify their physician if palpitations, syncope, edema, weight gain, or decreased exercise tolerance occurs. The presence of comorbidities including lung disease, renal disease, and diabetes may influence the postoperative course and the needs at discharge.

Care of the Fetal Cardiology Patient with Prenatal Diagnosis

Over the past 30 years, the field of fetal cardiology has grown, largely due to advances in prenatal imaging and diagnosis. Although, in some large tertiary care centers, nearly 2,000 fetal echocardiograms are performed each year, only approximately 50 % of CHD is prenatally diagnosed. Most pregnant women have an anatomical fetal ultrasound at approximately 18–20 weeks. This allows for early detection of CHD and expedites the need for referral. Women are referred for fetal echocardiograms when their fetus has a suspected heart problem or other anomalies. Expectant mothers are also referred for a fetal echocardiogram if maternal conditions are present that increase the risk of having a baby with congenital heart disease, such as family history of congenital heart disease, maternal diabetes, maternal drug exposure, and maternal autoimmune disease. The first fetal echocardiogram should be performed at approximately 18 weeks; however, fetal echocardiograms may be performed up to 40 weeks. As gestational age advances, fetal size and positioning may cause suboptimal images; thus, earlier imaging is ideal.

In the field of fetal cardiology, the team provides care for expectant parents and the fetus; however, the patient is defined as the expectant mother. Care of the fetal cardiology patient is complex and multifaceted and requires excellent

Table 74.1 Initial assess of the fetal cardiology patient

Components of maternal health records	Review to determine the following
Echo report	Type and severity of CHD
	Reliability of diagnosis
	Most appropriate site for delivery
Ultrasound report	Need for additional imaging or pediatric specialty consultation, if other anomalies or concerns are present (e.g., two-vessel cord, increased nuchal thickness, echogenic bowel, clenched hands, single kidney, cleft lip and palate, club feet, neural tube defect, growth problems, and hydrops)
	Risk of increased morbidity or mortality with presence of extra cardiac anomalies or evidence of fetal distress
Due date (EDC)	Gestational age and size and impact on cardiac imaging
	Gestational age and impact pregnancy decision making
Genetics	Presence of abnormal early screening or risk assessment
	Presence of abnormal chromosomes or genetic markers (e.g., chromosomes or markers for trisomy 21 (Down syndrome), trisomy 13 or 18, Turner syndrome, DiGeorge syndrome (22q11.2 deletion), or Noonan syndrome)
	Family history of CHD, birth defects, or other genetic problems
Obstetric history	Gravida and parity
	History of infertility
	History of assisted reproductive technology
	History of prematurity
	History of prenatal, postnatal, or childhood loss
Maternal past medical and surgical history	Maternal health issues or medications which may impact pregnancy or delivery
Psychosocial history	Maternal and paternal psychosocial and mental health history which may impact coping or parenting
	Ability to understand, to cope, and to care for a child with congenital heart disease
	Level of education and occupation
	Religious beliefs

organization and communication between a multitude of specialists and disciplines. Fetal cardiology care team members include fetal care center, cardiac intensive care, interventional cardiology, cardiac surgery, cardiac genetics, referring and local obstetric teams, maternal fetal medicine (high-risk obstetrics), neonatology, and many other specialists. The role of the nurse on the fetal cardiology care team is usually filled by a nurse practitioner or an advanced practice nurse. This nurse is the designated point person and the liaison for communication between all of the care team members. Prenatal counseling, education, and family preparation are enhanced by the nurse's knowledge and clinical expertise in longitudinal pediatric cardiac care. The care may even extend beyond delivery.

Important components of the nursing care are outlined below and include initial assessment, fetal cardiology consultation, follow-up care, delivery preparation, and cardiac triage planning.

The initial assessment of a fetal cardiology patient begins at the time of referral. The first step is to carefully review the maternal health records. Table 74.1 outlines the aspects to include in a complete assessment of the maternal health records.

Following a detailed review of the maternal records, the nurse contacts the expectant mother and completes an initial assessment. The patient is asked why she has been referred for a fetal echocardiogram. It is important to clarify knowledge of the reason for referral as occasionally patients referred for fetal echocardiogram are not aware of the suspected diagnosis of CHD. The patient is informed that there is concern regarding the baby's heart and a fetal echocardiogram will help confirm or exclude CHD. Confirmation may mean an alteration in the diagnosis; therefore, the prognosis might be better, worse, or similar to what was previously expected. In some cases, more detailed information may be able to be provided regarding the typical course and prognosis of the diagnosis. Recognizing that many patients seek information via the Internet, patients are counseled to wait until the diagnosis is confirmed to avoid misinformation. Sometimes even a straightforward diagnosis may have a subtle nuance that could impact the treatment and prognosis.

After completion of a verbal history and confirmation of the maternal health history, other questions and issues are addressed. Patients are questioned if they are considering termination of pregnancy – every effort is made to see these patients as quickly as possible and prior to the state legal limit for termination. Patients are reassured that they will be supported regardless of the decision made regarding care. The initial fetal care visit is then described.

On the day of the fetal cardiology consultation, following completion of the fetal echocardiogram, the expectant parents meet with the team in a private room. The fetal cardiologist describes and illustrates normal cardiac anatomy, fetal cardiac anatomy, and the specific congenital heart defect diagnosis. Neonatal and lifelong surgical options and prognosis are presented to the family.

Other important factors addressed during the consult include neurodevelopmental issues, nutrition and feeding issues, potential impact of the diagnosis upon future exercise capacity and quality of life, and the need for lifelong cardiology care and potential for unexpected hospitalizations or illnesses throughout life. Parents are given generous estimates for the length of stay for the initial hospitalization so they are prepared and not disappointed that their stay is longer than expected. The nurse participates in the discussion and notes important highlights of the consult for the patient to later take home.

After the consultation with the cardiologist is complete, the nurse reviews the diagnosis, illustrations, and care pathway options that were discussed in the consult. Further discussions include transfer of care to a high-risk obstetrician or maternal fetal medicine physician, when and what to expect at delivery, and plans for follow-up care during pregnancy. Notes from the consultation are reviewed and given to the patient with other educational material, including a fetal cardiology care checklist. This patient education packet is provided so that the patient may review the details of the visit and prognosis at home. Patients often have difficulty remembering all the information discussed during the initial consults due to the stressful nature of hearing the diagnosis.

Fetal cardiology consults may be prolonged and intensified by extreme parental anxiety and grief surrounding the "loss of the idealized child" and the potential for prenatal and postnatal morbidity and mortality. Many families are referred to the fetal care social worker following the cardiology consultation for further discussions around coping with the unexpected diagnosis or decision making regarding continuation of pregnancy.

Depending on the gestational age of the fetus at diagnosis and the type of CHD, most patients will be scheduled for one or more fetal echocardiograms and consultations. Every attempt is made to schedule these follow-up visits with the same cardiologist to promote continuity of care. Many large centers have an existing referral network, and it is a priority for the patient to meet their pediatric cardiologist prior to delivery to ease the transition. Identification of a local pediatrician who feels comfortable for caring for a baby with CHD is also strongly recommended.

A cardiac geneticist will be consulted if there is a known or suspected chromosome abnormality, additional birth defects, or a family history of congenital heart disease. An amniocentesis and a FISH for 22q11.2 deletion (DiGeorge syndrome) are recommended for all CHD diagnosis.

Additional imaging, such as MRI, may also be warranted to further investigate other anomalies. Other pediatric specialists are consulted as needed.

The family will meet the fetal care social worker to learn more about resources provided by the hospital, including a lactation consultant, and to discuss additional questions about accommodations and travel. Any psychosocial or coping concerns will be addressed. The family also tours the pediatric cardiac intensive care unit.

Mothers of babies with ductal-dependent CHD are advised to transfer their care to a maternal fetal medicine doctor. When possible, delivery should occur at a tertiary hospital adjacent to the neonatal cardiac surgical program. This will allow for a smooth and timely transfer of the baby and will allow for the parents to more easily visit her baby.

In most cases, mothers may deliver vaginally; a cesarean section delivery is not usually required due to the baby's CHD diagnosis; however, the mother's obstetric team will decide the best mode and timing of delivery. If the mother does not live close to the neonatal cardiac surgical program, relocation to the delivery location around 36–37 weeks is recommended. In most cases, a planned induction will generally occur at approximately 39 weeks. Inductions prior to 39 weeks are reserved for unique medical circumstances.

Each week, the fetal cardiology nurse creates and maintains a list of all fetal cardiology patients due to deliver, a "Cardiac Baby Delivery List." Weekly meetings with the maternal fetal medicine team, as well as daily dialogues with the cardiology and obstetric teams, provide the most updated and current information possible. Delivery alerts are sent out weekly or emergently as needed to the pediatric and obstetric teams.

The "Cardiac Baby Delivery List" includes important patient information organized in an excel spreadsheet by EDC as well as planned date and mode of delivery. Details include updated fetal cardiac diagnosis, other anomalies or concerns, amniocentesis or genetic testing results, relevant psychosocial information, name of fetal and pediatric cardiologist, name of maternal fetal medicine physician, and

delivery hospital. Also included in the cardiac triage plan are instructions for initiation of PGE_1 if the baby has a ductal-dependent congenital heart defect, specification of the unit where the baby should be transferred to, anticipated need for urgent catheterization, or additional instructions for the care of the critically ill neonate with CHD.

The role of the nurse is to optimize the care of the fetal cardiology patient. This role requires clinical expertise, sound clinical judgment, and a highly developed knowledge of normal and abnormal cardiac anatomy and physiology as well as fetal circulation. The nurse is a facilitator of learning, providing comprehensive prenatal education within a robust system of clinical inquiry. Care is enhanced when the nurse is a proactive systems thinker who remains in continual communication and collaboration with all members of the care team. Above all, advocacy and caring practices are integral to the care of the fetal cardiology patient. The fetal cardiology advanced practice nurse is a novel role that is dedicated to the unique issues of each patient and care team with the overall goal of providing safe, timely, effective, and efficient patient and family-centered care.

Cardiac Surgery Same-Day Admission Patient

The patient with congenital heart disease is part of an evolving patient population. The process of preparing these patients for surgical repair is potentially complex, as this population may require a myriad of medical procedures over their lifetimes.

Congenital heart disease is the most common type of birth defect, afflicting approximately 40,000 infants a year in the United States [56]. Cardiovascular surgery and cardiac catheterization techniques and interventions have enhanced quality of life and added substantive years to these patients' lives. Between the 1979 and 1997, mortality rates have decreased by 40 %. Eighty-five percent of infants with congenital heart disease are expected to reach adulthood [57].

It is estimated that there are over one million adults with congenital heart disease. Approximately 66 % of adults with congenital heart disease are considered to have complex congenital heart disease, with half of those patients diagnosed with moderately severe defects. This wide age range of patients adds complexity from both a medical and physiological perspective and also has social and life style impact, as this was once thought to be an essentially childhood problem [58, 59].

Cardiologists spend a significant amount of time with the family and patient reviewing the normal heart anatomy and patient-specific cardiac pathophysiology in order that all understand the indications for a procedure or surgery. Due to multiple stress-related factors, patients and families may only assimilate limited amounts of information and often arrive at their preoperative/pre-procedural assessments with many questions [60, 61].

Preoperative evaluation for the patient with congenital heart disease begins when the patient's cardiologist recommends the patient for a procedure or surgery. Once the clinicians in the preoperative area are notified, the medical and surgical review must allow sufficient time to prepare for the patient and adequately plan for any additional consultations that may be required. Timing of preparation is especially important for complex patients who may have a lengthy medical history, are from other institutions, or have additional medical problems that may need to be addressed prior to the preoperative appointment and procedure [61, 62]. The preoperative process should begin with an understanding of the underlying cardiac physiology, discussion of the procedure, as well as the indications for the procedure [62]. For planning purposes, it is necessary to be aware of any other procedures to be performed at the same time to anticipate logistical plans for allied clinician preparation and support. Additional procedures are often done at the same time either because supplementary information is necessary for the main procedure (i.e., bronchoscopy investigating extrinsic compression of the airway) or in the interest of economy of anesthesia exposure

(i.e., tympanic myringotomy at the time of a cardiac catheterization). A comprehensive review of the patient's medical history, anesthesia history, as well as a review of systems is done as this provides the key components needed to prepare the patient for their preoperative course. Ideally the scheduling of the preoperative evaluation should offer sufficient time to assess and account for the multiple variables that may affect the overall peri- and postoperative management [61, 62].

The preoperative day should be designed to allow a comprehensive evaluation and provide substantive teaching, anticipatory guidance, and explanation of expectations for hospitalization. This process is important and will clarify any misconceptions that might present misunderstandings during the hospitalization. It may also help decrease family and patient stress [61]. For patients and families that have been through the preoperative process recently or multiple times, teaching may be briefer in scope and still be effective in establishing a mutual understanding of the operation and hospitalization plan. The preoperative evaluation day offers an efficient mechanism to mitigate potential issues before they become larger problems. Used effectively, this process may decrease patient visit time, the need to reschedule operations, and repeated evaluations and testing. This may also work to decrease operating room "none-use" time, enhancing the day of surgery, as variables with the potential to affect peri- and post-procedure fluidity may be identified and addressed in a timely fashion [61].

Teamwork fully optimizes the preoperative process. Many preoperative clinics are staffed by nurses, nurse practitioners, and physician assistants as primary clinicians. The preoperative clinicians provide the primary medical and surgical history and physical assessment along with teaching and anticipatory guidance. To enhance the preoperative experience and offer the families and patients the full gamut of assistance, coping resources, and teaching, the preoperative service offers access to other key resources such as social work services and child life specialists. Additionally, administrative assistants and clinical assistants are essential to managing patient flow, coordinating the ordered testing as well as other important appointments. The preoperative clinicians collaborate with surgeons, interventional cardiologists, anesthesiologists, and referring cardiologists to implement the preoperative plan by coordinating and ensuring all tests and appointments are completed. During the preoperative day, surgeons and interventionalists meet with the patients and families to review the planned procedure, answer questions, and also obtain informed consent.

Once a thorough review of systems has been completed, other specialists may be consulted based on the specific patient care needs.

Patients with congenital heart disease or other forms of cardiac disease are often well studied and their cardiac pathophysiology is precisely documented. Depending on the patient's cardiac anatomy and physiology, past medical and surgical history, and perceived cardiac problems, the evaluation process may entail a myriad of testing. This includes cardiac catheterization with or without endomyocardial biopsy, electrophysiology studies with or without ablation, cardiac MRI, echocardiography, electrocardiogram, lung scan, cardiac/chest CT, exercise tolerance test, myocardial perfusion scans, chest x-ray, and laboratory testing [62].

Along with examination of the patient's cardiac problems, the referring cardiologist may also initiate inquiry of other medical issues which could potentially require management during the peri- and post-procedure period. The preoperative clinicians collaborate with the referring cardiologists as well as other members of team to account for and evaluate additional medical issues that might add complexity to the overall patient's care and management.

It is well documented that other physiological systems of patients with congenital heart disease are affected by their heart disease. A comprehensive assessment of all patients' organ systems is indicated and should be performed through review of available medical records, patient history, and physical exam.

A thorough respiratory system history is elicited. Special attention is given to central or obstructive sleep apneas, reactive airway disorders, chronic obstructive/restrictive lung disease, admission of use of inhaled tobacco and other substances, recent or current upper or lower respiratory illnesses, and mechanical airway conditions such as bronchomalacia, tracheomalacia, and other forms of extrinsic airway compression. It is essential to identify patients with tracheostomies or those with assistive ventilatory support requirements, such a continuous positive airway pressure, before hospital admission and incorporate these added complexities into the preoperative care planning [61, 62].

Planning and obtaining an endocrine consultation may also be essential. The potential diagnosis of type 1 and type 2 diabetes is an important variable to be considered. Endocrine consultation may assist with NPO guidelines and provide insulin management strategies pre- and perioperatively. Endocrine consultation may also help manage patients with various forms of adrenal insufficiency and provide effective corticosteroid replacement. Hyperthyroidism and hypothyroidism are also significant endocrine imbalances to identify, assess, and manage perioperatively [61, 62].

Patients with a history of prolonged bleeding times may need hematology consultation for either further assessment or perioperative management of blood product administration. Patients, whose history or genetic testing indicates a propensity for thrombosis, may need additional consultation for peri- and postoperative management. Also those patients receiving anticoagulation or antiplatelet therapy will require detailed preoperative guidance and planning depending on the indication for the therapies [62].

Patients with liver disease must have the nature of their pathophysiology and liver function clearly defined. Liver dysfunction affects the metabolism of many drugs, which may guide medication choices peri- and post-procedure. Additionally, liver disease may affect the synthesis of clotting factors and add to the complexity to peri- and postoperative hemostasis [61].

As with the liver, it is important to define the presence of renal dysfunction before surgery. Altered renal function may guide peri- and postoperative drug use and dosing. It may also indicate the need for preoperative IV hydration to enhance renal function. Patients with chronic renal failure or end-stage renal disease may need their operation coordinated with dialysis pre- and postoperatively. Any electrolyte imbalances are also identified and evaluated with a treatment plan [61].

Past anesthesia encounters should be reviewed. Patients with abnormal airway anatomy or a history of difficult intubation must be identified and examined and an appropriate intubation strategy developed. Those patients with diagnosis or family history of malignant hyperthermia are identified so suitable anesthesia management may be planned. Patients with the potential for the occurrence of bronchospasm must also be identified and this factored into the anesthesia approach [61].

Patients with dental caries may need dental clearance prior to cardiac surgery. Patients, particularly adolescents, who have an orthodontic apparatus (i.e., palate expanders) may present a challenge in maintaining satisfactory airway management. Oral infections are treated prior to cardiac surgery [61].

Regardless of age, patients with psychiatric illness, cognitive deficits, and behavioral issues must be identified ahead of time to allow for evaluation and development of pre-, peri-, and postoperative management strategies with appropriate consultation. Parental custody issues should be defined and the necessary legal documentation in place. Additionally, other parental legal issues (i.e., restraint orders) or faith-based issues requiring legal consultation (i.e., Jehovah's Witness) must be recognized.

Patients may require or request social work consultation to assist with emotional as well as concrete needs throughout the hospitalization. Child life specialists provide a wealth of support to both parents and children and may also be a tremendous resource in preparing families and young patients for the hospitalization [60, 61].

During the preoperative/pre-procedural preparation, time is spent in educating the parents and patients. The goal of this interaction is to promote interactive communication between the preoperative clinician, usually a nurse practitioner, and the patient/parents so all are comfortable asking questions. Increased education may aid in coping with changes in health status and increase compliance/assistance with perioperative care.

On the day of surgery, routine and anticipated recovery course (intensive care and hospital stay) are reviewed. This includes nothing by mouth or NPO guidelines and time frames for arrival to the hospital. Patients are instructed to arrive a few hours prior to the actual operation start time to provide anesthesia and nursing ample time for assessment and preparation for surgery.

Personal considerations, such as appropriate clothing to wear, use of jewelry and makeup, personal items to bring (toy/blanket/electronic device, movies), and the importance of leaving valuables at home, are discussed. Siblings' presence is discouraged on day of surgery, and a limitation on the number of visitors in the critical care areas is clarified.

All patients receive instructions regarding the technique for preoperative skin preparation or a "scrub" to be done the evening before their scheduled surgery, including materials and written instruction, during the preoperative visit. Cleansing the chest area has been shown to reduce the risk of skin infection.

For patients over 18 years of age, advance directive information is reviewed as required, and documentation of healthcare proxy is assured.

On the day of surgery, most patients receive premedication (usually oral; however, intravenous or intramuscular routes may be utilized) in the operating room holding area with the parents present. This is done in an attempt to minimize the stress of separation.

The intensive care atmosphere is reviewed with the parents and patients. Ventilators/monitoring lines are explained. Families are offered a tour of the cardiac intensive care and ward by the child life therapist. If the patients/parents are reluctant to participate in a tour, the child life team utilizes a book of pictures for the family to review. The intensive care visiting policy is discussed emphasizing the importance of self-care and breaks for parents during this stressful time.

Table 74.2 Preoperative pediatric cardiac surgery patient medications

Type of medication	Intraoperative concerns	Management	Discontinuation issues
Diuretics	Hypokalemia, hypovolemia	Monitor potassium levels preoperatively and maintain hydration	Morning dose held Rare problems
Anticoagulation/ antiplatelet drugs	Impaired platelet function – bleeding	Aspirin, *clopidogrel*, *enoxaparin*, Coumadin	Risk of increased bleeding if not discontinued
ACE inhibitors	Hypotension with or without bradycardia, intolerance to hypovolemia	*Captopril, enalapril,* lisinopril	Brief interruption for patients is usually well tolerated
Antiarrhythmics	Cardiac depression, prolonged neuromuscular blockade, amiodarone-induced hypotension and atropine-resistant bradycardia requiring pacing	Propranolol, *procainamide, flecainide*	Discontinuation rarely recommended as usually not prescribed for benign arrhythmias
Antireflux	Risk of aspiration	Ranitidine, PPIs (*omeprazole, lansoprazole, pantoprazole*)	
Other meds		Sildenafil, asplenia/ polysplenia prophylaxis (Bactrim, amoxicillin)	Sildenafil is given to prevent pulmonary hypertension. No concerns if prophylaxis medications held

The most common medications taken by cardiac surgery preoperative clinic patients are diuretics; medications for reflux, afterload reduction, arrhythmias, anticoagulation, pulmonary hypertension; and/or antibiotic prophylaxis for asplenia. Antiplatelet drugs such as aspirin and Plavix are stopped 7–10 days prior to cardiac surgery. Warfarin is usually stopped 3–5 days prior to the surgery. Depending on the indication for anticoagulation (low risk vs. high risk), some patients may need to be bridged with Lovenox or admitted for intravenous heparin prior to surgery. The surgical schedulers instruct patient regarding medications when they notify the patient/family of the surgical date. Angiotensin-converting enzyme (ACE) inhibitors are not given for 24 h prior to surgery. Diuretics are not administered for 12 h prior to surgery. Antireflux medications, beta-blockers, antiarrhythmic medications, and medications for pulmonary hypertension are usually taken prior to surgery. See Table 74.2 below.

Occasionally cases are canceled during the preoperative day. Some reasons for cancellation are patient illness (this is determined after discussion with the surgeon and anesthesiologist) or active dental caries.

The majority of the patients complete the preoperative day as an outpatient. On the day of surgery, they are admitted as a same-day admission. Some patients are admitted to the ward before surgery. These are patients with increased hematocrit requiring intravenous hydration prior to surgery or those with high risk for the development of blood clots if anticoagulation is discontinued and require IV heparin once their international normalized ratio (INR) is below a certain value. Another group of patients that may require preoperative hospital admission are infants who were born premature or patients who received sedation on the preoperative day and, because of sedation criteria, require overnight observation.

References

1. Knowles R, Griebsch I, Dezateux C et al (2005) Newborn screening for congenital heart defects: a systemic review and cost-effectiveness analysis. Health Technol Assess 9(44):iii–xi
2. Sawdowski S (2009) Congenital cardiac disease in the newborn infant: past, present and future. Crit Care Nurs Clin North Am 21:37–48

3. Killian K (2006) Left sided obstructive congenital heart defects. Newborn Infant Nurs Rev 6(3):128–136

4. Fleiner S (2006) Recognition and stabilization of neonates with congenital heart disease. Newborn Infant Nurs Rev 6(3):137–150

5. Witt C (1997) Cardiac embryology. Neonatal Netw 16(1):43–49

6. Karl TR (2001) Neonatal cardiac surgery: anatomic, physiologic, and technical considerations. Clin Perinatol 28:159–185

7. Borowski A, Schickendantz S, Mennicken U, Korb H (1997) Open heart interventions in premature low and very low birth weight neonates: risk profile and ethical considerations. Thorac Cardiovasc Surg 45:238–241

8. Numa A, Butt W, Mee RBB (1997) Outcome of infants with birthweight 2000 g or less who undergo major cardiac surgery. J Paediatr Child Health 28:318–320

9. Parkman S, Woods S (2005) Infant who have undergone cardiac surgery: what can we learn about lengths of stay in the hospital and presence of complications? J Pediatr Nurs 20(6):430–440

10. Marino B, Bird G, Wernovsky G (2001) Diagnosis and management of the newborn with suspected congenital heart disease. Clin Perinatol 28:91–136

11. Brousseau T, Sharieff G (2006) Newborn emergencies: the first 30 days of life. Pediatr Clin North Am 53:69–84

12. Colletti J, Homme J, Woodridge D (2004) Unsuspected neonatal killers in emergency medicine. Emerg Med Clin North Am 22:929–960

13. Schelonka R, Carlo W (2010) The oxygen conundrum for infants with suspected congenital heart disease. Neonatology 97:163–164

14. Johnson B, Ades A (2005) Delivery room and early postnatal management of neonates who have prenatally diagnosed congenital heart disease. Clin Perinatol 32:921–946

15. Yee L (2007) Cardiac emergencies in the first year of life. Emerg Med Clin North Am 25:981–1008

16. Theilan U, Shekerdemian L (2005) The intensive care of infants with hypoplastic left heart syndrome. Arch Dis Child Fetal Neonatal Ed 90:F97–F102

17. Talosi G, Katona M, Turi S (2007) Side effects of long term prostaglandin E1 treatment in neonates. Paediatr Int 49:335–340

18. MIMS online (2011) Retrieved 21 July 2011, from https://www.mimsonline.com.au/Search/FullPI.aspx?ModuleName=Product%20Info&searchKeyword=Prostaglandin+E1&PreviousPage=~/Search/QuickSearch.aspx&SearchType=&ID=2780001_2

19. Merle C (2001) Nursing considerations of the neonate with congenital heart disease. Clin Perinatol 28:223–233

20. Howley L, Kaufman J, Thureen P, Magouirk J, McNair B, da Cruz E (2011) Enteral feeding in neonates with prostaglandin-dependant congenital cardiac disease; international survey on current trends and variations in practice. Cardiol Young 2011. doi:10.1017/S1047951111001016 Available on CJO

21. Castillo S, McCulley M, Khemani R, Jeffries H, Thomas D, Peregrine J et al (2010) Reducing the incidence of necrotizing enterocolitis in neonates with hypoplastic left heart syndrome with the introduction of an enteral feed protocol. Pediatr Crit Care Med 11:373–377

22. McElhinney D, Hedrick H, Bush D, Pereira G, Stafford P, Gaynor JW et al (2000) Necrotizing enterocolitis in neonates with congenital heart disease: risk factors and outcomes. Pediatrics 106:1080–1087

23. Medoff-Cooper B, Irving S (2009) Innovative strategies for feeding and nutrition in infants with congenitally malformed hearts. Cardiol Young 19(suppl2):90–95

24. Upham M, Medoff-Cooper B (2005) What are the responses and needs of mothers of infants diagnosed with congenital heart disease? Matern Child Nurs 30(1):24–29

25. Landzberg M (2011) Introduction: adult congenital heart disease. Prog Cardiovasc Dis 53:237–238

26. Betz C (2010) Approaches to transition in other chronic illnesses and conditions. Pediatr Clin North Am 57:983–996

27. Daniels C (2008) The young adult with congenital heart disease. In: Allen H, Driscoll D, Feltes T, Shaddy R (eds) Moss and Adams' heart disease in infants, children, and adolescents, including the fetus and young adult, 7th edn. Lippincott Williams & Wilkins, Philadelphia

28. Marelli A, Therrien J, Mackie A et al (2009) Planning the specialized care of adult congenital heart disease patients: from numbers to guidelines; an epidemiologic approach. Am Heart J 157(1):1–8

29. Marelli A, Mackie A, Lonescu-Ittu R et al (2007) Congenital heart disease in the general population: changing prevalence and age distribution. Circulation 115(2):163–172

30. Webb C, Jenkins K, Karpawich P et al (2002) Collaborative care for adults with congenital heart disease. Circulation 105:2318–2323

31. Guleserian K (2011) Adult congenital heart disease: surgical advances and options. Prog Cardiovasc Dis 53:254–264

32. Allan CK (2011) Intensive care of the adult patient with congenital heart disease. Prog Cardiovasc Dis 53:274–280

33. Abadia S, Khairy P (2011) Electrophysiology and adult congenital heart disease: advances and options. Prog Cardiovasc Dis 53:281–292

34. Boris S, Lowe MB, Therrien J et al (2011) Diagnosis of pulmonary hypertension in the congenital heart disease adult population. J Am Coll Cardiol 58:538–546

35. Mackie A, Ionescu-Ittu R, Therrien J et al (2009) Children and adults with congenital heart disease lost to follow-up: who and when? Circulation 120:302–309

36. Moons P, Pinxten S, Dedroog D et al (2009) Expectations and experiences of adolescents with congenital heart disease on being transferred from pediatric cardiology to an adult congenital heart disease program. J Adolesc Health 44:316–322

37. Kovacs A, Verstappen A (2011) The whole adult congenital heart disease patient. Prog Cardiovasc Dis 53:247–253

38. Berdat P, Immer F, Pfammatter J et al (2004) Reoperations in adults with congenital heart disease: analysis of early outcome. Int J Cardiol 93:239–245

39. Moons P, Van Deyk K, Marquet K et al (2005) Individual quality of life in adults with congenital heart disease: a paradigm shift. Eur Heart J 25:298–307

40. Baslaim G, Bashore J (2009) A unique milieu for perioperative care of adult congenital heart disease patients at a single institution. Ann Thorac Cardiovasc Surg 15(3):150–154

41. Karamlou T, Diggs B, Person T et al (2008) National practice patterns for management of adult congenital heart disease: operation by pediatric heart surgeons decreases in-hospital death. Circulation 118:2345–2352

42. Kim Y, Gauvreau K, Bacha E et al (2011) Risk factors for death after adult congenital heart surgery in pediatric hospitals. Circ Cardiovasc Qual Outcomes 4:433–439

43. Metter B, Peeler B (2001) Congenital heart disease surgery in the adult. Surg Clin North Am 89:1021–1032

44. Warnes C, Williams R (co-chair) et al. (2008) ACC/AHA guidelines for adults with CHD. J Am Coll Cardiol. 52(23): 143–263

45. Deanfield J, Thaulow E, Warnes C et al (2003) Management of grown up congenital heart disease. Eur Heart J 24:1035–1084

46. Meadows J, Landzbery M (2011) Advances in transcatheter interventions in adults with congenital heart disease. Prog Cardiovasc Dis 53:265–273

47. Nordmeyer J, Khambadkone S, Coats L et al (2007) Risk stratification, systematic classification, and anticipatory management strategies for stent fracture after percutaneous pulmonary valve implantation. Circulation 1115:1392–1397

48. Giamberti A, Chessa M, Abella R et al (2009) Morbidity and mortality risk factors in adults with congenital heart disease undergoing cardiac reoperations. Soc Thorac Surg 88:1284–1290

49. Warnes CA (2006) Transposition of the great arteries. Circulation 114:2699–2709

50. Tanel R (2011) Preventing sudden death in the adult with congenital heart disease. Curr Cardiol Rep 13:327–335

51. Warnes C, Sommerville J (1987) Transposition of the great arteries: late results in adolescents and adults after the mustard procedure. Br Heart J 58:148–155

52. Cetta F (2009) Atrioventricular septal defects. In: Warnes C (ed) Adult congenital heart disease. Wiley-Blackwell, Dallas

53. Perloff J, Warnes C (2001) Challenges posed by adults with repaired congenital heart disease. Circulation 103:2637–2643

54. Marx G, Fyler D (2006) Endocardial cushion defects. In: Keane J, Fyler D, Lock J (eds) Nadas' Pediatric cardiology, 2nd edn. WB Saunders/Elsevier, Philadelphia

55. Kovacs A, Bendell K, Colman J et al (2009) Adult congenital heart disease: psychosocial needs and treatment preferences. Congenit Heart Dis 4:139–146

56. www.cdc.gov/features/heartdefects/

57. Moodie D (2010) Adult congenital heart disease. Tex Heart Inst J 38(6):705–706

58. Kovacs A (2011) The whole adult congenital heart disease patient. Prog Cardiovasc Dis 53(4):247–253

59. Khairy P, Landzberg MJ (2008) Editorial: toward prospective risk assessment of a multisystemic condition. Circulation 117:2311–2312

60. Hazinski M (1992) Nursing of the critically ill child. Mosby-Year Book, Salem

61. Nagelhout J, Plaus K (2010) Nurse anesthesia. Saunders Elsevier, St. Louis

62. DiNardo J (1998) Anesthesia for cardiac surgery. Simon & Schuster, Stamford

63. Curley MA, Maloney-Harmon P (eds) (2001) Critical care nursing of infants and children, 2nd edn. W.B. Saunders, Philadelphia

64. Rodriguez F, Moodie D, Parekh D et al (2011) Outcomes of hospitalization in adults in the United States with atrial septal defect, ventricular, septal defect, and atrioventricular septal defect. Am J Cardiol 108:290–293

Pediatric Cardiac Intensive Care – Cardiovascular Management: Nursing Considerations

75

Patricia Lincoln, Dorothy Beke, Nancy Braudis,
Elizabeth Leonard, Sherry Pye, and Elisabeth Smith

Abstract

Cardiac care of the patient in the PCICU is a complex process. This chapter describes salient aspects of nursing care associated specifically with cardiovascular management, delayed sternal closure, and the use of extracorporeal membrane oxygenation. Also included is discussion regarding implications of fast-track pathway of care. Additionally, this chapter will incorporate examples of communication tools utilized during patient handoffs to foster improved care and safety, in specific centers.

P. Lincoln (✉) • D. Beke • N. Braudis
Clinical Nurse Specialist, Cardiac Intensive Care Unit,
Boston Children's Hospital, Boston, MA, USA
e-mail: patricia.lincoln@childrens.harvard.edu;
Dorothy.beke@childrens.harvard.edu;
nancy.braudis@childrens.harvard.edu

E. Leonard
Critical and Cardiorespiratory Unit, Great Ormond Street
Hospital for Children NHS Foundation Trust, London,
England, UK
e-mail: elizabeth.leonard@gosh.nhs.uk

S. Pye
Pediatric heart Transplant Coordinator, Department of
Pediatric, Cardiology, University of Arkansas for
Medical Sciences, Arkansas Children's Hospital,
Little Rock, AR, USA
e-mail: sepye@uams.edu

E. Smith
Great Ormond Street Hospital for Children NHS
Foundation Trust, London, England, UK
e-mail: smithe1@gosh.nhs.uk; liz.smith@gosh.nhs.uk

Introduction

Cardiac care of the patient in the PCICU is a complex process. This chapter describes salient aspects of nursing care associated specifically with cardiac vascular management, delayed sternal closure, and the use of extracorporeal membrane oxygenation. Also included is discussion regarding implications of fast-track pathway of care.

E.M. da Cruz et al. (eds.), *Pediatric and Congenital Cardiology, Cardiac Surgery and Intensive Care*,
DOI 10.1007/978-1-4471-4619-3_196, © Springer-Verlag London 2014

Keywords

Admission process • Arrhythmias • Cardiac output • Delayed sternal closure • EMCO • Fast-track protocols • Hemodynamic monitoring • Low cardiac output syndrome (LCOS) • Patient handoffs • Pulmonary hypertension

Introduction

Cardiac care of the patient in the PCICU is a complex process. This chapter describes salient aspects of nursing care associated specifically with cardiovascular management, delayed sternal closure, and the use of extracorporeal membrane oxygenation. Also included is discussion regarding the implications of a fast-track pathway. Additionally, this chapter will incorporate examples of communication tools utilized during patient handoffs to foster improved care and safety.

Postoperative Admission to the Pediatric Cardiac Intensive Care Unit

Much work has led to the development of a system for admissions to the PCICU in which the nurse is supported, the patient safe, the family is informed, and all members of the multidisciplinary team receive the handover information needed to optimize the patient's stay in intensive care. It is important to explain how this has been achieved, so this information may be transferred to multiple units and situations.

One of the most important factors is the knowledge base and preparation of the family and patient that is to be admitted. The fetal care team will work with families during pregnancy and ensure seamless communication between time of delivery and admission to the PCICU, preparing the family and ensuring the clinical team is updated on baby's condition. For the same day admission (SDA) patient, the nursing team endeavors to meet the parents and child beforehand. Often, there will be a visit to the PCICU on a preadmission visit for all families. This allows for assessment of individual needs and to ensure that the family is familiar with their potential pathway of care. For the SDA patient, on the morning of the operation, the PCICU nurse may visit and introduce themselves to the child and family. Research has shown that this may significantly reduce stress for parents, as well as for the child [1].

The preadmission visit has high importance for the SDA patient, allowing the parents to discuss any worries and permitting observation of the child for age-appropriate behavior and level of activity, presence of cyanosis or respiratory distress, or any concerns that would contraindicate surgery. A recent initiative in England is nurse-led developmental neurological scoring before surgery to flag potential problems and discuss these with the family. A second follow-up developmental neurological score is performed prior to postoperative discharge to note the development of new areas of support needed for the child or family at a local level (unpublished). Also, preoperatively, patient information leaflets are distributed (an example may be found on www.gosh.nhs.uk/gosh_families/information_sheets), and expected dates of discharge from PCICU, intermediate care area, and the ward to home are discussed [2]. Planning the estimated days of intensive care admission allows the family to ensure they have local arrangements and when they should anticipate discharge.

Admission to the PCICU requires focused planning and preparation. The bed space, equipment, and needed supplies are obtained in anticipation of an emergency situation as well as ensuring the availability of the tools required to deliver effective and timely care. Oxygen, suction, and other safety equipment are checked and available in the bed space. Standardized fluids and medications are prepared, and early entry into the computerized electronic charting is established. The mechanical ventilator is set up with settings from the operating room, allowing the system to be pre-checked.

Safety underlines all care in the PCICU – from the most junior member of staff to the unit lead. This is illustrated in the unit handover policy, developed from the pit stop process of Formula 1 motor racing where handover, safety, and teamwork were observed and those transferable skills to the healthcare setting were noted. Each individual has a defined role, reducing variability and therefore potential error within the system [3].

Phases of clinical handover

Phase	Event	Action
0	Patient transfer form from the operating room	Check list of ventilator settings and monitoring lines recorded for set up/update for unit team and needed equipment
1	Equipment and technical handover	Handover of all equipment and monitoring
2	Information phase	Defined role for each team member. Anesthetist reviews events of intubation, ventilation, and bypass and any observations during the operation. The surgeon comments on the surgical procedure and any intraoperative problems
3	Discussion phase	The anticipated recovery plan is verbalized by the intensive care physician. A decision on the appropriate pathway or other care/intervention is discussed. Two nurses assist – one concentrates on the verbal report from the operating room team and the other performs the initial patient assessment and admission of the patient to the PCICU (obtaining vital signs and laboratory blood specimens and connects and records drainage from chest drains)

Once the handover is completed, the bedside nurse's main concern is on ventilation and the hemodynamic status of the patient. A full physical examination is completed – assessment of equal breath sounds, bilateral chest movement,

presence of air leak around the endotracheal tube, and amount and characteristics of chest drainage. Hemodynamic assessment includes heart rate, blood pressure, heart filling pressures, peripheral pulses, and color/temperature of peripheral limbs. Prolonged capillary refill and cool extremities may indicate a low cardiac output state [4]. A chest radiograph (CXR), 12-lead electrocardiogram (ECG), and sometimes an additional echocardiogram (ECHO) are required within the first hour postoperatively to help support direction of care.

Mindful of the anxiety of the waiting parents, they are permitted to be with their child at the bedside. Families may stay for as long as they wish [5]. Recent research [6] highlighted the immediate postoperative period as one of the most stressful times for parents. The management of pain is of great concern to families, and continual assessment using an appropriate comfort/pain scale [7] ensures adequate pain relief and the administration of prescribed medications. Distress may be minimized using comfort measures suitable to the patient's age and condition, and there is also access to the hospital pain control team and ongoing anesthesia staff support.

Communication is of vital importance in the patient care process. All handovers, including the nursing handover, use a standardized communication tool, SBARD [8, 9]:
- Situation
- Background
- Assessment
- Recommendation
- Decision

Many institutions use a similar tool.

To ensure vital information is relayed with each patient, a handover mnemonic MINDER is used. The benefit of a structured formulaic handover is that the major concerns are addressed in a consistent and standardized approach across the clinical team.
- M (mechanical – is the endotracheal tube secure)
- I (infection – are bundles being followed)
- N (nutrition – is the child feeding by mouth or receiving TPN)
- D (drugs – are levels appropriate)

- E (emergency – resuscitation status)
- R (reduce – may any medication or mechanical ventilation strategy be weaned)

After the patient has been admitted and stabilized, it is the role of all team members to ensure the child and family progress through to recovery [10–12].

"Fast-Track" Pediatric Cardiac Surgery

Fast-track cardiac surgery has been defined as a reduction in the patient journey time from admission to discharge [13, 14]. This encompasses a reduction in ventilation time, possible same day discharge to an intermediate care unit from the PCICU, and early de-intensifying. This pathway, however, is dictated by the clinical condition of the child, safety being of paramount importance.

Working in emerging economies has provided insights and an "informal" evidence base for fast-track-type service delivery, within a health provision system where resources and time may be constrained. In addition, exposure to the success of these programs by the multiprofessional team has been a positive influence on the development of this service within pediatric cardiac services in the National Health Service (NHS) in England. Other factors for support are:

- Cardiac Nurse Practitioner (CNP) role development
- Joint cardiac conferencing and agreed multiprofessional criteria
- Anticipated recovery pathways, to standardize care delivery
- Preadmission assessment
- Timing of surgery
- Use of modern anesthesia agents
- Improvements in surgical techniques
- Improvements in cardiopulmonary bypass techniques, including ultrafiltration at the end of cardiopulmonary bypass [15]
- Parental presence during recovery
- Intensive care developments, including short acting opiates and advanced pain management skills

Collectively, these factors have led to a reduction in pediatric mortality and morbidity with subsequent cost reduction implications. The delivery of cost-efficient care is now an additional variable when measuring and comparing surgical outcomes [16–18]. Below is one example of a "fast-track model":

Eligibility for the fast-track pathway requires:

- Low-complexity cardiac surgery, for example, repair of atrial septal defect (ASD), ventricular septal defect (VSD), subaortic stenosis
- No major comorbidities that may involve a higher postoperative risk
- Patient otherwise in good general health and asymptomatic
- Patient over 6 months of age

Limiting criteria for the fast-track pathway include:

- Small infant with increased potential to fail early extubation
- Complex surgery or staged palliation surgery
- The presence of other noncardiac issues

Candidates for fast track will be done as first cases in the operating room (OR) and transitioned by a specific time to an intermediate care unit. The preadmission assessment is obtained within 1 month of the planned surgery. Patient and family teaching done preoperatively is essential in reducing postoperative anxiety and enabling the children to more easily accept their subsequent medical care [2]. On the day of surgery, a presurgery, clinical assessment is performed by the CNP and anesthesiologist. This meeting also ensures that the anesthetist and clinical team are aware of the plans for fast-track surgery, including mode of operative sedation and analgesia.

Although a large component of fast-track surgery is the reduction of mechanical ventilation time and early extubation, it is important to recognize that fast track and early extubation are not synonymous [17]. Extubations performed in the recovery room before return to the PCICU do not necessarily decrease recovery time in that unit.

The majority of the postoperative care for the fast track patient does not differ from our standardized cardiac postoperative care. Excellent clinical assessment skills and knowledge of the individual child are important for continued progress through the care pathway. This supports the provision of a dedicated team to lead this care pathway, staff that is familiar with the differences in parameters and timing of events.

Prior to leaving the operating room, the surgeon or the anesthetist infiltrates the sternal wound with local anesthetic. This provides additional pain relief with reduced use of opiates and may be effective for up to 8 h, potentially contributing to early extubation. A continuous incisional infusion of local anesthetic has been reported by the Congenital Heart Institute of Miami Children's Hospital and Arnold Palmer Hospital for Children, Miami, Florida, to reduce the length of stay, amount of sedation, and antiemetics [19]. The child will also receive intravenous non-opioid pain medication until tolerating oral intake, then oral pain medication and nonsteroidal anti-inflammatory [20, 21].

If the child is not extubated prior to leaving the operating room, experience demonstrates that extubation occurs within 4 h postoperatively. These patient decisions utilize advanced nursing education and assessment skills, increased autonomy of nursing practice, and caseload management combined with communication briefings with relevant nursing and medical teams. At 4 h postoperatively, the child is assessed for same day discharge to an intermediate care unit.

Events that may prevent discharge to intermediate care unit:

- Post-extubation stridor/respiratory compromise
- Bleeding from chest drains
- Arrhythmia
- Bed availability

A Children's Early Warning System (CEWS) [22] and a standardized communication tool such as SBARD (situation, background, assessment, recommendation, and decision) should be used to alert teams to early changes in a child's clinical condition and ensure accurate, consistent, and safe communication between teams. These tools clarify what and how information is communicated between members of the team and also help develop teamwork and foster a culture of patient safety.

On postoperative day 2, the child is rapidly assessed for de-intensification from the intermediate care unit. Strong clinical assessment skills, knowledge of the process, and decision-making are key to the safety of this process. An arterial blood gas review with no concerns allows the arterial line to be removed. Transthoracic pacing wires are removed without an additional ECG if there is no evidence of arrhythmia or need for external cardiac pacing. Peripheral IV access is assured. Chest drain removal is assessed on predefined criteria from the anticipated care pathway and local guidelines. No routine pre- or post-chest drain removal CXR is performed unless there is clinical reason [23].

It is the responsibility of the advanced practice nurse to assess the child's suitability for discharge home and to ensure they have all relevant discharge information, education, and emergency contact information. Prior to the child's discharge, usually on postoperative day 3, there is a review and agreement from the multiprofessional team, as well as the child and family, regarding discharge suitability and any ongoing medical concerns.

As a safety net to a rapid process of care, a follow-up phone call will be placed to the family within 48 h of discharge. This early communication and update with the child and family is a critical safety step in a rapid discharge process. Assessment is made of family management of care, and any questions regarding medications, analgesia, surgical wounds, feeding, or general concerns that may have arisen since discharge are addressed. Any acute issues will continue to be monitored until the next clinic appointment.

Cardiac Postoperative Care

The nursing considerations involved providing exceptional postoperative care of the pediatric cardiac surgery patient necessitate a full understanding of the patient's cardiac defect, the impact of the defect on other body systems, and the patient's treatment, repair, or palliation. Nursing focus is on vigilant patient monitoring, anticipating potential problems, and providing care with a proactive preventative approach.

Cardiac output is defined as the amount of blood ejected from the heart in 1 min. It is a function of heart rate multiplied by stroke volume. Stroke volume consists of preload, afterload, and contractility. Cardiac index, often used in pediatrics, is calculated as cardiac output divided by body surface area and expressed as liters/minute/meter^2 [24]. Assessment of cardiac output includes evaluating heart rate and rhythm, blood pressure, intracardiac filling pressures, core temperature, peripheral perfusion, urine output, acid–base balance, lactic acid excretion, and oxygen consumption [25].

Preload is the volume of blood in the left ventricle prior to ejection and may be indirectly assessed by monitoring atrial filling pressures. Preload may be decreased with excessive fluid loss or inadequate volume replacement. This may occur during rewarming and subsequent vasodilation, postoperative bleeding, diuresis, or capillary leak syndrome following cardiopulmonary bypass (CPB) [26]. Bleeding and abnormal coagulation factors may be corrected by giving fresh frozen plasma, cryoprecipitate, or other blood products. Packed red blood cells may be given to correct a low hematocrit and stabilize intravascular volume. Hypovolemia resulting from rewarming, capillary leak, or diuresis may be managed with colloid or crystalloid replacement. Fluid boluses are administered cautiously while assessing atrial filling pressure, arterial blood pressure, peripheral edema, liver distention, and fontanel fullness. Preload may be increased from myocardial dysfunction, intravascular overload, tamponade physiology, tachyarrhythmia, or increased pulmonary vascular resistance (PVR) and systemic vascular resistance (SVR).

Afterload is resistance to ejection of blood from either or both ventricles predisposing the myocardium to elevations in PVR and/or SVR. Common causes of increased PVR and SVR in the postoperative cardiac surgical patient are multifactorial and may include hypoxemia, acidosis, hypothermia, pain, or obstruction to blood flow from the ventricles. Systemic vascular resistance may increase in response to a low cardiac output state or as a result of high-dose inotropic medications. Increased PVR may result from both acute and chronic states. Neonates in particular often have a highly reactive pulmonary vascular bed resulting in elevations in PVR. Treatment strategies to decrease afterload resistance include avoidance of common triggers and manipulation of mechanical ventilation to reduce PVR, administration of sedatives and analgesics to blunt the stress response, and use of vasodilating agents.

In addition to preload and afterload, other determinants of cardiac output include heart rate, conduction, and contractility. Ventricular rate varies according to size, age, and patient condition and may be influenced by autonomic, humeral, and environmental stimuli [27]. Cardiac output is more dependent on heart rate due to limited stroke volumes in smaller, pediatric patients as compared with adults. Though a neonate may tolerate an elevated heart rate, decreased myocardial compliance predisposes the neonatal heart to increased sensitivity to SVR and limited response to elevations in preload [25]. Tachycardia may limit ventricular filling and decrease cardiac output when heart rate exceeds 220 beats per minute in the neonate or 180 beats per minute in the pediatric patient [27].

Cardiac contractility refers to the ability of the myocardium to produce force based on preload and alterations in sympathetic stimulation of the ventricles [27]. Postoperative factors leading to impaired myocardial contractility include medications and anesthetic agents, hypoxemia, acidosis, ischemic insult, cardiac tamponade, ventriculotomy incision, and residual anatomic cardiac lesions [28]. Inotropic support and afterload reduction should be optimized to support impaired cardiac contractility and low cardiac output. Decreased contractility from cardiac tamponade requires prompt intervention including maintaining patency of chest tubes and possible emergent mediastinal exploration.

Low cardiac output syndrome (LCOS) has been reported in approximately 24 % of neonates following congenital heart surgery [29]. The lowest cardiac index occurred 6–12 h after CPB. The decrease in cardiac index was associated with a significant rise in SVR and PVR over baseline values. Signs of LCOS include tachycardia, hypotension, decreased urine output, poor systemic perfusion, increased core temperature, elevated lactate, and decreased mixed venous oxygen saturation [25, 30]. Potential sources of low cardiac output include (1) residual cardiac defect, (2) myocardial ischemia, (3) inadequate myocardial protection during CPB, (4) inflammatory response, (5) increased SVR and PVR, (6) arrhythmias, (7) cardiac tamponade, and (8) ventriculotomy [28, 31, 32]. Early recognition and management of a low-output state is essential to minimize morbidity and mortality.

Measures to improve cardiac output include volume management to maintain adequate preload, vasoactive infusions to improve cardiac contractility, and afterload reduction to minimize the stress on the myocardium. Dopamine or low-dose epinephrine may be used for inotropic support to improve myocardial contractility and reverse hypotension related to LCOS. However, catecholamine infusions are not without risk and may cause a tachyarrhythmia, increased myocardial oxygen consumption, and increased end-diastolic pressure and afterload [31]. Milrinone is a phosphodiesterase inhibitor that has both inotropic effects and afterload-reducing properties and may prevent or improve the management of LCOS. In a multicenter study, infants receiving a high-dose infusion of Milrinone (0.75 mcg/kg/min) were found to have a 64 % relative risk reduction in the development of LCOS in the postoperative period following congenital heart surgery [32].

Efforts to manipulate SVR and PVR are crucial to maintaining hemodynamic stability in the postoperative period. Factors that may contribute to an increase in SVR and PVR such as inadequate pain control, hypoxia, acidosis, and hypothermia should be effectively treated to further reduce the risk of developing LCOS. Adjunct therapies include mechanical ventilation, neuromuscular blockade, adequate sedation, and arrhythmia management. Atrioventricular (AV) synchrony is critical to maintaining adequate cardiac output in the postoperative period. Treatment includes pacing strategies and the use of antiarrhythmic medications to optimize cardiac function.

The use of extracorporeal membrane oxygenation (ECMO) is indicated for progressive myocardial dysfunction refractory to conventional therapies, failure to wean from CPB, or cardiac arrest [33, 34]. ECMO may be used to provide short-term support for the myocardium or as a bridge to transplant.

Pediatric patients with congenital heart disease are prone to developing arrhythmias from underlying cardiac disease, surgical techniques, medical management, and electrolyte imbalance [35]. The incidence of arrhythmias in pediatric patients ranges from 8 % to 29 % in the postoperative period [35–37]. The loss of atrioventricular (AV) synchrony associated with many arrhythmias may result in a 20–30 % reduction in cardiac output [28]. Poor heart rate variability or cannon waves on a left atrial (LA) tracing may be important indicators of an abnormal rhythm. Temporary epicardial pacing wires are often placed following congenital heart surgery for the diagnosis and management of arrhythmias [38, 39]. Accurate diagnosis and prompt management are essential to reduce the effects of low cardiac output related to an arrhythmia.

Common arrhythmias identified in the postoperative period following pediatric heart surgery are supraventricular tachycardia, ventricular tachycardia, junctional ectopic tachycardia, and complete heart block [40]. Supraventricular tachycardia (SVT) is a reentry tachycardia with an abrupt onset and regular rate. It is often poorly tolerated in infants but may resolve with vagal maneuvers or overdrive pacing. Adenosine is a first-line drug for SVT in a stable patient [41]. However, synchronized cardioversion may be necessary in hemodynamically unstable patients. Ventricular arrhythmias are less common in young children but increase in frequency in teenagers and young adults. The risk for developing ventricular arrhythmias increases with acidosis, low cardiac output, electrolyte imbalance, and myocardial ischemia [42]. Sustained ventricular tachycardia (VT) is emergently treated with lidocaine as a first-line drug in a hemodynamically stable patient. Synchronized cardioversion is the treatment of choice for compromised patients. Torsades de pointes, another form of VT, typically occurs in the setting of QT prolongation. Initial treatment is with magnesium sulfate.

Junctional ectopic tachycardia (JET) usually occurs in the first 24–48 h after surgery and is the most common postoperative arrhythmia in infants and children less than 2 years of age [18]. The ventricular rate is generally greater than 160 with a slower atrial rate that may cause hypotension and increased filling pressures. Complete heart block (CHB) results from the complete dissociation of the atria and ventricles leading to a low-output state. It is usually transient in the postoperative period and is treated with external AV sequential pacing.

Although normothermia is the general goal of temperature regulation, a mild degree of hypothermia may be beneficial in the immediate postoperative period. There may be a brief period of temperature instability following congenital heart surgery and efforts should be aimed at limiting wide fluctuations in body temperature. Induced hypothermia may reduce oxygen consumption, limit the effects of tachyarrhythmias, and improve neurological outcomes [43, 44]. However, a decrease in body temperature may cause an elevation in SVR and PVR, decrease cardiac output, and potentially increase the risk of bleeding [26, 42]. Infants are especially vulnerable to cold stress because of the large body surface area and a limited ability to regulate body temperature. Rewarming should occur gradually with close monitoring.

Increased body temperature may result from activation of the inflammatory response after CPB or from low cardiac output. Hyperthermia increases oxygen consumption and may increase the risk of arrhythmias and neurological injury. Active cooling strategies may be implemented to limit the deleterious effects of hyperthermia in the immediate postoperative period.

The use of intracardiac monitoring catheters provides quantitative data for hemodynamic assessment in the postoperative patient. Knowledge of the patient's specific cardiac anatomy and details pertaining to the surgical repair or intervention are necessary to correctly interpret any information obtained. The catheters are placed transthoracically into the right atrium (RA), left atrium (LA), and/or pulmonary artery (PA). These intracardiac catheters provide information on heart chamber and great vessel pressures and saturations. This hemodynamic information also assists in evaluating responses to pharmacological therapies, mechanical ventilation changes, and fluid administration. Chest radiograph confirmation of catheter location is required, with waveform assessment and the presence of blood return, to assure functionality. Precise interpretation of pressures or oxygen saturation depends on catheter location and specific patient anatomy.

Reported risks of intracardiac catheter use include malposition, thrombus formation, and infection [45]. The LA and PA catheters are usually removed 24–48 h postoperatively, unless continued monitoring for LA or PA hypertension is required. The RA catheter may remain in place for an extended period to provide access for nontraumatic blood sampling and administration of vasoactive infusions, parental nutrition, or volume. Complications associated with removal of these catheters are hemorrhage, entrapment, or fragmentation [45, 46]. Following guidelines in regard to evaluation of hematological status, patient hemodynamics, use of chest drains, and availability of blood products for removal of intracardiac catheters will decrease the occurrence of complications and associated risks.

Right atrial (RA) or central venous monitoring catheters provide information about systemic venous return, vascular volume, and right ventricle function. These catheters are placed directly into the right atrium or internal jugular vein or superior vena cava. Right atrial pressure (RAp) or central venous pressure (CVP) are recorded as mean pressure, and the value reflects patient preload or right ventricle end-diastolic pressure (RVEDP) if the tricuspid valve is competent [42]. The average range of RAp or CVP is 1–5 mmHg, though these may have a slight normal elevation in the cardiac postoperative patient of 6–8 mmHg. Elevated RAp or CVP may indicate fluid overload, right ventricle (RV) dysfunction or hypertrophy, problems with the tricuspid valve, left to right intracardiac shunting, increased pulmonary vascular resistance, cardiac tamponade, or a pericardial effusion. Decreased RAp or CVP usually indicates hypovolemia [24, 42]. Measurement of blood oxygen saturation from these catheters will estimate systemic venous or mixed venous oxygen saturation and assist in evaluation of cardiac output [1].

Left atrial (LA) monitoring catheters provide information about pulmonary venous pressure, left heart preload, and left ventricle function. These catheters are usually threaded through a superior pulmonary vein across into the left atrium. The average left atrial pressure (LAp) is usually 1–2 mmHg greater than RAp. Of note, LAp measuring less than 12–14 mmHg is frequently tolerated in the postoperative patient [24, 42]. LAp is recorded as mean pressure and the value reflects left ventricle end-diastolic pressure if the mitral valve is competent. Elevated LAp may indicate left ventricle (LV) dysfunction or hypertrophy, problems with the mitral valve, increased systemic vascular resistance, right to left intracardiac shunting, volume overload, or cardiac tamponade [24]. Persistently elevated LAp may indicate the development of LA hypertension. Decreased LAp may indicate hypovolemia. Normal oxygen saturation of the blood in the LA is 100 % [26]. Blood shunting from the RA to the LA or the presence of pulmonary vein desaturation will decrease this value [24].

Cannon waves occurring in RA or LA recordings usually indicate the loss of normal sinus rhythm, as these waves occur when the atria contracts against a closed valve [47].

Pulmonary artery (PA) monitoring catheters provide information about mixed venous oxygen saturations, RV function, right ventricular outflow tract patency, pulmonary vascular reactivity, and mean filling pressures on the left side of the heart [1]. These catheters are threaded through the muscular wall of the RV, across the RV outflow tract, and into the main pulmonary artery. From there, it may migrate into a branch pulmonary artery. The pulmonary artery pressure (PAp) is recorded as mean, systolic, and diastolic, with the systolic value equal to the RV systolic pressure and the diastolic value equal to the LAp if pulmonary hypertension or mitral valve problems are not present. The PAp usually measures 1/4 to 1/3 of systemic blood pressure. The average mean PAp is 15 mmHg, with a range of 10–20 mmHg. During the postoperative period, PAp as high as 25 mmHg may be tolerated [24, 26, 46]. Elevated PAp may indicate an obstruction in the pulmonary embolus, pulmonary hypertension, pulmonary vascular obstructive disease, reactive airway, lung disease, the presence of acidosis, a large left to right intracardiac shunt, increased LAp, or mechanical obstruction of the airway. Decreased PAp may indicate hypovolemia, decreased cardiac output, or obstruction to pulmonary blood flow [24]. Continuous recordings done as the PA catheter is pulled back from the pulmonary artery into the right ventricle may indicate the pressure of a residual right ventricle outflow tract obstruction in patients post-Tetralogy of Fallot repair [47]. Oxygen saturation values obtained from the pulmonary arteries are true mixed venous saturations, with a normal value of slightly less than 80 %. High PA oxygen saturation values may indicate the presence of a significant left to right intracardiac shunt, possibly a ventricular septal defect [26].

Mean PAp greater than 25 mmHg at rest constitutes pulmonary hypertension (PHTN) [48]. After surgery, the effect of PAp on patient outcome depends upon many factors, especially the preoperative RV pressure and the postoperative circulation physiology. For example, a patient with systemic level PAp preoperatively may tolerate ½ to ¾ systemic RV pressure well after operation; however, a patient with Fontan physiology will be seriously compromised by PAp greater than ~15–17 mmHg. Patients with increased PVR preoperatively are more likely to present with postoperative pulmonary hypertension than those with normal PVR [49].

The cause(s) of postoperative PHTN are not well understood. Pulmonary vascular endothelium dysfunction may be important in some cases, and abnormality of vascular smooth muscle and circulating vasoactive substances may all be relevant. Injury related to the effects of cardiopulmonary bypass (CPB) and activation of pulmonary endothelial vasoconstricting mediators, pulmonary leukosequestration, microemboli, hypothermia, lung disease, blood product administration, and certain medications such as protamine may all play a role [50]. During an acute pulmonary hypertensive crisis, PAp exceeds systemic blood pressure resulting in progressive right ventricular dysfunction, reduced cardiac output, and sometimes hypoxemia. In the patient with Fontan physiology, increased PAp causes decreased cardiac output and high central venous pressure. During an acute crisis, patients with existing intracardiac shunts may present with an initial decrease in oxygen saturation [51]. Other signs include tachycardia, hypotension, and elevated end-tidal carbon dioxide ($EtCO_2$) levels associated with lack of sufficient pulmonary blood flow. Early intervention is required to avoid bradycardia and impending cardiac collapse. Acute interventions include mechanical hyperventilation with 100 % oxygen, administration of sedation and analgesia that may be combined with pharmacologic paralysis, the use of inhaled nitric oxide (iNO), and promoting a situation of respiratory alkalosis [48].

Postoperative PHTN from increased pulmonary vascular resistance may be transient, but in some case persist. Treatment strategies should focus on proactive measures to prevent an acute pulmonary hypertensive crisis and avoiding precipitatory factors including hypoxia, hypoventilation, acidosis, alpha-adrenergic inotropes, sympathetic stimulation, and environmental stress. Administration of analgesics and sedation prior to stressful procedures such as endotracheal tube suctioning may be helpful in decreasing a pulmonary vasoreactive response. Measures to decrease pulmonary reactivity include maintaining an alkalotic pH (which promotes pulmonary vasodilation), providing sufficient right atrial preload and cardiac output, managing RV failure, ensuring patient comfort and analgesia, and providing optimal mechanical ventilation and oxygenation [51]. Adequate positive end-expiratory pressure (PEEP) will assist in preventing atelectasis and pulmonary vasoconstriction, though excessive PEEP may be detrimental by causing hyperinflation and elevated PVR [49, 51, 52]. Pulmonary vasodilator therapy with pharmacologic agents may assist in decreasing pulmonary vasoreactivity. Inhaled nitric oxide, a quick-acting, selective pulmonary vasodilator, is currently the agent of choice, although it is not always effective [53, 54]. Rebound PHTN associated with abrupt discontinuation of iNO may be avoided by very slowly weaning iNO (especially below 5 ppm) and a single dose of a dose of oral sildenafil citrate.

Delayed Sternal Closure

Clinical and surgical management strategies that maximize and promote cardiac output after pediatric cardiac palliative or corrective surgery are essential in decreasing morbidity and promoting positive outcomes in the ongoing struggle with congenital heart disease. One such strategy is the surgical use of an open sternotomy followed by delayed sternal closure (DSC) during the postoperative period in the PCICU. This technique was first described in 1978 in a pediatric case report and has continued to be utilized [55].

After an extensive cardiac surgical procedure, the myocardium may undergo a process of inflammation and swelling. Due to the limited anatomical space in the pericardiomediastinal area in infants and children, cardiac compression may occur in this closed sternum environment. This compression leads to a low cardiac output state due to decreased ventricular compliance, filling, and preload [56]. This phenomenon has been described by different terms in the literature such as tight mediastinal syndrome, cardiac compression, and typical and atypical tamponade [55, 57–59].

The cardiovascular (CV) surgeon will either electively or emergently leave the sternum open to allow the patient to undergo recovery and achieve an adequate state of cardiac output and hemodynamic stability. Additionally, some patients with an open sternum may require the use of a rib spreader or a splinting device to lift the sternal edges off the heart to further decrease any remaining cardiac compression. A sterile occlusive dressing is placed over the open sternum by the CV surgeon to prevent mediastinal contamination and infection.

After the patient has achieved hemodynamic stability and recovery, DSC will be surgically performed either at the bedside or in the operating room (OR). The time frame for the use of an open sternum is patient dependent; however, a range of 18–40 h with a median time of 21 h has been reported [60]. Clinical issues that may prevent DSC include, but are not limited to, implantation of a mechanical support device thru the open sternum or mediastinitis. In these situations, the sternum will remain open with a sterile occlusive dressing in place until the device is surgically removed, or ongoing mediastinitis management may include the use of a vacuum-assisted device for DSC.

Experienced and technically advanced nurses are required to provide the minute to minute bedside care for these critically ill pediatric patients. There are two specific periods of recovery that require special attention and focus. The patient recovery periods are initially after returning from the OR with an open sternum and immediately after undergoing DSC.

After returning from the OR, the nurse's ongoing bedside assessments and interventions are very system focused. Achieving and maintaining optimal cardiac output is the key goal in this recovery phase. The different indicators of cardiac function, which may include heart rate, blood pressure, filling pressures such as RAp, LAp, or CVP, pulse oximetry, urine output, near-infrared spectroscopy readings (NIRS), capillary refill, and central and peripheral perfusion, are monitored closely. The CV surgeon or intensive care medical team will order interventions that are aimed at improving any deficit in cardiac performance. The nurse is responsible for administering the intravenous fluid, medications, or ventilator changes as ordered and providing the important follow-up patient clinical assessments. Monitoring for complications such as postoperative bleeding is especially important. Patients who have undergone cardiopulmonary bypass may return from the OR with a potential for a coagulopathy problem and may require monitoring of clotting factors and the administration blood products. This recovery period is very busy and stressful. The nurse demonstrates effective time management and multitasking skills to meet the ongoing clinical needs of these patients.

The guidelines for the care of the pediatric postoperative cardiac surgery patient (see Table 75.1) provides a summary of different specialized nursing interventions and considerations for the initial recovery period [61].

Immediately after DSC, the nurse must be aware of the physiological cardiopulmonary changes that occur at the time of sternotomy closure and monitor for the corresponding hemodynamic clinical indicators. With sternal closure, the intrathoracic pressure increases which in turn causes increased pressure and compression on the heart and lungs. Multiple hemodynamic changes have been demonstrated to occur at the time of sternal closure [62, 63]. The cardiac changes will be reflected in the patient's blood pressure, mean arterial pressure, and filling pressures. Depending on the clinical indicators and assessed markers of cardiac output, the patient may require additional fluid administration and initiation and/or titration of inotropic medication infusions to assist and manipulate the patient's cardiac performance during this transition period. From a respiratory standpoint, the patient will experience decreased chest wall compliance at the time of sternal closure, and this will in turn impact patient oxygenation and ventilation. Monitoring of breath sounds, chest wall excursion during the phases of inspiration and expiration, pulse oximetry trends, and follow-up chest radiograph after closure will provide the nurse with important information about the patient's oxygenation and ventilation status. Ventilator changes may have to be utilized to compensate for this acute change in chest wall compliance and improve overall patient oxygenation and ventilation. Below is a summary of the hemodynamic changes associated with chest closure (see Table 75.2) [61].

The bedside nurse is the key individual in providing ongoing clinical assessments and interventions for the patient undergoing open sternotomy and DSC. Open and clear communication strategies utilized by the nurse and the managing intensive care team and/or cardiovascular surgeon are critical. The postoperative use of open sternotomy and delayed sternal closure has become a proven strategy in the surgical

Table 75.1 Guidelines for care of the pediatric postoperative cardiac surgery patient

Patient identification
Bag/mask at bedside with fractional inspired oxygen (FiO_2) set appropriately for patient diagnosis
Suction available
Monitor alarm limits on and set appropriately for age and diagnosis
Paced setting on/off as appropriate
NBP cuff of appropriate size
Emergency medications and vasoactive infusions dose information
Vital signs monitored – heart rate, arterial blood pressure (ABP)/noninvasive blood pressure (NBP), RAp, LAp, Pap and CVP are recorded
Review heart rate and rhythm – note regularity and assess for bradycardia/tachycardia, arrhythmias
Temperature recorded every 2–4 h (consider continuous temperature monitoring for labile neonates or patients actively being cooled)
Review invasive line waveforms and placement on CXR – interpret values
Four extremity NBP on admission of newborn, and then every shift and prn for patients with obstruction to systemic blood flow lesions
Obtain and document PR interval (every shift and prn)
12-lead ECG on admission and with arrhythmias; consider need for atrial wire tracing prn
Pacemaker setting checked every hour and prn – knowledge of underlying rhythm
Assessment of heart sounds for presence of murmurs (continuous murmur with patient on prostaglandin E_1 (PGE_1) infusion and patent ductus arteriosus (PDA) or patient with Blalock-Taussig shunt (BTS))
Assessment of perfusion – warmth of extremities, capillary refill time, presence of differential between core and peripheral temperature
Assessment of central and peripheral pulses (0 absent, 1+ barely palpable, 2+ normal, 3+ full volume, 4+ bounding)
Record amount and characteristics of all chest tube drainage hourly as needed
Assess respiratory rate and depth, evidence of distress, and quality of breath sounds every 2 h and with change in clinical status
Check endotracheal tube (ETT) placement on CXR
Identify patients at high risk for decompensation with ETT suctioning (patients with sensitive PVR)
Suction ETT once a shift and when clinically indicated: document breath sounds before and after intervention
Assess and document ventilator settings and monitored parameters every 2 h and when arterial blood gas (ABG) drawn or ventilator changes made
Assess and document $EtCO_2$ hourly and with ABG analysis
Ventilator FiO_2 set no lower than .30 to .40 for all patients except:
Patient with a BTS or ductal-dependent lesion
Ambu bag set at 100 % for all patients except:
Patient with BTS or ductal-dependent lesion – room air or 10 % greater than vent
Assess level of consciousness (LOC), orientation, and baseline behavior on admission and hourly as indicated
Assess movement and strength off all extremities
For patients <2 years of age – head circumference on admission
Auscultate bowel sounds
Assess and document abdominal girth on patient <1 year of age on admission, once a shift, and every 4 h while advancing feeds
Assess stool for color, consistency, and presence of blood
Daily calorie calculation for patients <1 year of age, NPO patients, patients receiving IV nutrition or tube feeding supplementation
Monitor serum laboratory results
Hourly documentation of all intake and output
Assess response to diuretic therapy
Skin assessment (including back and gluteal fold) on admission and with each turn
Turn/reposition patient every 2 h
Assess skin under medical devices prn as needed
Assess all surgical sites and need for dressings

Table 75.2 Hemodynamic changes associated with chest closure

Cardiac		
Blood pressure	No change or decrease	Administration of fluids
		Initiation or titration of infusion(s) of inotropic medications
		Monitor for signs and symptoms or markers of decreased cardiac output
		Obtain echocardiogram to assess for function and tamponade
Mean systemic arterial pressure	No change or decrease	Administration of fluids
		Initiation or titration of infusion(s) of inotropic medications
		Monitor for signs and symptoms or markers of decreased cardiac output
Filling pressures	Increases	Monitoring for changes in preload
Central venous pressure		Administration of fluids
Right atrial pressure		Administration of diuretic
Left atrial pressure		Monitor for signs and symptoms of tamponade
Respiratory		
Decreased chest wall compliance	Changes in ventilation	Manipulate minute ventilation by changing rate or title volume
		Obtain follow-up arterial blood gas analysis to assess patient response
	Changes in oxygenation	Manipulate with change in positive end-expiratory pressure or oxygen percentage
		Obtain follow-up arterial blood gas analysis to assess patient response

Based on data from Main et al. [62] and McElhinney et al. [63]

palliation and/or repair for infants and children with congenital heart disease.

Use of Venoarterial Extracorporeal Membrane Oxygenation (VA-ECMO)

In patients with cardiogenic shock that are failing conventional medical therapies, mechanical circulatory support should ideally be initiated early to improve survival and prevent end-organ dysfunction. Common indications for VA-ECMO in the cardiac patient include failure to wean from CPB, progressive low cardiac output, cardiopulmonary arrest, profound cyanosis from intracardiac shunting, pulmonary hypertension, intractable arrhythmias, and respiratory failure [64, 65]. VA-ECMO may be used for short-term support of the heart until return of intrinsic myocardial function, as a bridge to transplant or as a bridge for longer-term support with a ventricular assist device when myocardial recovery duration is greater than expected or not anticipated. A system for rapid deployment of ECMO during

resuscitation, or extracorporeal cardiopulmonary resuscitation (ECPR), necessitates the appropriate resources and personnel for full time in hospital coverage. This requires a skilled team including nurses, cardiac surgeons, ECMO therapists, cardiac intensivists, and respiratory therapists and consultation with specialty services that include hematology, neurology, cardiac transplantation, social services, child life, and pastoral care. The ECMO specialist works directly with the bedside nurse and members of the interdisciplinary team and is responsible for maintaining the circuit, minimizing circuit-related complications, and managing circuit emergencies.

Once the patient is stabilized on ECMO and adequate flow is established, it is necessary to identify any possible causes for patient decompensation. A chest radiograph is obtained to evaluate cannula placement, and blood tests are performed to assess tissue perfusion and end-organ function. Laboratory tests include evaluation of acid–base balance, serum lactate, mixed venous saturation, renal and hepatic function tests, and hematological studies as well as evaluation of urine output [65]. Patients may benefit from a mild degree of hypothermia in the first 24 h to prevent the progression of further neurologic injury [66]. Temperature is adjusted accordingly via the heat exchanger from the ECMO circuit, and a continuous temperature monitoring may be initiated. The patient should be evaluated for increased LV wall stress and left atrial hypertension from aortic cannula position and poor LV function predisposing the patient to excessive LV dilation, pulmonary edema or hemorrhage, and prolonged myocardial recovery [67, 68]. Echocardiography and clinical analysis are indicated to diagnose this problem. Left atrial decompression may be accomplished with a vent placed from the LA to the venous side of the circuit in the patient with an open sternotomy incision or by transcatheter approach to create an intra-atrial communication [68]. While supported with ECMO, patients are at risk for significant complications including bleeding, thromboembolic injury, neurological insult, infection, renal dysfunction, and multisystem organ failure [69–71].

Monitoring of cardiac output and hemodynamic parameters is accomplished with continuous assessment of heart rate, rhythm, arterial and venous blood pressures, and tissue perfusion. Despite adequate tissue perfusion in the presence of unstable arrhythmias while on ECMO, measures to restore atrioventricular synchrony should be taken since myocardial distension and poor recovery of ventricular function may otherwise ensue. This may be achieved with stabilization of electrolytes, antiarrhythmic therapies, cardiac pacing, and defibrillation or cardioversion [72]. Typically, mean arterial and venous pressures are monitored since ECMO flow is relatively non-pulsatile causing pressure waves to dampen. Venous and intracardiac pressures are generally low. Elevated filling pressures are suggestive of cardiac tamponade or decreased myocardial function [72]. Mean arterial pressure (MAP) varies according to size and age of the patient and is generally adequate if 35–45 mmHg in neonates or greater than 60–70 mmHg in larger pediatric and adult patients [72]. ECMO circulation is dependent on adequate preload and avoidance of increased afterload. Fluid should be

Table 75.3 Therapeutic hematologic values for the patient on VA-ECMO

PT <17 s
aPTT 60–80 s
ACT 180–210 s
Fibrinogen >100 mg/dl
Unfractionated heparin 0.3–0.7 IUnits/ml
Antithrombin III >70 %
Platelet count >100,000
Hematocrit ≥35 %

readily available to manage hypovolemia along with blood products to treat abnormal hematologic parameters (see Table 75.3). Providing a level of inotropic support may assist with assisting intrinsic cardiac ejection and maintaining adequate blood pressure if needed [73]. Increased SVR may inhibit forward flow of ECMO and inhibit tissue perfusion. Excessive use of inotropes, hypothermia, tamponade, or mechanical problems may all contribute to increased afterload and should be avoided. Pharmacologic measures for afterload reduction may be accomplished with phosphodiesterase inhibitors such as milrinone, vasodilators, and beta-adrenergic blockers [65]. Analgesics and sedatives are often used to manage patient pain and agitation as well as to minimize the effects of pulmonary and systemic vascular resistance.

Once on full ECMO support, mechanical ventilation should be adjusted to maintain adequate pulmonary venous saturation and coronary oxygenation [72]. Physical exam, lung compliance, arterial blood gas analysis, and chest radiograph results are used to manipulate ventilatory support. If increased PVR is present, vasodilator therapy or iNO may be helpful as indicated. Generalized opacification of the lungs often develops within 24 h following cannulation as a result of capillary leak and inflammation from blood contact with ECMO surfaces. This can also be a consequence of left atrial hypertension and requires urgent decompression of the left atrium. The airway should be maintained as needed with routine pulmonary toilette with gentle endotracheal tube suctioning. Caution is required to prevent pulmonary hemorrhage.

Hemorrhage and thromboembolic events are common complications while on mechanical circulatory support [73]. Blood contact with the foreign surfaces of the ECMO circuit stimulates complement and clotting cascades causing the activation of multiple blood components. This predisposes the patient to a chronic inflammatory state and thromboembolic events [72]. An immature hematologic system may complicate the anticoagulation course in the pediatric patient on mechanical circulatory support. Routine monitoring includes assessment of activated partial thromboplastin time (aPTT), prothrombin time (PT), fibrinogen, unfractionated heparin level, hematocrit, platelet count, activated clotting time (ACT), and antithrombin III levels (AT III) (see Table 75.1). Heparin is the anticoagulant that is commonly used to avoid complications related to coagulopathy. Heparin binds to AT III to suppress the coagulation effects of factor X and fibrin. If AT III levels are inadequate, heparin response may be suboptimal. Treatment with AT III or fresh frozen plasma (FFP) assists in maintaining therapeutic AT III levels. In addition, thromboelastograph (TEG) analysis is used to assess time to clot formation as well as specific properties of thrombus and may be helpful in monitoring and diagnosis of coagulation issues during ECMO support [72]. An anticoagulation monitoring protocol may be helpful to provide a standardized approach to managing hematological parameters, decrease circuit interventions, and minimizing complications of bleeding and clotting.

Patients are at significant risk for hemorrhage related to coagulopathy and anticoagulation requirement. Those who are cannulated in the perioperative phase are especially at risk due to fresh suture lines, dilution of clotting factors, hypothermia, low oxygenation, and acidosis [72]. Unfractionated heparin levels, aPTT, ACT, and other anticoagulation tests may need to be adjusted accordingly if significant bleeding is present. Bleeding may occur from surgical incisions and drains as well as within major organ systems including the cranium, abdomen, and lungs. Hypertension should be avoided to minimize bleeding. Venipuncture and arterial punctures as well as invasive or potentially traumatic procedures should be avoided whenever possible. In order to avoid bleeding, caution should be taken with endotracheal tube suctioning and when inserting nasogastric (NG) or nasojejunal (NJ) tubes. The appropriate blood products, including platelets, packed red blood cells, FFP, and cryoprecipitate, are used to treat nontherapeutic levels and coagulopathy (see Table 75.3). Exposure to blood products should be limited in order to avoid sensitization of the patients and the formation of associated antibodies that may compromise future organ transplantation compatibility.

Postcardiotomy patients are at greater risk for cardiac tamponade, inhibiting venous return to the ECMO circuit and compromising systemic circulation. Chest tubes must remain patent to allow for drainage of blood from the chest cavity, and patients with open sternotomy incisions require continuous assessment of the site to ensure a concave appearance. Signs of cardiac tamponade include tachycardia and elevated intracardiac and central venous filling pressures and convex appearance of open sternotomy dressing with subsequent hypotension. These signs may present with increased chest tube output or sudden cessation of drainage. Immediate surgical exploration of the chest is required.

Neurologic injury, including brain death, infarction, or intracranial hemorrhage, is a common complication of ECMO support [74–76]. Careful assessment of the patient's neurologic status including hourly pupil response in the sedated and anesthetized patient, level of consciousness, and assessment for seizure activity is warranted. Infants with an open fontanel should have a routine head ultrasound performed every 2 days or more frequently as needed to assess for intracranial hemorrhage [65]. Routine neurology consult following ECMO cannulation is indicated for both short- and long-term assessment of neurological status.

While analgesics and sedatives are used to provide patient comfort, it is necessary to avoid pharmacologic muscle relaxants as possible to promote optimal neurological exams and spontaneous respiratory effort as appropriate. Analgesics such as morphine and benzodiazepines are often used to promote comfort and decrease pain and anxiety while on ECMO support. Inhaled anesthetic agents, such as isoflurane, may also be used [77]. Once the patient is weaned from muscle relaxants and anesthetic agents, developmentally and physiologically appropriate pain scales are helpful in pain management.

Cardiac patients on ECMO support are at high risk for infection from multiple central and peripheral venous and arterial access sites, surgical incisions, prolonged mechanical ventilation, invasive catheters and tubes, and immune-compromised state [70]. Antibiotic and fungal prophylaxis is indicated to prevent infection while receiving mechanical circulatory support. Typical signs of infection may be unreliable while on ECMO support since temperature is regulated by the heat exchanger, and thrombocytopenia may occur as a result of platelet destruction by the ECMO circuit. Routine complete blood count and cultures while on support may be indicated to rule out infection [65].

Once on ECMO, aggressive fluid management is warranted for most patients due to fluid overload from resuscitation, low cardiac output, renal dysfunction, or capillary leak from CPB prior to cannulation [72, 77]. Fluid overload is managed with pharmacologic therapies including furosemide, fenoldopam, renal range dopamine, and other diuretic agents. Renal dysfunction is a common complication of mechanical circulatory support and a predictor of mortality for patients on ECMO [70, 78, 79]. Accurate assessment of urine output, correction of electrolyte imbalance, and monitoring renal function tests are indicated. Efforts should be directed at promoting intrinsic urine output. Ultrafiltration, continuous venovenous hemofiltration or dialysis may otherwise be indicated.

Children with complex congenital heart disease are at high risk for growth failure [80]. Traditionally, parental nutrition has been the preferred method of optimizing nutrition in pediatric cardiac patients supported on VA-ECMO because of the risks associated with inadequate gut perfusion. The effects of high-dose vasopressors on the gastrointestinal system prior to initiating ECMO [81] and the alteration in gut function secondary to CBP [82] may increase the risk of developing necrotizing enterocolitis. Use of enteral nutrition in neonates on VA-ECMO was found to be well tolerated with few complications [81].

Patients on ECMO support are at risk for pressure ulcers (PU) and decreased circulation from immobilization, potential compromised tissue perfusion, and poor nutrition. Patient position should be changed every 2 h, and skin and pressure points are assessed routinely. Due to size and distribution of mass, infants and smaller patients are at risk for developing pressure ulcers on the occipital area, while older patients are at greater risk for pressure-related wounds on sacral areas [83]. Despite site of cannulation, the patients head and body should be turned slightly at routine intervals as possible to decrease the incidence of a PU. In the patient with femoral ECMO cannulas, body alignment should be maintained enough to maintain ECMO flow and to avoid potential nerve damage to the lower extremities. In these patients, distal perfusion may be compromised enough to consider a jump graft to provide adequate distal limb circulation.

Parents with critically ill children requiring invasive life support are predisposed to feelings of helplessness and anxiety related to fear of their child's suffering, neurologic injury, or death [84]. The bedside nurse is in a critical position to provide information and organize communication with the interdisciplinary team especially during a time of uncertainty regarding patient prognosis and survival. Honest and open dialogue with families is crucial for building trust and to assist in guiding decisions. Support from social work, child life, and pastoral care services play a valuable role in assisting families in crisis.

Time on ECMO is variable and dependent on myocardial recovery or decision to transplant, transition to a longer-term mechanical support with a ventricular assist device, or withdrawal of support for severe, irreversible, end-organ dysfunction. Decannulation from ECMO support is attempted after signs of myocardial recovery are apparent with trials on decreased ECMO flow rates. Echocardiography, evaluation of pulsatile blood pressure, hemodynamic status, acid–base balance, serum lactate, and mixed venous saturation are used to determine readiness for decannulation [72]. Mechanical ventilatory support should be adjusted to provide optimal oxygenation and ventilation, and vasoactive infusions are in line and administered as needed to support cardiac output. The patient should receive adequate analgesia, sedation, and muscle relaxants to decrease stress. If the patient tolerates low flow of less than 15 % prior to clamping and adequate tissue oxygenation and perfusion for at least 60 min with the circuit clamped, decannulation may be attempted [72].

References

1. Balluffi A, Kassam-Adams N (2004) Traumatic stress of parents of children admitted to the pediatric intensive care unit. Pediatr Crit Care Med 5(6):546–553
2. Jawahar K, Scarisbrick AA (2009) Parental perceptions in pediatric cardiac fast-track surgery. AORN J 89(4):725–731
3. Catchpole KP, de Leval MR, McEwan A, Pigott N, Elliott MJ, McQuillan A, MacDonald C, Goldman AJ (2007) Patient handover from surgery to intensive care using Formula 1 pit-stop and aviation models to improve safety and quality. Paediatr Anaesth 17(5):470–480
4. Leonard P, Beattie T (2004) Is measurement of capillary refill time useful as part of the initial assessment of children? Eur J Emerg Med 11(3):158–163
5. Franck LS, McQuillan A, Grocott MP, Goldman A (2010) Parent stress levels during children's hospital recovery after congenital heart surgery. Pediatr Cardiol 31(7):961–968
6. Colville G, Cream P (2009) Post traumatic stress in parents after a child's admission to intensive care: maybe Nietzsche was right? Intensive Care Med 35(5):919–923
7. Franck LS, Ridout D, Howard R, Peters J, Honour JW (2011) A comparison of pain measures in newborn infants after cardiac surgery. Pain 153(8): 1758–1765
8. Christie P, Robinson H (2009) Using a communication framework at handover to boost patient outcomes. Nurs Times 105(47):13–15
9. NHS (2011) National Patient Safety Agency. http://www.npsa.nhs.uk/. Last viewed 12 Aug 2011
10. Lachman P, Yuen S (2009) Using care bundles to prevent infection in neonatal and paediatric ICUs. Curr Opin Infect Dis 22(3):224–228
11. Department of Health (2007) Saving lives: reducing infection, delivering clean and safe care. http://webarchive.nationalarchives.gov.uk/+/www.dh.gov.uk/en/Publicationsandstatistics/Publications/PublicationsPolicyAndGuidance/DH_078134. Last viewed 21 Nov 2011
12. Galvin P (2009) Cultivating quality: reducing surgical site infections in children undergoing cardiac surgery. Am J Nurs 109(12):49–55
13. Howard F, Brown KL, Garside V, Walker I, Elliott MJ (2010) Fast-track paediatric cardiac surgery: the feasibility and benefits of a protocol for uncomplicated cases. Eur J Cardiothorac Surg 37(1):193–196
14. GOSH Clinical Guidelines (2010) Fast track cardiac surgery. http://www.gosh.nhs.uk/gosh_families/information_sheets/cardiac_surgery_fast_track/cardiac_surgery_fast_track_families.html. Last viewed 4 Aug 2011
15. Jonas RA, Elliott MJ (eds) (1994) Cardiopulmonary bypass in neonates and young children. Butterworth Heinemann, Oxford
16. Aps C (2006) Adopting a fast track approach to cardiac surgery. Br J Card Nurs 1(4):175–179
17. Laussen PC, Roth SJ (2003) Fast tracking: efficiently and safely moving patients through the intensive care unit. Prog Pediatr Cardiol 18:149–158
18. NHS Institute for Innovations and Improvements (2006) www.institute.nhs.uk/safer_care/safer_care/Situation_Background_Assessment_Recommendation.html. Last viewed 10 Aug 2011
19. Tirotta CF, Munro HM, Salvaggio J, Madril D, Felix DE, Rusinoswki L, Tyler C, Decampli W, Hannan RL, Burke RP (2009) Continuous incisional infusion of local anesthetic in pediatric patients following open heart surgery. Paediatr Anaesth 19(6):571–576
20. GOSH clinical guidelines (2011) Pain assessment. http://www.gosh.nhs.uk/gosh/clinicalservices/Pain_control_service/Custom%20Menu_02. Last viewed 10 Aug 2011
21. GOSH clinical guidelines (2010) Postoperative pain management. http://www.gosh.nhs.uk/clinical_information/clinical_guidelines/cmg_guideline_00005. Last viewed 10 Aug 2011
22. Pearson G, Duncan H (2011) Early warning systems for identifying sick children. Pediatr Child Health 21(5):230–233
23. Bosse K, Krasemann T (2009) Is routine chest X-ray indicated before discharge following paediatric cardiac surgery? Cardiol Young 19(4):370–371
24. Roth SJ (1998) Postoperative care. In: Chang AC, Hanley FL, Wernovsky G, Wessel DL (eds) Pediatric cardiac intensive care. Lippincott, Williams, and Wilkins, Philadephia
25. Wessel DL, Laussen PL (2006) Intensive care unit. In: Keane JF, Lock JE, Fyler DC (eds) Nadas' pediatric cardiology, 2nd edn. Elsevier, Philadelphia
26. Laussen P (2004) Pediatric cardiac intensive care unit. In: Jonas RA (ed) Comprehensive surgical management of congenital heart disease. Arnold, London

27. McCance KL (2006) Structures and function of the cardiovascular and lymphatic system. In: McCance KL, Huether SE (eds) Pathophysiology: the biologic basis for disease in adults and children, 5th edn. Elsevier, St. Louis

28. Backer CL, Badden HP, Costello JM et al (2003) Perioperative care. In: Mavroudis C, Backer CL (eds) Pediatric cardiac surgery, 3rd edn. Mosby, Philadelphia

29. Wernovshy G, Wypij D, Jonas RA et al (1995) Post-operative course and hemodynamic profile after the arterial switch operation in neonates and infants: a comparison of low-flow cardiopulmonary bypass and circulatory arrest. Circulation 92:2226–2235

30. Stocker CF, Shekerdemian LS (2006) Recent developments in the perioperative management of the paediatric cardiac patient. Curr Opin Anaesthesiol 19:375–381

31. Wessel DL (2001) Managing low cardiac output syndrome after congenital heart surgery. Crit Care Med 29(10):S220–S230

32. Hoffman TM, Wernovsky G, Atz AM, Kulik TJ, Nelson DP, Chang AC et al (2003) Efficacy and safety of Milrinone in preventing low cardiac output syndrome in infants and children after corrective surgery for congenital heart disease. Circulation 25:996–1002

33. Laussen PC, Roth SJ (2005) Mechanical circulatory support. In: Sellke FW, del Nido PJ, Swanson SJ (eds) Sabiston and Spencer: surgery of the chest, vol 2, 7th edn. Elsevier, Philadelphia

34. Wessel DL, Almodovar MC, Laussen PC (2001) Intensive care management of cardiac patients on extracorporeal membrane oxygenation. In: Duncan B (ed) Mechanical circulatory support for cardiac and respiratory failure in pediatric patients. Marcel Dekker, New York

35. Hoffman TM, Wernovsky G, Wieand TS et al (2002) The incidence of arrhythmias in a pediatric cardiac intensive care unit. Pediatr Cardiol 23:598–604

36. Delaney JW, Moltedo JM, Dziura JD et al (2006) Early postoperative arrhythmias after pediatric cardiac surgery. J Thorac Cardiovasc Surg 131:1296–1300

37. Yildirim SV, Tokel K, Saygili B, Varan B (2008) The incidence and risk factors of arrhythmias in the early period after cardiac surgery in pediatric patients. Turk J Pediatr 50:549–553

38. Moltedo JM, Rosenthal GL, Delaney J et al (2007) The utility and safety of temporary pacing wires in postoperative patients with congenital heart disease. J Thorac Cardiovasc Surg 134:515–516

39. Skippen P, Sanatani S, Froese N et al (2010) Pacemaker therapy of postoperative arrhythmias after pediatric cardiac surgery. Pediatr Crit Care Med 11:133–138

40. Beke DM, Braudis NJ, Lincoln P (2005) Management of the pediatric post-operative cardiac surgery patient. Crit Care Nurs Clin North Am 17:405–416

41. Perry JC, Walsh EP (1998) Diagnosis and management of cardiac arrhythmias. In: Chang AC, Hanley FL, Wernovsky G, Wessel DL (eds) Pediatric cardiac intensive care. Lippincott, Williams, and Wilkins, Philadelphia

42. Craig J, Fineman LD, Moynihan P, Baker AL (2001) Cardiovascular critical care problems. In: Curley MAQ, Moloney-Harmon P (eds) Critical care nursing of infants and children, 2nd edn. WB Saunders, Philadelphia

43. Tabbutt S, Ittenbach RF, Nicolson SC et al (2006) Intracardiac temperature monitoring in infants after cardiac surgery. J Thorac Cardiovasc Surg 131:614–620

44. Moat NE, Lamb RK, Edwards JC et al (1992) Induced hypothermia in the management of refractory low cardiac output states following cardiac surgery in infants and children. Eur J Cardiothorac Surg 6:579–585

45. Flori HR, Johnson LD, Hanley FL et al (2000) Transthoracic intracardiac catheters in pediatric patients recovering from congenital heart defect surgery: associated complications and outcomes. Crit Care Med 28(8):2997–3001

46. Gold JP, Jonas RA, Lang P et al (1986) Transthoracic intracardiac monitoring lines in pediatric surgical patients: a ten-year experience. Ann Thorac Surg 42:185–191

47. Elixson ME (1989) Hemodynamic monitoring modalities in pediatric cardiac surgical patients. In: Rotondi P, Gould KA (eds) Critical care nursing clinics of North America. WB Saunders, Philadelphia

48. Humpl T, Schulze-Neick I (2010) Pulmonary vascular disease. In: Anderson RH, Baker EJ, Penny D et al (eds) Pediatric cardiology, 3rd edn. Churchill, Livingstone/Elsevier, Philadelphia

49. Kulik TJ (1998) Pulmonary hypertension. In: Chang AC, Hanley FL, Wernovsky G et al (eds) Pediatric intensive care. Lippincott, Williams, and Wilkins, Philadelphia

50. Odegard KC, Laussen PC (2005) Pediatric anesthesia in critical care. In: Sellke FW, del Nido PJ, Swanson SJ (eds) Surgery of the chest, vol 2. Elsevier, Philadelphia

51. Taylor MB, Laussen PC (2010) Fundamentals of management of acute postoperative pulmonary hypertension. Pediatr Crit Care Med 11(2):S27–S29

52. Kulik TJ (2010) Pathophysiology of acute pulmonary vasoconstriction. Pediatr Crit Care Med 11(2):S10–S14

53. Adatia I, Atz A, Jonas RA (1996) Diagnostic use of inhaled nitric oxide after neonatal operations. J Thorac Cardiovasc Surg 112(5):1403–1405

54. Russell IA, Zwass MS, Fineman JR et al (1998) The effects of inhaled nitric oxide on postoperative pulmonary hypertension in infants and children undergoing surgical repair of congenital heart disease. Anesth Analg 87:46–51

55. Ott DA, Cooley DA, Norman JC, Sandiford FM (1978) Delayed sternal closure: a useful technique to

prevent tamponade or compression of the heart. Cardiovasc Dis 5(1):15–18

56. McElhinney DB, Reddy VM, Parry AJ, Johnson L, Fineman JR, Hanley FL (2000) Management and outcomes of delayed sternal closure after cardiac surgery in neonates and infants. Crit Care Med 28(4): 1180–1184

57. Riahi M, Tomatis LA, Scholosser RJ, Bertolozzi E, Johnston DW (1975) Cardiac compression due to closure of the median sternotomy in open heart surgery. Chest 67(1):113–114

58. Ziemer G, Karck M, Muller H, Luhmer I (1992) Staged chest closure in pediatric cardiac surgery preventing typical and atypical cardiac tamponade. Eur J Cardiothorac Surg 6(2):91–95

59. Shore DF, Capuani A, Lincoln C (1982) Atypical tamponade after cardiac operation in infants and children. J Thorac Cardiovasc Surg 83(3):449–452

60. Riphagen S, McDougall M, Tibby SM et al (2005) "Early" delayed sternal closure following pediatric cardiac surgery. Ann Thorac Surg 80(2):678–685

61. Pye S, McDonnell M (2010) Nursing considerations for children undergoing delayed sternal closure after surgery for congenital heart disease. Crit Care Nurse 30(3):50–62

62. Main E, Elliott MJ, Schindler M, Stocks J (2001) Effect of delayed sternal closure after cardiac surgery on respiratory function in ventilated infants. Crit Care Med 29(9):1798–1802

63. McElhinney DB, Mohan RV, Johnson LD et al (1997) Open Sternotomy and delayed sternal closure following cardiac surgery in neonates: outcomes of a strategy for managing critical ill patients [abstract 202]. Presentation at annual meeting of the American Pediatric Society and the Society for Pediatric Research, May 1997, Washington, DC

64. Salvin JW, Laussen PC, Thiagarajan R (2008) Extracorporeal membrane oxygenation for postcardiotomy mechanical cardiovascular support in children with congenital heart disease. Pediatr Anesth 18: 1157–1162

65. Cooper DS, Jacobs JP, Moore L et al (2007) Cardiac extracorporeal life support: state of the art in 2007. Cardiol Young 17(2):104–115

66. Tabbut S, Ittenbac RF, Nicolso SC et al (2006) Intracardiac temperature monitoring in infants after cardiac surgery. J Thorac Cardiovasc Surg 131:614–620

67. Fuhrman B, Hernan L, Rotta AT et al (1999) Pathophysiology of cardiac extracorporeal membrane oxygenation. Artif Organs 23(11):966–969

68. Blume ED, Laussen PC (2008) Cardiac mechanical support therapies. In: Moss AJ, Adams FH (eds) Heart disease in infants, children and adolescents, vol 1, 7th edn. Wolters, Klubner/Lippincott, Williams, and Wilkins, Philadelphia

69. Chan T et al (2008) Survival after extracorporeal cardiopulmonary resuscitation in infants and children with heart disease. J Thorac Cardiovasc Surg 136:984–992

70. Susheel Kumar TK et al (2010) Extracorporeal membrane oxygenation in postcardiotomy patients: factors influencing outcome. J Thorac Cardiovasc Surg 140(8):330–336

71. Raymond TT, Cunnyngham CB, Thompson MT et al (2010) Outcomes among neonates, infants, and children after extracorporeal cardiopulmonary resuscitation for refractory inhospital pediatric cardiac arrest: a report from the national registry of cardiopulmonary resuscitation. Pediatr Crit Care Med 11(3):362–371

72. Short BL, Williams L (2010) ECMO specialist training manual, 3rd edn. ELSO, Ann Arbor

73. delNido P (1996) Extracorporeal membrane oxygenation for cardiac support in children. Ann Thorac Surg 61:336–339

74. Barrett CS, Bratton SL, Salvin JW et al (2009) Neurological injury after extracorporeal membrane oxygenation use to aid pediatric cardiopulmonary resuscitation. Pediatr Crit Care Med 10(4):445–451

75. Alsoufi B, Al-Radi OO, Gruenwald C (2009) Extracorporeal life support following cardiac surgery in children: analysis of risk factors and survival in a single institution. Eur J Cardiothorac Surg 35:100401011

76. Hamrick S et al (2003) Neurodevelopmental outcome of infants supported with extracorporeal membrane oxygenation after cardiac surgery. Pediatrics 111: e671–e675

77. Carberry KE, Gunter KS, Gemmato CJ et al (2007) Mechanical circulatory support for the pediatric patient. Crit Care Nurs Q 30(2):121–142

78. Thiagarajan RR, Laussen PC, Rycus PT et al (2007) Extracorporeal membrane oxygenation to aid cardiopulmonary resuscitation in infants and children. Circulation 9:1693–1700

79. Kane DA et al (2010) Rapid-response extracorporeal membrane oxygenation to support cardiopulmonary resuscitation in children with cardiac disease. Circulation 122(suppl 1):S241–S248

80. Peterson RE, Wetzel GT (2004) Growth failure in congenital heart disease: where are we now? Curr Opin Cardiol 6(3):275–279

81. Hanekamp MN, Spoel M, Sharman-Koendjbiharie I et al (2005) Routine enteral nutrition in neonates on extracorporeal membrane oxygenation. Pediatr Crit Care Med 6(3):275–279

82. Ohri SK, Somasundaram S, Pathi V et al (1994) The effect of intestinal hypoperfusion on intestinal absorption and permeability during cardiopulmonary bypass. Gastroenterology 106:318–323

83. Quigley SM, Curley MAQ (1996) Skin integrity in the pediatric population: preventing and managing pressure ulcers. J Soc Pediatr Nurs 1(1):7–18

84. Hickey P, Atz T (1998) Nursing perspective in the cardiac intensive care unit. In: Chang AC, Hanley FL, Wernovsky G et al (eds) Pediatric cardiac intensive care. Lippincott, Williams, and Wilkins, Philadelphia

Pediatric Cardiac Intensive Care – Postoperative Management: Nursing Considerations

76

Patricia Lincoln, Jeanne Ahern, Nancy Braudis, Loren D. Brown, Kevin Bullock, Janine Evans, Yong Mein Guan, Wenyi Luo, Nanping Sheng, and Margaret Schroeder

Abstract

Care of the patient in the pediatric cardiac intensive care involves focus on the whole patient. This chapter describes nursing care and assessment related to the impact of congenital heart disease on the other organ systems. Transition of the patient to the ward and then home is discussed, together with care of the patient undergoing cardiac catheterization. It is important that cardiovascular nurses have a broad understanding of patient progression through the cardiac care continuum. This chapter will assist staff in the education of patients and their families on the healing process and aid in setting appropriate expectations.

P. Lincoln (✉) • N. Braudis
Clinical Nurse Specialist, Cardiac Intensive Care Unit,
Boston Children's Hospital, Boston, MA, USA
e-mail: patricia.lincoln@childrens.harvard.edu;
nancy.braudis@childrens.harvard.edu

J. Ahern
Staff Nurse III, Cardiac Operating Room, Boston
Children's Hospital, Boston, MA, USA
e-mail: jeanne.ahern@childrens.harvard.edu

L.D. Brown
Clinical Educator, Cardiac Catheterization Laboratory,
Boston Children's Hospital, Boston, MA, USA
e-mail: loren.brown@childrens.harvard.edu

K. Bullock
Supervisor, Respiratory Therapy Department, Boston
Children's Hospital, Boston, MA, USA
e-mail: kevin.bullock@childrens.harvard.edu

J. Evans
Clinical Nurse Consultant, Royal Children's Hospital,
Melbourne Parkville/Victoria, Australia
e-mail: janine.evans@rch.org.au

Y.M. Guan
Head Nurse, Cardiac Intensive Care Unit, Shanghai
Children's Medical Center, Pudong,
Shanghai, China
e-mail: lilyhsu@projecthope.org.cn

W. Luo
Clinical Staff Nurse, Cardiac Intensive Care Unit,
Shanghai Children's Medical Center, Pudong, Shanghai,
China
e-mail: sally.lwy@hotmail.com

N. Sheng
Vice Director of the Nursing Department, Nursing
Department, Shanghai Children's Medical Center,
Pudong, Shanghai, China
e-mail: vivianshenying@yahoo.com

M. Schroeder
Nurse Practitioner Inpatient Cardiology, Boston
Children's Hospital, Boston, MA, USA
e-mail: margaret.schroeder@cardio.chboston.org

Keywords

Analgesia/sedation • Cardiac catheterization • Discharge instructions •
Endotracheal tube suctioning • Feeding the infant with congenital heart
disease • Gastrointestinal system • Hematological system • Mechanical
ventilation • Necrotizing enterocolitis (NEC) • Neurological system •
Postoperative bleeding • Postoperative care of the pediatric cardiac surgery
patient • Renal system • Respiratory system • Thromboembolism concerns

Introduction

Care of the patient in the pediatric cardiac
intensive care involves focus on the whole
patient. The chapter describes nursing care and
assessment related to the impact of congenital
heart disease on the other organ systems.
Transition of the patient to the ward and then
home is discussed, together with care of the
patient undergoing cardiac catheterization. It is
important that cardiovascular nurses have a broad
understanding of patient progression through the
cardiac care continuum. This chapter will assist
staff in the education of patients and their families on the healing process and aid in setting
appropriate expectations.

Respiratory Postoperative Care

Careful management of mechanical ventilation is
essential in the postoperative pediatric cardiac surgery patient. The use of positive pressure
ventilation produces changes in intrathoracic pressure and lung volumes, which may alter
myocardial function as well as pulmonary blood
flow. Therefore, the goals of ventilatory management and gas exchange must be tailored to an
individual patient's cardiovascular physiology.
Vigilant assessment of patient-ventilator interaction during the onset of spontaneous ventilation
will limit drastic changes in intrathoracic
pressure, while reducing work of breathing, both
of which may have detrimental effects on
hemodynamic stability. For clinicians, balancing
patient sedation needs and optimizing nutrition
and oxygen carry capacity will facilitate weaning

and eventual separation from mechanical
ventilation. Throughout the postoperative course,
pulse oximetry, and when available, continuous
end-tidal carbon dioxide ($EtCO_2$) monitoring,
should be employed to guide the ventilatory
management plan.

Under normal circumstances, spontaneous ventilation produces negative intrathoracic pressure,
drawing air into the lungs. This negative intrathoracic pressure augments systemic venous return
and ventricular filling while maintaining adequate
lung volume. Positive pressure ventilation, especially the use of high levels of positive end-
expiratory pressure (PEEP), may impede systemic
venous return and raise right ventricular after load
by increasing pulmonary vascular resistance
(PVR). Conversely, positive pressure may
improve left ventricular ejection by altering the
pressure gradient between intra- and extra-thoracic
blood vessels [1]. This gradient, in effect, pushes
blood out of the intrathoracic vessels, increasing
their capacitance during systole.

Maintenance of adequate lung volume near
functional residual capacity (FRC) will optimize
ventilation-perfusion matching and subsequently,
gas exchange. PVR is affected by alterations in
blood pH, alveolar oxygen tension, and lung volumes. At low lung volumes, alveoli collapse leading to hypoxic vasoconstriction and loss of radial
traction on blood vessels, resulting in increased
PVR. Alternatively, overdistention of alveoli
may lead to mechanical impedance of blood
flow, which also elevates PVR [1]. Alterations in
pulmonary mechanics or diminished pulmonary
blood flow may cause respiratory acidosis, which
will further exacerbate pulmonary vasoconstriction. In contrast, hyperoxia, respiratory alkalosis,

or alkalosis through administration of sodium bicarbonate will lead to dilation of pulmonary vasculature with a subsequent drop in PVR [2–4]. Dilation of the pulmonary vasculature will also occur with the use of inhaled nitric oxide [3, 4]. Alterations in PVR play a major role in the management of the postoperative patient with congenital heart disease (CHD), especially those with intracardiac shunting.

When intracardiac shunting is present or the surgical repair involves creating abnormal pulmonary arterial pathways, clinicians must work to balance pulmonary blood flow (Qp) and systemic blood flow (Qs), normally a 1:1 ratio. Blood flow follows the path of least resistance which generally favors the pulmonary vasculature. Excessive pulmonary blood flow will increase blood volume to the pulmonary vasculature and may damage the intima of the blood vessels leading to thickening in the vessel walls and, over time, increase resistance to flow. Also, increased pulmonary blood flow occurs at the expense of systemic perfusion. Alternatively, an imbalance toward Qs will lead to inadequate Qp, worsening ventilation and oxygenation. Careful management of PVR, systemic vascular resistance (SVR), gas exchange, and cardiopulmonary interactions will optimize Qp:Qs, thereby preserving systemic output and pulmonary function [5].

Generally, pediatric cardiac surgery patients do not have significant lung disease that complicates their postoperative course. However, the inflammatory response to cardiopulmonary bypass may affect pulmonary compliance, pulmonary interstitial fluid, and PVR [6, 7]. Moreover, poor left ventricular function, residual mitral or aortic valve disease, pulmonary venous obstruction, and fluid overload will manifest itself in the lungs with ventilation difficulties, secondary to increased pulmonary capillary volume and pressure. When pulmonary capillary pressure/volume exceeds the natural capacitance of the vessels, fluid will leak into the lung interstitium and the alveoli, causing pulmonary edema. This may exhibit as respiratory distress, decreased oxygenation, and carbon dioxide (CO_2) retention, all requiring escalation of mechanical respiratory support. The clinicians caring for the postoperative pediatric cardiac surgery patient must fully understand each individual's cardiopulmonary physiology and its impact on mechanical ventilation and gas exchange, along with the effects from cardiopulmonary bypass.

In the immediate postoperative period, clinicians determine goals for ventilation and oxygenation. Assessment of pulmonary compliance, pulmonary vascular reactivity, and arterial to $EtCO_2$ gradients will aid in patient management. $EtCO_2$ monitoring should be employed throughout the ventilation course to allow clinicians to monitor for acute changes in pulmonary blood flow and trend overall ventilation [8]. Volumetric CO_2 monitoring is preferred for its sensitivity to changes in pulmonary capillary blood flow during ventilator manipulation. Volumetric CO_2 monitoring enables clinicians to serially quantify the amount of ventilation taking place in the absence of perfusion, known as dead space, to tidal volume ratios (Vd/Vt). Vd/Vt calculations give clinicians the ability to gauge the efficacy of ventilatory and pharmacologic interventions on pulmonary blood flow. Vd/Vt calculations may also allow clinicians to predict the need for prolonged mechanical ventilation and the possibility of successful extubation [9, 10]. Moreover, $EtCO_2$ monitoring during cardiopulmonary resuscitation is an excellent indicator of the adequacy of chest compressions and return of spontaneous circulation [11].

In the patient that has undergone a complete repair, a PEEP level of $5 cmH_2O$ will maintain adequate lung volume and have little effect on hemodynamics. Gas exchange and tissue oxygenation should be optimized at the lowest possible mean airway pressure (mPaw). Pressure-controlled ventilation is a preferred mode in the postoperative period as it limits peak inspiratory pressure (PIP) and its contribution to mPaw. PIP may be adjusted to maintain tidal volumes (Vts) in the 6–8 ml/kg (mL/kg) range, with a respiratory rate that normalizes partial pressure of carbon dioxide ($PaCO_2$). Fraction of inspired oxygen (FiO2) should be titrated to achieve normal oxygen saturations.

Patients with single ventricle physiology undergo numerous palliative procedures. Due to their resultant systemic to pulmonary shunts and passive pulmonary blood flow, managing Qp:Qs is of the utmost importance. These patients are the most effected by mechanical ventilation and its alterations in hemodynamics. PEEP may be reduced to 3–4cmH$_2$O with a widened delta pressure to maintain tidal recruitment of alveoli. PIP adjustments targeting mechanical Vts in the 8–12 mL/kg range will enable clinicians to use lower ventilation rates which may lead to a marked reduction in mPaw. In addition, large tidal volumes make patients less likely to develop atelectasis and subsequent hypoxic pulmonary vasoconstriction while employing low PEEP levels. FiO2 should be maintained as close to room air as possible, in an effort to minimize the potent pulmonary vasodilatory effects of high alveolar oxygen concentrations. For clinicians to minimize FiO2 and accept oxygen saturations in the 70–80 % range, the patient's hematocrit should be maintained above 40 % to optimize the oxygen carry capacity of the blood. Utilizing these ventilation strategies while supporting myocardial contractility and systemic vascular resistance (SVR) with inotropic agents will aid in balancing Qp:Qs. Once hemodynamic stability is achieved, the patient goal should be spontaneous ventilation.

Supporting early spontaneous ventilation with the use of pressure support ventilation (PSV) allows clinicians to unload the work of breathing and normalize ventilation physiology as soon as possible. Gradual reduction in ventilator mandatory respiratory rate will facilitate increased spontaneous ventilation, culminating in a trial of straight PSV. PSV allows the patient to determine their own inspiratory time, respiratory rate, and Vt, generally leading to improved patient-ventilator synchrony and the need for less sedation. Early extubation may be successfully achieved in postoperative cardiac surgical patients; however, timing of extubation should be determined on a case by case basis due to the complexity of surgical techniques and patient physiology [12].

Ensuring patency of the endotracheal tube requires clinicians to periodically suction the airway. Suctioning an endotracheal tube is not a benign procedure and may cause bradycardia/tachycardia, loss of lung volume, acidosis and/or hypoxia, elevations in PVR, mucosal damage, and pain [13]. Any of these are capable of causing a serious event in the postoperative pediatric cardiac patient. The goal for clinicians should be to reduce the occurrence of these effects and facilitate a rapid respond to any adverse events resulting from a patient being suctioned.

Routine suctioning should be delineated to once per shift for the purpose of ensuring endotracheal tube patency. Any other instances of suctioning should take place only when clinically indicated. These patient indications include decrease in tidal volume or saturations, increased EtCO$_2$, visible secretions in the endotracheal tube, or prior to procedures that may make urgent suctioning difficult and extubation. Exposing patients to the noxious stimuli of suctioning should be limited as much as possible.

Communication regarding patient concerns begins upon arrival of the patient to the unit or following a clinical event. The goal of this communication is to ensure the entire patient care team recognizes the fragility of the patient when exposed to noxious stimuli. It is vital to determine if the patient is hyper- or hypotensive, prone to arrhythmias, or intolerant of tachycardia or bradycardia. It is also important to anticipate if the patient's oxygen saturations leave little reserve for any further desaturation or if the patient may be intolerant of hyperoxia. Other preliminary key elements are (a) to define the patient's pulmonary blood flow indicated by arterial to EtCO2 gradients; (b) to understand how reactive the patient's pulmonary vasculature may be; (c) to clarify if sedation, paralysis, or preoxygenation is necessary; and (d) to understand if inhaled nitric oxide should be preemptively available. These are questions that must be answered to determine the safest plan for managing the patient.

The patient that is susceptible to adverse events associated with suctioning is deemed "high risk" and warrants special considerations. Other examples of "high-risk" patients may be those diagnosed with pulmonary hypertension, patients with shunted single ventricle physiology, all patients less than 1 year of age for the first 24 hours following cardiopulmonary bypass, and patients with or at risk for left atrial hypertension.

Some high-risk patients may have hypercarbia or hypoxemia, require inhaled nitric oxide, be in a low cardiac output state, or need high-frequency ventilation.

Once the team has acknowledged a patient's fragility, a multidisciplinary discussion should take place at the bedside to determine any concerns related to endotracheal tube suctioning and what precautions are necessary to prevent any adverse events. These discussions must take place prior to suctioning the patient and daily during rounds. Precautions may include the need for sedation or paralysis prior to suctioning, endotracheal instillation of lidocaine to lessen the stimulation of the airways during suctioning, bronchodilator medications, and pre-/post-oxygenation for patients on inhaled nitric oxide. Determination of a suctioning schedule for patients on high-frequency ventilation and the need for a medical provider to be present for the suctioning procedure are also considerations for "high-risk" patients.

Suctioning is never done as a single clinician procedure. This is especially true for units that utilize open suctioning rather than in-line suction catheters. Open suctioning enables pre-/post-oxygenation as well as manual pre-/post-ventilation with slightly higher ventilatory pressures to maintain and reestablish alveolar recruitment. All appropriate equipment must be at the bedside. Clinicians assess adequate oxygen flow to the anesthesia bag and that the manometer is functioning properly. For the patient on inhaled nitric oxide, the manual ventilation system with correct dosage is verified. For the patient at risk for pulmonary hypertension, a nitric oxide delivery system must be available for emergencies. Appropriate size suction catheter is selected; this should be no larger than half the size of the endotracheal tube's inner diameter. $EtCO_2$ monitoring, when available, should be used in line with manual ventilation as a monitor of pulmonary blood flow. Suction pressure is set at the lowest setting for patient size, to effectively clear secretions. This is usually 80–100 mm Hg (mmHg) for infants, increasing as high as 150 mmHg for adults [13].

Normal saline should be available at the bedside for instillation. Instill saline only if necessary and use minimum instill volume. The first pass of the suction catheter should be done without saline instillation to assess secretions and ease of their removal. Suggested volumes for saline instillation are based on patient size: 0.25–0.5 mL for neonates and infants, 0.5 mL for children 1–8 years old, and 1–2 mL for children older than 8 years.

The patient is determined to be high risk or low risk for suctioning. For the low-risk patient, a two person team may perform the procedure without additional precautions. For the high-risk patient, additional discussion takes place with the medical providers to determine necessary precautions and arrange for them to be at the bedside. Ensure all appropriate personnel and necessary equipment are present at the bedside.

Pre-oxygenate the patient for 30–60 s on 100 % $FiO2$. For the shunted single ventricle patient, blend the $FiO2$ to 21–40 %. Suction the endotracheal tube using sterile technique to minimize airway contamination. Utilize measured depth suctioning to decrease stimulation by only passing the catheter to 0.5 cm beyond the end of the endotracheal tube. If the suction catheters used have measurements, match the number on the catheter to the number on the endotracheal tube plus 0.5 cm. If the catheters do not have numbers, measure the length of the tube from the last numerical marking to the end of the endotracheal tube adaptor, then add this length plus 0.5 cm to the last numerical marking. Limit each pass of the suction catheter to 10–15 s.

After each pass, manually or mechanically ventilate the patient with the previously determined $FiO2$ for 30–60 s before the next pass. Always ventilate between suctioning, especially if normal saline instillation is necessary. Prolonged instances without ventilation may lead to adverse events. Perform up to three passes of the suction catheter, assessing the need for an additional pass after each time.

When the patient requires no further suctioning, post-oxygenate at the higher FiO_2 for at least sixty seconds before returning to the original FiO_2. If in-line suctioning was utilized, consider a temporary increase in ventilatory support to aid in the post-suction recovery. Clinicians must be vigilant and remember to decrease the ventilatory support to its original level following the recovery period. Upon completion of the suctioning procedure, clinicians should assess breath sounds, color, respiratory effort, visual evidence of secretions, $EtCO_2$, V_T, hemodynamics, and oxygen saturation to determine patient tolerance. The procedure and patient response should be documented in the medical record and discussed daily during rounds. Pediatric cardiac patients are a fragile population that requires vigilant assessment and specific ventilator management. When necessary, procedures with increased risk may need to be conducted; however, specific plans must be in place to expedite treatment and minimize the potential for adverse events.

Neurological Postoperative Care

Children undergoing surgery for congenital heart disease (CHD) have a reported incidence of neurological complications of 2–25 % [14, 15]. Postoperative neurological complications commonly seen include seizures, cerebral infarctions, periventricular leukomalacia [15], and hemorrhage. Associated risk factors for neurological injury are complex surgery, metabolic acidosis, elevated lactate levels [16], and young age [17]. Neurological care post-cardiac surgery involves the identification of complications and management to prevent or reduce neurological injury, thus improving neurodevelopmental outcomes [18]. The focus of care includes assurance of adequate cardiac output, neurological examination, observation for seizures, and the use of neuromonitoring devices.

Neurological complications may be a result of preoperative brain abnormalities or injury from intraoperative or postoperative events [19]. Preoperative neurological abnormalities include brain or brain blood vessel malformations [14], which are more common in complex lesions such as hypoplastic left heart syndrome (HLHS) [19], genetic defects [14], embolic events from right to left shunting, or brain abscess formation in older children with cyanotic CHD [15]. Intraoperative and postoperative events may result in injury due to cerebral hypoxia/ischemia or cardiac reperfusion complications [15]. Causative factors include the use of cardiopulmonary bypass, deep hypothermic cardiac arrest, low cardiac output states, impaired cerebral autoregulation post-circulatory arrest [18, 19], hypoglycemia, and electrolyte imbalances [14, 15, 20].

Postoperative neurological care must ensure that effective cerebral perfusion is maintained via adequate cardiac output. This also reduces secondary injury to any cells that have been damaged during the surgery. Elevated serum lactate levels and metabolic acidosis are markers of inadequate tissue perfusion and also associated with poor neurological outcomes [16].

The patient should receive a thorough neurological examination on arrival from operating room and then after at regular intervals. The exam involves assessment of consciousness state, pupillary size and reaction, fontanel fullness, the appearance of posturing, and limb movement and strength. Sedatives and paralysis will limit the effectiveness of the clinical exam to some extent [18]. Lower motor deficits after surgery to repair coarctation of the aorta may be attributable to the rare risk of spinal cord ischemia.

Seizures are a common postoperative problem [15, 20]; however, up to half are unable to be detected clinically [19]. Evidence of seizures should be observed for closely. In the muscle relaxed or heavily sedated patient, seizures may be difficult to identify; however, changes in heart rate, blood pressure, and pupils may be observed. Electroencephalogram (EEG) monitoring may be used in some units to help identify seizures. If the child exhibits seizure activity, blood levels of glucose, calcium, magnesium [20], as well as blood oxygen and carbon dioxide must be checked, to identify correctible causes. Anticonvulsants may be ordered, though these must be administered with caution as some have a myocardial depressant effect.

Neuromonitoring is a relatively new area in postoperative management, with most reported experience during the perioperative period. Neuromonitoring, which is applied and interpreted at the bedside, allows for identification of problems that may be hidden by sedation and paralysis. Available techniques in the intensive care areas include cerebral tissue oxygenation and simple EEG monitoring. Near-infrared spectroscopy (NIRS) monitors regional cerebral tissue oxygenation (rSo_2i) via a probe attached to the forehead. The exact baseline reading for rSo_2i will differ depending on individual patient cardiac defects [16], thus trends are more important. Some studies demonstrate a correlation between central venous saturations and rSo_2i; however there are wide limits of agreement [21]. Early evidence appears to reveal a link between a low rSo_2i, ischemic changes on magnetic resonance imaging (MRI) [18, 19, 21], and poor neurological outcomes [14], though the threshold for injury occurrence is undefined [16]. Bispectral Index (BIS) is another form of neuromonitoring. It is simplified EEG monitoring involving electrodes placed on the forehead and temple that converts raw EEG data to an index score via an algorithm. It is used commonly to monitor depth of anesthesia [14]. The BIS will decrease in the presence of cerebral ischemia [22]; however, readings may also be affected by medications, and its effectiveness in infants and children is still unclear [14]. It may be that multimodal neuromonitoring is more effective than one type alone [14].

Gastrointestinal, Genitourinary, and Hematological Postoperative Care

The incidence of gastrointestinal (GI) complications is low among children undergoing the cardiac surgery; however, its occurrence may lead to serious outcomes in these fragile patients, especially neonates. The knowledge of potential GI complications is essential to promote pediatric cardiac surgery recovery. The most common GI complications following surgery for congenital heart disease include upper digestive tract bleeding, necrotic enteritis (NEC), and intestinal tract dysfunction.

The source of upper digestive tract bleeding is usually the development of a stress ulcer.

This condition presents as dark coffee-colored GI drainage fluid. Melena will develop as bleeding continues. If severe bleeding occurs, this may lead to hypovolemic shock [23].

Nursing management of GI bleeding includes monitoring the amount and characteristics of the patient's continuous GI drainage via an oral gastric or nasogastric tube, assuring the patient remains having nothing by mouth (NPO), and the use of normal saline (room temperature or iced) stomach lavage to control the bleeding. Pediatric patients requiring extended hemodynamic and respiratory support should be prescribed with histamine$_2$ (H$_2$) blockers and/or antacids for prophylactic use to reduce the risk of stress ulceration and gastritis [24]. Nurses should monitor the coagulation status and prepare appropriate blood products if bleeding is excessive. Intravenous medications and fluids are recommended to substitute oral intake when patients experience GI bleeding.

Necrotizing enterocolitis (NEC) is an acute inflammation of the small and large intestine by the bacterium *Clostridium perfringens* which may lead to perforation of the intestinal wall [25]. Infants with CHD are susceptible to develop NEC during both the pre- and postoperative periods. The risk of developing NEC in infants with CHD was reported at 3.5 % or 10 times the rate in normal infants [26]. The risk increased to 7.6 % for infants with single ventricle physiology. Clinicians are often reluctant to initiate and advance enteral feedings in infants with complex CHD because of this increased risk. Clinical signs and symptoms vary and include temperature instability, lethargy, abdominal distention, vomiting, bloody stools, metabolic acidosis, and presence of pneumatosis intestinalis on abdominal radiograph [27]. Neonates are more susceptible to decreased gut perfusion, especially those with low cardiac output or an interruption in systemic perfusion, such as the preoperative infant receiving an intravenous (IV) infusion of prostaglandin E_1 (PGE$_1$) to maintain their PDA or a postoperative infant with a systemic to pulmonary shunt.

Key issues of nursing management for infants with NEC include maintaining the patient as NPO, initiation of hyperalimentation nutritional support, and institution of antibiotic therapy. Serum electrolyte levels are monitored and imbalances corrected as needed. Abdominal girth is measured every 4–6 h to observe for distention. The head of bed is elevated at a 30° angle to assist with ventilation if abdominal distention is present. Serial radiographs of the abdomen are obtained to assess disease progression. All stools are tested for the presence of blood. Fluid resuscitation and inotropic support may also be needed in these patients, depending on the severity and timing of the NEC diagnosis.

Alteration in hepatic function may occur in the patient with a low perfusion state after cardiopulmonary bypass [28]. In addition, the presence of elevated right-sided heart pressure may add to hepatic congestion. Liver function tests are monitored in any high-risk patient. Medication doses may be adjusted for the patient with altered hepatic function. Some infants may develop hyperbilirubinemia. Phototherapy is initiated for those neonates with severe jaundice.

Intestinal dysfunction is common in infants following CHD surgery. This is related to mucosal edema of the intestinal wall results from use of cardiopulmonary bypass, decreased perfusion of GI tract with low cardiac output, and administration of sedation and muscle relaxants which may decrease intestinal peristalsis. Clinical symptoms of intestinal dysfunction are abdominal distention, vomiting, and diarrhea.

Acute genitourinary (GU) dysfunction may develop as a complication at post-cardiopulmonary bypass due to low cardiac output and decreased kidney perfusion. Hypovolemia will promote vasopressin and antidiuretic hormone production to increase the amount of fluid reabsorbed in the body. Decreased body temperature will further reduce renal blood flow. Since neonates have immature GU systems and decreased glomerular filtration, any factors that affect the renal flow will also impact to their GU function.

Adequate cardiac output and organ perfusion status may be evaluated through many methods including renal blood flow and urinary volume. At first, urinary volume may be adequate due to the additional fluids infused during the intraoperative period. Subsequently, urine volume becomes less as blood glucose increases as a stress response to surgery and cardiopulmonary bypass, postoperative fluid shifts occur, and cardiac output decreases. For patients after cardiac surgery, the minimal acceptable urinary volume is 0.5–1 mL/kg/h for the pediatric patients and 30 mL/h for adults. Diuretics are recommended beginning late on the day of surgery or on the first postoperative day to prevent fluid overload. Strict and hourly measurement of intake and output is necessary to assess patients' fluid balance. Fluid needs and evaluation of diuretic effects are based on reviewing daily fluid balances during the postoperative period. Adverse effects of diuretic therapy include the loss of sodium, potassium, and chloride and may result in the development of metabolic alkalosis or possible cardiac arrhythmias. The decision to provide electrolyte supplement depends on the results from serum electrolyte monitoring [23]. Blood urea nitrogen, creatinine, and specific gravity of urine are important data to evaluate the GU function and intravascular volume. Also hemoglobinuria is common during the immediate postoperative period, resulting from erythrocyte damage from the use of cardiopulmonary bypass. Hemoglobinuria presents as red or brown colored urine [23]. This discoloration will clear slowly over the first few hours postoperatively.

Bleeding after pediatric cardiac surgery includes both active bleeding and diffuse oozing. Active bleeding occurs rapidly. The speed of diffuse oozing is comparatively slower and typically results from coagulation or platelet dysfunction due to the cardiopulmonary bypass, lack of available clotting factors, or presence of unneutralized heparin. Cyanotic patients experience diffuse oozing more frequently after cardiac surgery, due to abnormal coagulation.

Chest drains must remain patent to evacuate blood, thus protecting the patient's heart and lungs from fluid accumulation. Chest drainage > 10 mL/kg over 1 h or 3 mL/kg/h over 3 h is of concern. Characteristics of the fluid from chest drains must be observed and recorded accurately. Laboratory tests for hemoglobin, hematocrit, and platelet count are done when the patient is admitted to intensive care unit after surgery. If excessive bleeding is present, clotting factors should be assessed at that time. Otherwise, once the patient's temperature is stable and the hematologic effects of cardiopulmonary bypass are controlled, clotting factors are evaluated 6–8 h postoperatively.

Blood products are administered to correct any abnormal laboratory values. An acyanotic patient with hematocrit < 40% is treated with red blood cells/μl (RBC/mcL) is usually treated with 10–15 mL/kg of packed red blood cells (PRBCs), whereas the cyanotic patient with hematocrit < 40 RBC/mcL is treated with the same approach. Platelet replacement is considered for a platelet count < 50,000 platelets × 10^3 cells/mcL; however, patients with CHD and a platelet count < 100,000 platelets × 10^3 cells/ mcL that are experiencing bleeding need immediate attention and proper treatment. The administration of cryoprecipitate and fresh frozen plasma depends on the status of abnormal clotting factor values and the presence of bleeding. Special considerations for allosenitized or children being considered for organ transplantation may override these recommendations.

Other interventions to control bleeding include the administration of sedation and pain medications in an effort to keep the patient comfortable and to decrease oxygen consumption. If the patient presents with blood pressure instability or hypotension, fluids are administered, including blood products, colloids, or crystalloids, to maintain adequate blood pressure and filling pressures. A PEEP of 4–6 cmH2O for the mechanically ventilated patient is recommended to stanch bleeding through elevation of intrathoracic pressure. All bleeding is carefully monitored and recorded accurately to compare actual blood loss with total blood volume.

Nutritional Concerns for Infants Within the Postoperative Period

Infants with CHD are at high risk for malnutrition and growth failure related to inadequate caloric intake, decreased gastrointestinal absorption, and increased energy expenditure [29–32]. Clinicians are often reluctant to initiate and advance early enteral nutrition because of the increased risk of NEC [26, 33, 34]. Other risk factors for poor nutritional intake in the postoperative period include swallowing dysfunction, vocal cord paralysis, gastroesophageal reflux, and chylothorax [35].

Neonates with complex CHD require at least 120–150 cal/kg/day to achieve significant growth [36]. If these infants are unable to tolerate enteral feeds, goal calories for total parenteral nutrition (TPN) are recommended to reach at least 80–90 cal/kg/day [37]. Standardized feeding algorithms are used to optimize nutritional intake and limit interruptions and complications associated with the initiation and advancement of enteral nutrition. Feeding protocols have been safely used in high-risk pediatric cardiac populations and found to improve nutritional outcomes and reduce the incidence of NEC [38, 39].

Transitioning to oral feedings is particularly challenging in infants with CHD. Mothers are encouraged to breastfeed infants with complex CHD; however, these children may require enteral supplementation based on growth indices. Postoperative feeding difficulty has been described as a prolonged time to reach goal oral feeds, prolonged transition to oral feeds requiring tube feeds at time of discharge, and the need for additional procedures to facilitate feeding [40]. The exact etiology of oral feeding problems is not entirely understood and likely related to a combination of factors that spread across the continuum of care including preoperative, intraoperative, and postoperative factors.

Gestational age, low birth weight, hypoxia, poor pulmonary function, and comorbidities present several of the preoperative risk factors. Operative factors such as surgical procedure, severity of illness score, and utilization of transesophageal echocardiography have been noted to contribute to feeding problems [40]. In addition, cyanotic patients tend to have delayed time to first oral feed [41].

Cardiorespiratory issues have a strong impact on attainment of full oral feeding. Infants who exhibit signs of increased work of breathing have an inhibited ability to achieve adequate oral feeding. Cardiorespiratory instability often leads to delayed initiation of oral feeds; however, these patients are often able to engage in a regimen of oromotor exercises such as nonnutritive sucking to promote oromotor strength and decrease signs of oral aversion in the long term [42].

The effects of prolonged intubation have contributed to the symptoms of oral aversion, dysphagia, and delayed oromotor coordination [43]. Traumatic intubation and reintubation may contribute to vocal cord injury and laryngopharyngeal dysfunction. These procedures place infants at an increased risk for swallowing dysfunction and aspiration, a serious clinical concern that contributes to morbidity and could lead to serious cardiorespiratory sequelae. Following the Norwood procedure, the risk of laryngopharyngeal dysfunction reached as high as 48 % and aspiration was noted in 24 % of this population [44]. This serious complication, which often can be detected through close clinical assessment and feeding team involvement, requires the need for enteral tube placement and may increase interstage mortality among single ventricle patients.

Gastrointestinal issues such as gastroesophageal reflux, formula intolerance, malabsorption, constipation, and delayed gastric emptying affect the infant's ability to feed. Advancements in oral feeding are challenging when these issues arise, and early detection and intervention is essential to optimize the patient's clinical status and feeding readiness and ability.

Neurological sequelae that contribute to feeding delays include prolonged sedation, presence of a genetic syndrome, occurrence of a stroke, or central nervous system abnormalities. Long-term sedation alters gut motility and perfusion as well as causes a neurological state suboptimal to breast or bottle feeding [41]. In addition, symptoms of withdrawal perpetuate the cycle of feeding intolerance. Infants with CHD, especially cyanotic heart disease, are prone to developmental delay which often first presents as inability to orally feed. An estimated 29 % of children with hypoplastic left heart syndrome (HLHS) have congenital defects of their central nervous system, highlighting the need for particular attention to this population [45]. Genetic syndromes such as DiGeorge and Down's syndrome are highly associated with CHD and also an increased risk of feeding difficulties [46].

Abnormal feeding development may continue into later childhood. A 22 % prevalence of feeding disorders has been found in children with CHD at 2 years of age as opposed to a 1.4 % in the general population [46]. Patients with a univentricular repair had a higher risk of later feeding disorders than patients having a biventricular repair.

Feeding is an active social interaction between the infant and feeder and consequently is affected by psychosocial factors such as parental involvement, stress, and coping. It has been reported that mothers of children with congenital heart disease have less emotional and social interactions with their infants during feeding, which may be related to fear and stress during the feeding process [47]. Oral aversion may be generated by intubation and surgery, repeated stressors, and negative stimuli, which ultimately lead to the refusal of the infant to orally feed [48].

Definition of risk factors for oral feeding difficulties in neonates undergoing cardiac surgery is crucial, given the importance of nutrition related to postoperative healing and long-term outcomes. Nursing interventions must be implemented to decrease overall length of stay related to oral feeding problems. Nurses play a vital role in facilitating the feeding process by evaluating cues for feeding readiness, assessing feeding progress, identifying feeding issues/concerns to be addressed by the medical team, and supporting and educating families with this challenging task.

Integumentary Concerns

Pressure ulcers continue to be a significant and expensive complication that increases length of stay, morbidity, hospital readmission, and healthcare costs. The Institute for Healthcare Improvement (IHI) estimates that nearly 2.5 million people develop pressure ulcers annually and IHI's "5 Million Lives Campaign" chose the prevention of pressure ulcers as one of the 12 interventions by reliably using science-based guidelines for their prevention [49]. Breaks in skin integrity serve as vehicles for the development of infections, cause pain management challenges, psychological distress, and a significant increase in length of stay. Pressure ulcers are typically perceived as a problem for adult and elderly patients, with research and reporting related to pressure ulcer prevention primarily focusing on the adult population. However, infants and children do develop pressure ulcers, and recent studies have identified the need for pressure ulcer prevention in the pediatric patient population [50–53].

Risk factors identified in the pediatric studies were similar to those of adult patients. Pediatric cardiac surgery patients are considered especially at risk for tissue injury. Children with congenital heart disease may have lower oxygen saturations and experience altered nutritional status. In addition, these patients may have periods of decreased tissue perfusion and decreased systolic blood pressure while on cardiopulmonary bypass during their surgical repair.

The operating room environment adds additional challenges to maintaining skin integrity and preventing tissue damage. A patient under anesthesia experiences long periods of immobility without the sensation of pain or discomfort. Surgical drapes limit the nurse's ability to assess the patient. Equipment used intraoperatively may create unrealized pressure on skin surfaces. Postoperative ventilation and care in the intensive care unit also increase risk for pressure ulcer development. Identifying and addressing these risk factors in pediatric cardiac surgical patients is a cornerstone for a pediatric pressure ulcer prevention initiative [54, 55].

Ensuring that appropriate skin assessments are performed before surgery in the preoperative clinic and upon hospital admission is a component of pressure ulcer prevention. Although there does not appear to be clear consensus in the literature for completing a skin assessment, there is a document used by hospital surveyors that supports quality and is available for healthcare institutions. This document contains five key parameters relevant to skin assessment: temperature, turgor, moisture, integrity, and color [56].

Reducing the incidence of pressure ulcers in children with congenital heart disease is a nursing challenge. Strategies that involve comprehensive prevention as part of a quality improvement project have demonstrated successful reduction in prevalence and incidence of pressure ulcers. Education, engagement of the interdisciplinary team, and use of clinical expert resources have also demonstrated efficacy/value [57].

Prevention of pressure ulcers begins with identification of patients at risk. The Braden Q Scale demonstrates high sensitivity and specificity in identifying infants and children at high risk for developing pressure ulcers [58]. A valid pressure ulcer risk assessment scale facilitates the implementation of treatment options for high-risk patients such as specialty beds, nutrition plans, and redistribution mattress surfaces as well as other decisions that minimize length of stay and costs. Assessing pressure ulcer risk does not reduce the incidence of pressure ulcers; it increases awareness of the need for preventative measures and interventions [50].

If a pressure ulcer occurs, it is helpful if families have prior knowledge of preventative care processes that were in place. Proactive family education on admission helps families avoid unrealistic expectations relevant to treatment, prognosis, and staging. Content for family education includes information about redistributing mattress surfaces, importance of turning, moisture management, nutrition, and medical device management.

Skin assessment begins in the cardiac preoperative and clinic areas. Nurse practitioners facilitate the implementation of a skin assessment on all cardiac medical and surgical patients seen in these areas. Parents are questioned regarding any unusual skin conditions and encouraged to participate in pressure ulcer prevention strategies during their child's hospitalization. Perioperative nursing interventions targeting pressure ulcer risk reduction include assessment and identification of patients at risk, documentation of a thorough skin assessment, and the communication of skin alterations.

Targeted systematic interventions such as "bundles" may be effective in preventing and reducing the incidence of pressure ulcers. An evidence-based pressure ulcer prevention bundle for immobilized patients might include repositioning every 2 h and elevating heels off the bed to be implemented with support surface guidelines for at-risk patients. Compliance with a care bundle is tracked through documentation and observation audits.

For critically ill patients in the pediatric cardiac intensive care unit, the skin assessment is completed on admission and reassessment is repeated every 12 h. Clinical documentation in the patient's medical record includes skin assessment, pressure ulcer risk assessment, pressure ulcer measurement when present, turning, patient or family teaching relevant to pressure ulcers, and use of specialty mattresses or supportive structures.

Skin assessments differ from pressure ulcer risk assessments. Both need to be completed and documented in the medical record. With a skin risk assessment, a validated risk assessment tool is used to document the risk score and does not necessarily indicate that a skin assessment was completed. To validate the completion of a skin assessment, visual audits need to be completed as well as documenting the words anterior and posterior to demonstrate that the patient was turned and examined.

Clinicians assessing patients for the presence of pressure ulcers should be familiar with their institution's pressure ulcer risk assessment process and tool. The pressure ulcer risk assessment is more than just a tool with a number. The risk assessment tool is a clinical instrument that prompts a decision and possible intervention to prevent a pressure ulcer [56].

Pressure ulcer documentation also includes the presence of a condition upon admission, and the frequency of documentation is dependent upon the care setting. The pressure ulcer documentation should include wound measurement, description, pressure redistribution surfaces in place, turning schedules, and wound treatments [56].

Evaluation of staff current knowledge and education addressing skin issues is a first step in pressure ulcer prevention. Education and resources around use of risk assessment tools, proper skin assessment, pressure ulcer staging, and nursing interventions that direct prevention and treatment of pressure ulcers should be available for all nurses caring for pediatric cardiovascular patients across the continuum of care.

Education and knowledge of pressure ulcers is essential in promoting best practices. Staff competency relevant to pressure ulcer staging and skin assessments should be evaluated and ongoing education needs to be in place. Education should be repeated at regular intervals as the guidelines are modified.

Documentation and nurse-to-nurse reporting of skin issues are also essential. All aspects of nursing care and surveillance should be reviewed for staff in the cardiac operating room, intensive care unit, cardiac catheterization laboratory, and inpatient cardiovascular unit, focusing on support surfaces, skin protection, and patient positioning protocols during procedures [59].

A pressure ulcer prevention plan alone does not assure successful outcomes. A program-wide interdisciplinary team is crucial for success. Monitoring of pressure ulcer data to improve consistency and methodologies, development and implementation of appropriate strategies to attain and maintain intact skin, creative education with staff and families, and careful assessment of early signs of pressure ulcer development are all keys for success [57]. The greatest number of pressure ulcers occurs in the first 12–24 h of patient admission. Nursing shares responsibility with the interdisciplinary team and all members are charged with prioritizing and maintaining pressure ulcer prevention plans [60].

Use of Analgesia and Sedation in the Postoperative Period

The assessment and treatment of pain and anxiety is a difficult and important aspect of care for the pediatric cardiovascular intensive care patient. With the administration of pharmacological paralysis in an unstable, critically ill patient, this assessment becomes increasingly challenging. Observation of physiologic patient responses, such as hypertension, tachycardia, diaphoresis, and pupil size and reaction, may be helpful [61]; however, these may also be symptoms of withdrawal. Once the effects of muscle relaxants are no longer present, response to painful stimuli, fluctuations in respiratory movements, presence of guarding, and facial grimacing may offer more insight on patient comfort levels. Developmentally appropriate pain scales are utilized to assess degree of discomfort and effectiveness of any pain treatments [62]. The patient's level of sedation and degree of agitation may also be measured [63]. However, the use of objective measurement continues to be difficult.

In some institutions, combining opioid analgesics, such as morphine, with benzodiazepines, such as midazolam, provides effective analgesia and sedation in the pediatric postoperative cardiac patient [24, 61]. However, since opioid analgesics may cause histamine release, with resultant vasodilation and elevations in PA pressure, the use of shorter-acting, synthetic opioids, like fentanyl, may be utilized to provide analgesia without stimulating a histamine response [24]. In many situations, insufficient or excessive sedation, tachyphylaxis, dose dependence, and withdrawal associated with pain and sedative medications are potential problems. Acetaminophen and short-term nonsteroidal anti-inflammatory drugs (NSAIDs), such as ketorolac or ibuprofen, may be effective adjutants to pain therapies and are generally not associated with adverse effects of opioids and benzodiazepines. NSAIDs may cause nephrotoxicity and inhibition of platelet aggregation, therefore may be contraindicated in the presence of existing renal insufficiency or postoperative

bleeding [63]. Multimodal therapies such as Tylenol and a NSAID alternated every 6 h may be helpful. Likewise, managing nausea and encouraging the transition to enteral opioids are also important.

The introduction of dexmedetomidine for sedation in the pediatric cardiac ICU has become more widespread due to the drug's ability to provide cooperative sedation; the patient is awake and calm [64]. This may be helpful in managing the child that requires an extended period of intubation.

For the pediatric cardiac patient that is to be extubated soon after surgery, a short-acting continuous infusion sedative or anesthetic, such as propofol, may be administered until the effects of anesthesia are cleared. After a specific time frame, the medication is discontinued; the patient awakens and is successfully extubated [65, 66]. Propofol has no pain control effects so it is important to consider a pain control plan. Some centers may administer an opioid approximately 1 h before the planned discontinuation of propofol to assist in comfort management.

Developmentally, appropriate, non-pharmacological management of patient comfort is an important consideration. Massage therapy, acupressure/acupuncture, swaddling, sucrose, nonnutritive sucking, biofeedback, and use of heat/cold are examples of interventions that may be helpful in managing comfort in the PCICU. Sleep and quiet programs are also useful in promoting overall comfort of these patients and their families.

Transfer of the Patient from the Pediatric Cardiac Intensive Care Unit to the Acute Care Setting and Discharge

After the patient is safely past the critical postsurgical period, they are transferred from the intensive care unit to the ward where medications are optimized, nutrition maximized, and, with good pain control, activity slowly resumed. Steps are taken toward a safe and timely discharge to home. The complexity of the discharge of a child post-cardiac surgery varies tremendously according to the age of the patient, complexity of the disease and surgery, length of hospital course, and, of course, the needs and resources of the family. Despite the wide spectrum of complexity in the discharge process for each patient, the key topics remain the same: medications and medication teaching, nutrition, wound care, activity, follow-up visits, and primary care issues. In addition, congenital heart disease is often associated with non-cardiovascular complications, chromosomal abnormalities, and genetic syndromes, e.g., Down's syndrome, DiGeorge syndrome, Holt-Oram syndrome, Turner syndrome, and Williams syndrome among others. These patients will have additional concerns involving other disciplines that will need to be addressed during and after the discharge process.

Most patients are typically discharged on at least one or two medications, and many go home receiving multiple medications. For each medication, the bedside nurse provides verbal and written instruction on administration, side effects, and dietary restrictions as appropriate. For the infant and younger child, the parents are taught how to measure the correct dose, how to administer the dose, and at what time(s). With some supervision, the school age and adolescent patients may begin to take on this responsibility. Many medications are not made as a liquid preparation, and only a small number of pharmacies have the capability to compound, i.e., specially make a liquid preparation. Table 76.1 outlines the most common medications that patients typically discharged home are on after cardiac surgery and which of these require compounding (see Table 76.1).

In addition, specific medicines require ongoing monitoring outside of the hospital, such as enoxaparin, warfarin, and some anti-arrhythmia medications. A follow-up plan is established at the time of discharge to outline when and where blood levels will be drawn and which healthcare provider will monitor these levels.

Nutrition plays a significant role in the recovery of the child after cardiac surgery. Caloric needs and subsequent metabolic demands vary

Table 76.1 Home discharge medications (medications that require compounding are in italics)

Type of medication	Most commonly used
Diuretics	Furosemide, chlorothiazide, *spironolactone*
Anticoagulation	Aspirin, *clopidogrel, enoxaparin*, Coumadin
Afterload reduction	*Captopril, enalapril*, lisinopril
Antiarrhythmics	Propanolol, *procainamide, flecainide*
Pain	Acetaminophen, ibuprofen, codeine, oxycodone, Percocet
Anti-reflux	Ranitidine, PPIs (*omeprazole, lansoprazole, pantoprazole*)
Other meds	Sildenafil, asplenia/polysplenia prophylaxis (Bactrim, amoxicillin)

greatly according to the age of the patient and the type of heart defect. Newborns, particularly with single ventricle anatomy, complex congenital heart disease, and/or a protracted intensive care stay, have a higher metabolic demand and require additional calories beyond the recommended dietary allowance to establish growth [67]. Parents are given a recipe for the advanced calorie formula/breast milk and are shown how to mix the higher calorie formulation. Of note, breast milk varies in the amount of kilocalories per 100 mL. This should be kept in mind as calories are added to the breast milk [68]. Many of these infants are unable to meet their metabolic demands strictly through oral feeding and require enteral supplements either through a temporarily placed nasogastric tube or surgically placed gastrostomy tube.

Beyond the infant year, children with similar criteria – single ventricle anatomy and complex heart disease including heart failure and transplantation – require additional calories. High-calorie nutritional drinks are encouraged and in extreme cases, nighttime enteral tube feedings are utilized. For most post-cardiac surgical patients, a regular diet is resumed during the recovery period. A healthy, well-balanced diet that is low in salt, fat, and sugar is encouraged.

Parents and age-appropriate patients are instructed to monitor the surgical incision daily and to watch for signs of infection – increased redness, swelling, or drainage. Many surgeons use a glue-like substance, DERMABOND® along the incision, which will come off by itself, usually within 2–3 weeks. When used, sutures and staples are typically removed while the patient is still in the hospital. The sutures which approximate the chest drain openings, however, are removed at the outpatient follow-up visit. In the infant, it is not uncommon for the baby to have a low grade temperature and increased redness along the incision within the first 24 h after suture/staple removal. Steri-Strips® are sometimes applied to chest drain sites and/or the surgical incision after removal of staples or sutures, and these generally come off 7–10 days after application. No lotions, ointments, sunscreen, or powder should be applied to the incision. Itching is a normal sign of healing. To reduce the risk of infection, patients should wear a shirt over the chest area and keep fingernails short. Sun exposure darkens the scar and should be avoided after surgery, especially in the first year.

Bathing and showers are usually allowed about 1 week after surgery but scrubbing or soaking off the surgical area should be avoided to prevent possible infection. If showering, the patient should stand with his/her back to the showerhead in order to avoid direct pressure and excess water on the incision. After bathing/showering, the incision is gently patted dry.

Upon discharge home, the school age and adolescent patient are instructed to take it slow and easy for at least 2 weeks after leaving the hospital and to avoid strenuous activity for 6 weeks after surgery. During the initial few weeks, plenty of time should be allowed to accomplish tasks, and the patient should pace him/herself with return to regular activity. At the first follow-up appointment, the cardiologist will inform the patient when he/she can return to school as well as any ongoing restrictions, such as participation in gym and team sports. Rest and activity periods should be balanced and long periods of inactivity should be avoided. The sternum takes about 6 weeks to heal after open heart surgery. During this time, any activities that might cause injury to the chest or interfere with the healing of the sternum, such as bicycle riding, skating, gymnastics, swimming, or contact sports, are avoided as well as heavy lifting, pushing, pulling, or twisting movements. For the patient who is of driving age, the cardiologist will indicate when the patient may resume driving at the follow-up appointment. Once home, the patient may notice that he/she tires more easily and needs frequent rest periods. This is normal after surgery, however should improve over time. Finally, for the adolescent who is sexually active, sexual activity places a demand on the heart and the patient is advised to talk with the cardiologist about safety and resumption of sexual activity. Typically, the use of oral contraceptive pills is temporarily suspended following open heart surgery due to the increased chance of clotting complications. If the patient is using oral contraceptive pills for contraception, barrier methods should be discussed as an alternative.

Restricting activity in the toddler is very difficult; however, this age child will self-limit their activity and require minimal external limitation on the part of the parent. For infants and toddlers, parents should avoid lifting the child under the arms for 6 weeks, to allow the sternum time to heal. For the infant, there is little concern regarding activity restrictions. At the follow-up appointment, the cardiologist will indicate when the infant may re-initiate belly time. If the infant resumes belly time of his/her own accord after surgery, parents should pay attention to the cues indicating pain or tiredness.

Typically, the patient sees the cardiologist within the first 2 weeks of going home. For the infant and toddler, it is also recommended that he/she be seen by their pediatrician within the first 2 weeks. The newborn is seen by the pediatrician within the first couple of days after discharge from the hospital. Single ventricle and high-risk infants undergoing the three-staged single ventricle repair are closely followed at home between the first and second stages of the single ventricle repair (Box 76.1). For all patients who have undergone open heart surgery, at the time of discharge, parents are given a list of guidelines for calling the physician or nurse practitioner (see Table 76.2).

There are a number of primary care questions that arise as the patient is prepared for discharge

Box 76.1: Home-Monitoring Surveillance

Infants with single ventricle lesions, such as HLHS, are extremely vulnerable to even mild changes in their physiologic state following Stage I palliation, and interstage mortality may reach 10–15 %. It has been shown that certain physiologic variables such as decreased arterial saturation or poor weight gain may foretell the presence of serious anatomic lesions or intercurrent illness and that early detection would allow for life-saving intervention [69]. Many pediatric cardiac centers currently have a home-monitoring program in place that closely follows these at-risk infants between their first- and second-stage palliations. Families are provided a pulse oximeter for twice daily checks and a digital infant scale for daily weights. In addition, a logbook is provided to document oxygen saturations, heart rate, daily weights, and feeding trends. Following discharge, nurse practitioners make weekly follow-up phone calls to assess the infant's progress and discuss parental concerns.

home after cardiac surgery, including subacute bacterial endocarditis (SBE) prophylaxis, vaccine schedules coupled with palivizumab, and influenza vaccine, and general growth and development concerns. For the newborn who has never been home and the older patient who has had a complex postoperative course, a call is placed to the primary care provider's office to facilitate the transition of care.

Routine and elective dental procedures should be avoided for 4–6 months. If it is unavoidable, SBE prophylaxis is necessary. The American Heart Guidelines for SBE prophylaxis indicate that antibiotics be given prior to a dental procedure only to those at highest risk for problems resulting from SBE [70]. Prior to any dental procedures, the cardiologist should be contacted to inquire if the patient should take antibiotics before the dental appointment.

Table 76.2 When to call the physician or nurse practitioner

Temperature greater than 101.5°F (38.5°C) if > 1 year of age; temperature greater than 100.5°F (38°C) if < 1 year of age
Flu-like symptoms
Color changes (pale, blue, gray)
Increased work of breathing, excessive shortness of breath, or trouble breathing while at rest
Increased puffiness of ankles, feet, or hands
Abnormal drainage, increasing redness, or tenderness of incision
Pain not controlled by pain medication
Chest pain
Persistent bowel problems
Persistent nausea
Change in level of activity
Extreme fatigue

Vaccination for the infant prior to cardiac surgery is very important, and the vaccine schedule should be maintained according to the Centers for Disease Control and Prevention (CDC) recommendations. However, if the infant/child is to undergo open heart surgery within 1–2 weeks, vaccination is delayed until after the surgery so that antibodies are not washed out in bypass. After surgery, there is some variation regarding the timing of vaccines relating to cardiologist practice. Typically, if the infant/child underwent cardiac surgery requiring bypass, it is recommended that vaccines be delayed for a minimum of 1 month so that once given, the infant/child will be able to mount a strong antibody response. Occasionally, the type of congenital heart defect and subsequent surgery play a role in the timing of vaccines. For example, some cardiologists will not administer any vaccinations to the single ventricle infant between the first- and second-stage surgeries.

The exceptions to vaccination for the postsurgical cardiac infant/child are palivizumab for respiratory syncytial virus (RSV) and the influenza vaccine. During RSV season, palivizumab is provided to those patients who meet the criteria according to the Red book: infants and children less than 2 years of age with unrepaired heart defects, cyanotic lesions, pulmonary hypertension, or history of prematurity should receive the vaccine for RSV monthly [71]. The vaccination is administered prior to discharge from the hospital and is continued to be administered monthly during RSV season (November to April in North America). Similarly, if the infant/child meets the criteria for the influenza vaccine and has not received it prior to the admission for surgery, he/she should be given the vaccine before going home. Furthermore, members of the patient's household should be vaccinated, especially if the infant is too young to receive the influenza vaccine.

Infants and children who have serious heart disease are at risk for developmental delays. Multiple factors influence neurodevelopmental outcomes in the child with congenital heart disease. In addition to genetic and family background, preoperative factors such as prematurity, presence of cyanosis, and shock; intraoperative factors such as the use of cardiopulmonary bypass and deep hypothermic circulatory arrest; and postoperative factors such as hemodynamic instability, hypoxia, acidosis, cardiac arrest, stroke, and ischemic events all impact developmental delay [72, 73]. While severe neurologic problems such as cerebral palsy, epilepsy, and mental retardation are uncommon, there is a relatively high prevalence of other developmental issues including gross and fine motor delays, learning disabilities, inattention, hyperactivity, and speech and language difficulties [74]. The occurrence of these problems underlines the importance of community resources starting with early intervention during infancy and continuing through the child's school years to assist the child and their family struggling with neurodevelopmental delays.

As described above, congenital heart disease is often associated with chromosomal abnormalities and genetic syndromes [75]. Furthermore, many infants and children with congenital heart disease who have undergone open heart surgery, while not having a known chromosomal abnormality, have non-cardiovascular problems such as significant reflux that require additional services beyond the scope of the cardiovascular team. These patients will have additional concerns that will need to be addressed during and after the discharge process and, depending on the syndrome, may require multiple consulting services such as genetics, gastroenterology, neurology, endocrinology, and immunology.

Care of the Patient with Congenital Heart Disease Undergoing Cardiac Catheterization

Indications for a pediatric cardiac catheterization may include hemodynamic evaluations (preoperatively or pre-transplant), catheterization procedure which offers less invasive means to improve circulation (pulmonary artery dilations), repair of a congenital defect (dilation and stenting of a coarctation, device closure of an atrial septal defect (ASD)), or a palliative procedure until surgery is able to be performed (placing a covered stent in a weakened vessel, balloon atrial septostomy in a patient with HLHS) (see Table 76.3). Prior to a scheduled cardiac catheterization, pre-procedural history, physical assessment and, if necessary, anesthetic consultation are obtained. Chest radiograph, blood laboratory studies, 12-lead ECG and echocardiography may also be performed. Blood laboratory studies include a complete blood count, pregnancy test for female patients 12 years or greater or who are post-menarche, electrolytes, clotting times, and type and crossmatch. Blood type and crossmatch are necessary for most interventional procedures and infants under 5 kg. For the patient undergoing an interventional catheterization, many cardiac catheterization laboratories have a unit of packed red blood cells available in the room for the procedure.

Pre-procedural preparation for both parents and child will greatly reduce their anxiety. This is accomplished with a visit to the nursing unit and the cardiac catheterization laboratory while discussing anticipated time frames, availability of updates, and expectations from admission through post-catheterization recovery. Written information regarding the pre-catheterization

Table 76.3 Common reasons for pediatric cardiac catheterization

Diagnostic	Interventional
Preoperative assessment of cardiac defect anatomy	Device placement for defect closure (ASD/patent ductus arteriosus (PDA))
Hemodynamics in pre-Glenn/pre-Fontan anatomy	Blood vessel or valve dilations (aortic stenosis, pulmonary stenosis, peripheral pulmonary stenosis (PPS), coarctation of the aorta (CoA))
Hemodynamics in the setting of pulmonary hypertension	Blood vessel stenting (CoA, PPS)
Biopsy in the pre- or posttransplant setting	Blood vessel occlusion (collaterals)
Postoperatively for patients failing to progress	Balloon atrioseptostomy (HLHS, tricuspid atresia, pulmonary atresia/intact ventricular septum (PA/IVS), complete transposition of the great arteries (TGA))

teaching should be available to the family for reinforcement. A list of whom and where to call if questions arise, with telephone numbers, should be part of the information packet [76, 77].

Complications such as device embolization, cerebral emboli, or heart perforation are rare, however very serious, and must be considered when catheterization is performed. Meticulous neurological assessments are critical. It is imperative that the nurse be able to differentiate between an altered level of consciousness related to anesthesia or sedation and an altered blood flow to the brain from an embolized device. Cerebral emboli may cause neurological changes such as slurred speech, altered level of consciousness, decreased movement or strength on one side of the body, or unequal pupillary response. The occurrence of air emboli is another patient risk during cardiac catheterization. Frequent flushing of the procedure catheters and the use of a contrast medium injection pump during angiography are two potential entry points where an air embolus may be introduced. The symptoms of

an air emboli are similar to a cerebral emboli if the patient has right to left shunting within the heart or if the air is delivered on the systemic side of the heart [78].

The most common complication after cardiac catheterization is thrombus development in the cannulated vein or artery. This will affect the circulation to that extremity. Frequent palpation and documentation of peripheral pulses, capillary refill, and temperature of the catheterized extremity and observation of the puncture site used for access are an integral part of the post-catheterization nursing care plan.

The impact on a patient's fluid and electrolyte status caused by excessive catheter flushing and the use of contrast media for angiography should also be considered and monitored during and after the procedure. Blood laboratory specimens, including electrolytes, are obtained frequently during the catheterization procedure and are corrected with specific electrolyte replacements or IV fluid adjustments as necessary. Large quantities of injected contrast media may cause excessive diuresis, and the nurse must carefully monitor the patient's intake and output totals [78].

Blood loss may occur during the catheterization procedure from multiple access attempts, through sheath changes, and with repeated saturation sampling, and will be reflected in a decreased hematocrit level. This is also a risk of post-catheterization bleeding, which may occur externally or internally. The use of a dry sterile dressing covered with a transparent dressing allows direct visualization of the catheterization site and is more comfortable to remove than an elasticized tape pressure dressing. The nurse must monitor the vascular access dressing site and the surrounding area for the development of a hematoma. In patients with groin access for catheterization, the flank area must be monitored for possible retroperitoneal blood collection. Post-catheterization hematocrit is obtained 6–8 h after the procedure to assure homeostasis.

The temperature in the catheterization laboratory and the size of a patient may increase the risk of hypothermia during a procedure. Lowered body temperature may lead to bradycardia and could compromise patient stability. Hypothermia may be prevented by utilizing a warming device on or under the child during the procedure and controlling the temperature in the room. The nurse must monitor, during and post-catheterization, for other warning signs of potentially serious issues. Symptoms, such as tachycardia, hypotension, unexplained chest, abdominal or flank pain, or abdominal rigidity, may be indicative of internal bleeding [78].

Depending on the facility, the patient may be cared for both pre- and post-catheterization by the same nurse. This nurse completes an initial assessment of the patient before the procedure and is familiar with the child's baseline condition and the patient's medical history. Report regarding the catheterization procedure should include a description of procedure performed, identification of venous and arterial catheter sites, significant hemodynamic values, explanation of interventions performed, the amount and timing of any medications administered, the condition of the patient during the procedure, and any specific problem areas or complications noted. The administration of a continuous heparin infusion may be necessary in patients with specific cardiac device placements, post-peripheral pulmonary artery dilation, or a situation in which a narrow systemic/pulmonary shunt was explored with a catheter. Homeostasis should be established before the heparin infusion is begun. Although post-catheterization care may vary between institutions, the plan should include strict bed rest with the affected extremity maintained in extension for 4 h for venous access and 6 h for arterial access use. Vital signs, including heart rate, blood pressure, pulse oximetry, and respiratory rate, along with post-procedural sedation scoring are checked every 15 min for at least 1 h post-catheterization, decreasing to every 30 min, and then to every hour as the child becomes more alert and their condition returns to the pre-procedural baseline. Catheter insertion sites and surrounding areas must be assessed for bleeding, edema, or discoloration during the vital sign monitoring intervals along with the quality of pulses and peripheral perfusion in the catheterized extremity. Use of a Doppler device may be helpful in locating difficult-to-palpate peripheral pulses and monitoring the tone quality of the pulse for possible stenosis.

Catheterization site dressings are typically removed the morning following the procedure, and the site is then covered with a Band-Aid. Discharge teaching post-catheterization includes dressing the access site with a clean Band-Aid and avoiding tub baths and swimming for 3 days. Families should be instructed to call their physician if increased bruising or swelling is noted at the access site or there is a change in temperature from the non-affected leg. Diet is advanced as tolerated. Quiet activities are encouraged for the day of procedure, but most patients are able to return to school or their normal activities the day after catheterization [76].

References

1. Pinsky M (2005) Cardiovascular issues in respiratory care. Chest 128:592S–597S
2. Moriss K et al (2000) Comparison of hyperventilation and inhaled nitric oxide for pulmonary hypertension after repair of congenital heart disease. Crit Care Med 28(8):2974–2978
3. Winberg P et al (1994) Effect of inhaled nitric oxide on raised pulmonary vascular resistance in children with congenital heart disease. Br Heart J 71(3): 282–286
4. Azeka E et al (2002) Effects of low doses of inhaled nitric oxide combined with oxygen for the evaluation of pulmonary vascular reactivity in patients with pulmonary hypertension. Pediatr Cardiol 239(1):20–26
5. Cooper S et al (2008) Current challenges in cardiac intensive care: optimal strategies for mechanical ventilation and timing of extubation. Cardiol Young 18(suppl 3):72–83
6. Stayer S et al (2000) Changes in respiratory mechanics in infants after cardiac surgery. Anesth Analg 98:49–55
7. Shulze-Neick I et al (2001) Pulmonary vascular resistance after cardiopulmonary bypass in infants: effect on post-operative recovery. J Thorac Cardiovasc Surg 121:1033–1039
8. Walsh B et al (2011) Capnography/Capnometry during mechanical ventilation: 2011. Respir Care 56(4):503–509

9. Ong T et al (2009) Higher pulmonary dead space may predict prolonged mechanical ventilation after cardiac surgery. Pediatr Pulmonol 44(5): 457–463

10. Hubble C et al (2000) Dead space to tidal volume ratio predicts successful extubation in infants and children. Crit Care Med 28(6):2034–2040

11. Kleinman M et al (2010) Part 14: pediatric advanced life support: 2010 American heart association guidelines for cardiopulmonary resuscitation and emergency cardiovascular care. Circulation 122(18 Suppl 3):S876–S908

12. Alghamdi A et al (2010) Early extubation after pediatric cardiac surgery: systematic review, meta-analysis and evidence-based recommendations. J Card Surg 25:586–595

13. AARC clinical practice guideline (2010) Endotracheal suctioning of mechanically ventilated patients with artificial airways. Respir Care 55(6):758–764

14. Andropoulos D, Stayer S, Diaz L, Ramamoorthy C (2004) Neurological monitoring for congenital heart surgery. Anesth Analg 99:1365–1375

15. Chang T, Jonas R (2006) Neurologic complications of cardiovascular surgery. Curr Neurol Neurosci Rep 6:121–126

16. Kussman B, Wypij D, DiNardo J, Newburger J, Mayer J, del Nido P et al (2009) Cerebral oximetry during infant cardiac surgery: evaluation and relationship to early outcome. Anesth Analg 108:1122–1131

17. Trittenwein G, Nardi A, Pansi H, Golej J, Burda G, Hermon M et al (2003) Early postoperative prediction of cerebral damage after pediatric cardiac surgery. Ann Thorac Surg 76:576–580

18. Hoffman G (2005) Detection and prevention of neurological injury in the intensive care unit. Cardiol Young 15(Suppl 1):149–153

19. Cooper D, Nichter M (2006) Advances in cardiac intensive care. Curr Opin Pediatr 18: 503–511

20. Curley MA, Maloney-Harmon P (eds) (2001) Critical care nursing of infants and children, 2nd edn. W.B.Saunders, Philadelphia

21. McQuillen P, Nishimoto M, Bottrell C, Fineman L, Hamrick S, Glidden D et al (2007) Regional and central venous oxygen saturation monitoring following pediatric cardiac surgery: concordance and association with clinical variables. Pediatr Crit Care Med 8:154–160

22. Hayashida M, Kin N, Tomioka T, Orii R, Sekiyama H, Chinzei M et al (2004) Cerebral ischaemia during cardiac surgery in children detected by combined monitoring of BIS and near-infrared spectroscopy. Br J Anaesth 92:662–669

23. Ding W, Su Z (2009) Handbook of pediatric cardiac intensive care. World Publishing Corporation, Shanghai

24. Laussen P (2004) Pediatric cardiac intensive care. In: Jonas RA (ed) Comprehensive surgical management of congenital heart disease. Arnold, London

25. Chen S, Ruan H, Cheng Y (2007) Modern practical nursing. University Press, Shanghai

26. McElhinney DB, Hedrick HL, Bush DM et al (2000) Necrotizing enterocolitis in neonates with congenital heart disease: risk factors and outcomes. Pediatrics 106(5):1080–1087

27. Kalhan SC, Price PT (2001) Nutrition and selected disorders of the gastrointestinal tract. In: Klaus MH, Fanaroff AA (eds) Care of the high-risk neonate, 5th edn. WB Saunders, Philadelphia

28. Xu Z (2006) Pediatric cardiac surgery. People's Military Medical Press, Beijing 1:203-205

29. Kelleher DK, Laussen P, Teixeira-Pinto A et al (2006) Growth and correlates of nutritional status among infants with hypoplastic left heart syndrome after stage I Norwood procedure. Nutrition 22: 237–244

30. Peterson RE, Wetzel GT (2004) Growth failure in congenital heart disease: where are we now? Curr Opin Cardiol 19:81–83

31. Medoff-Cooper B, Irving SY, Marino BS et al. (2010) Weight change in infants with a functionally univentricular heart: from surgical intervention to hospital discharge. Cardiology in the young 21(2):136–144

32. St. Pierre A, Khattra P, Johnson M et al (2010) Content validation of the infant malnutrition and feeding checklist for congenital heart disease: a tool to identify risk of malnutrition and feeding difficulties in infants with congenital heart disease. J Pediatr Nurs 36(1):63–67

33. Jeffries HE, Wells WJ, Starnes VA et al (2006) Gastrointestinal morbidity after Norwood palliation for hypoplastic left heart syndrome. Ann Thorac Surg 81:982–987

34. Cribbs RK, Heiss KF, Clabby ML et al (2008) Gastric fundoplication is effective in promoting weight gain in children with severe congenital heart defects. J Pediatr Surg 43:283–289

35. Anderson RH, Baker EJ, Penny DJ et al (eds) (2010) Paediatric cardiology, 3rd edn. Elsevier, Churchill Livingstone

36. Norris MK, Hill CS (1994) Nutritional issues in infants and children with congenital heart disease. Crit Care Nurs Clin North Am 6(1):153–163

37. Jaksic T, Shew SB, Keshen TH et al (2001) Do critically ill surgical neonates have increased energy expenditure. J Pediatr Surg 36(1):63–67

38. Braudis NJ, Curley MAQ, Beaupre K et al (2009) Enteral feeding algorithm for infants with hypoplastic left heart syndrome post stage I palliation. Pediatr Crit Care Med 10:460–466

39. DelCastillo SL, Moromisato DT, Dorey F et al (2009) Reducing the incidence of necrotizing enterocolitis in neonates with hypoplastic left heart syndrome with the introduction of an enteral feed protocol. Pediatr Crit Care Med 11:373–377

40. Kogon B, Ramaswamy V, Todd K et al (2007) Feeding difficulty in newborns following congenital heart surgery. Congenit Heart Dis 2:332–337

41. Jadcherla S, Vijayapal A, Leuthner S (2008) Feeding abilities in neonates with congenital heart disease: a retrospective study. J Perinatol 29:112–118

42. Field T, Ignatoff E, Stinger S et al (1982) Non-nutritive sucking during tube feeds: effects on preterm neonates in an intensive care unit. Pediatrics 70:381–384

43. Einarson K, Arthur A (2003) Predictors of oral feeding difficulty in cardiac surgical infants. Pediatr Nurs 29(4):315–319

44. Skinner M, Halstead L, Rubinstein C, Atz A, Andrews D, Bradley M (2005) Laryngopharyngeal dysfunction after the Norwood procedure. J Thorac Cardiovasc Surg 130(5):1293–1301

45. Glauser T, Rorke L, Weinberg P et al (1990) Congenital brain anomalies associated with the hypoplastic left heart syndrome. Pediatrics 85(6):984–990

46. Maurer I, Latal B, Geissmann H (2011) Prevalence and predictors of later feeding disorders in children who underwent neonatal cardiac surgery for congenital heart disease. Cardiol Young 21:303–309

47. Lobo D, Sarkar A, Marwaha N, Singh G, Khanna SK (1992) Enteral nutrition in surgical patients. Natl Med J India 5(2):55–59

48. Imms C (2001) Feeding the infant with congenital heart disease: an occupational performance challenge. Am J Occup Ther 55(3):277–284

49. McCannon CJ (2007) Miles to go: an introduction to the 5 million lives campaign. Jt Comm J Qual Saf 33 (8):477–484

50. Bolton L (2007) Which pressure ulcer risk assessment scales are valid for use in the clinical setting? J Wound Ostomy Continence Nurs 34(4):368–381

51. Noonan C, Quigley S, Curley MA (2011) Using the Braden Q scale to predict pressure ulcer risk in pediatric patients. J Pediatr Nurs 26(6):566–575

52. Pasek TA, Geyser A, Sidoni M, Harris P, Warner JA, Spence A, Trent A, Lazzaro L, Balach J, Bakota A, Weicheck S (2008) Skin care team in the pediatric intensive care unit: a model for excellence. Crit Care Nurse 28(2):125–135

53. Curley MAQ, Quigley SM, Lin M (2003) Pressure ulcers in the pediatric intensive care unit: incidence and associated factors. PCCM 4(3):284–290

54. Butler C (2007) Pediatric skin care: guidelines for assessment, prevention and treatment. *Dermatology Nursing* 19(5):471–485. Courtney BA, Ruppman JP 22. 22

55. Cooper HM (2006) Save our skin: initiative cuts pressure ulcer incidence in half. *Nursing Management.* www.nursingmanagement.com

56. Ayello E, Capitulo K, Fife C et al (2009) Legal issues in the care of pressure ulcer patients: key concepts for health care providers: a consensus paper from the international expert wound care advisory panel. J Palliat Med 12(11):995–1008

57. Elliot R, McKinley S, Fox V (2008) Quality improvement program to reduce the prevalence of pressure ulcers in an intensive care unit. Am J Crit Care 17(4):328–334

58. Curley MAQ, Razmus IS, Roberts KE, Wypij D (2003) Predicting pressure ulcer risk in pediatric patients. Nurs Res 52(1):22–23

59. De Laat E, Pickkers P, Schoonhoven L, Verbeek A, Feuth T, Van Achterberg T (2007) Guideline implementation results in a decrease of pressure ulcer incidence in critically ill patients. Crit Care Med 35(3):815–820

60. Buckland SEM (2005) Pressure ulcer risk in the perioperative environment. Nurs Stand 20(7):74–86

61. Odegard KC, Laussen PC (2005) Pediatric anesthesia and critical care. In: Sellke FW, delNido PJ, Swanson SJ (eds) Sabiston and Spencer: surgery of the chest, vol 2. Elsevier, Philadelphia

62. Merkel SI, Voepel-Lewis T, Shayevitz JR et al (1997) The FLACC: a behavioral scale for scoring postoperative pain in young children. Pediatr Nurs 23(3):293–297

63. Jacobi J, Fraser GL, Coursin DB et al (2002) Clinical practice guidelines for the sustained use of sedatives and analgesics in the critically ill adult. Crit Care Med 30(1):119–141

64. Gerlach AT, Dasta JF (2007) Dexmedetomidine: an updated review. Ann Pharmacother 41:245–254

65. Teng SN, Kaufman J, Czaja AS, Friesen RH, DaCruz EM (2011) Propofol as a bridge to extubation for high-risk children with congenital heart disease. Cardiol Young 21(1):46–51

66. Cray SH, Holtby HA, Kartha VM, Cox PN, Roy WL (2001) Early tracheal extubation after paediatric cardiac surgery: the use of propofol to supplement low-dose opioid anaesthesia. Paediatr Anaesth 11(4):465–471

67. Quinn N (2005) Cardiac disease. In: Hendricks KM, Duggan C (eds) Manual of pediatric nutrition, 4th edn. BC Decker, London

68. Czank C, Mitoulas LR, Hartmann PE (2007) Human milk composition – nitrogen and energy content. In: Hale TW, Hartmann PE (eds) Textbook of human lactation, 1st edn. Hale Publishing L.P, Texas

69. Ghanayem NS, Hoffman GM, Mussatto KA et al (2003) Home surveillance program prevents interstage mortality after the Norwood procedure. J Thor CT Surg 126:1376–1377

70. Wilson W, Taubert KA, Gewitz M et al (2007) Prevention of infective endocarditis: guidelines from the American Heart Association. Circulation 116(15):1736–1754

71. Pickering L (ed.) (2009) American academy of pediatrics, committee on infectious diseases, red book: 2006 report of the committee on infectious diseases, ed. 28727, Elk Grove Village, IL

72. Newburger JW, Jonas RA, Soul J et al (2008) Randomized trial of hematocrit 25 % versus 35 % during hypothermic cardiopulmonary bypass in infant heart surgery. J Thorac Cardiovasc Surg 135:347–354

73. Wypij D, Jonas RA, Bellinger DC et al (2008) The effect of hematocrit during hypothermic cardiopulmonary bypass in infant heart surgery: results from the

combined Boston hematocrit trials. J Thorac Cardiovasc Surg 135:355–360

74. Wernovsky G (2006) Current insights regarding neurological and developmental abnormalities in children and young adults with complex congenital cardiac disease. Cardiol Young 16(Suppl 1):92–104

75. Ferencz C, Neill CA, Boughman JA et al (1989) Congenital cardiovascular malformations associated with chromosome abnormalities: an epidemiologic study. J Pediatr 114:79–86

76. Monett ZJ, Roberts PJ (1995) Patient care for interventional cardiac catheterization. Nurs Clin North Am 30:333–345

77. Roberts PJ (1989) Caring for patients undergoing therapeutic cardiac catheterization. Crit Care Nurs Clin North Am 1:275–288

78. Arpagaus-Lee M, Brown LD, Watson S, Gorski KA (eds) (2011) Invasive cardiology: a manual for cath lab personnel, 3rd edn. Jones and Bartlett Learning, Mississauga

Chronically Critically Ill Pediatric Cardiac Patient: Nursing Considerations

77

Sandra Staveski, Elizabeth Price, Esther Liu, Aileen Lin, Elisabeth Smith, and Michelle Ogawa

Abstract

The syndrome of the chronically, critically ill patient is emerging as life-sustaining technologies advance healthcare delivery. The occurrence of such syndrome may include long-stay pediatric cardiac intensive care unit patients, patients on ventricular assist devices as a bridge to transplant or destination therapy, complicated heart failure patients requiring home milrinone infusions, or the advanced technologies used to support pulmonary hypertension patients in the hospital and at home. This section will describe the syndrome of the chronically, critically ill patients and their complex, interdisciplinary care needs.

Keywords

Advanced practice nurses • Cardiac rehabilitation • Chronically • Critically ill patient (CCI) • Complementary therapies • Heart failure • Home infusion therapies • Interdisciplinary communication • Long-stay PCICU patients • Primary nursing • Pulmonary hypertension • Ventricular assist devices

S. Staveski (✉) • E. Price
Pediatric Cardiovascular Intensive Care Unit, Lucile
Packard Children's Hospital at Stanford, Palo Alto,
CA, USA
e-mail: sstaveski@lpch.org; elprice@lpch.org

E. Liu • A. Lin
Heart Failure Program, Lucile Packard Children's
Hospital at Stanford, Palo Alto,
CA, USA
e-mail: eliu@lpch.org; alin@lpch.org

E. Smith
Great Ormond Street Hospital for Children NHS
Foundation Trust, London, England, UK
e-mail: smithe1@gosh.nhs.uk; liz.smith@gosh.nhs.uk

M. Ogawa
Pulmonary Hypertension Program, Lucile Packard
Children's Hospital at Stanford, Palo Alto,
CA, USA
e-mail: mogawa@lpch.org

E.M. da Cruz et al. (eds.), *Pediatric and Congenital Cardiology, Cardiac Surgery and Intensive Care*,
DOI 10.1007/978-1-4471-4619-3_85, © Springer-Verlag London 2014

Introduction

Advancement in surgical interventions, technology, and medical management has improved survival outcomes of children with complex heart disease. Many will require numerous medical interventions, multiple surgeries, diagnostic procedures, and frequent clinic visits throughout their lives. The *syndrome of the chronically, critically ill patient* (CCI) is emerging as life-sustaining technologies advance healthcare delivery. The occurrence of CCI may include long-stay pediatric cardiac intensive care unit (PCICU) patients, patients on ventricular assist devices as a bridge to transplant or destination therapy, complicated heart failure patients requiring home milrinone infusions, or the advanced technologies used to support pulmonary hypertension patients in the hospital and at home.

Long-Stay Patients

Long-stay PCICU patients often face multiple episodes of instability and prolonged interventions in efforts to save their lives. Many will have resulting comorbidities from these periods of instability that require management by numerous providers. Extended stays in a PCICU require that healthcare team provide psychosocial and educational supports which may not be routine in standard care delivery. In addition, there are multiple psychosocial responses and mood alterations that accompany the physical issues associated with long stays in the ICU [1]. CCI symptom identification and management is an essential aspect of nursing care delivery. Interventions to standardize care, ameliorate symptoms, and improve communication for the patient and their families are important to minimize stressors and optimize outcomes.

The occurrence of CCI has social and emotional burdens on these children, their parents, caregivers, and the healthcare systems [2]. Relationship-focused care is an important aspect of providing a holistic approach to this complex

patient population. Primary nursing teams and advanced practice nurses (APNs) are in an excellent position to manage and coordinate plans to reduce care fragmentation, enhance communication, and minimize morbidity and mortality for these patients. Early and ongoing patient and family meetings with the interdisciplinary team provides a structured process for communication between the family and care team, helps to establish important milestones to guide patient and families, and enables the family and clinicians to tailor interventions to meet the needs of the child [3]. Detailed patient care plans should be developed in these meetings and posted prominently to improve adherence with the plan of care. Complementary and adjunct therapies such as spiritual care, music therapy, massage therapy, pet visitation, and reengagement with school are important aspects of care delivery to be considered [4]. Physical activity and formal cardiac rehabilitation programs for CCI children have emerged as required patient care for this population.

Cardiac Rehabilitation

Cardiac rehabilitation has been identified as a mechanism to optimize functional capacity. Physical therapy (PT) and occupational therapy (OT) are integral providers for assisting with early mobilization. Many benefits are associated with early mobilization, such as enhanced cardiovascular function, decreased depression, improved cognition, and preserved musculoskeletal and neuromuscular integrity. Depression and anxiety may hinder rehabilitation, and thus early psychological and emotional support is paramount to the success of cardiac rehabilitation.

At the initiation of cardiac rehabilitation, an assessment must be performed to identify specific goals associated with recovery, safety plans to be considered, and any precautions/limitations related to the disease process. The following is an example of the implementation of a cardiac rehabilitation program in a CCI patient:

Hailey is a 9-year-old girl with cardiomyopathy who is admitted to the hospital due to decompensation after an exacerbation of her congestive heart failure. She requires intravenous vasoactive infusions, aggressive diuretic therapy, and supplemental oxygen to maintain her marginally compensated physical status. She spends most days in her hospital bed because she is fatigued, even at rest. Hailey has no appetite and has lost 4 kg during this hospitalization. Although she is waiting on the transplant list for a donor heart, it may be months before one becomes available. The interdisciplinary team meets first with Hailey's family, and a smaller fraction of the team meets with Hailey to collaboratively develop a cardiac rehabilitation plan.

Cardiac rehabilitation is initiated with the overall goal of optimizing Hailey's physical, functional, and emotional status in anticipation of heart transplantation. A program is developed, which incorporates the goals of rebuilding Hailey's strength, resumption of activities of daily living, and attending the hospital school. The PCICU nutritionist performs a calorie count; Hailey's diet is adapted to meet her nutritional needs, and she now receives nasojejunal tube feedings overnight. PT, OT, and the child life specialist develop a daily schedule of activities and therapy sessions for Hailey. A large, brightly colored poster is created, which details Hailey's daily schedule. The poster is taped to the wall in her hospital room. Hailey's primary nurse and APN help keep the team and Hailey on this plan.

At a weekly interdisciplinary meeting, Hailey's progress is reviewed. She is now walking with assistance and attending the hospital school daily. The nutritionist reports that Hailey is gaining back weight appropriately. If Hailey did not meet her milestones, this would be an opportunity for the members of Hailey's care team to revise her cardiac rehabilitation program and enlist additional resources.

Given the unique nature of the CCI pediatric patient, collaboration among multiple disciplines is an important component of an effective cardiac rehabilitation program. Although cardiac rehabilitation is often initiated in the critical care setting, it should follow the patient throughout the healthcare system.

Pediatric Heart Failure

Pediatric heart failure is a complex clinical syndrome resulting from a wide array of etiologies and contributory mechanisms. It may affect children of all ages – from neonates to young adults – and present with diverse clinical manifestations. The spectrum of disease severity ranges from the asymptomatic, well-compensated child to one in heart failure with hemodynamic compromise. In end-stage disease, definitive treatment to improve long-term survival and quality of life has historically been limited to heart transplantation. However, due to limited donor organ availability, children awaiting heart transplantation face prolonged waiting list time and inpatient hospital stays with risk for hospitalization-related complications.

Recently, select patients requiring advanced heart failure therapy have been successfully managed in outpatient settings. While advanced outpatient therapies, including continuous intravenous inotropic medication administration and ventricular assist devices, offer patients and families a respite from hospitalization, they must be managed with caution. They demand tremendous patient and family education and participation, frequent communication with healthcare providers, as well as regular comprehensive clinical assessments. As a result, nurses play a critical role in ensuring the delivery of safe and effective care.

For all heart failure patients, ongoing patient and family education regarding signs and symptoms of worsening heart failure as well as side effects of therapy are paramount to maintain optimal outpatient care. For example, patients and caregivers need to recognize and report common symptoms such as respiratory distress, palpitations, dizziness, growth failure, edema, exercise intolerance, and fatigue. Infants and young children are more likely to exhibit respiratory distress and poor weight gain, while older children often have symptoms of exercise intolerance and gastrointestinal discomfort (nausea, vomiting, and decreased appetite).

Nurses must take the lead in teaching patients and families concerning medications and compliance monitoring. First-line heart failure medications include diuretics, which are primarily used for symptom relief and to maintain euvolemia. Angiotensin-converting enzyme (ACE) inhibitors (e.g., captopril and enalapril) and angiotensin receptor blockers (e.g., losartan) have been shown to improve symptoms and increase ventricular remodeling and survival. Beta-blockers (e.g., carvedilol) – which antagonize the harmful effects of sympathetic activation on the myocardium – may be beneficial. However, side effects, such as bradycardia, hypotension, and worsening heart failure, may result. Aldosterone antagonists (e.g., spironolactone) may prevent cardiac fibrosis and are used in concert with ACE inhibitors and beta-blockers.

Outpatient intravenous inotropic therapy is an option for children who are unable to be weaned from inotropic support and are otherwise stable for hospital discharge. Milrinone is the more common agent although case reports describe successful therapy with dobutamine as well [5]. These inotropes are initiated in the intensive care unit with close monitoring for hypotension, electrolyte abnormalities, and arrhythmias. If the medication is tolerated with improved heart failure symptoms, patient and caregiver education is initiated and an indwelling central venous catheter is placed. Among children requiring continuous inotropic therapy, priority status on the transplant waiting list depends on medication dosage.

Milrinone is usually dosed between 0.25 and 0.75 mcg/kg/min and has a half-life of about 2 h; the dose is adjusted for renal impairment. In the outpatient setting, specialty pharmacies are able to constitute this medication so that a single bag runs over 72 h. This is desirable to minimize frequency of medication bag and pump tubing changes; however, patient age, fluid restriction, and adequate flow rate to maintain catheter patency should be considered. For example, younger children may have difficulty carrying a large volume bag and may be more comfortable with smaller bags that require more frequent changing.

Patients and caregivers must be taught standard infusion pump functions such as priming the cassette, troubleshooting alarms, and switching batteries. Other functions, such as titrating medication flow rates, may only be performed by qualified staff. Children generally place the home pump (about the size of two large cell phones placed side by side) in a small backpack. Patients with central venous catheters are at increased risk of catheter-related bloodstream infections, so particular attention is given to teaching about sterile dressing changes, saline and heparin flushes, and signs of infection. Patient and caregivers must demonstrate core competencies prior to discharge from the hospital.

During the initial transition from the hospital to outpatient settings, patients and families should be housed in local accommodations until clinical stability is assured; this interval typically lasts for several weeks to months. Children are seen at a minimum of once a week with phone management as frequently as multiple times each day. Common complications resulting from outpatient therapy include infection, reduced catheter patency, and heart failure progression.

Nursing Delivery of a Mechanical Circulatory Support Program

Pediatric mechanical circulatory support as a bridge to cardiac transplantation for children and young people in end-stage heart failure refractory to conventional therapy was introduced to reduce the number of complications and deaths on the cardiac transplant waiting list [6].

These programs have grown and evolved, and now many are using the Berlin Heart EXCOR Pediatric® ventricular assist device (VAD) on small children and infants, providing a longer duration of support for a wide age range of children (greatest time on device worldwide to date is 1,041 days [7]). It also provides an improved quality of life during support, allowing patients to be self-ventilating, mobile, and active and optimizing recovery time post-cardiac transplantation (Great Ormond Street Hospital data, 2004–2008 [8]).

Over 50 % of patients supported with the device worldwide required bridging as a result of dilated cardiomyopathy. Other reasons for support include myocarditis and end-stage congenital heart disease [7].

Explantation of the Berlin Heart EXCOR is possible, and thus a bridging to recovery strategy may be instituted should recovery of myocardial function be observed. Destination therapy has been widely used in the adult population [9].

The use of a mechanical heart device places huge pressures on families. Consenting to implantation not only requires adaptation to the device and acceptance of the risks associated with the therapy but also requires the family to live at the hospital for a potentially lengthy period with the associated disruptions to work, parental roles, and family life. Thorough preparation of the family and child must therefore commence at the earliest possible point, ideally prior to admission to the VAD center.

Children referred fall largely into two categories, those with chronic heart failure, who may be relatively well prepared for this course of treatment, and those in acute failure for whom the discussions around transplantation and mechanical support are an enormous shock. Preparation for this second group can be especially difficult as having a sick, potentially unstable child in PCICU severely restricts the time period available for families to absorb such large volumes of information and make such critical decisions.

The families' experience should be optimized through the provision of timely, accurate, individualized, and consistent information [10]. This includes information about their child's condition, the heart transplantation process, explanations and demonstrations of the device itself, and what the family can expect over the coming days/months. Booklets [11], web-based media, and other family's experiences are invaluable to the family. The risks of the device must be conveyed and understood as part of the consent process, particularly bleeding, infection, and stroke. Cultural and religious requirements should be established and facilitated.

Where the child is of an age and development to have a suitable level of understanding, information appropriate to their level of cognitive development should be provided and they must be included in any decision-making. Family and child should be encouraged to meet existing families with children on or with experience of the Berlin Heart.

In addition to the core skills and knowledge required by all cardiothoracic practitioners working within nursing [12] an additional set of competencies are required in order to safely care for children on mechanical heart support. These incorporate the nursing roles unique to caring for patients on this type of support and are tailored to the nurse's clinical area of work. Learning takes place in both formal group sessions and individualized bedside training. Additional multimedia learning resources may effectively facilitate training.

Best practice promotes annual staff updates to ensure skills are maintained, either in group training or via multimedia web-based learning and assessment. A functioning Berlin Heart mannequin is invaluable for helping staff to gain confidence in managing the Ikus® console and also for allowing the simulation of emergency situations within a safe and supportive environment.

Implantation of the Berlin Heart takes place on cardiopulmonary bypass (CPB); therefore, children return directly to the PCICU. If only a left ventricular assist device (LVAD) is implanted, the nurse should anticipate a degree of right ventricular failure, potentially requiring support with inotropes and inhaled nitric oxide.

The priorities for the child immediately postimplantation are, as for any child post-CPB procedure, the following: to achieve hemostasis, stable hemodynamics and tissue perfusion, appropriate ventilation, and prevention of sepsis. Optimal functioning of the VAD is an essential component of this, and thus nurses caring for these patients at any stage in their course must have completed additional competency-based training.

Proactive nursing care facilitating early intervention is fundamental in optimizing patient outcomes. Specific nursing roles unique to this group of patients include the ongoing assessment of pump function, appreciation of factors that affect this, knowledge of possible consequences, and the actions required. If untreated, poor pump function severely compromises cardiac output and tissue perfusion and may encourage pump thrombus formation with associated complications.

Surveillance of the pump chamber for thrombus deposits is instrumental in preventing patient thromboembolic events, one of the largest risks to the patient on a VAD. The nurse regularly inspects the pump with a bright light source, documenting and reporting any changes noted which might necessitate the device chamber to be electively changed. Effective nursing knowledge and management of anticoagulation with adherence to guidelines is crucial in minimizing the incidence of thrombus occurrence, thus maintaining patient safety.

Although rare, prompt management of any VAD-related emergencies, including mechanical pump failure and membrane rupture, is vital in order to prevent serious harm. Regular child and device safety checks are carried out in order to anticipate problems before they escalate into emergency events, and emergency equipment is kept with the patient at all times.

Children are anticipated to require 2 weeks of PCICU support prior to ward transfer. As ongoing monitoring of organ function and anticoagulation are keys to care, a long-term venous access device should be secured during this period to enable needle-free laboratory draws once on the ward, reducing patient anxiety and infection risks.

Once the child has moved through the initial postimplantation phase of recovery, a coordinated multidisciplinary approach to rehabilitation is required, with the goal of achieving maximal restoration of physical, spiritual,

psychological, and recreational well-being [13]. This involves:

- Facilitating psychological adjustment to the device and diagnosis
- Maximizing the child's physical health through physiotherapy, mobilization, and good nutrition
- Promoting normal social interactions, play, and education
- Minimizing the incidence of complications

Often patients are too sick preimplantation to receive any significant psychological preparation and must have to adjust to the Berlin Heart device and their prognosis when they regain consciousness postimplantation. Their needs should be fully assessed by a dedicated psychologist and relevant specialist teams.

Younger children who are unable to communicate their anxieties verbally may display behavioral signs of stress such as regression or mood changes. The family needs guidance in how best to manage this. A targeted therapeutic play program is an effective strategy to assist children's acceptance of their device and should be part of the patient's pathway of care [14].

With intensive physiotherapy and nutritional support, even children who have been in chronic heart failure for some time are rapidly mobilized and quickly move beyond the confines of their hospital bed space. Caring for the active child on the Berlin Heart requires the continuous evaluation of "reasonable risk." Though the safest place to be for the child on the device is in their hospital bed surrounded by a highly skilled team, this does not necessarily promote well-being and quality of life for the child.

Instead, children are encouraged to be mobile and active, to eat and drink normally, to leave the ward area to attend the hospital school or playroom, and to participate in normal developmental activity and interactions (Fig. 77.1a–d). When the weather is dry, and the child is stable, they may venture outside of the hospital building. Practice guidelines and patient assessment must be completed for moving outside of the ward area.

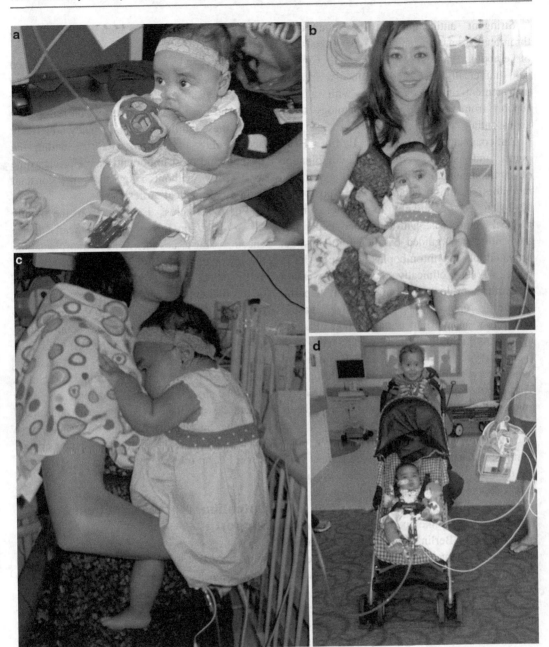

Fig. 77.1 (a–d) A child convalescing from the implantation of an LVAD

Although children are encouraged to be active, patient safety is paramount with each extension of the boundaries being fully risk-assessed and supported with identified safety procedures.

Few countries have the resources to have a dedicated Mechanical Heart Center, and consequently these patients tend to be absorbed into general or cardiothoracic critical care units and cardiothoracic wards, with the large numbers of medical, nursing, and biomedical staff that this affords. Consistency in care is established and reenforced with the use of agreed protocols, care pathways, and checklists.

Stringent anticoagulation is required if thrombus formation and the associated risk of embolus is to be diminished. Concise and universally accepted protocols for the management of anticoagulation, with ongoing support from the specialist hematology team, are essential.

Anticoagulation of the Berlin Heart pump and patient requires a combination of anticoagulants and platelet aggregation inhibitors. Anticoagulation is postponed 12–24 h postoperatively to promote initial surgical hemostasis. Unfractionated heparin is then introduced, guided by the protocol target activated plasma thromboplastin time (APTT) range. When clinically stable, conversion to warfarin or low molecular weight heparin, depending upon the patient's size, gastric absorption, and current dietary intake. Platelet aggregation inhibition is achieved with both acetylsalicylic acid and dipyridamole and monitored with platelet aggregation testing [15]. Thromboelastograms are of great value in guiding the management of mechanical heart anticoagulation.

Where vitamin K antagonists are administered, child and family should meet with the dietician or nurse specialist for support in making appropriate diet and menu choices.

VAD cannulae implantation sites must initially be treated like open wounds to decrease infection risks. Berlin Heart 2008 recommends that a consistent approach wound care be maintained. A wound care protocol will develop standardized care and assessment by nursing staff and parents [16]. Parents and other caregivers of the child are ideal to perform consistent wound care as well as providing a step into caring for their child on a mechanical heart device.

Specialists in tissue viability should be involved at early signs of any wound breakdown.

Parents are encouraged to participate in their child's care through a parent-specific skills program. This addresses skills such as moving and handling the child while on the device to emergency management and basic life support. Each family member will be supported and assessed individually on their progress in this program.

Parents and caregivers who have been assessed as competent in these skills are able to leave the ward area independently with their child and have a dramatic effect on the quality of life these families can attain. They now freely access play and school facilities within the hospital and most importantly have private time as a family without being under the constant scrutiny of medical professionals.

Enormous stress is placed on the family of a child on a mechanical heart device encompassing issues such as heart transplantation, the uncertainty of waiting times, and potential assist device complications. Consideration of other children, parental relationships, work, and financial difficulties contribute to the stress experienced. A structured psychosocial multiprofessional support system is needed to provide support the many aspects of family life. Consistent supportive communication regarding the child's clinical course is essential, and regular updates should be provided by a specified consultant/attending and clinical nurse specialist/nurse practitioner [13]. The family has regular contact with the heart transplant team.

Outpatient Mechanical Circulatory Support

With the advent of totally implantable axial pumps, mechanical circulatory support for the advanced heart failure patient is now more feasibly possible in the outpatient setting. Similar to intravenous inotropic therapy, VADs may be used as a bridge to transplantation or considered as palliation for those children where immediate heart transplantation is not an option. VAD therapy unloads the failing ventricle and maintains adequate blood flow to the vital organs. The newer generations of VADs allow patients to participate fully in rehabilitation, return to school, and overall improve quality of life. However, the success of VAD therapy hinges on patient selection, patient and family education, and ongoing follow-up.

VAD patient selection and evaluation mirrors heart transplantation evaluations. The second generations of VADs (Heartmate II, HeartWare) are continuous flow pumps designed to be more durable and totally implantable. This limits its use to a minimum body surface area of 1.2 m^2. These VADs are also only indicated for left ventricle support. Thus, body habitus, degree of potential right heart failure, and surgical risk mortality must be assessed prior to implantation. Nurses play a crucial role in providing preimplant device education, expectations of care, and assessment of psychosocial limitations. During evaluation, patients and families need to be prepared for a significant lifestyle change. VAD therapy will likely improve the child's debilitating heart failure symptoms; however, adjustment to altered body image, device care, activity restrictions, and dependence on caregivers need to be addressed. Patients and family must also have a clear understanding of the VAD risks – including potential right heart failure, arrhythmias, bleeding, stroke, infection, and device malfunction.

Immediately postimplantation, the patient and family should be integrated into the daily routine care of the VAD, thus reinforcing confidence and the capabilities of the patient and caregiver. Postimplant nursing considerations include early mobilization and physical therapy, good nutrition for optimal healing, and thorough wound care to prevent infections. The nurse will assess to what degree of autonomy can be assigned to the child in regard to VAD device care. However, ultimately the care, responsibility, and maintenance lie with the primary caregiver. Restrictions while on VAD therapy include contact sports, excessive jumping, sitting in the front seat with frontal air bags, or any activity where chest impact may dislodge the inflow cannula, water submersion as the device is dependent on electrical power, and vacuuming or build up of excessive static energy. Diagnostic tests such as a magnetic resonance imaging (MRI) are contraindicated. Changes to daily living include incorporating the use of a shower bag to protect the electrical components of the device, maneuvering with the device at all times, and performing driveline dressing changes.

Discharging Mechanical Support Patients

Some children on VADs will be discharged to home. Vital to a patient's discharge is community reintegration. This begins once the patient and family demonstrate VAD device and emergency competencies. The child and family go on excursions outside the hospital to face real-life challenges such as curbs, crowds, and chaos. A home assessment is then completed by the family before discharge to detect and remedy any tripping hazards, to clearly identify one area for all VAD supplies and equipment, to evaluate the need for assistive device needs such as shower chair, and to ensure proper electrical grounding and supply for the device. Dependent on the patient's heart failure symptoms and comorbidities, he or she may elect to return to school. Reintegration into school requires careful planning with the school nurse to ensure a safe environment.

In the event of an emergency, a VAD patient requires deviation from standard protocol. Therefore, proper notification and VAD education for the emergency medical services (EMS) are imperative. EMS must first quickly identify a VAD patient in order to prevent potential damage to the driveline site located in the abdomen. Then, utilize other physical assessments such as color, capillary refill, temperature, and the "hum" of the device when assessing an unconscious event to determine its etiology. A child with a second-generation VAD may or may not have palpable pulses due to the continuous flow of the pump. Chest compressions are generally not recommended as they can dislodge the inflow cannula causing hemorrhage. However, all other forms of advanced life support are indicated including defibrillation. A hand pump is only available for first-generation VADs.

Ongoing care and follow-up for a child and family on VAD therapy includes frequent phone triage, clinic visits, and device interrogation. Signs and symptoms of progressive heart failure, medication compliance, and driveline dressing change technique are heavily reinforced as the most common outpatient complications include infection, progression of heart failure, stroke, bleeding, and device malfunction.

Advanced heart failure therapies such as intravenous inotropic medications and VAD therapy may be administered safely in the outpatient setting. Ongoing patient education and close monitoring and assessment are paramount to its success. Patients on outpatient therapy face many challenges – physiologic, pharmacologic, and psychosocial – and depend on nursing care for successful outcomes.

Care of Children with Pulmonary Arterial Hypertension

Pulmonary arterial hypertension (PAH) is a rare, progressive, and fatal disease in which elevated pulmonary artery pressure causes increased workload on the right ventricle, leading to right heart failure and eventually the need for lung or heart-lung transplant. Currently approved PAH therapies target the pathophysiologic mechanisms that the disease may compromise. Although these therapies do not provide a cure, survival outcomes for children with PAH have improved since they became available [17]. Chronic management of pediatric patients with PAH, especially those on intravenous (IV) prostacyclin therapy, presents unique challenges to the clinician, requiring constant education and guidance for the patient and family.

Patient and family education at the time of diagnosis is vital to ensure that caregivers properly monitor the child at home and know when to contact the clinician for further medical assistance. Possible symptoms associated with PAH may include dizziness, chest pain, palpitations, shortness of breath, fatigue, and pre-syncope. These symptoms are usually exhibited with exercise or physical exertion. Syncope is a highly concerning symptom that should be cause for alarm, as it may be life-threatening. Children and caregivers are counseled to contact the clinician immediately when new onset or worsening of symptoms occurs.

Once cardiac catheterization confirms the diagnosis and severity of PAH, the child will likely be started on one or more therapies in a stepwise fashion. All PAH therapies are targeted to cause pulmonary vasodilation. However, these drugs, some more than others, can cause systemic vasodilation as well. Common side effects of these drugs can include dizziness, headache, flushing, nausea, and emesis. Intravenous and subcutaneous prostacyclin therapies may additionally cause diarrhea, lower extremity pain, and jaw pain with the first bite of food. Patients and caregivers are advised of these potential side effects. If the child becomes symptomatic when starting a new therapy or when increasing the dose, the caregiver contacts the clinician to determine if the medication dose should be adjusted or possibly changed or discontinued.

For patients on continuous intravenous prostacyclin therapy, safe medication administration at home is paramount. A minimum of two caregivers and the patient, if appropriate, must be independent in medication preparation, management of the home pump (Fig. 77.2), and changing the central venous catheter dressing. If possible, a specialty pharmacy nurse provides intensive hands-on education at home before the therapy is initiated in the hospital. Otherwise, training occurs during the child's hospitalization when the IV therapy is initiated. The patient will not be discharged from the hospital until two caregivers demonstrate their capabilities. If necessary, a specialty pharmacy nurse provides additional support at home once the patient is discharged. The clinician also maintains close follow-up and guidance as well, especially directly after hospital discharge and during times of dose titration at home.

The use of a central venous catheter with IV prostacyclin therapy increases the child's risk of acquiring a catheter-related bloodstream infection (BSI). Intravenous treprostinil use has been associated with a higher rate of BSIs, specifically from gram-negative bacteria, than epoprostenol [19, 20]. Caregivers are instructed in the use of a closed-hub system and maintaining a dry catheter-to-tubing connection when the

Fig. 77.2 Home infusion pump options for intravenous prostacyclin therapy. Treprostinil can be delivered by all three pumps. Epoprostenol can be delivered by pump in center of photo (Courtesy of Ogawa et al. [18])

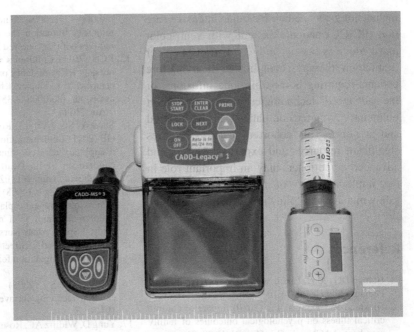

child is bathing, as these measures have been shown to reduce the incidence of BSIs among pediatric patients on IV treprostinil [21].

If a child on chronic IV or subcutaneous therapy requires hospitalization, the clinician should pay special attention to the dose, dose weight, concentration, and rate of the drug at the time of hospital admission, especially if transitioning from a home pump to a hospital pump. Incorrect dosing may cause significant hemodynamic changes, which may be life-threatening. Each hospital has its own policy regarding the use of the home pump in the hospital. Some institutions will require the child to use a hospital syringe pump for IV prostacyclin therapy. For patients receiving IV treprostinil, the drug is stable at room temperature for 48 h and has a half-life of approximately 4 h. In contrast, epoprostenol (Flolan; GlaxoSmithKline, Research Triangle Park, NC) is stable at room temperature for 8 h or requires use of ice packs to keep it stable for 24 h. This drug has a half-life of approximately 6 min. Extreme caution must be taken when administering these continuous IV and subcutaneous prostacyclin therapies, as these are life-sustaining medications and the patient may not tolerate medication interruption.

Management of these children also includes psychological support for the family unit, as they face the devastating impact of this life-limiting disease. Daily care of the child, especially one on IV therapy, places a tremendous responsibility on the caregiver. A clinically trained social worker, child psychologist, and child life specialist are integral members of a multidisciplinary team and will provide essential psychological support and guidance to help families cope with the stress of a chronic disease.

Chronic and safe medical management of children with PAH requires the clinician to understand and address the unique challenges related to the care of these patients. Expert consensus documents [22, 23] strongly urge that these children be referred to a PAH center for management or comanagement to ensure access to all types of existing and research-based therapies, family support, and best outcomes.

Conclusion

The occurrence of CCI is increasing as multidisciplinary teams achieve better survival rates and outcomes. Chronically, critically ill patient may include long-stay pediatric cardiac intensive care unit (PCICU) patients, patient with ventricular assist devices as a bridge to transplant or destination therapy, complicated heart failure patients requiring home milrinone infusions, or the advanced technologies used to support pulmonary hypertension patients in the hospital and at home. This cohort of patients requires significant resources and expertise. Nurses and advanced practitioners play an important role in the implementation of efficient programs to safely manage and follow-up these patients.

References

1. Human DG (2009) Living with complex heart disease. Pediatr Child Health 14:161–166
2. Hickman RL, Douglas PA (2010) Impact of chronic critical illness on psychological outcomes of family members. AACN Adv Crit Care 21(1):80–91
3. Lily C, De Meo D, Sonna L et al (2000) An intensive communication intervention for the critically ill. Am J Med 109:469–475
4. Lee D, Higgins PA (2010) Adjunctive therapies for the chronically, critically ill. AACN Adv Crit Care 21(1):92–106

Heart Failure

5. Berg A, Snell L, Mahle W (2007) Home inotropic therapy in children. J Heart Lung Transplant 26(5):453–457
6. Goldman AP, Cassidy J, De Leval M, Haynes S, Brown K, Whitmore P, Cohen G, Tsang V, Elliott M, Davidson A, Hamilton L, Bolton D, Wray J, Hasan A, RadleySmith R, Macrae D, Smith J (2003) The waiting game: bridging to heart transplantation. Lancet 362(9400):1967–1970
7. Berlin Heart (2011) Excor pediatric update, June 2011, Berlin Heart
8. Great Ormond Street Hospital NHS Trust (2008) - Berlin HEART database. (Internal database)
9. Long J, Kfoury A, Slaughter M, Silver M, Milano C, Rogers J, Delgado R, Frazier O (2005) Long-term destination therapy with the heart mate XVE left ventricular assist device: improved outcomes since the REMATCH study. Congest Heart Fail 11(3):133–138
10. Davidson JE (2009) Family centred care; meeting the need of patients' families and helping families adapt to critical illness. Crit Care Nurse 29(3):28–34
11. Great Ormond Street Hospital NHS Trust, Berlin Heart Mechanical Heart Assist – Information for families (2009) http://www.gosh.nhs.uk/gosh_families/information_sheets/berlin_heart/berlin_heart_families.pdf (Last viewed 20 Nov 2011)
12. RCN (2011) Children's and young people's cardiac nursing: RCN guidance on roles, career pathways and competence development. http://www.rcn.org.uk/__data/assets/pdf_file/0006/393513/004121.pdf (Last viewed 7 Aug 2011)
13. Staveski SL, Avery S, Rosenthal D, Roth SJ, Wright GE (2011) Implementation of a comprehensive interdisciplinary care coordination of infants and young children on Berlin Heart ventricular assist devices. J Cardiovasc Nurs 26(3):231–238
14. Li HCW, Lopez V (2008) Effectiveness and appropriateness of therapeutic play intervention in preparing children for surgery: a randomized controlled trial study. J Spec Pediatr Nurs 13(2):63–73
15. Great Ormond Street Hospital NHS Trust (2010) Anticoagulation for Berlin Heart Excor. (Internal protocol)
16. MacQueen S (2005) The special needs of children receiving intravenous therapy. Nurs Times 101(8):59
17. Yung D, Widlitz AC, Rosenzweig EB et al (2004) Outcomes in children with idiopathic pulmonary arterial hypertension. Circulation 110:660–665
18. Ogawa M, Albrecht D, Liu E (2009) Medical and non-medical considerations for the outpatient management of children with pulmonary arterial hypertension. Progress in Pediatric Cardiology 27:57–61
19. Kallen AJ, Lederman E, Balaji A et al (2008) Bloodstream infections in patients given treatment with intravenous prostanoids. Infect Control Hosp Epidemiol 29:342–349
20. Center for Disease Control (2007) Bloodstream infections among patients treated with intravenous epoprostenol or intravenous treprostinil for pulmonary arterial hypertension – seven sites, United States, 2003–2006. Morb Mortal Wkly Rep 56:170–172
21. Ivy DD, Calderbank M, Wagner B et al (2009) Closed-hub systems with protected connections and the reduction of risk of catheter-related bloodstream infection in pediatric patients receiving intravenous prostanoid therapy for pulmonary hypertension. Infect Control Hosp Epidemiol 30:823–829
22. McLaughlin VV, Archer S, Badesch DB et al (2009) ACCF/AHA expert consensus document on pulmonary arterial hypertension: a report of the American College of cardiology foundation task force on expert consensus documents and the American heart association developed in collaboration with the American College of chest physicians; American Thoracic Society, Inc; and the Pulmonary Hypertension Association. J Am Coll Cardiol 53:1573–1619
23. Galie N, Hoeper MH, Humbert M et al (2009) Guidelines for the diagnosis of pulmonary arterial hypertension. Eur Heart J 30:2493–2537

Acquired Heart Disease, Arrhythmias and Transplantation: Nursing Considerations

78

Cecila St. George-Hyslop, Kelly Kirby, Deborah Gilbert, and Bethany Diamond

Abstract

Many infants, children, and adolescents with congenital heart disease may develop heart failure and/or arrhythmias over the course of their lifelong illness. Alternatively, healthy children may acquire these issues. The pediatric patient with cardiovascular issues is a diverse and challenging patient population. Some of these children may go on to require advanced therapies such as device placement, chronic therapies (see ► chronically, critically ill section), and/or heart transplantation. This section will describe nursing care of patients with acquired heart disease, electrophysiology issues, and heart transplantation.

Keywords

Acute rheumatic fever • Acute RV dysfunction/failure • Arrhythmias • Cardiac pacemaker • Cardiac transplantation • Cardiomyopathies • Cardioversion • Immunosuppression (in cardiac transplantation) • Internal defibrillator • Kawasaki disease • Myocarditis • Postcardiotomy ventricular failure • Rejection (in cardiac transplantation)

C. St. George-Hyslop (✉)
Advanced Nursing Practice Educator, Hospital for Sick Children, Canada, Toronto, ON, Canada
e-mail: cecilia.hyslop@sickkids.ca

K. Kirby
Heart Rhythm Service, Lucile Packard Children's Hospital at Stanford, Palo Alto, CA, USA
e-mail: kkirby@lpch.org

D. Gilbert
Nurse Practitioner Cardiac Surgery, Children's Hospital of Colorado, Aurora, CO, USA
e-mail: deborah.gilbert@childrenscolorado.org

B. Diamond
Children's Hospital of Colorado, Aurora, CO, USA
e-mail: bethany.diamond@childrenscolorado.org

Introduction

Many infants, children, and adolescents with congenital heart disease will develop heart failure and/or arrhythmias over the course of their lifelong illness. Healthy children may also acquire these problems. The pediatric patient with cardiovascular issues is a diverse and challenging patient population. However, these children all share a propensity to have potential difficulties with regulation of their cardiac performance and resultant inadequate tissue perfusion. Some of these children may require advanced therapies such as device implantation, chronic therapies (see ▶ chronically, critically ill section) and/or heart transplantation. This section will describe nursing care of patients with acquired heart disease, electrophysiology issues, and heart transplantation.

Acquired Heart Disease

Acquired pediatric cardiac disease covers a broad spectrum of complex diseases, including cardiomyopathies, Kawasaki disease, endocarditis, myocarditis, and acute rheumatic fever. Dilated cardiomyopathy and myocarditis are the most common of these. Other causes of acquired disease include postcardiotomy ventricular failure, pulmonary hypertension, valvular disease, tumors, and arrhythmias [1]. This chapter will review categories of disease, signs and symptoms, invasive and noninvasive assessment of hemodynamic and cardiovascular function, and appropriate management. The conditions discussed in this chapter were chosen due to their frequency and because they illustrate the principles related to the care of patients with acute acquired cardiac disease.

Damage to myocardial cells will result in a low cardiac output state, ranging from mild hypotension to cardiac arrest. A child's hemodynamic status may rapidly deteriorate from myocardial damage, resulting in significant morbidity and mortality. Sudden cardiac collapse may occur from primary ventricular failure or lethal cardiac arrhythmias. Nurses must clearly understand the disease etiology, pathophysiology, clinical presentation, and management of the different acquired cardiac issues. Sharp clinical assessment skills will support early identification of even subtle signs of cardiac failure. This assessment is paramount to optimizing patient outcomes. Nursing vigilance in monitoring as well as anticipation of acute adverse events improves rapid recognition and prompts immediate intervention.

Generally children with acquired cardiac disease are previously healthy. Onset of disease brings a range of signs and symptoms. A diagnosis of acquired heart disease may be devastating for patients and families. Nurses share the responsibility of assessing knowledge gaps and tailoring care to the child and family's specific needs. Listening and respecting different opinions and providing compassionate family-centered care, with individualized support, are essential elements for enhancing family trust in the health-care team. Offering information and resources, organizing consultation, and acknowledging cultural and spiritual needs are also crucial. Facilitating the parental role in the hospital environment is necessary for healthy family adaptation. A child's angst is heightened by the fears and anxieties of their parents. Assessment of family dynamics and reducing unnecessary stressors assist the child and family along their journey toward recovery, palliation, or death.

A program's model of providing patient care is an important factor to be considered while optimizing outcomes for these patients. Given the high patient acuity, nurses "in-charge" positions should consider patient-nurse synergy when planning assignments. Careful consideration of each patient's unique characteristics (i.e., "stability, complexity, predictability, resiliency, vulnerability, participation in decision making, participation in care and resource availability"), and matching these with nurses' clinical skill mix and competencies, may optimize outcomes [2]. Providing consistency in caregivers or establishing a "core" care team supports family adjustment. Nursing expertise coupled with effective team

Table 78.1 Cardiac assessment

Cardiac assessment	
Assessment of perfusion	Assess for warm extremities, capillary refill (< 2 s), adequate mean arterial blood pressure, alterations in level of consciousness. Identify a differential between the core and peripheral temperature of perfusion Identify abnormalities, i.e., pulsus paradoxus (fall in blood pressure on inspiration due to pericardial effusion, constrictive pericarditis, or severe airway obstruction) and pulsus alternans (alternating strong and weak beats indicating poor LV function)
Pulse quality	Assess central and peripheral pulses: [0 absent; 1+ diminished barely palpable; 2+ normal, 3+ full volume, 4+ bounding] [3]
Cardiac rhythm	Heart rate and rhythm: assess for bradycardia or tachycardia and note regularity of rhythm
	Consider effects of drugs on heart rate, rhythm, and perfusion. Inspect apical pulse for normal placement (4th intercostal space, midclavicular line). Assess for cardiomegaly (pulsation displaced to the left of normal position). Assess for forceful quality (left ventricular hypertrophy) or evidence of parasternal heave (right ventricular hypertrophy)
Assessment of heart sounds	Assess for the presence of murmurs, ejection clicks, a pericardial friction rub, or gallop rhythm
Hemodynamics	Review invasive arterial and central line waveforms. Interpret values, i.e., mean arterial (MAP) and central venous (CVP) pressures
Hydration status	Monitor hydration (i.e., dry, edematous). Assess fluid balance. Strict intake and output measurement. Urine output goal of 1–2 mL/kg/h. Urinary output < 1 ml/h for two consecutive hours warrants notifying MD. Assess urine output in relation to diuretics
Laboratory work	Monitor blood work. Interpret values for arterial blood gases, electrolytes, lactate levels, mixed venous oxygen saturations, CBC, WBC and differential, ESR, viral polymerase chain reaction (PCR) and troponin I levels (marker of necrosis) [4]

crisis resource management (CRM) skills during critical events supports favorable outcomes.

Care of these children mandates close monitoring of their cardiovascular status. Hourly assessments are advisable during acute stages, when the risk of hemodynamic compromise is high. The clinician should perform a complete initial head-to-toe assessment, with frequent reassessments and comparison. A systematic assessment of neurological function provides a window to patient well-being, and an abnormal neurologic status may indicate a serious new problem such as a stroke or critically low cardiac output. Neurologic status is evaluated by assessing the level of consciousness (LOC), use of the Glasgow Coma Scale (GCS) Score, and pupil size and reaction, as well as cognitive and motor function. It is also important to determine differences from patient baseline as reported by the family. Agitation may be a "red flag" and sign of impending deterioration. Respiratory assessment includes observation of skin color (i.e., pale, ashen, cyanosis), including nail beds and mucous membranes. Oxygen requirements (FiO_2) are determined. The respiratory rate is counted for 1 min and assessment made of work of breathing and symmetry of chest wall movement. Breath sounds are auscultated for adventitious sounds (i.e., crackles, wheezes).

Evaluation of the child's cardiovascular status requires a thorough cardiac assessment. Identification of clinical changes, however slight, by the nurse, patient, or family should trigger a closer examination by the medical care team. Please see Table 78.1.

Nursing's understanding of the unique characteristics of each of the acquired cardiac diseases facilitates favorable management. The primary diseases of cardiomyopathy, myocarditis, Kawasaki disease, and acute rheumatic disease will be reviewed.

Cardiomyopathy is a disease of the myocardium that leads to abnormalities in structure and function. Causes include idiopathic, viral, and familial/genetic origins. There are four main types of cardiomyopathy: dilated, restrictive, hypertrophic, and arrhythmogenic right ventricular dysplasia [4]. These classifications are based on certain anatomic features detectable by echocardiogram, MRI, or pathologic examination. There are numerous and sometimes overlapping genetic, metabolic, and/or physiologic causes of each type of cardiomyopathy.

The most common type, the dilated cardiomyopathy, is characterized by progressive cardiac dilatation with thinning of the myocardial walls and systolic dysfunction [5]. Nurses should recognize the signs of progressive systolic dysfunction, which are manifested by cardiomegaly, pulmonary venous congestion, and severe congestive heart failure. "Red flag" characteristics include respiratory distress or failure, tachycardia, weak pulses, delayed capillary refill, low mixed venous saturations (<70 %), rising serum lactate levels (> 2.0 mmol/L), and an enlarging liver. An increasing serial serum lactate level >3 mmol/L is associated with increased morbidity and mortality and warrants close monitoring. Children also frequently present with gastrointestinal signs and symptoms including pain, nausea, and vomiting. Prompt administration of pharmacologic support may assist the failing myocardium. Vasoactive medications should be administered through centrally inserted IV catheters due to concerns of drug potency and extravasation. Nurses must validate drug compatibility when medications are administered simultaneously through the same lumen of the central line. The more potent medications will infuse in the port closest to the patient. Nurses safely titrate medication doses according to medical orders and continuously assess hemodynamic response to each dose change. When discontinuing a medication, the IV tubing should remain attached to the patient intravenous line for up to 4 h, ensuring that the medication may be readily restarted if sudden cardiac compromise occurs.

Vigilant monitoring of response to volume administration or medications includes a thorough patient assessment, coupled with appropriate laboratory monitoring [6]. Nurses must utilize caution when volume is administered to patients with dilated cardiomyopathy. Judicious volume administration is key, and as little as 5–10 mL/kg IV will likely achieve a positive response if indeed the patient is volume responsive. A large volume bolus of 20 mL/kg IV, or volume that is administered too quickly, may prove harmful. Overstretching the ventricle beyond its contractile capacity results in reduced function, hypotension, and possibly cardiac arrest [2]. Assessment of blood pressure is a poor marker of low cardiac output. Better markers to assess perfusion are core and extremity temperature, pulse quality, and capillary refill. Monitoring for ischemia (ST segment or T wave changes) on the bedside monitor is fundamental.

Diagnostic testing (echocardiogram, ECGs, CTs, MRIs) helps to determine the degree of cardiac dilation, wall motion, ejection fraction, and the possibility of ischemia. [6]. Sometimes mural thrombi are detected, and as these may lead to embolization, nurses should monitor the patient for respiratory distress, seizures, change in LOC, or cognitive/motor function deficits [5]. Cardiac catheterization may be necessary to assess left ventricular filling pressure and/or pulmonary vascular resistance.

Hypertrophic cardiomyopathy involves regional or global thickening of the left ventricular wall and intraventricular septum causing diastolic dysfunction and poor ventricular compliance. Septal hypertrophy may obstruct the left ventricular outflow tract during systole. The cause of hypertrophic cardiomyopathy is thought to have a genetic/familial basis, although 74 % of cases are idiopathic [4, 7]. Failure of the muscle to relax properly will result in impaired ventricular filling leading to a decrease in stroke volume and poor cardiac output [4]. Progression of the disease may cause lethal cardiac arrhythmias, and nurses must assess and anticipate rhythm disturbances. An implanted cardioverter-defibrillator may be necessary for repeated episodes of ventricular tachycardia or ventricular fibrillation. About 25 % of children with hypertrophic cardiomyopathy have left ventricular outflow tract obstruction with a pressure gradient of > 30 mmHg across the subaortic region [4]. There is increased risk of left ventricular outflow obstruction and sudden death during exercise when increased contractile force induces acute obstruction to left ventricular outflow. Nurses must share clear concise information regarding the need for moderate exercise restriction [4]. Teaching families to watch for signs of fatigue, difficulty breathing, or palpitations is imperative [8].

Restrictive cardiomyopathy, the least common of the cardiomyopathies, produces stiff, non-compliant ventricular walls, which impair ventricular filling while preserving systolic function. Cardiac failure follows and may include progressive pulmonary hypertension. Its cause is thought to be genetic or familial; however, it may also be idiopathic. Patients develop signs of respiratory distress including dyspnea, orthopnea, and usually repeated respiratory tract infections [4]. They may present with right-sided heart failure, including edema and syncope, signs of increased CVP, atrial dilation, and hepatosplenomegaly. They may experience myocardial ischemia with symptoms of chest pain. These patients are at high risk for intracardiac thrombus formation. With a 25 % risk of thromboembolism, nursing care includes the administration of anticoagulation and monitoring of therapeutic anticoagulation levels [8]. This disease has a poor prognosis related to congestive heart failure or sudden death. The threat of high mortality requires consistent family support. Early listing for cardiac transplantation may be presented as a treatment option for these patients.

Myocarditis is a disease marked by inflammatory infiltrates which accumulate in the cardiac muscle causing the cells to become injured or necrotic. Causes may be infectious, immune mediated, or related to the presence of toxins [5]. Of the infectious etiology (viral, bacterial, fungal, rickettsial, protozoal, spirochetal), viral myocarditis (i.e., Coxsackie B, enteroviruses) is the most common type of myocarditis in pediatrics [9]. Patient history usually reveals the onset of congestive heart failure, without any identifiable cause. The family may relay a recent episode of gastroenteritis or flu-like symptoms including malaise, fever, muscle aches, and fatigue and then signs such as tachypnea, dyspnea, and tachycardia [5]. Children may be asymptomatic or present with signs of congestive heart failure.

Others develop a fulminant form of myocarditis, with severe dysfunction and an ejection fraction of <35 %, which rapidly evolves into a state of shock. Malignant ventricular arrhythmias may severely depress cardiac function and lead to cardiac arrest. The definitive diagnostic test for myocarditis is an endomyocardial biopsy; however, biopsy carries significant risk of perforation, and the patchy areas of inflammation may result in false-negative transcatheter biopsy results. Consequently, biopsies are now less commonly performed at many centers, and tests such as MRI are being used to aid in diagnosis.

Nursing care of myocarditis patients involves early assessment and recognition of actual or impending hemodynamic compromise. Changes in cardiac rhythm or congestive heart failure may cause pre-syncope or syncopal episodes. ECG monitoring for ST segment changes, inverted T waves, or low voltage QRS, which may indicate possible myocardial ischemia or injury, is important for timely intervention. Supraventricular tachycardia (SVT), premature ventricular contractions (PVCs), and ventricular tachycardia (VT) are common types of cardiac arrhythmias [4]. If these arrhythmias occur, ordered medical therapy must be quickly implemented, and the child's clinical status and response to treatment must be evaluated. Cardiogenic shock from dysrhythmias requires pharmacological or electrical intervention (cardioversion/defibrillation) including a possible rapid fluid bolus (10 mL/kg) with 0.9 NaCl or 5 % albumin. The previously described caution regarding fluid administration in dilated cardiomyopathy applies to myocarditis patients as well.

Supportive care is the primary treatment for myocarditis. Vasoactive infusions of inotropes, inodilators, and/or vasodilators are administered. Patient hemodynamic status may be highly dependent on these vasoactive medications, and changes to infusion doses must be monitored closely. Nurses play an active role in the assessment of effectiveness of vasoactive therapy. Care is taken when changing medication syringes and IV tubing and adding or discontinuing medications, to minimize interruptions in delivery and prevent inadvertent boluses, which may lead to hemodynamic instability. Other beneficial medications used in the treatment of myocarditis are anticoagulants, diuretics, and beta-blockers, although beta-blockers are generally avoided in the setting of acute ventricular dysfunction [4]. In fulminant myocarditis, children may require advanced life support by extracorporeal membrane oxygenation (ECMO). Some children develop chronic dilated cardiomyopathy and require cardiac transplantation [4], others experience sudden death despite aggressive efforts for stabilization, and some recover in full.

Kawasaki disease causes inflammation of the microvascular circulation. Although thought to have an infectious etiology, its cause remains unknown, though genetic factors may play a role in this disease. White blood cells (WBCs) infiltrate the heart muscle, causing myocarditis and possibly pericarditis. Inflammation affects the conduction system and causes heart rhythm disturbances [8]. Myocardial infarction, from coronary artery aneurysm and thromboembolic development, may produce chest pain, malignant ventricular arrhythmias, and cardiac arrest [9]. Children classically present with high fever > 5 days, and any four of the following: cutaneous rashes, lymphadenopathy, conjunctivitis, inflamed lips/strawberry tongue and oral mucosa, redness/edema, and desquamation of palms of the hands and soles of the feet. Atypical cases may not exhibit all of these findings. The coronary arteries become dilated in the early phase of the disease due to WBC infiltration of the blood vessel walls, and this may progress to aneurysm development. In the acute stage, anemia, increased WBC, C-reactive protein, ESR, and thrombocytosis may be present. Aspirin is administered for its antiplatelet properties to prevent coronary thrombosis, as well as its antipyretic effects [4]. High dose IV immune gamma globulin (IVIG) is administered to decrease inflammatory effects and prevent coronary artery aneurysm development [11]. Most patients recover from this illness; however, some will develop coronary artery aneurysms, conduction problems, and/or myocardial infarction. There is concern related to thrombosis occurrence in the dilated coronary arteries; therefore, patients need to be monitored for chest pain and observed for changes in Q wave, ST segments, and T waves on ECG. Upon discharge, nurses coordinate follow-up appointments and ensure family understanding of the long-term follow-up requirements. Complications from Kawasaki disease (i.e., coronary aneurysms and thrombosis) may continue to be problematic into adulthood [10, 11].

In acute rheumatic fever, children of school age present with fever; arthritis of the hands, knees, and ankles; and pancarditis (pericarditis, endocarditis, and myocarditis). Rheumatic fever is usually caused by an antecedent group A, β-hemolytic streptococcus infection [4]. Patient history will reveal complaints of a sore throat, tonsillitis, and pharyngitis, about 1–5 weeks ago. This is followed by a latent period, in which the child begins to feel better. Subsequently, the symptoms of rheumatic fever develop, termed Jones Criteria: fever, arthritis, carditis, valvular regurgitation, subcutaneous nodules, chorea, and erythema marginatum (a characteristic pinpoint circular rash).

Similar to the other diseases noted in acquired heart disease, treatment is supportive. During the initial acute stage, the tonsillar pharyngitis is treated with antibiotics. Pain medications are administered, together with corticosteroids for the inflammatory carditis. This disease primarily affects the left-sided heart valves (aortic and mitral). The valves become regurgitant or stenotic, possibly requiring repair later in life. The need for bed rest is reinforced, the length of time of which depends on the degree of congestive heart failure and cardiomegaly.

The supportive nature of treatment for all of these acquired cardiac diseases requires an understanding of the complex relationship between oxygen supply (delivery) and the body's metabolic demand and consumption. Knowledge of principles of *cardiac output (CO)* = *heart rate (HR) X stroke volume (SV)* assist nurses to think critically regarding changes in a patient's hemodynamic status. Is the change a result of decreased oxygen delivery, increased oxygen

Table 78.2 Factors decreasing oxygen delivery to the tissues

Assessment	Nursing and medical management CO = HR X SV
Inspired oxygen Ventilation	Administer O_2 to keep oxygen saturations between 94 % and 99 %. Assess need for suctioning. Monitor for signs of atelectasis, consolidation, pneumothorax, and lung pathology
	Assess need for intubation/mechanical ventilation. Reassess appropriateness of ventilator settings as condition changes. Consult physician and respiratory therapist (RRT)
Hemoglobin (Hb) level: Oxygen carrying capacity	If Hb > 70 g/L and patient is clinically well, continue to monitor for changes in Hb. Minimize frequent blood sampling if possible
	If Hb < 120 g/L and patient is clinically unwell, administer blood products as ordered to increase oxygen carrying capacity. Assess for anemia, hemodilution, and overt or occult bleeding
Heart rate	Assess cardiac rate/rhythm: Is it too fast, too slow, or irregular? Evaluate tolerance of rate and rhythm. Monitor and treat cardiac arrhythmias with antiarrhythmic medication, synchronized cardioversion, defibrillation, or pacing as the condition warrants
Stroke volume (Contractility)	Once fluid status has been optimized, administer inotropic drugs (i.e., dobutamine, epinephrine), which increase the force of contraction; inodilators (i.e., milrinone); or electrolytes (i.e., calcium)
Stroke volume (Preload)	Assess volume status and optimize preload: central venous pressure (CVP) is usually 5–10 mmHg. CVP value should be individualized to patient's own normal values and specific physiology. Consider fluid shifting into interstitial spaces and/or bleeding. Give 5–10 mL/kg fluid bolus as per order, unless hemorrhaging, in which case match losses
	Know ordered total fluid intake (TFI). Restrict fluids to 70–80 % of maintenance, when in congestive heart failure or mechanically ventilated. Assess effects of diuretics
Stroke volume (Afterload)	*Assess systemic vascular resistance (SVR)*: If SVR is low (vasodilated), administer ordered vasoconstrictors (i.e., epinephrine, norepinephrine, phenylephrine, and vasopressin). Note that increasing SVR can decrease stoke volume and cardiac output
	If SVR is high (cool, mottled, dusky), administer ordered vasodilators (i.e., nitroprusside, nitroglycerin, phentolamine, captopril) or inodilators (i.e., milrinone, amrinone, dobutamine)
	Assess pulmonary vascular resistance (PVR). Evaluate effects of hypoxemia, hypercapnia, and acidosis on PVR. Monitor for signs of right-sided failure such as high CVP. Administer drugs that relax PVR, i.e., inhaled nitric oxide, prostacyclin, and sildenafil. Use caution in administration of pulmonary vasodilators to patients with high left atrial pressure as acute pulmonary edema may result

consumption, or both? Intermittent measurement to trend serum lactic acid levels and mixed venous oxygen saturations will assist in evaluating the degree of illness. Rising serum lactate levels greater than 2.0 mg/dL are of concern. Normal central venous oxygen saturation or mixed venous saturation values are 70–80 %; values < 70 % or > 80 % indicate cardiocirculatory dysfunction. Advancements in noninvasive monitoring such as near-infrared spectroscopy (NIRS) are beneficial for continuous assessment of regional perfusion. Normal cerebral regional NIRS (rSO_2) value is 60–80 %. In patients with structurally normal hearts, values < 50 % or a 20 % change from original set baseline is considered a critical value. Factors affecting oxygen delivery to the tissues

and oxygen consumption should be reviewed, and alternate management strategies should be initiated. Please see Tables 78.2 and 78.3.

Regardless of the etiology of acquired pediatric cardiac disease, these patients share a common risk of developing cardiogenic shock. Treatment, in most cases, is supportive until the disease completes its course. Pharmaceutical measures alone may be insufficient to maintain hemodynamic stability, and some patients may require more advanced forms of therapy. Intubation, mechanical ventilation, and mechanical circulatory support may be necessary with worsening clinical status. Nursing support will intensify as the child's clinical needs change. ECMO may be utilized to support patients in the acute phase of illness when refractory myocardial

Table 78.3 Factors increasing oxygen consumption (metabolic rate)

Assessment	Nursing and medical management
Work of breathing (WOB)	Excessive WOB increases O_2 consumption by 40 % [7]. Assess need for mechanical ventilator or other noninvasive support
Fever/sepsis Shivering	For each 1° rise in temperature, oxygen consumption increases by 10 % [7]. Treat with antipyretics for temp ≥ 38.0 deg. Apply ice to head. Initiate cooling on cooling blanket if fever refractory. Physician's order should state desired degree of cooling. Assess for infection/sepsis. Obtain cultures and administer antibiotics if infectious etiology, as per physician orders. Severe infection increases oxygen consumption 60 % [7]
	Shivering increases metabolic rate. O_2 consumption increases 50–100 % [7]
Drug infusions that increase O_2 consumption	Assess vasoactive supports (inotropes) for their role in contributing to increased myocardial oxygen consumption. Note that epinephrine 0.1 mcg/kg/min (high dose) increases consumption by 23–29 %. Norepinephrine increases O_2 consumption by 10–21 % 7. Reassess if medication doses may be reduced or discontinued
Pain	Assess pain scores using age appropriate tools (i.e., PIPP, FLACC; Numeric Rating Scale; FACES) [2]. Determine quality, location, aggravating and alleviating factors, radiation, severity, and timing of pain. Treat pain with pharmacological and non-pharmacological methods. Reassess pain frequently
Anxiety/ agitation	O_2 consumption rises by 16 % with agitation [7]. Administer ordered sedatives. Use alternative comfort measures. Agitation may be a sign of poor cardiac output
Overstimulation Activity	Assess tolerance to nursing interventions – i.e., bathing, turning, and suctioning. Allow for periods of rest. Minimize unnecessary handling. O_2 consumption increases with dressing changes (10 %), nursing assessment (12 %), bathing (23 %), ETT suctioning (27 %), and turning (31 %) [8]
	Critically ill patients may require a muscle relaxant to decrease muscular activity (i.e., Pavulon, rocuronium)
Seizures	Monitor for clinical seizures. Ensure patient safety. Administer antiseizure medication as ordered and reassess

failure occurs. This may be transitory as a bridge to recovery or may become a bridge to transplantation [1, 6]. Univentricular and biventricular assist devices that are pulsatile (i.e., Berlin Heart Excor, Thoratec) and non-pulsatile (i.e., Heartware) may also be utilized as a bridge to cardiac transplantation, though recovery has been reported with use of these devices in adults and rare pediatric cases.

Anticoagulant administration (i.e., heparin, coumadin, enoxaparin) for disease treatment or advanced life support is a shared responsibility between nursing and other team members. Nurses are involved in monitoring desired anticoagulation levels (i.e., activated clotting times (ACTs), international normalized ratio (INR), aPT, partial thromboplastin time, thromboelastograms (TEG), and antithrombin III levels). Vigilant monitoring for the development of blood clots or excessive bleeding

is essential [6]. Frequent communication between health-care professionals helps ensure anticoagulation is tailored to specific patient needs and that program-specific protocols are understood and followed. Team preparedness to monitor for and respond to adverse events such as hemolysis, strokes, seizures, infection, and bleeding is vital.

Acquired heart disease is associated with considerable morbidity and mortality. These diseases share a potential common path of cardiogenic shock, lethal arrhythmias, cardiac arrest, and death. The trajectory of illness may be complete recovery, chronic disability, cardiac transplantation, or palliation and death. Nurses have a significant role as an advocate for these children and their families, as health-care needs often continue over many years. Nurses must combine sharp assessment skills with intuition and anticipation. They must recognize even subtle of signs of failure, and be prepared to initiate early aggressive therapy as ordered. It is the combination of astute clinical assessments, good communication, and effective crisis resource management skills that may save the lives of these acutely and/or critically ill children.

Pediatric Arrhythmias

Pediatric arrhythmia patients are a complex and diverse population of children that are cared for across all levels of health-care settings. Children with normal cardiac anatomy, structural heart defects, and primary electrical diseases may have a wide variety of normal heart rates and rhythms, which also vary with patient age and activity [11]. Pediatric electrocardiogram (ECG) parameters, such as PR interval, QRS duration, QRS and T wave axis, are all age specific as well [12].

Swift recognition of rhythm changes and fluctuations in patient symptoms, efficient communication with the medical team, and timely response with intervention are key to providing care for children with arrhythmias. A thorough knowledge of normal pediatric cardiac anatomy, cardiac physiology, and the electrical conduction system is vital. Awareness of the specific patient's diagnosis, the surgical procedure, and a baseline head-to-toe assessment may aid in early recognition and rapid response to arrhythmias during the postoperative period. A comprehensive summary of general nursing considerations and specific nursing interventions for the care of the pediatric arrhythmia patient is found in Table 78.4.

Cardiac monitoring and telemetry is a crucial diagnostic tool for children with arrhythmias in the hospital setting. Audible monitor alarms should be set with appropriate parameters for age and diagnosis. Also, ensure that the monitor is set in the paced or non-paced mode depending on patient pacing activity. It is important to assess the patient by palpating a radial or brachial artery pulse rate if a heart rate discrepancy is noted

between the child's pacemaker and cardiac monitor reading. Recordable telemetry is essential and must be set to record and print at all times. Documentation of arrhythmias is important to allow the medical team to evaluate the intervals and rates.

Supraventricular tachycardia (SVT) is the most common arrhythmia experienced by the pediatric population [13]. SVT generally describes a regular, narrow complex tachycardia that originates above the level of the bundle of His, though some wide complex and irregular forms of this rhythm may be experienced. SVT may be ectopic in nature or may result from a reentrant circuit such as AV nodal reentrant tachycardia (AVNRT) or an accessory pathway mediated tachycardia, known as atrioventricular reentrant tachycardia (AVRT). Children with Wolff-Parkinson-White (WPW) syndrome have an accessory pathway that is classically diagnosed by a short PR interval and slurred upstroke of the QRS complex, known as a delta wave, on ECG. Children with WPW may be asymptomatic or experience intermittent episodes of SVT. Although rare, the child with WPW is at risk of sudden death if atrial fibrillation occurs and the accessory pathway supports conduction to the ventricle with a 1:1 ratio.

Treatment of SVT in the hospital setting may include the use IV adenosine which blocks electrical conduction through the AV node. First, obtain a 12-lead ECG to confirm the diagnosis of SVT. Always remember the five rights of medication administration, to run a continuous rhythm strip before/during/after IV adenosine administration and to have emergency cart in the patient room with defibrillator and emergency airway equipment readily accessible. Due to the short half-life of adenosine, it is essential to administer IV adenosine via rapid IV push followed by an immediate IV saline flush. It is important to remember that a transient sinus pause will occur. The dose may be repeated and increased if needed. Vagal maneuvers may also be utilized to treat SVT. Vagal maneuvers are an effective and useful tool in the treatment for SVT and may be tailored to the age of the child. These special maneuvers stimulate the vagus nerve in

Table 78.4 Nursing care for pediatric arrhythmia patients

General nursing considerations	Specific nursing interventions
Know your patient	Become familiar with patient status to enhance recognition of change in condition
	Document rhythm strip and record any noted arrhythmia events
	Always perform a careful assessment before and after administration of medication
Inform your patient	Educate patient and family about the heart, conduction system, arrhythmia, and treatments
	Provide anticipatory guidance at a cognitively and behaviorally appropriate level
	Ensure that education is provided at an appropriate time with adequate time allotted for questions and reinforcement of information
	Prepare child and family for noninvasive testing and invasive procedures
	Ensure child and family understanding of the diagnosis, treatment options, and the plan of care
Communicate effectively about your patient	Communicate changes in patient status and rhythm to medical team
	Collaborate with multidisciplinary team to provide teaching and education for patient and family
Comfort and advocate for your patient	Reduce anxiety and facilitate effective coping strategies for patients and family members during times of stress
	Ensure safe, optimal, and effective use of diagnostic and therapeutic procedures
	Increase sense of mastery and preserve personal control for patients and family members
	Enhance trust between child, family, and health-care providers

an attempt to decrease heart rate and include ice to face, blowing on thumb, doing a headstand, and bearing down.

Pediatric arrhythmia patients cared for on the general pediatric floor include children with refractory SVT who are admitted for oral medication initiation or titration, such as sotalol or flecainide therapy. Nurses should be familiar with the administration and side effects of oral and IV antiarrhythmic medications. These patients require cardiac monitoring and close observation.

Pediatric patients with SVT and WPW may undergo an electrophysiology study and catheter ablation to eliminate the abnormal electrical circuit in the heart. These procedures are not without risk, and it is imperative that pediatric nurses be familiar with this population of pediatric arrhythmia patients as they may be admitted post-procedure to either the general pediatric floor or ICU. Prior to the scheduled procedure, nurses may instruct patients and families regarding strategies to stop an episode of SVT through the use of vagal maneuvers. Following the ablation procedure, nurses must monitor the patient for post-procedure complications: hematoma, arrhythmia recurrence, AV block, premature

atrial contractions, bleeding from catheter site, and pericardial effusion/tamponade.

Patients who have undergone surgical repair of congenital heart disease and develop arrhythmias require careful observation and rapid intervention. These patients may be critically ill and hemodynamically unstable. Knowledge of the surgical repair, potential mechanisms for possible arrhythmia development, diagnostic tools, and planned interventions is necessary. Early and accurate recognition may aid in restoration of hemodynamic stability [14]. Documentation of the child's baseline rhythm in the immediate postoperative period is vital. Knowledge of potential arrhythmias that may occur based on diagnosis and surgical repair will help in preparing for urgent intervention or emergency treatment. Postoperative junctional ectopic tachycardia (JET), ectopic atrial tachycardia (EAT), and multifocal atrial tachycardia (MAT) may cause significant hemodynamic compromise [15].

JET is a common arrhythmia after cardiac surgery. It is an automatic narrow complex rhythm with heart rates from 150 to 300 bpm. The ectopic focus resides in the AV node and results in AV dissociation, which further alters hemodynamics. A slower JET rate, AV synchrony, and subsequent stable hemodynamics may be achieved by decreasing the patient's temperature, decreasing stimulation of circulating catecholamines, and utilizing external AV sequential pacing above JET rate.

EAT is an atrial ectopic tachycardia that appears as a result of an automatic focus within the atrium. There is minimal beat-to-beat variation in heart rate, and this rhythm may be monotonous and incessant in nature. There is characteristic warm-up and cooldown to the tachycardia. When EAT occurs, correction of any electrolyte imbalance is a priority.

MAT is a chaotic rhythm that varies considerably in rate and has irregular PP intervals. Characterized by three or more distinct p wave morphologies, this tachycardia is triggered by multiple premature beats originating from several sites within the atrium. For patients in MAT, limiting catecholamine release or administration and minimizing patient stimulation may be useful. These patients are hemodynamically labile and typically are refractory to pacing termination of the arrhythmia, so may require urgent treatment with IV flecainide or amiodarone [13]. All arrhythmia patients require close observation and cardiac monitoring.

Defibrillation is the emergency treatment for pulseless ventricular tachycardia (VT) and ventricular fibrillation (VF). This potentially lifesaving therapy is often delivered in the very high-stress setting of emergency resuscitation. Nurses must be familiar with the emergency cart and proper use of the defibrillator. Adhering to established roles during an emergency situation is essential. Precise documentation of medication and defibrillation doses and times, including rhythm strips, is critical to assess effectiveness of treatment and the need for changes in plan of care.

Atrial flutter or stable VT may require direct current (DC) cardioversion for treatment. Atrial flutter is a rapid atrial rhythm with classic saw-toothed p waves with intermittent ventricular conduction up to 150 bpm. Ventricular tachycardia is a wide complex tachycardia originating in the ventricle that results in a series of three or more ventricular contractions. DC cardioversion is used in the treatment of atrial flutter or stable VT with the goal of conversion to normal sinus rhythm. Key nursing responsibilities when utilizing DC cardioversion are to ensure adequate patient sedation/pain control, provision of continuous cardiac monitoring, and access to emergency PCICU care. The emergency cart must be available with defibrillator and airway equipment readily accessible. DC cardioversion requires the synchronization of the charge to the patient's ECG to avoid delivery of the shock on the T wave.

Another therapy that may be required in the postoperative period is overdrive atrial pacing. This involves burst atrial pacing through the use of a temporary pacemaker delivered at a rate above the patient's own atrial rate. This intervention is used in atrial tachycardia to restore normal sinus rhythm. It is important to remember that this treatment may also be proarrhythmic, and resuscitation equipment should be readily available.

Temporary cardiac pacing is used in the immediate postoperative period to treat surgical atrioventricular (AV) block or sinus node dysfunction. A temporary pacing system may also be used by the Electrophysiology Service to conduct pacing studies or diagnose potential cardiac conduction problems. Epicardial pacing wires are placed on the surface of the atrium and ventricles during cardiac surgery. Typically, the atrial wires exit the right side of chest, and the ventricular wires exit the left side of chest. Temporary pacing wires should be looped and secured to the patient to prevent dislodgement. These wires are unipolar; therefore, there must be two wires to complete the electrical circuit. If only one wire is present, a skin lead/wire must be inserted. Ideally, pacing wires may be used for 10–14 days [16].

Temporary pacemaker settings should reflect the physician orders. The external pacemaker box should always be visible and secured to the bed. It may be helpful to record a rhythm strip at the beginning of every shift and with changes to pacemaker settings. Sensing and capture thresholds are to be checked daily by a physician, and a backup pacemaker programmed to current settings with new batteries should be available at bedside. Program-specific policies on frequency and procedures for battery changes and care of the temporary pacing wires should be available.

Some patients have a permanent pacemaker or internal cardiac defibrillator (ICD) placed. It is important to know the patient's underlying rhythm and pacemaker device settings. A special piece of equipment, called a programmer, is used to evaluate and program the settings of permanent pacemakers and ICDs. Programmers are specific to the device's manufacturer.

With all pediatric pacemaker and ICD patients, knowledge of their underlying rhythm is important. However, special care is required for pacemaker-dependent children who have no underlying heart rhythm. Routine interrogation of the device including threshold testing requires extra vigilance to avoid prolonged periods of loss of capture. Careful long-term device follow-up may assist in avoiding potentially fatal issues such as ventricular lead fracture, device malfunction, and depletion of battery life. Awareness of electromagnetic interference is essential to maintain pacemaker function and avoid oversensing and subsequent loss of capture. Reprogramming of the pacemaker to an asynchronous mode in pacemaker-dependent children undergoing surgical procedures involving the use of cautery is crucial.

Pediatric patients with normal cardiac anatomy who have undergone transvenous placement of a pacemaker or ICD will recover in the PACU and spend one night on the general pediatric floor. Specific care plans will vary by institution, though typically include CXR immediately upon arrival in the PACU and repeat 2-view CXR the following morning to assess heart and lung fields, to assess lead and generator placement, and to rule out pneumothorax. Pain medication and intravenous antibiotics are routine management strategies. Knowledge of your patient's underlying rhythm as well as the pacemaker or ICD settings is important to their care. For newly implanted devices, a sling to the affected arm is suggested for the first 48 h. Close monitoring of the wound site is also important to assess for bleeding, hematoma, or signs of infection. Cardiac monitoring should be set up according to the patient's device settings.

Discharge teaching is an important part of caring for children who have undergone pacemaker or ICD implant. The patient and family must be provided enough time to understand the information. It is important to discuss return to school and sports participation/restriction. Schools often require written notes describing the plan of care in case of emergency. Major concerns such as depression, anxiety, change in body image, and quality of life changes following device implant are appropriate to discuss, and a child psychiatry referral is often appropriate [17]. Establishing psychosocial support via support groups, summer camps, and social networking may be very helpful to the child's recovery. For children with inherited arrhythmias, the Sudden Arrhythmia Death Syndromes (SADS) Foundation is a powerful educational and networking tool [18]. Parents are also empowered and reassured by taking CPR classes and purchasing medical ID bracelets and chest protectors. Discharge planning for a pediatric patient with a newly implanted pacemaker or ICD is a complex process that is greatly enhanced by a multidisciplinary approach.

Inherited arrhythmias are complex diagnoses that may be a source of great stress and concern for the entire family. Families are often diagnosed at the time of a sudden catastrophic arrhythmic event. Throughout the diagnostic process, the uncertainty for the health and safety of the child and siblings is an overwhelming stressor. Once a diagnosis is determined, genetic testing may cause parental guilt. Testing is now widely available, and genetic counselors are an essential part of caring for families with inherited arrhythmias. The treatment for some inherited arrhythmias is life changing, involving placement of an ICD, beginning lifelong medical therapy, and possible restriction of activities. It is essential to involve psychosocial support early.

Nurses should be aware of the special considerations required for some children based on their specific diagnosis. For example, children with Brugada syndrome are at high risk for lethal arrhythmias during times of febrile illness. Brugada syndrome is an inherited mutation of the sodium channel and causes sudden death in structurally normal hearts [19]. Parents should be instructed on fever reduction strategies and when to seek emergency medical care. Another potentially lethal inherited arrhythmia is long QT syndrome. A defect in the ion channels in the heart results in a prolonged QT interval, risking development of torsades de pointes, a life-threatening form of VT. For children with long QT syndrome, a comprehensive list of medications to avoid is found online at the University of Arizona Center for Education and Research on Therapeutics website (http://www.azcert.org) where potentially lifesaving information is continuously updated [20].

While providing excellent care for pediatric patients with arrhythmias is a challenge, nurses have great opportunities to improve outcomes. Nurses must be aware of their patient's anatomy and physiology, hemodynamics, impact of medications, and interventions on the patient and the arrhythmia, all while being cognizant of the psychosocial status of the patient and family. The bedside nurse must be able to recognize postoperative rhythm changes and intervene quickly if hemodynamic compromise is present. Nurses play an essential role in establishing trust between the patient, family, and multidisciplinary medical care team. Nurses are also responsible for informing the patient and family of rhythm changes and any required interventions.

Children with congenital heart defects now survive complex surgical repairs and live well into adulthood. Arrhythmias are a common and predictable concern for this growing population. Nursing care has changed with the significant medical advances for treatment of children with arrhythmias. Proficiency in nursing considerations for pediatric arrhythmia patients is an integral part of providing exceptional care for this complex population of children.

Heart Transplantation

Resources for Families and Health-Care Professionals

http://www.azcert.org/ http://www.sads.org/ Pediatric Heart Transplantation.

Heart transplantation is an accepted treatment for acquired or congenital end-stage heart failure in pediatric patients. After a referral for transplantation, the transplant program completes a comprehensive evaluation that includes medical, psychosocial, and financial aspects. The medical aspect establishes the medical need for transplant with no absolute contraindications. The psychosocial aspect involves social work who evaluates the needs of the patient and family, and a psychologist or psychiatrist who helps evaluate emotional readiness and response to the transplant process. Due to the expense related to transplant, financial/insurance company approval must also be in place. As transplantation is not curative, discussions with the patient and family must include need for lifetime medication administration, long term follow-up, and risk of rejection of the donor heart. Infection and the potential for malignancy risks related to lifelong immunosuppression, the financial implications of transplant, and medication side effects involving other organ systems must also be reviewed.

Once approved for transplantation, the patient is placed on a national wait list with the United Network of Organ Sharing (UNOS) and becomes a candidate for heart transplant. Candidates are listed as Status 1A, 1B, 2, or 7 (Table 78.5). Hearts are matched to awaiting candidates by blood type and size first. Additionally, donations of pediatric (under age of 18 years old) hearts are allocated to pediatric candidates before being offered to adult patients. Hearts are also allocated to candidates at local transplant centers first then outward from the donor hospital in zones of 500-mile radius to aid in minimizing ischemic times [22, 23].

Postoperative management of a pediatric heart transplant recipient involves understanding the

Table 78.5 Heart transplantation wait list determinants

Status	Definition
1A – A candidate listed as Status 1A meets at least one of the following criteria	(a) Requires assistance with a ventilator
	(b) Requires assistance with a mechanical assist device (e.g., ECMO)
	(c) Requires assistance with a balloon pump
	(d) A candidate less than six months old with congenital or acquired heart disease exhibiting reactive pulmonary hypertension at greater than 50 % of systemic level. Such a candidate may be treated with prostaglandin E (PGE) to maintain patency of the ductus arteriosus
	(e) Requires infusion of high dose (e.g., dobutamine $>/=$ 7.5 mcg/kg/min or milrinone $>/=$ 0.5 mcg/kg/min) or multiple inotropes (e.g., addition of dopamine at $>/=$ 5 mcg/kg/min)
	(f) A candidate who does not meet the criteria specified in (a), (b), (c), (d), or (e) may be listed as Status 1A if the candidate has a life expectancy without a heart transplant of less than 14 days, such as due to refractory arrhythmia. Qualification for Status 1A under this criterion is valid for 14 days and may be recertified by an attending physician for one additional 14-day period. Any further extension of the Status 1A listing under this criterion requires a conference with the applicable Regional Review Board
	Qualification for Status 1A under criteria (a) through (e) is valid for 14 days and must be recertified by an attending physician every 14 days from the date of the candidate's initial listing as Status 1A to extend the Status 1A listing
1B – A candidate listed as Status 1B meets at least one of the following criteria	(a) Requires infusion of low dose single inotropes (e.g., dobutamine or dopamine $</=$ 7.5 mcg/kg/min)
	(b) Less than 6 months old and does not meet the criteria for Status 1A
	(c) Growth failure, i.e., <5th percentile for weight and/or height or loss of 1.5 standard deviations of expected growth (height or weight) based on the National Center for Health Statistics for pediatric growth curves
2	A candidate who does not meet the criteria for Status 1A or 1B is listed as Status 2
7	A candidate listed as Status 7 is considered temporarily unsuitable to receive a thoracic organ transplant

UNOS policy 3.7

care of the pediatric patient having undergone open heart surgery and cardiopulmonary bypass. Other essential knowledge includes current techniques for hemodynamic monitoring and systems-based assessment for observation of complications such as arrhythmias, increased risk of bleeding related to resection of adhesions from previous surgeries, respiratory compromise, renal dysfunction, and infection. The bedside nurse must be familiar with the patient's medical and cardiac history, as well as details of the transplant surgical procedure, including anesthesia course, concerns related to cardiopulmonary bypass and circulatory arrest, and ischemic times of the allograft to provide care to the recipient [23, 24].

Postoperatively, critical information is necessary to optimize patient management. Central venous access will allow direct assessment of cardiac hemodynamics. The placement of an arterial line permits arterial blood pressure measurement and collection of arterial blood gases and other serum laboratory measurements. A Swan-Ganz catheter, if inserted, will estimate central venous blood pressure, pulmonary artery blood pressure, and pulmonary capillary wedge pressure (an estimate of left atrial or left ventricular end-diastolic pressure) [24]. The noninvasive use of a near-infrared spectroscopy (NIRS) cerebral oximeter will assess changes in cerebral perfusion [25]. The combination of these measurement tools will provide the bedside nurse with a better understanding of the recipient's condition including cardiac output, pulmonary status, and electrolyte and fluid balance as well as end-organ function. Careful monitoring of heart rate and rhythm in the post-transplant period is important. Sinus node dysfunction is common after heart transplantation. Chronotropic support for bradycardia with either external pacing or continuous infusion of isoproterenol may be necessary [23]. Denervation in the transplanted heart may occur from the location of the atrial suture line, resulting in the heart's inability to respond to stimuli from the sympathetic nervous system. Pediatric patients usually depend on heart rate to increase cardiac output and since denervation makes it difficult to increase heart rate, stroke volume must be utilized instead. Adequate preload, and the use of Starling mechanism, will increase stroke volume. Circulating catecholamines will also assist with this response [26, 27].

More specific issues related to the postoperative transplant patient are primary graft failure, right heart failure, and elevated pulmonary pressures. Primary graft failure may be related to donor or recipient causes or from rejection. Donor heart issues include quality of the donor tissue, donor/recipient size mismatch, or organ ischemic time. Any of these will impact heart contractility and ventricular function and may cause death. Recipient issues include pre-transplant diagnosis, end-organ dysfunction, number of previous surgeries, the presence of elevated pulmonary pressures, and the use of pre-transplant ECMO or ventilatory support. Elevated pulmonary pressures may be a consequence of the pre-transplant diagnosis or pre-transplant congestive heart failure or left ventricular failure. This has postoperative implications as the donor right ventricle has not been previously exposed to high pulmonary pressures, and right ventricular failure may ensue [28]. Signs of right heart failure in the postoperative transplant patient are increased right atrial pressure, the presence of pulmonary edema, increased liver size, and decreased cardiac output. To rectify right heart failure, the cause must be determined. If pulmonary hypertension is suspected, inhaled nitric oxide may be utilized to decrease afterload on the right ventricle [29].

The bedside nurse must monitor for arrhythmias in the postoperative cardiac transplant patient. Due to denervation of the graft, common postoperative dysrhythmias are junctional rhythms or bradycardia [29]. Additionally, the patient may experience heart block. To maintain cardiac output, inotropic support or external pacing may be utilized to achieve adequate heart rate and improve cardiac output. Also arrhythmias, if present in the donor, may now present in the recipient. While the postoperative transplant patient has many of the same concerns as other postoperative cardiac patients, they do require special attention. Function of the graft, control of the immune response, and increased infection risk are the most important considerations in the immediate post-transplant period.

Rejection is a significant concern in the post-transplant patient. Rejection occurs when the recipient's immune system attacks the transplanted graft. The immunological forms of rejection include cellular and humoral (antibody-mediated) rejection. The rarest form of rejection is hyperacute rejection, which occurs in the first minutes following implantation of the donor organ and is thought to be caused by circulating preformed antibodies. Acute rejection is a more common phenomenon, and although risk is highest in the first year post-transplant, this may occur at any time. Acute rejection is the result of a cellular response, when T lymphocytes recognize the graft as foreign [30]. Acute rejection is responsible for nearly 20 % of deaths in the first year post-transplant, decreasing to less than 10 % at >10 years post-transplant [31].

In an attempt to prevent rejection from occurring, transplant recipients are placed on immunosuppressive medications. Immunosuppressive medications block the immune response that causes rejection. Corticosteroids (methylprednisolone and prednisone), calcineurin inhibitors (cyclosporine and tacrolimus), antiproliferative medications (azathioprine and mycophenolate mofetil), and TOR inhibitors (sirolimus) are the primary immunosuppressive agents used.

Initial immunosuppression is provided through induction therapy that is done in the immediate postoperative period to decrease the risk of acute rejection and, if necessary, allow maintenance immunosuppression to be postponed. Induction therapy is used by almost 70 % of pediatric heart transplant programs. The detailed induction regimens is program dependent; however, polyclonal (ATG and ATGAM) antibody or interleukin-2 receptor antagonist (Simulect) and corticosteroids are the primary agents currently used in induction [31]. Steroids help decrease inflammation and aid in suppressing the immune system by blocking the first phase of the immune response, including the production of interleukin-1. The polyclonal antibody/antilymphocyte antibody blocks both T cell and B cell surface antigens. Side effects of medications used for induction therapy are multiple and may be life threatening. The bedside nurse must monitor the patient for anaphylaxis, headache, rash, hypertension, hypotension, fever, dyspnea, nausea, chest pain, and headache. These symptoms may represent a reaction to the medication itself or are an implication that cell lysis is occurring. Many symptoms may be avoided or blunted if a histamine blocker or steroids are administered prior to the infusion of the antibody preparation [28].

During induction therapy, calcineurin inhibitor (CNI) therapy is often initiated at low doses. Calcineurin inhibitors may impact renal function; therefore, introduction of a CNI may be delayed if renal function concerns are present in the postoperative patient. The post-transplant patient on a CNI has daily trough levels drawn to monitor drug levels, optimizing immunosuppression and minimizing renal toxicity [28].

Maintenance immunosuppression consists of daily medications taken by a transplant patient over their lifetime to prevent rejection. These are usually initiated in the first week after transplant, once induction therapy is completed. Approximately 99 % of all post-transplant patients are on a CNI for primary immunosuppression [28]. The CNI inhibits T cell production. Often, the CNI is augmented by an antiproliferative agent and occasionally a corticosteroid.

Signs and symptoms of clinical rejection are generally vague and may mimic other illnesses. Symptoms of rejection are low-grade fever, lethargy, palpitations/aberrant heartbeats, shortness of breath with or without exertion, abdominal pain, and loss of appetite, nausea, vomiting, and fluid retention. Signs of rejection may present as echocardiogram changes, tachycardia,

arrhythmias, and pulmonary edema. Echocardiogram changes include increased AV valve regurgitation, pericardial effusion, diminished ventricular function, left ventricular wall thickening, and unusual septal wall motion. The degree of rejection, together with the extent of hemodynamic compromise of the patient, determines how aggressively the patient should be treated.

Treatment of rejection depends on the type of acute rejection that occurs. With cellular rejection, which is T-cell-mediated rejection, steroids (oral or IV) are generally administered and treatment may be augmented with an antilymphocytic antibody such as ATG, ATGAM, or anti-CD52 agents (Campath). These antilymphocytic antibodies lyse the T cells causing cell death. Antibody-mediated rejection (AMR) is B-cell-mediated rejection; these are antibodies specific to the donor heart. With evidence of AMR, treatment usually includes the antilymphocytic antibodies and photopheresis or plasmapheresis to target the B cells [30].

The risk of infection is closely monitored in the post-transplant patient. In their immunosuppressed status, these patients are at higher risk for acquiring an infection. Timely removal of indwelling lines, drains, and tubes is recommended to decrease iatrogenic infections. With careful planning, medication administration and central line access may be timed to minimize infection risks. Risk of death related to infection is highest in the first few months after transplant [32]. Issues that affect infection susceptibility in the post-transplant patient are the amount of immunosuppression prescribed, previous infectious exposures (recipient and/or donor), surgical procedures, invasive devices, and metabolic factors [33]. Induction therapy for immunosuppression may also be postponed if the patient has delayed sternal closure or is supported on ECMO, due to the inherent infection risk in both of these situations.

Opportunistic infections such as cytomegalovirus (CMV), Epstein-Barr virus (EBV), and Pneumocystis carinii pneumonia (PCP) are generally prevented in the postoperative period, as well as topical, fungal infections such as thrush. The risk of occurrence of these infections is highest in the immediate postoperative period due to the amount of immunosuppression the patient is receiving. There is an increased risk for CMV infection if the donor is CMV positive and the recipient is CMV negative [32].

Antiviral, antibiotic, and antifungal medications are administered to treat infection and prophylaxis against infection. Specific immunoglobulins are also administered for prophylaxis, such as IVIG for general coverage, Cytogam for CMV, and Synagis for RSV. Routine immunizations are not administered for 3–6 months after transplantation to allow for an adequate antibody response to the vaccine for proper protection. Live virus vaccines are generally avoided in transplant recipients [32].

Coronary allograft vasculopathy (CAV) is a late complication post-transplant. CAV in the post-transplant patient differs from typical atherosclerosis in that CAV is a concentric thickening of the intimal lining of the coronary artery wall as opposed to isolated areas of plaque buildup. This concentric thickening occurs throughout the entire coronary artery and may be more severe in some areas than others. CAV is most likely an immune response; however, usually there are other contributing factors. Due to denervation at the time of transplant, the patient may be asymptomatic. Occasionally, patients experience angina, abdominal pain, and arm pain, symptoms consistent with classic myocardial infarction [34]. A second transplant is often the treatment for severe CAV.

Another late complication post-transplant is post-transplantation lymphoproliferative disorder (PTLD). PTLD is a variety of lymphomas that develop in the transplant patient due to their immunocompromised state [35]. Most commonly, an overgrowth of Epstein-Barr virus infected B cells cause the lymphoma. The immunosuppression medications taken to prevent donor heart rejection also cause T cell's inability to control proliferation [36]. Approximately 5 % of pediatric heart transplant recipients acquire PTLD. Survival is 67 %, 7 years after diagnosis of PTLD. Signs and symptoms of PTLD vary greatly and depend on where PTLD manifests. Most commonly, symptoms are fever, lymphadenopathy, lethargy, and splenomegaly. PTLD may present anywhere in the body where there is lymphoid tissue [37]. Treatment of PTLD includes reduction of maintenance immunosuppression or chemotherapy depending on the type and severity of the PTLD [34].

Due to a shortage of donor hearts, there have been initiatives to increase the donor pool. One way this may be achieved is through ABO mismatch. Babies less than 2 years of age may be listed with UNOS for a donor heart with an otherwise incompatible blood type. The immune system in infants is immature and has no "natural" antibodies against other blood group antigens, therefore making transplantation across blood types possible in the very young. Usually these isoagglutinins do not form until around 6 months of age [38]. Another effort to increase to donor pool is donation after circulatory death (DCD). DCD is organ donation after cessation of cardiac activity as opposed to the traditional donation after brain death is declared. These donors generally have experienced a devastating brain injury; however, they have not been declared brain dead [39]. These donors' families have decided to withdraw support prior to being approached for organ donation.

Heart transplantation is a psychologically and physically challenging endeavor. The families and patients must commit to lifelong medications and health care. These patients and families will need continued nursing support throughout each step of the transplant process.

Summary

Cardiovascular compromise may result from acquired heart disease, electrophysiologic disturbances, or sequelae of cardiac transplantation. Children with these cardiovascular problems require specialized care for optimal results. Nurses are in an excellent place at the bedside to make a strong impact on care of children with these cardiovascular concerns.

References

1. Webber S (2008) New-onset heart failure in children in the absence of structural congenital heart disease. Circulation 117:11–12, American Heart Association
2. Curley M, Moloney-Harmon P (2001) Critical care nursing of infants and children. W.B. Saunders, Philadelphia
3. Canobbio M (1990) Cardiovascular disorders. Mosby's Clinical Nursing Series, St. Louis
4. Anderson R, Baker E, Penny D, Redington A, Rigby M, Wernovsky G (2010) Pediatric cardiology, 3rd edn. Churchill Livingstone/Elsevier, Philadelphia, PA
5. Chang A, Hanley F, Wernovsky G, Wessel D (1998) Pediatric cardiac intensive care. Lippincott Williams & Wilkinson, Philadelphia
6. Sharma M, Webber S, Morell V, Gandhi S, Wearden P, Buchanan J, Kormos R (2006) Ventricular assist device support in children and adolescents as a bridge to heart transplantation. Ann Thorac Surg 82:926–932
7. Darovic G (1995) Hemodynamic monitoring: invasive and noninvasive clinical application. W.B. Saunders Co, Philadelphia
8. Park M (2010) The pediatric cardiology handbook, 4th edn. Mosby/Elsevier, Philadelphia, PA
9. Keane J, Lock J, Fyler D (2006) Nadas' pediatric cardiology, 2nd edn. Saunders, Elsevier, Philadelphia
10. Allen H, Gutgesell H, Clark E, Driscoll D (2001) Moss and Adams' heart disease in infants, children, and adolescents: including the fetus and young adult, vol 1. Lippincott Williams & Wilkins, Philadelphia
11. Burns J (2007) The riddle of Kawasaki disease. N Engl J Med 356:659–661
12. ArizonaCERT (Center for education and research on therapeutics). http://azcert.org/, Web. 7 May 2012
13. Boville B, Young L (eds) (2011) Quick guide to pediatric cardiopulmonary care. Edwards Life Sciences, Irvine
14. Collardey K, Bradley D (2011) Care of the pediatric patient with SVT. In: Tsiperfal A (ed) Cardiac arrhythmia management: a practical guide for nurses and associated professionals. Wiley-Blackwell, Chichester
15. Dick M (ed) (2006) Clinical cardiac electrophysiology in the young. Springer, New York
16. Dubin A (2004) Cardiac arrhythmias. In: Behrman R, Kliegman R, Jenson H (eds) Nelson textbook of pediatrics, 17th edn. Saunders, Philadelphia
17. Hanisch D (2011) Care of the pediatric patient with a device. In: Tsiperal A (ed) Cardiac arrhythmia management: a practical guide for nurses and associated professionals. Wiley-Blackwell, Chichester
18. Park M (2003) The pediatric cardiology handbook, 3rd edn. Mosby, Philadelphia
19. Payne L, Zeigler V, Gillette P (2011) Acute cardiac arrhythmias following surgery for congenital heart disease: mechanisms, diagnostic tools, and management. Crit Care Nurs Clin North Am 23:255–272
20. Sudden Arrhythmia Death Syndromes (SADS Foundation). http://www.sads.org/, Web. 7 May 2012
21. Zeigler V, Gillette P (eds) (2001) Practical management of pediatric cardiac arrhythmias. Futura, Armonk
22. UNOS policy 3.7 retrieved on 5/20/2012 from http://optn.transplant.hrsa.gov/PoliciesandBylaws2/policies/pdfs/policy_9.pdf
23. Kirklin J, Young J, McGiffin D (2002) Heart transplantation. Churchill Livingstone, New York
24. Costanzo M, Dipchand A, Starling R (2010) Task force 1: peri-operative care of the heart transplant recipient. In: The international society of heart and lung transplantation guidelines for the care of heart transplant recipients. Retrieved from http://www.ishlt.org/ContentDocuments/ISHLT_GL_TaskForce1_080410.pdf
25. Adnan T, Jesse W, James G et al (2007) Noninvasive cerebral oximeter as a surrogate for mixed venous saturation in children. Pediatr Cardiol 28:34–41
26. Funk M (1986) Heart transplantation – postoperative care during the acute period. Crit Care Nurs 6:27–45
27. Nottingham A, Rambo A (1986) Electrocardiographic phenomena in the transplanted human heart. Focus Crit Care 13:641–646
28. Huddleston CB, Alejos JC, Thus JM (2007) Postoperative management: early graft failure, pulmonary hypertension and initial immunosuppression strategies. In: Canter CE, Kirklin JK (eds) Pediatric heart transplantation. Elsevier, Philadelphia
29. Gazit AZ, Fehr J (2011) Perioperative management of the pediatric cardiac transplantation patient. Curr Treat Options Cardiovasc Med 13:425–443
30. Dodd DA, Cabo J, Dipchand AI (2007) Acute rejection: natural history, risk factors, surveillance, and treatment. In: Canter CE, Kirklin JK (eds) Pediatric heart transplantation. Elsevier, Philadelphia
31. Kirk R, Edwards L, Kucheryavaya AY et al (2011) The registry of the international society for heart and lung transplantation: fourteenth pediatric heart transplantation report – 2011. J Heart Lung Transplant 30:1095–1103
32. Schowengerdt KO, Azeka E (2007) Infection following pediatric heart transplantation. In: Canter CE, Kirklin JK (eds) Pediatric heart transplantation. Elsevier, Philadelphia
33. Renoult E, Buteau C, Lamarre V et al (2005) Infectious risk in pediatric organ transplant recipients: is it increased with the new immunosuppressive agents? Pediatr Transplant 9:470–479
34. Pahl E, Caforio ALP, Kuhn MA (2007) Allograft vasculopathy: detection, risk factors, natural history, and treatment. In: Canter CE, Kirklin JK (eds) Pediatric heart transplantation. Elsevier, Philadelphia

35. Webber SA, Naftel DC, Fricker FJ et al (2006) Lymphoproliferative disorders after paediatric heart transplantation: a multi-institutional study. Lancet 367:233–239

36. Manlhiot C, Pollock-BarZiv SM, Holmes C et al (2010) Post-transplant lymphoproliferative disorder in pediatric heart transplant recipients. J Heart Lung Transplant 29:648–657

37. Addonizio LJ, Boyle GJ (2007) Postransplant malignancy: risk factors, incidence, diagnosis, treatment. In: Canter CE, Kirklin JK (eds) Pediatric heart transplantation. Elsevier, Philadelphia

38. West LJ, Shaddy RE, Balfour IC (2007) Special immunologic issues in pediatric heart transplantation. In: Canter CE, Kirklin JK (eds) Pediatric heart transplantation. Elsevier, Philadelphia

39. Yoo PS, Olthoff KM, Abt PL (2011) Donation after cardiac death in pediatric organ transplantation. Curr Opin Organ Transplant 16(5):483–488

Pediatric Cardiac Intensive Care: Nursing Education and Leadership

Sandra Staveski, Patricia Lincoln, Heather Freeman, Debra Morrow, and Christine Peyton

Abstract

Nurses, nurse educators, and advanced practice nurses (APNs) are in an excellent position to provide leadership in the pediatric cardiac intensive care unit (PCICU). Nursing leadership roles include quality improvement, consultation, education, development and implementation of evidence-based practices, and research. This is especially true as more and more APNs are pursuing doctoral education. Many centers have nursing shared leadership with unit-based councils. Also included in this section is a summary of recommendations for orientation and education for the bedside nurse working in the pediatric cardiac intensive care unit. These recommendations provide a structured professional development program for newly hired nurses that maximize critical thinking abilities and

S. Staveski (✉)
Pediatric Cardiovascular Intensive Care Unit, Lucile
Packard Children's Hospital at Stanford, Palo Alto,
CA, USA
e-mail: sstaveski@lpch.org

P. Lincoln
Clinical Nurse Specialist, Cardiac Intensive Care Unit,
Boston Children's Hospital, Boston, MA, USA
e-mail: Patricia.Lincoln@childrens.harvard.edu

H. Freeman
Lucile Packard Children's Hospital at Stanford, Palo Alto,
CA, USA
e-mail: hfreeman@lpch.org

D. Morrow
Cardiac Intensive Care Unit, Boston Children's Hospital,
Boston, MA, USA
e-mail: debra.morrow@cardio.chboston.org

C. Peyton
Cardiac Intensive Care Unit, Clinical Nurse Specialist,
Children's Hospital Colorado, Aurora, CO, USA
e-mail: christine.peyton@childrenscolorado.org;
peyton.christine@tchden.org

E.M. da Cruz et al. (eds.), *Pediatric and Congenital Cardiology, Cardiac Surgery and Intensive Care*,
DOI 10.1007/978-1-4471-4619-3_109, © Springer-Verlag London 2014

acquiring complex skills. Ongoing education after onboarding is essential to the success of bedside nursing professional development. APNs and nurse leaders are essential to the development of a strong nursing team.

Keywords

Clinical nurse specialists • Critical thinking • Evidence-based practice • Hospital-acquired infections • Infection prevention bundles • Mentors • Nurse practitioners • Nursing education • Orientation • Quality improvement • Research

Introduction

Nurses, nurse educators, and advanced practice nurses (APNs) are in an excellent position to provide leadership in the pediatric cardiac intensive care unit (PCICU). Nursing leadership roles include quality improvement, consultation, education, development and implementation of evidence-based practices, and research. This is especially true as more and more APNs are pursuing doctoral education. Many centers have nursing shared leadership with unit-based councils. Also included in this section is a summary of recommendations for orientation and education for the bedside nurse working in the pediatric cardiac intensive care unit. These recommendations provide a structured professional development program for newly hired nurses that maximize critical thinking abilities and acquiring complex skills. Ongoing education after onboarding is essential to the success of bedside nursing professional development. APNs are essential to the development of a strong nursing team.

Advanced Practice Nursing in the Pediatric Cardiac ICU

Advanced practice nurses (APNs) have had specialized graduate-level nursing education and their role can include comprehensive health assessment, diagnosis, patient management, pathophysiology, care coordination, research, and education. These expert nurses stay close to patient care delivery and function in expanded nursing roles such as clinical nurse specialists (CNSs) and nurse practitioners (NPs) [1]. Consultation and leadership functions are essential aspects to the success of these roles in clinical practice. Moreover, the roles are evolving due to increases in patient acuity, care fragmentation from trainee work hour restrictions, shortages of trained personnel, and cost-containment strategies. Historically, the PCICU APN role was predominantly clinical nurse specialists (CNSs). In fact, the CNS role was developed to keep expert PCICU nurses at the bedside and improve patient care delivery. The focus of the CNS role is on expert clinical practice, consultation, education, and research. However, over the course of the past 10 years, pediatric nurse practitioners (PNPs) have become more abundant in Pediatric Cardiac Intensive Care Units (PCICUs) due to changes in healthcare delivery systems and cost-containment necessities.

Clinical Nurse Specialist

The CNS in the PCICU is an APN with clinical expertise in the care of the pediatric patient with heart disease. These nurses partner with the nurse at the bedside providing different levels of support, depending on the situation. Both the new graduate nurse and the experienced nurse may be a novice in the care of the pediatric cardiac intensive care patient. The novice nurse will require the CNS's expertise in patient/family assessment or implementation of care. Most PCICU patients have little reserve and decompensate quickly. The CNS assists the novice nurse to fully appreciate the fragility of these patients. As the CNS works with the nurse at the bedside in improving physical assessment skills, the nurse becomes more familiar in noting subtle patient changes. As assessment skills strengthen, the CNS then turns efforts toward supporting the novice nurse in nursing care decisions and the evaluation of patient outcomes. Assistance with family assessment may also be needed. Many units permit family to be at the patient bedside around the clock. The family of a PCICU patient is in need of much reassurance and education. The CNS may perceive understated cues from the family regarding this, which the novice nurse occupied with patient care may not pick up. The CNS could aid with de-escalation techniques for family members or additional education or clarification, if that is needed.

The more experienced nurse will profit from CNS involvement in other areas of nursing practice. The CNS may provide consultation regarding various patient concerns, for example, skin alteration or preservation measures, pain or sedation plans, and nutrition concerns. The CNS helps maintain focus on a multidisciplinary approach to patient care, with knowledge of resources and the necessary teambuilding skills. For the experienced nurse, the CNS may act as a "sounding board" for patient care concerns and obtain needed resources for the patient, the family, or the bedside nurse. When the nurse caring for the patient is unable to leave the bedside, the CNS may relieve the bedside nurse for patient care responsibilities. The CNS also mentors the experienced nurse in projects involved with patient care, for example, teaching classes within the hospital, abstract development for conferences, the use of evidence-based practice, quality improvement projects, and interpreting and collaborating in research. As an expert, the CNS has the ability to critically examine a situation and the confidence to implement a change and evaluate outcomes: taking full responsibility to integrate patient care modifications into practice.

The support of the bedside nurse by the CNS in the PCICU provides an environment that encourages questions and discussions, one that engages nurses in professional and educational opportunities, and also inspires the development of clinical excellence. This is the type of environment which contributes to work satisfaction and nursing recruitment and retainment.

The PCICU NP is educated and trained to provide direct patient care to critically and chronically, critically ill children with heart disease. The focus of their clinical practice is on restoration of optimal health status and is inclusive of patient stabilization, provision of comprehensive physical and psychosocial care, and harm reduction. PCICU NPs perform direct patient care to a cadre of patients; foster continuity for those patients and their families; and are liaisons between various members of the interdisciplinary team, consultants, case managers, leaders, and researchers. PCICU NPs examine and perform health assessments on their specific cohort of patients, write medical orders, perform diagnostic and therapeutic procedures, interpret laboratory and diagnostic testing, manage their patients, prescribe medications, counsel patients and families, and foster patient/family teaching in collaboration with physicians [2, 3]. A focus on health promotion and holistic care, an advanced understanding of pathophysiology, and a strong background in general nursing practice place the PCICU NP in an excellent position to minimize and/or prevent risks for patients inherent with a PCICU admission.

There are several models for PCICU NP practice and they include the following:

1. *PCICU PNP model*. This model provides comprehensive care by mid-level providers in order to fill in gaps where trainee hour restrictions and have presented opportunities to expand nursing presence and practice in the PCICU. This model provides holistic care delivery for patients in the PCICU; focuses on preventive services and harm reduction; provides stability and continuity for the PCICU patients, families, and team; and provides expert clinical practice and consultation

services specific for critically ill children with heart disease and their families. Chronically, critically ill patients and their families are well served by this model with the continuous, on-unit PCICU NP presence. Clinical privileges, role autonomy, broad scope of practice, and collaborative practice are the benefits of this model.

2. *Acute care pediatric nurse practitioner (ACPNP) case management model.* The goal of this model is to facilitate and coordinate a patient's hospital stay in order to provide quality, cost-contained care. Managed care and cost-containment can prompt early discharges, and ACPNPs in a case management model can play important roles in addressing these pressures through outpatient clinical visits, telephone triage, and liaisoning with primary care providers. Broader clinical knowledge base (than specific PCICU) and care continuity through the care continuum are the benefits of this model.

While CNS and PNP roles within the PCICU are very different, they share significant clinical nursing leadership functions while staying close to their patients. They share important roles in education, quality improvement, evidence-based practice, and research activities. Universally, APNs have important roles in facilitating teamwork and communication among the interdisciplinary team, optimizing staff, patient, and family experiences; fostering patient safety and minimizing the potential for harm; and promoting exceptional patient outcomes.

Advanced Practice Nurse's Role in Quality Improvement

Leadership, specifically "clinical, professional, and systems leadership" is a core competency of the advanced practice nurse (APN) [4]. The APN system leader role is a crucial one. APNs are uniquely trained and equipped to determine how the healthcare system functions and how it is designed. As noted in the IOM's Future of Nursing report: "Nurses' regular, close proximity to patients and scientific understanding of care processes across the continuum of care give them a unique ability to act as partners with other health professionals and to lead in the improvement and redesign of the health care system and its many practice environments" [5].

In the Crossing the Quality *Chasm, the IOM's Committee on Quality of Health Care in America's* second report, the IOM provided six aims for improvement: patient care should be "safe, effective, patient-centered, timely, efficient, and equitable" [6]. The role of the APN in system leadership is to lead, guide, and participate in the work to improve patient care within the six aims. A prerequisite to improving a system is to deeply understand the system.

Gaining System Knowledge

Deming repeatedly said, "There is no substitute for knowledge" [7]. Healthcare providers may assume that because they work daily within the system, they already know everything there is to know about the system. However, Deming also explained that a "system cannot know itself" and that an outside-in approach is required [8]. The way to gain knowledge about a system is to objectively observe elements and interactions within the system.

Nelson et al., the originators of clinical microsystem thinking, recommend studying five key elements, which they termed the "5Ps" [9, 10].

First, define the purpose of the care unit system to give clear direction for improvement work and clarify how work processes relate to patients' needs.

Next, seek to understand the patient population by studying elements such as age distribution, sex, common diagnoses, socioeconomic status, languages, and satisfaction with services.

Then describe the professionals working within the system by identifying all the types of professionals, their functions and how their function relates to the purpose, how staff use their time, how communication and collaboration occurs between staff, the resources available to provide daily care, and staff satisfaction/morale/engagement.

Processes are how professionals provide care, such as the admission process, the respiratory management processes, and the various processes to collaborate with and provide information to families. Each care process should be defined and steps within key processes identified in a flow chart. Directly observing and walking through key care processes, as they are experienced by patients, is necessary. Flow charts should include role of provider doing each step, how much time key steps take (cycle time) on average, and waiting/queues. Identifying steps in care processes provides the team with an opportunity to reduce wasteful, redundant steps and complexity. Care processes that are working well with little variability (according to standard) and those that are not working well and have high variability (not according to standard, or no standard in place) will be evident [9, 10].

The interaction of the former four "Ps" produces patterns. Patterns include census trends, and the key outcome and process metrics that result from care processes. Patterns, such as outcomes metrics, should be used to prioritize and guide improvement work [9, 10].

How to Improve: Applying Science to Improvement

Many improvement opportunities will be identified through the process of gaining system knowledge. The rigor applied to understanding the system is matched by the rigor required to improve the processes that make up the system.

The scientific method, developed 400 years ago by Sir Francis Bacon [11], is familiar to APNs: observation, hypothesis, intervention, results/reflection, revise hypothesis, new intervention, etc. Scientific method is iterative, reality and evidence based, and it starts with observation. Below are the basic steps to improve quality using a modification of the scientific method,

the Shewhart/Deming Plan-Do-Check-Adjust (PDCA) improvement cycle [9, 12]. The following paragraphs will include a fictitious problem to illustrate the improvement process.

Plan: Understanding the Problem(s) and Planning Changes

Upon reviewing outcomes data, a clinical unit finds that they have an unacceptably high central line–associated bloodstream infection (CLABSI) rate. The team began the three steps to understanding the problem: finding, clarifying, and determining the cause of the problem [13]. By reviewing data, the team *found* a problem. But, finding the problem is only the first step to understanding it.

It is tempting to plan changes as soon as a problem is found, but without clarifying and understanding the causes of the problem, changes will not be effective [13, 14]. *Clarifying* the problem requires observing the work: "Go and see for yourself to thoroughly understand the situation" [15]. Do detailed observations, involve staff in identifying problems, ask the questions "who, what, when, where, why and how" [13, 14]. An example, a team found that postoperative newborns (<8 weeks old) on parenteral nutrition located in a room of six patient beds comprised the greatest percentage (62 %) of the patient population that developed CLABSIs. This new information helped focus improvement energy toward the biggest problem.

The APN must ask "why" often to determine the cause(s) of a problem [12–14]. In the example, observations in the patient's room revealed that hand hygiene before patient contact was occurring 30 % of the time. Why: hand hygiene supplies were not located in close proximity to the patient, requiring care providers to walk across the room. Why: housekeeping did not put hand hygiene supplies at the bedside. Why: there were no devices for holding hand hygiene supplies at the bedside. Why: devices for holding hand hygiene supplies at the bedside had not been ordered or mounted.

After the problem is well understood, the next step is to identify what aim of the improvement work should be. The aim should be time specific and measurable. As Dr. Donald Berwick has said, "Some is not a number, soon is not a time" [16]. An example aim statement is, "We aim to decrease the CLABSI rate by 70 % in post-op newborn patients by July 15, 2014."

Next, establish measures in order to answer the question, "How will we know the change resulted in improvement?" [17]. For the above aim, the obvious metric is the CLABSI rate. Process measures, or measures that monitor whether changes are implemented consistently and are effective, should also be included. The example team included several process measures, one of them being compliance with the evidence-based hand hygiene protocol.

After the problem is well understood, the aim is set, and measures are selected, then it is time to develop changes. Proposed changes should directly address the causes of the problems that have been identified. Changes are not *solutions*. Changes are *potential solutions*. It is not possible to know if a change will produce the desired outcome without testing the change.

Do: Testing the Change

Change management is an art and science unto itself, rooted in psychology, sociology, and behavior science. In general, changes that have clear advantages are compatible with staff needs, have low complexity, and have a visible impact on outcomes are more readily adopted [18]. A good maxim is, "Make the right thing to do the easy thing to do." Changes that are tested and modified during testing are also more easily accepted [18]. The reason for trialing changes is twofold: to learn what changes are effective in addressing problems and to involve everyone in creatively and critically developing the new process [12, 13]. Motivation researcher Daniel Pink found that humans have an "innate need to direct our own lives, to learn and create new things, and to do better by our world" [19]. Giving staff the ability to contribute creatively to an important

cause is the most effective motivator for participation in and adoption of improvements.

In the example, the team decided to move hand hygiene supplies to the bedside and developed a plan to implement and test this change. Planning the test of change not only includes planning the actual change, such as ordering devices to hold hand hygiene supplies, but also includes planning education, communication, measurement to determine if the change is successful, and setting a trial period.

The team implemented, observed, and monitored the change. They found that compliance with the hand hygiene protocol increased to 75 % after the change. Other factors, such as communication and education, may have also contributed to increased compliance. Although this was a very successful intervention, the team realized that the change did not address all of the hand hygiene compliance problems because compliance was still less than 100 %. The team then had an opportunity to learn what other process problems existed and develop changes to address the other problems.

Adjust: Changing the Change

Adjust is the process of starting the improvement cycle over again, based on new knowledge gained by doing a test of change [12]. In this example, the team found that hand hygiene supplies were not reliably replenished. They therefore made a plan to ensure supplies were reliably replenished.

Eventually, after a number of change cycles, an effective process will emerge. However, sustaining the new, effective process is the next challenge.

Sustain

Creating and managing standards is the way to sustain a change [12]. If standards are not created and/or if a process to manage the new standards (e.g., a consistent process to check to see if the process is still working), the change succumbs to entropy and is not sustained [18]. In the example, compliance with hand hygiene will decrease again. The goal is to build highly reliable standard processes that are built into daily work and are routinely checked. How is this done?

Standards can take the form of checklists (e.g., order sets), visual controls (e.g., a marker on the floor to indicate where a code cart belongs), or involve mistake proofing which makes it impossible to do the wrong thing (e.g., oral syringes that are incompatible with IV tubing ports) [14, 20]. Again, the key to sustaining the change is to *make the right thing to do the easy thing to do.*

The APN is a system leader. Gaining knowledge of the system is the first step in improving the system. Successful, sustainable improvement processes are ones rooted in science and have the Plan-Do-Check-Act cycle at their core. Finding problems is just the first step in understanding the problem. Clarifying and identifying causes of problems is half the work of solving problems. Problems are not solved around the conference room table; they are solved at the place they occur. "Go and see" [13, 15]. Problems are not solved by individuals; they are solved by teams of people who are closest to the work.

> We need to be aware of problems and be passionate about being dissatisfied with the status quo; more importantly, we need to bond that dissatisfaction with our desire to improve. (Shingeo Shingo) [14]

Infection Prevention: An Example of Nursing Leadership Role in Quality Improvement Practices

Initiatives to decrease the incidence of healthcare-associated infections have been promoted by the Institute for Healthcare Improvement (IHI) [23, 25], the Child Health Corporation of America (CHCA) [24, 26], and the National Association of Children's Hospitals and Related Institutions (NACHRI) [29] since 2004. These initiatives endorse the implementation of practice "bundles" for the insertion and maintenance of indwelling venous and urinary catheters and medical devices such as endotracheal tubes. A "bundle" is a combination of evidence-based practices, which will improve patient outcomes when followed by every member of the healthcare team [25]. There are three areas of practice that are included in every bundle: hand hygiene, early removal of indwelling catheters and medical devices, and empowering staff to intervene when breaches in sterile technique are observed during the insertion and care of indwelling catheters and devices [22].

Hand hygiene is the cornerstone of all infection prevention initiatives. Studies have shown that the most common mode of transmission of infectious agents in hospitals is via the hands of healthcare workers. Hand hygiene should be performed before and after contact with a patient or patient's environment, before and after manipulating an invasive device, and before and after wearing gloves. The use of alcohol-based hand sanitizers is fast and effective, but hands should be washed with soap and water when visibly soiled, or when caring for a patient with infection from a spore-forming pathogen such as *Clostridium difficile.*

Indwelling venous and urinary catheters and temporary medical devices, such as endotracheal tubes, should be removed as soon as possible. Bacterial biofilm quickly builds up on the inner and outer surfaces of any indwelling catheter or tube. This biofilm can protect bacteria from antibiotics used to prevent or treat infections. Many intensive care units utilize a daily checklist to initiate a discussion on the need for each catheter or device, and what should be done to expedite its removal.

Nursing practices to prevent central line–associated bloodstream infections (CLABSIs) are as follows:

- Central venous catheters (CVCs) should be inserted by trained personnel using maximal sterile barriers (mask, cap, sterile gown, sterile gloves, and drape entire field) [35].
- Use >0.5 % chlorhexidine preparations containing alcohol for skin antisepsis before CVC insertion and during dressing changes [21, 28, 29, 35]. If there is a contraindication to chlorhexidine, the use of 70 % alcohol or povidone-iodine is acceptable [30].

Allow all agents to dry completely. A recent survey of neonatal ICUs revealed that many are using chlorhexidine on premature infants as young as 28 weeks gestation despite the FDA guidelines restricting use under 2 months of age [32].

- Use transparent, semipermeable dressings or sterile gauze on all CVCs. Do not place antiseptic agents on insertion site.
- Perform sterile CVC dressing change every 7 days or when damp, loose, or soiled. Change gauze and tape dressings every 48 h. Record date on dressings.
- Change CVC tubing no less than every 96 h, replace lipid emulsions tubing every 24 h. Record date on tubing.
- Perform a minimum 15 s scrub with friction of CVC cap prior to line access [33, 34]. Disinfectant agent can be 70 % alcohol, chlorhexidine/alcohol, or povidone-iodine preparations. All agents must dry before line access.
- Minimize CVC line access. Maintain a dedicated port for TPN infusions.
- Minimize connections; if stopcocks must be used, cap access port.
- Consider using antibiotic-coated catheters, and a chlorhexidine-impregnated sponge on the CVC insertion site, if CLABSI rates remain high after implementing a comprehensive program to decrease CLABSI rates [28].

Nursing practices to prevent ventilator-associated pneumonia are as follows:

- Use a cuffed endotracheal tube and elevate head of bed 30° for all intubated patients to prevent aspiration of oral secretions or gastric contents. Infants in isolettes should be positioned in reverse trendelenburg.
- Perform oral hygiene a minimum of every 12 h in all intubated patients. Brush teeth and gums with sterile water, using a toothbrush with toothpaste, to remove plaque. Gums of intubated infants should be cleaned with sterile water and gauze to prevent the buildup of plaque.
- Suction the posterior oropharynx before position changes to prevent oral secretions from entering the lower airway.

- Perform a daily sedation interruption and assessment of readiness to extubate when patient is stable

Nursing practices to prevent catheter-associated urinary tract infections are as follows:

- Urinary catheters should be inserted by trained personnel using sterile equipment.
- Maintain unobstructed urine flow in the collecting system and do not allow urine to reflux back into the bladder.
- Perform routine daily hygiene of the periurethral area. Daily urinary catheter care with antiseptic agents is not recommended.
- Do not break the urinary catheter-collecting system connection. Disinfect connection with 70 % alcohol prior to disconnecting and reconnect with a new collecting system.
- Utilize a bladder scanner to assess bladder volumes as part of the decision to catheterize for urinary retention. Intermittent catheterization decreases the risk of infection.

Nursing practices to prevent surgical site infections are as follows:

The prevention of surgical site infections begins in the operating room [23]. Chlorhexidine-alcohol preparations have been shown to decrease the incidence of surgical site infections as compared to povidone-iodine solutions [23, 32, 33] when used for the preoperative scrub. Antibiotic prophylaxis is delivered within 1 h before incision or within 2 h if vancomycin or a fluoroquinolone is used. When hair removal is needed, clippers or a depilatory agent should be used [22, 33].

Postoperative care of the surgical site

- Maintain a sterile, occlusive dressing on surgical site for first 48 h after surgery
- Maintain sterile occlusive dressings on all intracardiac lines, chest tubes, and pacing wires for duration of placement
- Delayed sternal closure: maintain sterile occlusive dressing and monitor patient closely for heat loss
- Discontinue postoperative prophylactic antibiotics be within 48 h of surgery [23, 25], however many centers continue prophylactic antibiotics until chest tubes are removed

Providing adequate enteral nutrition both pre- and postoperatively for the newborn with congenital heart disease is a challenge. Patients with ductal-dependant lesions are at risk for developing necrotizing enterocolitis, and many patients with CHD experience feeding intolerance and have a high incidence of gastroesophageal reflux. However, studies have shown that the implementation of early enteral feeds lowers infection rates, maintains normal gut flora, and decreases the duration of parenteral nutrition [34].

The APN Role in Evidence-Based Practice and Research

Education, quality improvement, evidence-based practice, and research are four pillars supporting excellence in nursing practice. Evidence-based practice (EBP) can be described as the integration of science and patient values into nursing clinical practice [36]. It is the goal of all healthcare institutions and a requirement of accreditation agencies. Thus, a systematic approach integrating existing nursing science into policies, procedures, and nursing practice is of the utmost importance. Research findings can be viewed as the "raw materials" that require transformation into the foundation of clinical protocols [37].

Many unit-based clinical practice councils and APNs are facilitators of EBP and are charged with this duty. Typically, a clinical practice council guided by their APN identifies a clinical issue, searches the literature via multiple databases, performs a best practice survey, and tailors nursing care delivery based on nursing science and best practice in lieu of existing research. Thus, EBP utilizes research to facilitate best clinical outcomes using proven information to inform nursing clinical decision-making. EBP defines quality, takes actions to improve care, and measures outcomes. A mechanism for determining clinical effectiveness of EBP is use of the clinical audit.

Barriers to EBP include staff nurse perceptions of their abilities, skills, and expertise to adequately analyze research studies, utilize search engines and databases, and integrate the

data into policy/procedure. Additionally, interfacing with various organizations can be challenging. Journal clubs can help to provide nurses and APNs with the resources to eliminate some of these barriers. Journal clubs promote the review and critique of published research studies and develop the skill sets of nurses to search, review, and critique the literature. Taking the next step and asking the correct question can also be challenging for novices, but it is an essential skill. One method for asking good questions can be to use the PICO template. P stands for patient problem, I stands for intervention, C stands for comparison, and O stands for outcome(s) [38].

Nursing research is the use of systematic, controlled, empirical, and critical investigations in order to confirm or discover scientific facts as they relate to nursing practice or an identified problem [39]. In other words, research is building knowledge and is a significant aspect of nursing practice. Research can be descriptive, exploratory, analytical, or evaluative. There are two main types of research studies: qualitative and quantitative. Qualitative studies are utilized to understand healthcare experiences, social settings, social interactions, and social processes. Data are collected by one of these mechanisms, namely, in-depth conversation, diaries, interviewing, focus groups, and observation. Quantitative methods are utilized to understand the workings of the world [39]. Nursing research phenomena can be people (e.g., patients, nurses, families), social, physical, interventions, and systems [39].

Research is a mechanism to determine how care can be best provided to improve outcomes, the impact of various aspects of nursing care; assess effectiveness of treatment modalities; assess cost-effective strategies; and/or advance the science of nursing. Making space and ensuring there is adequate time for performing nursing research is a challenge given the day-to-day workings of bedside nursing and advanced practice nursing. However, nurses and APNs can play an integral role advancing the practice and improving outcomes if they overcome barriers associated with performing research.

The Advanced Practice Nurse and Nursing Professional Development

The PCICU provides a challenging environment for the bedside nurse due to the complexity of patients with heart disease and wide age span housed therein. The nurse must have an excellent understanding of pathophysiology, congenital heart defects and their repairs, acquired heart disease, pulmonary hypertension, mechanical circulatory support, heart transplantation; hands-on skills set for managing premature, low-birth weight infants through adults with congenital heart disease and their comorbidities, critical care skills; and the capacity of dealing with patients and their families with a lifelong illness, which may require multiple admissions.

An orientation program for novice nurses can be overwhelming and needs to include the following elements: supported clinical experiences; didactic classroom education; simulation training; problem-based learning; introduction to policies, procedures, standards of care that guide practice; and computer-based instruction. Moreover, there must be a clear link between protocols, policies and procedures, didactic learning, competencies, and the nurses' practice. More advanced monitoring techniques and utilization of equipment have compounded competency validation challenges. Mentoring is a key element for novice and newly hired nurses to ensure their success as a PCICU nurse. A program that allows for supported experiences with complex patients after orientation is essential to excellence in practice and ongoing retention of nurses.

The current healthcare environment has led nursing staff professional development and education leaders to seek answers to the best strategies for recruiting and retaining nurses [40]. Orientation and ongoing education have played a key role in retaining nurses and require multiple resources. In the past, nurses with pediatric medical-surgical experience were preferable to be hired. However, critical care areas are utilizing a variety of registered nurses and novice nurses to reach desired staffing levels. Orientation programs in critical care areas require structured orientation plans to maximize the opportunities for all nurses and ensure they have the requisite knowledge and skills to care for this demanding patient population [41]. Thus, the same orientation plan may not work between groups (i.e., new graduate, experienced pediatric, experienced adult, experienced PICU, experienced adult ICU) and may need to be modified to be successful.

However, in general, nurses first entering the critical care environment will need a combination of didactic learning, simulation training, computer-based learning, and clinical experiences. Didactic learning incorporates topics to generate critical thinking when caring for patients with congenital and acquired heart disease. Problem-based learning has been found to be an effective mechanism for all entry nurses. A standard curriculum encompasses critical care nursing physical assessment skills including neurologic, cardiovascular, pulmonary, gastrointestinal, renal, hematologic, immunologic, endocrine, and infectious disease [42]. Congenital heart defects can be classified and presented in several ways such as: (1). lesions increasing pulmonary blood flow, lesions decreasing pulmonary blood flow, and obstructive lesions or (2). based on their acuity level one (RACHS-1 level 1 and 2), acuity level two (RACHS-1 level 3 and 4), and acuity level three (RACHS-1 level 5 and 6). Didactic education should include acquired heart disease topics such as cardiomyopathies, myocarditis, pediatric heart failure, pulmonary hypertension, mechanical circulatory support, and transplantation (see Table 79.1). Didactic learning should be incorporated with clinical experiences to enhance orientation and ongoing education.

Computer-based learning allows flexibility, interactive learning, and reduction orientation hours [41]. Computer training programs with interactive capabilities allow the learner to advance at their own pace and support the principles that adults have a variety of backgrounds and different learning styles; thus, they learn best when they are provided with various learning modalities [43]. The orientee should have dedicated hours for completing computer-based learning modules outside of their clinical hours.

Table 79.1 Didactic content for pediatric cardiac intensive care unit

Phase 1

Cardiac assessment

Respiratory assessment and basics of ventilation

Gastrointestinal assessment

Genitourinary assessment

Fluid and electrolyte management

Skin assessment and prevention of pressure injuries

Neurological assessment

Mechanical ventilation and positive pressure ventilation

Noninvasive ventilation

Cardiopulmonary interactions

Fetal circulation and cardiac embryology

Normal cardiac anatomy and physiology

EKG interpretation

Lesions with increased pulmonary flow or RACHS-1 level 1 and 2

Lesions with decreased pulmonary flow or RACHS-1 level 3 and 4

Right and left obstructive heart lesions or RACHS-1 level 5 and 6

Pediatric heart failure

Acquired heart disease

Cardiomyopathy

Single ventricle physiology

Heart transplantation

Pulmonary hypertension

Interventional cardiology

Invasive and noninvasive cardiac monitoring (EKG, arterial lines, venous central lines)

Cardiac pharmacology

Cardiopulmonary bypass

Nutrition in the critically ill patient

Pain assessment and management

Newborn assessment and developmental care

Interpretation of lab values

End of life care

Premature infant and their comorbidities

Adults and their comorbidities

Child development

Genetic syndromes

Introduction to the interdisciplinary team

Patient and family education

Phase 2

Advanced hemodynamic monitoring (Swan-Ganz, intracardiac line, cardiac outputs)

Temporary pacemakers

Defibrillations

Postoperative care and emergency procedures

(continued)

Table 79.1 (continued)

Mechanical circulatory support (ECMO, VAD)

CRRT

Case scenarios

PALS and ACLS certification

Multisystem organ failure

Septic shock

Cardiogenic shock

Hypovolemic shock

Catheterization lab hemodynamics

Reading radiographs

Neurodevelopmental considerations

Quality of life

Transitioning adolescents to adult services

Phase 3

Leadership training

  Preceptor

  Charge nurse

  Mentoring and coaching

Research basics

Presentation skills

Journal club

Nursing mortality and morbidity meetings

EKG electrocardiogram
ECMO extracorporeal membrane oxygenation
VAD ventricular assist device, *PALS* pediatric advanced life support, *ACLS* advanced cardiac life support
CRRT continuous renal replacement therapies

Computer-based learning should be assigned to the orientee throughout orientation which will reinforce critical thinking skills. Some examples of computer-based learning include arrhythmia recognition and acid-base balance. Quality improvement, evidence-based protocols, and patient safety initiatives can be effectively taught with a computer-based module. These initiatives need to be hardwired throughout orientation for sustainability. Clinical handoffs, medication administration errors, and central line infections are examples of quality improvement and patient safety initiatives that are essential for a newly hired nurse.

Clinical experiences need to take into account the acuity and complexity of patients in the pediatric cardiac intensive care unit to optimize learning for the newly hired nurse. Assignments should promote critical thinking and not

Table 79.2 Assignments for clinical experiences

First phase of clinical experience
Paired Assignments
Stable 1:1 patient on ventilator and/or vasoactive drips
All diagnosis with a minimum of 12–24 h postoperative
Diagnostic or interventional catheterization recovery
Preoperative patients
Newly diagnosed patients transferred from outlying hospital
Heart transplantation rejection
Cardiomyopathy patient
Second phase of clinical experience
Fresh postoperative congenital heart patients with the exception of Norwood or neonatal Ross procedure
Heart transplantation
Stabilization of the critically ill newborn
Third phase of clinical experience
ECMO patient
VAD patient
HLHS undergoing Norwood procedure
Neonatal Ross patient
CRRT patients

overwhelm the newly hired nurse (see Table 79.2). Daily journaling enhances clinical experience and includes documenting diagnosis, surgical and/or interventional procedure, medications, complications, and nursing skills performed for the patient. "Testing out" at various points in the orientation process can be beneficial. Progress meetings with the nurse educator, preceptor, and orientee are scheduled on a reoccurring basis throughout the initial clinical experience phase. Once the novice nurse completes initial orientation, they begin to take patient assignments independently to gain confidence.

The newly hired nurse will gain confidence over the next 4–6 months during the interval phase and continue to focus on organization and prioritization skills. The goal of orientation and the first 6 months of employment is to support the orientee into becoming a safe advanced beginner. A clinical nurse specialist can provide opportunities for the nurse to gain experience on skills they were not able to experience during their orientation. Tracking and progress meetings

should occur regularly between the newly hired nurse, nurse educator, and clinical nurse specialist. Simulation scenarios may provide additional clinical experiences as well. Emergency procedures and clinical deterioration of a patient are ideal simulation scenarios for the newly hired nurse. After completing the initial phase following orientation, the novice nurse can then be oriented to the next phase of their development such as recovering the immediate postoperative pediatric cardiothoracic patient or moving on to managing more complex patients with the support of expert nurses and clinical nurse specialists. The third phase will occur at various times but generally after 12 months of employment in the pediatric cardiac intensive care unit (see Table 79.2).

Journal clubs and nursing mortality and morbidity meetings offer alternative mechanisms for nursing education after the initial orientation. APNs are in an excellent position to assist with educational opportunities. Mentorship from APNs is crucial to the success of a professional development plan. Mentoring relationships offer support and professional development for nurses at all levels in the organization as well as foster a healthy work environment [40]. The novice nurse may focus on mastering identifying cardiac arrhythmias but may not effectively communicate with the family. In this situation, the mentor demonstrates how to attend to analyzing a cardiac arrhythmia while incorporating positive interaction with the patient and family. Mentoring relationships exist in an environment that is nurturing and supporting staff as they develop new skills, knowledge, and critical thinking [40].

The end of orientation should not halt staff development. Staff need to be encouraged to obtain CCRN certification; explore leadership training opportunities (e.g., preceptor training, charge nurse training, CRRT, VAD, and advanced pacemaker training); interact in nursing rounds; and attend unit-based, hospital-based, and community-based continuing education offering as well as completing computer-based learning modules. By utilizing didactic learning, simulation training, computer-based learning modules, and clinical experiences, the newly hired nurse can become successful in the pediatric cardiac intensive care unit.

The current challenge is educating and supporting nursing staff to manage and care for the diverse, complex specialty of pediatric cardiac critical care. Advanced practice nurses are key drivers in pushing autonomous nursing practice forward. Nurse educators, clinical nurse specialists, and nurse practitioners can educate, motivate, support, coach, and mentor bedside nurses. The next challenge for the specialty of pediatric cardiology nursing is to support patients and families living to their fullest potential with a lifelong illness. Frontline nursing staff are in an excellent position to make a significant positive impact on children with heart disease and their families' lives by putting them in the best place to heal and to return to their lives outside of the hospital in a holistic manner.

References

1. Bigbee JL, Amindi-Nouri A (2000) History and evolution of advanced nursing practice. In: Hamric AB, Spross JA, Hanson CM (eds) Advanced nursing practice. an integrative approach, 2nd edn. W.B. Saunders, New York
2. Rust DM, Magdic K (2000) The acute care nurse practitioner. In: Hamric AB, Spross JA, Hanson CM (eds) Advanced nursing practice: an integrative approach, 2nd edn. W.B. Saunders, New York
3. Schoenberg L, Gross BP (1998) The role of the advanced practice nurse. In: Chang AC, Hanley FL, Wernovsky G, Wessel DL (eds) Pediatric cardiac intensive care, 1st edn. Williams and Wilkins, Philadelphia
4. Hamrick A, Spross J, Hansen C (2009) Advanced practice nursing: an integrative approach, 4th edn. Saunders Elsevier, St. Louis
5. Committee on the Robert Wood Johnson Foundation Initiative on the Future of Nursing, at the Institute of Medicine (2011) The future of nursing: leading change, advancing health. The National Academy of Sciences, Washington, DC
6. Committee on Quality of Health Care in America (2001) Crossing the quality chasm: a new health system for the 21st century. The National Academy of Sciences, Washington, DC
7. Deming W (1982) Out of the crisis. The MIT Press, Cambridge, MA
8. Deming W (2000) The new economics, 2nd edn. The MIT Press, Cambridge, MA
9. Nelson E, Batalden P, Godfrey M (2007) Quality by design: a clinical microsystems approach. Jossey-Bass, San Francisco
10. Nelson E, Batalden P, Godfrey M et al (2011) Value by design: developing clinical microsystems to achieve organizational excellence. Jossey-Bass, San Francisco
11. Klein J (2011) Francis Bacon. In: Zalta E (ed) The Stanford encyclopedia of philosophy, summer 2011 edn. http://plato.stanford.edu/archives/sum2011/entries/francis-bacon/
12. Liker J, Franz J (2011) The Toyota way to continuous improvement. McGraw-Hill, New York
13. Shook J (2008) Managing to learn: using the A3 management process to solve problems, gain agreement, mentor and lead. The Lean Enterprise Institute, Cambridge, MA
14. Shingo S (2007) Kaizen and the art of creative thinking (English translation). Enna Products, Bellingham
15. Liker J (2004) The Toyota way. McGraw-Hill, New York, p 40
16. Berwick D (2005) Some is not a number, soon is not a time. In: Institute for Healthcare Improvement AHQA annual meeting and technical conference, San Francisco, 23 February 2005. www.ahqa.org/pub/uploads/BerwickKeynotePresentation.ppt
17. Associates in Process Improvement (2010) Model for improvement. http://www.apiweb.org/API_home_page.htm
18. Greenhalgh T, Robert G, MacFarlane F et al (2004) Diffusion of innovations in service organizations: systematic review and recommendations. Milbank Q 82(4):581–629
19. Pink D (2009) Drive: the surprising truth about what motivates us. Riverhead Books, New York
20. Gawande A (2009) The checklist manifesto. Metropolitan Books, New York
21. Costello JM, Graham D, Forbes Morrow D et al (2009) Risk factors for central line-associated bloodstream infection in a pediatric cardiac intensive care unit. Pediatr Crit Care Med 10(4):453–459
22. Levy I, Ovadia B, Erez E et al (2003) Nosocomial infections after cardiac surgery in infants and children: incidence and risk factors. J Hosp Infect 53:111–116
23. Costello JM, Graham D, Forbes Morrow D et al (2010) Risk factors for surgical site infection after cardiac surgery in children. Ann Thorac Surg 89:1833–1842
24. Grohskopf L, Sinkowicz-Cochrane R, Garrett D et al (2002) A national point-prevalence survey of pediatric intensive care unit-acquired infections in the United States. J Pediatr 140(4):432–438
25. Institute for Healthcare Improvement. http://www.ihi.org/
26. Jeffries H, Mason W, Brewer M et al (2009) Prevention of central venous catheter-associated bloodstream infections in pediatric intensive care units: a performance improvement collaborative. Infect Control Hosp Epidemiol 30:7

27. Miller MR, Griswold M, Harris JR et al (2010) Decreasing PICU catheter-associated bloodstream infections: NACHRI's quality transformation efforts. Pediatrics 125:206–213

28. O'Grady N, Alexander M, Burns L et al (2011) Guidelines for the prevention of intravascular catheter-related infections. http://www.cdc.gov

29. Maki DG, Stolz SS, Wheeler S et al (1991) Prospective randomized trial of povidone-iodine, alcohol and chlorhexidine for prevention of infection associated with central venous and arterial catheters. Lancet 338:339–343

30. Tamma P, Aucott S, Milstone A (2010) Chlorhexidine use in the neonatal intensive care unit: results from a national survey. Infect Control Hosp Epidemiol 31(8):846–849

31. Kaler W, Chinn R (2007) successful disinfection of needleless access ports: a matter of time and friction. JAVA 12(3):140–142

32. Soothill J, Bravery K, Ho A (2009) A fall in bloodstream infections followed by a change to 2% chlorhexidine in 70% isopropanol for catheter connection antisepsis. Am J Infect Control 37(8):626–630

33. Darouiche R, Wall M, Itani K et al (2010) Chlorhexidine-alcohol versus povidone-iodine for surgical site antisepsis. NEJM 362:18–26

34. Braudis N, Curley M, Beaupre K et al (2010) Enteral feeding algorithm for infants with hypoplastic left heart syndrome post stage 1 palliation. Pediatr Crit Care Med 10(4):460–466

35. Costello JM, Forbes Morrow D, Graham D et al (2008) Systematic intervention to reduce central line associated bloodstream rates in a pediatric cardiac intensive care unit. Pediatrics 121:915–923

36. Rickbiel P, Simones J (2012) Overcoming barriers to implementing evidenced-based practice: a collaboration between academics and practice. J Nurs Staff Dev 28(2):53–56

37. Brown SJ (2009) Evidenced-based nursing: the research-practice connection. Jones and Bartlett, Boston

38. Sackett DL, Richardson WS, Rosenberg W, Haynes RB (1997) Evidence-based medicine: how to practice and teach EBM. Churchill Livingston, New York

39. Schotfedt RM (1977) Nursing research: reflection of values. Nurs Res 26(1):4–8

40. Kanaskie M (2006) Mentoring – a staff retention tool. Crit Care Nurs Q 29(3):248–252

41. Square ND (2010) Modeling clinical applications in intensive care settings for nursing orientation. Adv Neonatal Care 10(6):325–329

42. McKane CL (1997) Professional advancement model for critical care orientation. J Nurs Staff Dev 13(2):88–92

43. Coffman S (1996) Applying adult education principles to computer education. J Nurs Staff Dev 12(5):260–263

Section XIV

Congenital Cardiovascular Diseases in Pediatrics

Eduardo M. da Cruz, Dunbar Ivy, James Jaggers, and Viktor Hraska

Spectrum of Congenital Cardiac Defects

80

Michael S. Schaffer

Abstract

The spectrum of congenital heart disease with its evolving science and treatment strategies involves recognizing the collaboration of the simultaneously developing sciences of descriptive anatomy, physiology, and surgical technique. It is the collaboration of these sciences and their simultaneous evolution which have led the field of congenital cardiovascular medicine from the early days of the description of the naturally malformed heart to today's advances offering a virtual cure to many congenital heart lesions. As increasing numbers of children survive and thrive into adulthood, the science of congenital heart disease is no longer only a pediatric issue but rather an area of science and discovery spanning prenatal life into adulthood.

Keywords

Adult congenital heart disease • Anderson, RH • Arterial switch operation • Atrial septal defect • Baille, M • Becker, AE • Blackstone, EH • Blalock, A • Blalock-Hanlon procedure • Castaneda, AR • Cardiac MRI • da Vinci, L • Edwards, JE • Edwards, SW • Evolution • Farre, JR • Foramen ovale • Grant, RP • Harvey, W • Ho, SY • Hypoplastic left heart syndrome • Interventional cardiology • Jatene, AD • Kirklin, JW • Lillehei, CW • Lister, RG • Mustard, WT • Odgers, PNB • Patten, BM • Rashkind balloon septostomy • Rudolph, AM • Shaher, RM • Senning, A • Spectrum • Strategy • Taussig, HB • Tissue characterization • Transposition of the great vessels • von Rogitansky C • Wood, P

M.S. Schaffer
Cardiology, Heart Institute, University of Colorado
School of Medicine, Children's Hospital Colorado,
Aurora, CO, USA
e-mail: michael.schaffer@childrenscolorado.org

The spectrum of congenital heart disease with its evolving science and treatment strategies involves recognizing the collaboration of the simultaneously developing sciences of descriptive anatomy, physiology, and surgical technique. Early descriptions of anatomy from Stensen-Neils [1], the eloquent characterizations of J.E. Edwards [2], and most recently the detailed descriptions of R.H. Anderson et al. [3] are paralleled by the developing science of cardiac physiology. The early descriptions and experiments from W. Harvey [4] and R.G. Lister [5] through the innovative work of P. Wood [6] gave way to the understanding of the cardiac output in the developing fetus and neonate, which were so beautifully described and picturesquely presented by A.M. Rudolph and associates [7]. Early cardiac surgeons developed the novel surgical treatments of congenital heart disease. The pioneering work of A. Blalock and H.B. Taussig [8] lead to the inspiring work of A.R. Castaneda and the beginning of neonatal repair [9] and the surgical results and outcomes research of J.W. Kirklin and E.H. Blackstone [10]. Their work could only have been undertaken with the simultaneous development of cardiopulmonary bypass by C.W. Lillehei and colleagues [11]. It is the collaboration of these sciences and their simultaneous evolution which have led the field of congenital cardiovascular medicine from the early days of the description of the naturally malformed heart to today's advances offering a virtual cure to many congenital heart lesions.

D-transposition of the great vessels and the evolution of its treatment beautifully demonstrate the progression of the science from the description and understanding to the management of a congenital heart lesion. In the presurgical era, the anatomic description of D-transposition of the great vessels was always made at postmortem, and transposition was virtually a 100 % fatal disease. In the late eighteenth and early nineteenth centuries, transposition of the great vessels was described by M. Baillie [12] and J.R. Farre [13]. More recently in the mid-twentieth century, transposition morphogenesis was further understood through the work of R.P. Grant [14] and

R.M. Shaher [15], yet surgery was still not a viable option. The obvious anatomic correction of an arterial switch with its coronary artery transfer could not be successfully performed at that time [16]. It was the imaginative, inaugural works of A. Senning [17] and W.T. Mustard [18] that these children could survive past early infancy. Even prior to their work, the operations of Blalock-Hanlon [19] and W.S. Edwards [20] could increase systemic and pulmonary venous mixing and provide the children with a chance to survive until they were larger and better candidates for the atrial redirection procedures. These palliative procedures could only have been performed with the simultaneous development of the understanding of the pathophysiology identified by A. M. Rudolph, J.I.E. Hoffman, and colleagues [21]. With the greater understanding of the neonatal pathophysiology and advancement in surgical techniques and neonatal cardiopulmonary bypass, the arterial switch operation was designed and introduced by Jatene and his associates [22, 23]. Today, the international pediatric cardiovascular community has collaborated to advance and modify the arterial switch operation, and children are being offered a return to near-normal life, albeit with concerns regarding late complications [24]. As these surgical treatments were evolving, so was the science of biotechnology with the advent of the balloon septostomy first reported by W. Rashkind [25] and the beginning of the era of interventional cardiology.

Atrial septal defects are another example of the evolution of the spectrum of congenital heart disease and its treatment. The first descriptions of atrial septal defects were reported by L. da Vinci [26] and C. von Rogitansky [27]. More recently the description of the anatomy of the atrial septum with the embryology pertaining to the formation and closure of the foramen ovale was described by B.M. Patten in 1931 [28]. P.N.B. Odgers further described the pathophysiology of the formation and an explanation for defects arising in the intra-atrial septum long before there was any type of surgical repair [29]. In the presurgical era, symptomatic children with an atrial septal defect were virtually committed to a lifetime of poor growth, exercise intolerance, and often early death secondary to either congestive heart failure or Eisenmenger syndrome. With the initial open-heart operations for atrial septal defect using the cross-circulation technique [30], the era of surgical repair began and has progressed to a state where an uncomplicated repair of an atrial septal defect is considered a cure with the children ultimately being discharged with minimal long-term cardiology follow-up. With the advances in biotechnology and bioengineering, uncomplicated atrial septal defects can now be cured through a transcatheter approach [31]. So now, as the field of congenital heart disease has progressed, a congenital heart defect, which had previously left children with exercise intolerance and a shortened life span, is virtually cured with a transcatheter approach, avoiding surgical invasion of the body.

Collaboration is a key factor in the advancement to the understanding and treatment of congenital heart disease. Hypoplastic left heart syndrome is the ultimate example of collaboration leading to successes which in the past were inconceivable [32]. Today, perinatologists identify hypoplastic left heart syndrome [33] and interventional cardiologists prenatally open restrictive intra-atrial septa reducing left atrial pressure relieving restriction to pulmonary venous return [34]. Prenatal balloon dilation of obstructive left ventricular outflow tracts is being performed intending to promote left ventricular growth and development [34]. Neonatal cardiovascular surgeons working in concert with interventional cardiologists [35] and pediatric cardiac intensivists [36] team together performing variations on the Norwood reconstruction and hybrid procedures in these neonates. The procedures can be scheduled and performed in a controlled fashion with aid from the fetal echocardiographers. It is these team efforts which have lead to the improved neonatal outcomes for these children with now an expectation of sports participation, albeit restricted, and mainstreamed school

attendance [37]. However, like many other forms of single ventricle, challenges for long-term survival and quality of life remain.

Pursuit to the descriptions of anatomy and physiology, the surgical and biotechnical advances and early intervention have lead to the prolonged survival of the patients. By the year 2020, it is expected that more adults than children will need open-heart procedures to correct congenital heart defects. As the previous morbidity and mortality of congenital heart treatment has been minimized, an entire new field of scientific investigation and treatment is now developing along with the appropriate resource allocation [38]. Again, as was done in the early stages of congenital heart disease, the description and understanding of the pathophysiology and subsequent structural remodeling has lead to the science of the unnatural history of the congenitally malformed heart. Cardiac magnetic resonance imaging with its precise detail of anatomy and tissue characterization is now an integral clinical tool for the planning of re-intervention and exercise prescriptions in adolescent and adult patients [39]. Treatment plans specific to the young and middle-aged adult with congenital heart disease have emerged into a new science of treatment and investigation [40]. As increasing numbers of the children survive and thrive into adulthood, the science of congenital heart disease is no longer only a pediatric issue but rather an area of science and discovery spanning prenatal life into adulthood.

References

1. Niels S. Acta medica et philosophica hafniencia 1671–1672; 1:202–203. Cited by Goldstein HI in discussion of Jarcho S: Giovanni Battista Morgagni. Bull Hist Med 1948; 22:503–527
2. Edwards JE, Carey LS, Neufeld HN, Lester RG (eds) (1965) Congenital heart disease: correlation of pathologic anatomy and angiography. WB Saunders, Philadelphia/London
3. Becker AE, Anderson RH (eds) (1982) Cardiac pathology: an integrated text and color Atlas. Gower Medical, London/New York

4. Exercitatio Anatomica du Moto Cordis et Sanguinis, Frankfort, Germany 1628 in Dempster JH (ed) (1914) Pathfinders of physiology. Detroit Medical Journal CO

5. O'Connor WJ (1988) Founders of British physiology: a biographical dictionary, 1920–1885. Manchester University Press, Manchester

6. Wood P (1958) The Eisenmanger syndrome or pulmonary hypertension with reversed central shunt. Br Med J 2:701

7. Rudolph AM (ed) (1974) Congenital diseases of the heart: clinical physiological considerations. Yearbook Medical Publishers, Chicago

8. Blalock A, Taussig HB (1945) The surgical treatment of malfunctions of the heart in which there is pulmonary stenosis or pulmonary atresia. JAMA 128:181–202

9. Castaneda AR, Lamberti J, Sade RW, Williams RG, Nadas AS (1974) Open-heart surgery during the first three months of life. J Thorac Cardiovasc Surg 63:719–731

10. Blackstone EH, Kirklin JW, Bradley EL, DuShane JW, Applebaum A (1976) Optimal age and results in repair of large ventricular septal defects. J Thorac Cardiovasc Surg 72:661–679

11. Lillehei CW (1957) Surgical treatment of congenital and acquired heart disease by use of total cardiopulmonary bypass; analysis of results of 350 patients. Acta Chir Scand 113:496–501

12. Baillie M (1797) The morbid anatomy of some of the most important parts of the human body, 2nd edn. Johnson and Nicol, London, pp 38–40

13. Farre JR (1814) Pathological researches. Essay 1: on malformation of the human heart. Longman, Hurst, Rees, Orme, Brown, London, pp 1–46

14. Grant RP (1962) The morphogenesis of transposition of the great vessels. Circulation 26:819–840

15. Shaher RM (1964) Complete and inverted transposition of the great vessels. Br Heart J 26:51–66

16. Evans WN (2009) The arterial switch operation before Jatene. Pediatr Cardiol 30:119–124

17. Senning A (1959) Surgical correction of transposition of the great vessels. Surgery 45:966–980

18. Mustard WT (1964) Successful two-stage correction of transposition of the great vessels. Surgery 55:469–472

19. Blalock A, Hanlon CR (1950) The surgical treatment of complete transposition of the aorta and pulmonary artery. Surg Gynecol Obstet 90:1–15

20. Edwards WS, Bargeron LM (1965) More effective palliation of transposition of great vessels. J Thorac Cardiovasc Surg 49:790–795

21. Rudolph AM (1966) Prenatal and perinatal influences of congenital heart disease III. Hemodynamic and biochemical abnormalities in the newborn with heart disease. In: Cassels DE (ed) The heart and circulation in the newborn and infant. Grune and Stratton, New York/London, pp 141–146

22. Jatene AD, Fontes VF, Paulista PP et al (1975) 1975 successful anatomic correction of transposition of the great vessels: a preliminary report. Arq Bras Cardiol 28:461–464

23. Jatene AD, Fontes VF, Souza LCB et al (1982) Anatomic correction of transposition of the great arteries. J Thorac Cardiovasc Surg 83:20–26

24. Lim HG, Kim WH, Lee JR, Kim YJ (2013) Long-term results of the arterial switch operation for ventriculoarterial discordance. Eur J Cardiothorac Surg 43:325–334

25. Rashkind WJ, Miller WW (1966) Creation of an atrial septal defect without thoracotomy: a palliative approach to complete transposition of the great arteries. JAMA 196:991–992

26. da Vinci L (1982) Excerpt from quadernia anatomic II. In: Rashkind WJ (ed) Congenital heart disease. Hutchinson Ross, Philadelphia, p 102

27. von Rogitansky C (1875) Die Defecte der Scheidewande des Herzens. Braunmuller, Vienna

28. Patten BM (1931) The closure of the foramen ovale. Am J Anat 48:19–44

29. Odgers PNB (1935) The formation of the venous valves, the foramen secundum and the septum secundum in the human heart. J Anat 69:412–422

30. Lewis FJ, Taufic M (1953) Closure of atrial septal defects with the aid of hypothermia, experimental accomplishments and the report of one successful case. Surgery 33:52–59

31. Bennhagen RG, McLaughlin P, Benson LN (2001) Contemporary management of children with atrial septal defects: a focus on transcatheter closure. Am J Cardiovasc Drugs 1:445–454

32. Feinstein JA, Benson DW, Dubin AM et al (2012) Hypoplastic left heart syndrome current considerations and expectations. J Am Coll Cardiol 59(1 Suppl S):S1–S42

33. Sivarajan V, Penny DL, Finlan P, Brizzard C, Sherekdemian LS (2009) Impact of antenatal diagnosis of hypoplastic left heart syndrome on the clinical presentation and surgical outcomes: the Australian experience. J Peadiatr Child Health 45:112–117

34. McElhinney DB, Tworetsky W, Lock JE (2010) Current status of fetal cardiac intervention. Circulation 121:1256–1263

35. Ringwald JM, Stapleton G, Suh EJ (2011) The hybrid approach – current knowns and unknowns: the perspective of cardiology. Cardiol Young 21(suppl 2):47–52

36. Wernovsky G, Kuijpers M, Van Rossem MC et al (2007) Postoperative course in the cardiac intensive care unit following the first stage of the Norwood reconstruction. Cardiol Young 17:652–665

37. Tabbutt S, Nord AS, Jarvik JP et al (2008) Neurodevelopmental outcomes after staged palliation for hypoplastic left heart syndrome. Pediatrics 121:476–483

38. Webb G (2010) The long road to better ACHD care. Congenit Heart Dis 5:198–205

39. Marcotte F, Poirier N, Pressacco J et al (2009) Evaluation of adult congenital heart disease by cardiac magnetic resonance imaging. Congenit Heart Dis 4:216–230

40. Warnes CA, Williams RG, Bashore TM et al (2008) ACC/AHA 2008 guidelines for the management of adults with congenital heart disease. A report of the American College of Cardiology/American Heart Association Task Force on Practice Guidelines (Writing Committee to develop guidelines on the management of adults with congenital heart disease). Circulation 118:e714–e833

Persistent Arterial Duct

81

Enrique García, Miguel A. Granados, Mario Fittipaldi, and Juan V. Comas

Abstract

The persistent arterial duct, also named persistent ductus arteriosus (PDA) or patent ductus arteriosus, was one of the first recognized congenital cardiac lesions. Although most cardiologists recommend closure of a moderate patent arterial duct before 1–2 years of age, controversy remains regarding treatment in the term and preterm infant. There are few randomized controlled trials in neonates, and there is a high rate of spontaneous closure. This chapter will review the history, pharmacology, and treatment of patent arterial duct.

Keywords

Endarteritis • Ibuprofen • Indomethacin • Interventional closure • Patent ductus arteriosus • PDA • Persistent arterial duct • Prematurity • Surgical closure • Thoracoscopic closure • Video assisted

Brief Historical Background

Although Galeno (AD 129) did not appreciate the blow flow and the circulation, he realized multiple aspects of fetal circulation, as some blood entered

Electronic Supplementary Material: The online version of this chapter (doi:10.1007/978-1-4471-4619-3_13) contains supplementary material, which is available to authorized users.

E. García (✉) • M.A. Granados • M. Fittipaldi • J.V. Comas
Pediatric Heart Institute, Hospital Universitario "12 de Octubre", Madrid, Spain
e-mail: enrique_huc@hotmail.com; magranadosr@hotmail.com; m.fittipaldi@me.com; jvcomas@gmail.com

the right ventricle and pulmonary artery and was then shunted into the aorta through a fetal "channel." In several dictionaries, the name of Botallo, an Italian physician born in 1513, still appears as an eponym for three cardiovascular anatomical structures: the foramen ovale, the ductus arteriosus (DA), and the ligamentum arteriosum [1]. As relevant historical background, it is important to mention Gipson's description in 1898 of the typical "machinery" murmur: "it begins softly and increases in intensity so as to reach its acme just about or immediately after the second sound and from that point gradually wanes till its termination. The second sound can be heard to be loud and clanging" [2]. No thought was given to the surgical treatment until 1907 when

Munro described a technique for the "ligation" of the ductus arteriosus. It was not until 1939, however, that Gross and Hubbard firstly described successful surgical ligation of a duct in a 7-year-old girl at Boston Children's Hospital [3]. Subsequently, the efficacy and safety of the surgical procedure improved, and excellent results were achieved even in infants. By the end of the 1970s, catheter-derived therapies had already begun to offer alternatives to the surgical approach. Then in 1979, the first successful catheter closure of a persistent arterial duct in a child weighing only 3.5 kg was made by Rashkind and colleagues who deployed a double-disc percutaneous device [4].

Introduction

PDA is a congenital heart abnormality defined as persistent patency of the lumen of the fetal ductus arteriosus in term infants beyond the neonatal period. Persistence implies that the duct is present after the time of its expected closure and, therefore, distinguishes a pathological from a physiological state. The concept of patency remains useful in the perinatal period, especially in the premature infant in whom the term can be used to signify a duct that is functionally open [5]. The ductus arteriosus is completely closed by 8 weeks of age. When the process is delayed, the term *prolonged patency* is the appropriate [6].

The factors that lead to persistent patency of the ductus arteriosus are incompletely understood. Due to physiological factors related to prematurity, premature birth increases the incidence of PDA. In term infants, however, persistent patency is related to inherent abnormality of the ductus. Most cases are sporadic, but there is increasing evidence that genetic factors are involved in many patients with PDA. Prenatal infection, such as rubella, may also play a role in some cases.

The incidence of PDA in infants and children that were born at full term is not precisely known due to the evolution of methods of detection and the fact that most infants with PDA are asymptomatic. The incidence of clinically evident persistent arterial duct was reported to be about 1 in 2,000 births. This accounts for approximately 5–10 % of all congenital heart disease. However, children are not infrequently found to have a clinically "silent" PDA discovered incidentally by echocardiography done for another purpose. The true incidence may therefore be as high as 1 in 500 [7].

The female-to-male ratio for PDA is about 2:1 in most reports. PDA also occurs with increased frequency in several genetic syndromes (Down syndrome, Holt-Oram syndrome, and others). Genetic linkage studies have also provided support for genetic etiology in some families (in a family having one sibling with a PDA, there is an approximately 3 % chance of a PDA in a subsequent offspring) [7].

Embryology and Anatomy

The DA arises from the distal portion of the left sixth embryonic aortic arch from which the pulmonary artery also originates. In the normal early embryonic stage, the arterial duct exists bilaterally on both right and left sides, but the right duct becomes atrophied at around 37–40 days postembryonic gestation.

The ductus arteriosus connects the proximal portion of the left pulmonary artery near its origin from the main pulmonary artery to the upper descending thoracic aorta just distal to the left subclavian artery (Fig. 81.1). In the presence of a right aortic arch, the ductus may be on the right. Anomalies in the development of aortic arch can be associated with an anomalous position of the PDA, or it can be part of a "vascular ring." The ductus arteriosus may persist in a variety of shapes and sizes. Most commonly, the aortic end of the ductus is larger than the pulmonary artery end, resulting in a somewhat funnel-shaped configuration. The size and shape of the PDA are important determinants of resistance to blood flow and also have important implications regarding the method of interventional closure.

Absence of ductus arteriosus was first described in 1671, in the autopsy of a patient with tetralogy of Fallot (TOF). Emmanoulides

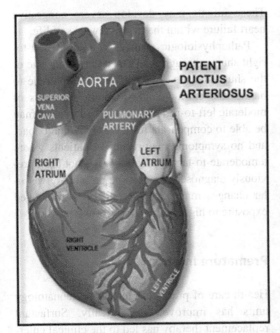

Fig. 81.1 Anatomy of usual PDA localization. Anterior heart view

et al. (1976) published a work of four children affected by TOF with absent pulmonary valve and absent ductus arteriosus [8]. Their hypothesis was that in the first phases of fetal development, the absence of a ductus could contribute to the massive dilatation of pulmonary artery; in the presence of high pulmonary resistance and high systolic volume of the right ventricle, the pulmonary arteries progressively distend. The ductus arteriosus is also absent in more than 75 % of patients with truncus arteriosus.

In RVOT (right ventricle outflow tract) obstruction lesions, the development of the ductus arteriosus is probably abnormal because of alteration in the normal flow patterns in fetal life. Because maintenance of a PDA is essential for maintenance of pulmonary blood flow, the constrictor response to an increase in PO_2 is undesirable. Despite the hypoxemia, the ductus arteriosus closes. Maintenance of systemic blood flow in lesions such as aortic atresia or interrupted aortic arch also may depend on a PDA and also takes an important role in infants with juxta-ductal aortic coartation; in these cases, if the ductus remains patent, obstruction may not occur or be lessened.

Histology and Anatomical Closure

The histology of the DA differs from that of other arteries. The wall of the normal DA is lined on its luminal aspect by an intimal layer of endothelial cells that overlies an internal elastic lamina. The elastic lamina is fragmented and interrupted by intimal cushions that lie underneath it. The media of the ductal wall mainly consists of longitudinally and spirally arranged layers of smooth muscle fibers [9].

The process of closure of the arterial duct occurs in two steps. Initially, medial smooth muscle contraction produces increased wall thickness and shortening and protrusion of the intimal cushions. This results in functional closure 10–15 h after birth in full-term infants. The second stage of the closure is due to proliferation of connective tissue in the intima and media. Atrophy of smooth muscle cells ultimately transforms the muscular vessel into a noncontractile ligament represented by a mass of dense elastic and fibrous tissue [9]. The arterial duct is completely closed by 8 weeks of age in 88 % of infants with a normal cardiovascular system [6].

Physiology and Pathophysiology

The DA plays a crucial role in fetal blood circulation, connecting the main pulmonary artery to the descending aorta. In utero, this vessel serves to divert right ventricular output away from the non-ventilated lungs and towards the placenta. Details may be found in a specific chapter that is dedicated to fetal circulation elsewhere in this textbook. Several factors, mainly low arterial PO_2, prostaglandins, and nitric oxide, contribute to the maintenance of ductal patency during fetal life. A key role in the regulation of the DA tone is played by prostaglandins and particularly by PGE_2. High circulating levels and ductal synthesis of PGE_2 are responsible for a strong vasodilator effect via specific receptors located on the ductal wall. Prostaglandins are detectable only in very low concentrations in adult plasma, and most are not thought to act as circulating hormones because of their rapid catabolism in the lung. The fetus, however, has high circulating concentrations of prostaglandins, probably owing to low fetal pulmonary blood flow and therefore decreased prostaglandin catabolism in the lungs, as well as to the fact that the placenta produces prostaglandins [10].

Immediately after birth at term, the loss of placenta and the increased pulmonary blood flow result in a reduced PGE_2-mediated vasodilation of the DA; the latter, in combination with a concurrent ductal constriction induced by a postnatal increase in PaO_2, will lead to functional closure of the DA by about 10–15 h postnatally.

The contraction of the ductus arteriosus results locally in a "hypoxic zone" and triggers cell death and synthesis of hypoxia-inducible growth factors. Accordingly, vascular remodeling and anatomic ductal closure occur.

In preterm infants, the insufficient constriction of the ductus may result in failure to generate the hypoxic zone, thus preventing true anatomic DA closure. In a term infant with a PDA, the structure of the ductal wall is abnormal. Histologically, the internal elastic lamina of the arterial duct is generally intact, and the internal cushions are absent or less well formed than usual [11].

Three major, interrelated factors control the magnitude of shunting: the diameter and length of the ductus arteriosus, the pressure difference between the aorta and the pulmonary artery, and the systemic and pulmonary vascular resistances. Because systemic vascular resistance does not change significantly after birth, changes in pulmonary vascular resistance are the major determinant in regulating the left-to-right shunting through a PDA [10].

In situations of persistent ductal patency, pathophysiology relates to reversal of ductal flow due to the normal decline in pulmonary vascular resistances (PVR) that occurs after birth. This results in a left-to-right shunt from the aorta to the pulmonary artery. Consequently, there is in an increased volume and workload on the left atrium and left ventricle. Left ventricular dilation will result in an increased left ventricular end-diastolic pressure with secondary increase in left atrial pressure. This may lead to signs of overt left heart failure with left atrial dilation and pulmonary edema.

These infants may develop severe congestive heart failure within the first 4–6 weeks of life.

Pathophysiologic changes caused by left-to-right shunts through the PDA relate to the size of the shunt and the ability of the left ventricle to handle the extra volume load. In situations of moderate left-to-right shunting, the left heart may be able to compensate for the extra volume load, and no symptoms may result. In patients where a moderate-to-large patent duct has not been previously diagnosed, irreversible pulmonary vascular changes may occur secondary to prolonged exposure to high pulmonary flow and pressure.

Premature Infants

Health care of premature infants in neonatology units has improved dramatically. Surfactant replacement therapy has led to the clinical emergence of a symptomatic PDA earlier and more frequently in preterm infants. As a result of this condition, the steal of aortic flow through the PDA with significant left-to-right shunt may lead to decreased perfusion in many organs, with potential negative clinical consequences, such as reduced cerebral blood flow, renal function, and myocardial and bowel perfusion.

Diagnosis

Clinical

The majority of the patients are usually asymptomatic. Infants with large PDA present with signs and symptoms of congestive heart failure (CHF) with pulmonary edema within the first 4–6 weeks of life. The main clinical signs are tachycardia, a continuous murmur, and full and bounding peripheral pulses. The continuous murmur is characterized by a late systolic accentuation and continuation through the second sound into diastole. As a consequence of the diastolic steal, the systemic pulse pressure is widened with a low diastolic pressure.

Preterm infants: The patterns that can be recognized relating to the evolution of pulmonary disease and pulmonary vascular resistances are [10]:

- *PDA with little or no lung disease*: Usually a systolic murmur can be heard 24–72 h after birth. If the shunt becomes sufficiently large, clinical evidence of left ventricular failure may appear. This includes tachycardia, tachypnea, and rales on auscultation.
- *PDA in infants recovering from lung disease*: The most common group of infants develops left-to-right shunting while recovering from respiratory distress syndrome. As this improvement continues, clinical evidence of a left-to-right shunt through a PDA appears. Deterioration in the ventilatory or hemodynamic status of an infant recovering from respiratory distress syndrome is often a strong indication of a significant left-to-right shunt through a PDA.

ECG

Patients with a significant volume overloading show left ventricular hypertrophy manifested by a deep Q wave and a tall R wave in leads II, III, aVF, and the left precordial leads. T waves in these leads are usually tall. Also, a widened P indicates left atrial enlargement.

Chest X-Ray

In infants with a large PDA, the chest roentgenogram shows enlargement of the left atrium and left ventricle with accentuated peripheral pulmonary vascular markings. As a consequence of the enlarged left atrium or pulmonary arteries, lobar collapse or emphysema owing to bronchial compression may occur. It is also possible to observe a horizontalization of the left bronchi secondary to the enlargement of the left atrium.

Echocardiography

Echocardiographic and Doppler evaluation is currently essential in the diagnosis and clinical assessment of the magnitude and direction of the shunt. Also, it is important to exclude other congenital cardiac lesions with similar clinical findings and, last but not least, any associated anomalies that

would reveal the need for ductal patency or dependency. The ratio of the left atrial (LA) diameter to the aortic root (Ao) diameter can be considered as useful parameter to determine the LA enlargement that may be proportional to the degree of the shunt; the normal LA:Ao ratio in infants is <1.2; a ratio >1.2 suggests left atrial enlargement; and a ratio >1.5 probably confirms a significant left-to-right shunt (Fig. 81.2; Videos 81.1 and 81.2). Direct visualization of the ductus arteriosus confirms the diagnosis. The usual echocardiography for PDA views are short axis and a high parasternal sagittal projection from the second left intercostal space parallel to the vertebral bodies (so-called ductus view) (Fig. 81.3; Video 81.3).

Cardiac Catheterization

Diagnostic cardiac catheterization is rarely required in patients with typical clinical and echocardiographic findings but should be considered when significant pulmonary vascular disease is suspected. Usually catheterization is limited to transcatheter therapies for occlusion of the duct. In this setting, ductal anatomy is usually defined with aortography (Fig. 81.4). The configuration of the ductus is demonstrated on the lateral angiogram [12].

Laboratory

Persistent metabolic acidosis observed in arterial blood gas in preterm infants may represent an early finding for suspected PDA with significant left-to-right shunt. Current studies are focusing on the follow-up of brain natriuretic peptide (BNP) as a marker of the PDA repercussion in this population [13].

Complications

Pulmonary Hypertension

A late complication of long-standing left-to-right shunts and increased pulmonary blood flow is the occurrence of fixed pulmonary vascular resistance

Fig. 81.2 Echocardiography in parasternal long axis view showing LA/AO ratio, in an infant with PDA with significant shunt

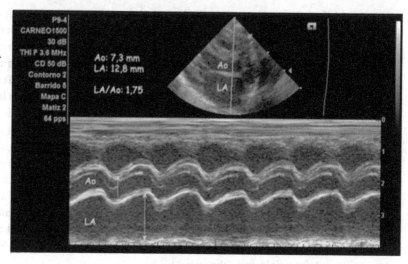

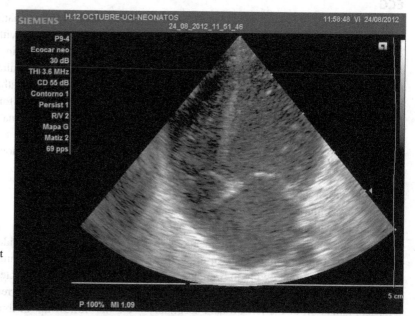

Video 81.1 **Apical four-chamber view**. Atrial and left ventricular enlargement of this infant with clinical diagnosis of ductus indicates a significant left-to-right shunt

and right-sided heart failure. This occurs primarily in patients with long-standing PDAs and ultimately results in right-to-left shunts at the ductal level. Thus, the delay in the PDA closure in patients with a large shunt must be avoided, in order to prevent pulmonary vascular disease [7].

Endarteritis

In the past, endarteritis was one of the leading causes of death in patients with PDA. This is now an extremely rare complication. Nevertheless, on occasions a case of ductus-related endocarditis

Video 81.2 Paraesternal long-axis view. Relation LA/Ao. To date there are no stringent echocardiographic criteria on the need for PDA closure. A relation LA/Ao ≥ 1,5 in the paraesternal long-axis view indicates a significant PDA shunt in infants

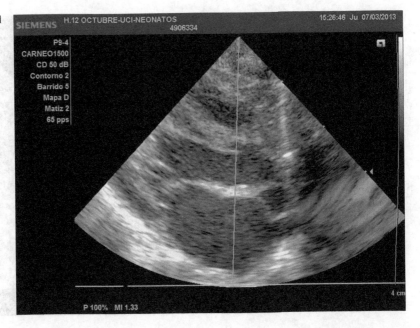

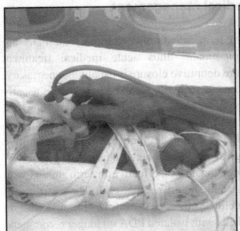

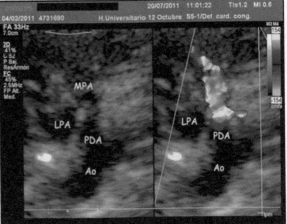

Fig. 81.3 Echocardiography demonstrating PDA. *Left*: Two-dimensional image of a PDA as seen in a high parasternal sagittal projection. *Ao* descending aorta, *MPA* main pulmonary artery, *LPA* left pulmonary artery. *Right*: Color Doppler image in the same view showing *left*-to-*right* shunting through the ductus

does occur. The vegetations related to this infection tend to occur on the pulmonic end of the ductus. This has prompted some centers to offer elective closure of the patent duct to all patients [14].

Calcification Formation

In adult patients, calcification of the PDA is frequent and may usually increase the surgical risk [6].

Video 81.3 High left parastemal sagittal view. Ductus view. The best views that allow study of the PDA anatomy and the flow patterns are the high left or right parastemal sagittal views, depending on wich side the PDAs is located. **Left**: View of descending aorta connecting through the ductus to the main pulmonary artery. **Right**: Color Doppler flow map of the left-to-right shunt across the PDA

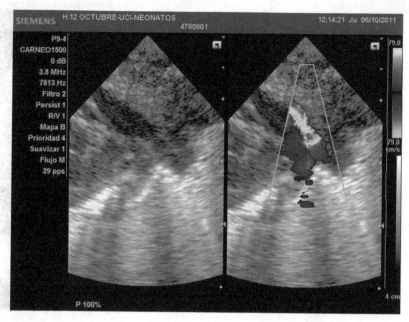

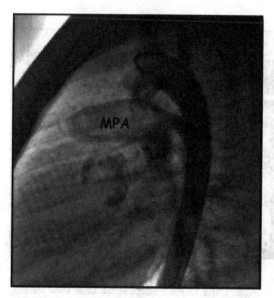

Fig. 81.4 Lateral angiogram demonstrating the typical anatomy of the PDA. Pulmonary end smaller than the aortic end. *PA* pulmonary artery, *Ao* aorta

Decision Making in Infants

An algorithm for decision making is provided in Fig. 81.5.

Medical Management

Most term infants and children with PDA are asymptomatic, thus acute medical treatment before definitive closure is usually not necessary. Those patients with symptoms, however, usually improve with a standard regimen of diuretics. Medical therapy for congestive heart failure due to PDA should be short term, until definitive surgical or transcatheter closure is performed. Indomethacin is ineffective in term infants with PDA and should not be used. The most recent guidelines for endocarditis prophylaxis in patients with isolated PDA no longer recommend pretreatment with antibiotics for risk procedures (class III, level C) [15].

Preterm Infants

Initial conservative management involves fluid restriction, diuretic therapy, and ventilator support. Indomethacin was introduced in 1976 as a pharmacological method for closing the ductus in the preterm infant. Both indomethacin and ibuprofen act as inhibitors of prostaglandin

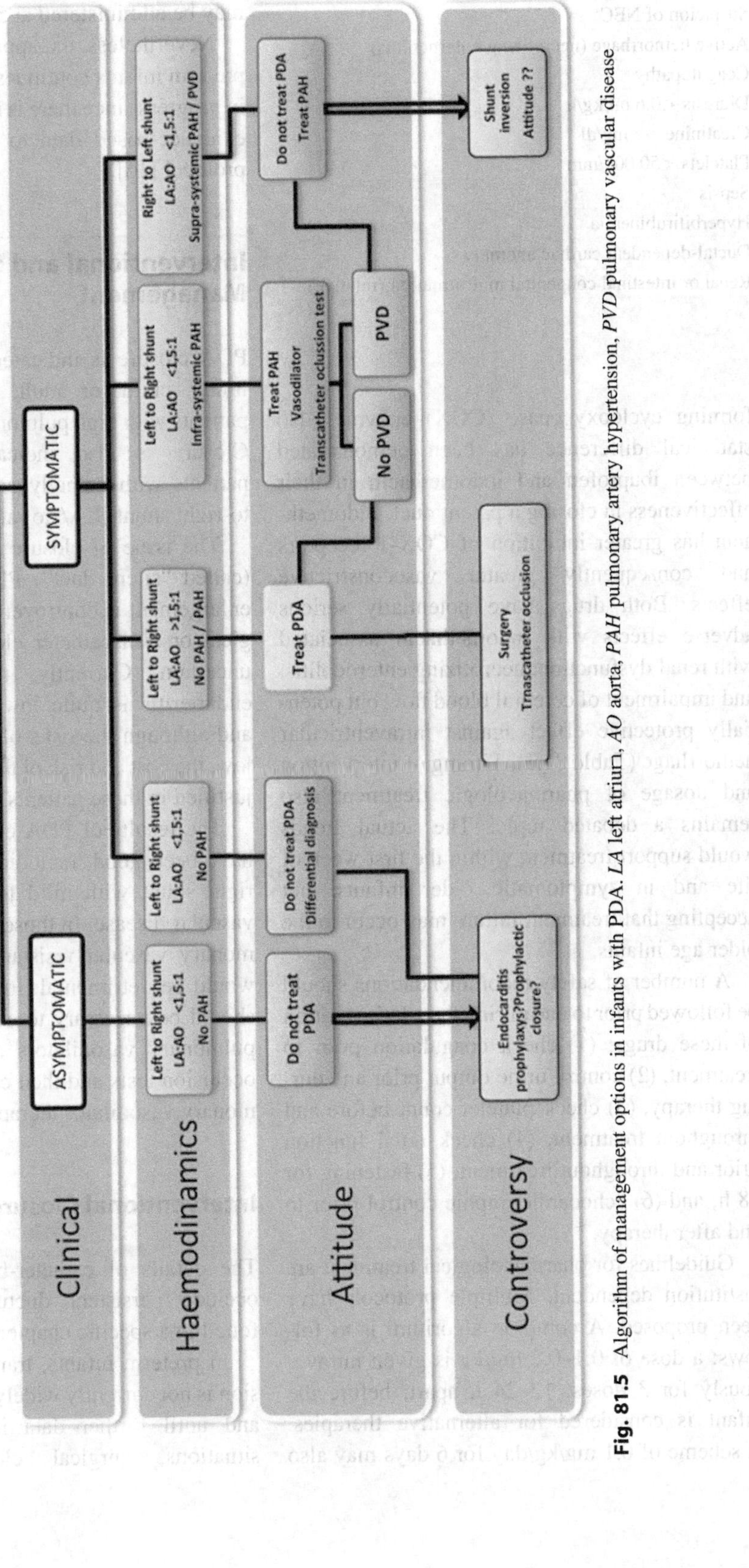

Fig. 81.5 Algorithm of management options in infants with PDA. *LA* left atrium, *AO* aorta, *PAH* pulmonary artery hypertension, *PVD* pulmonary vascular disease

Table 81.1 Contraindications to the use of indomethacin

Suspicion of NEC
Active hemorrhage (necrotizing enterocolitis)
Coagulopathy
Diuresis <0.6 ml/kg/h
Creatinine >2 mg/dl
Platelets <50,000/mm^3
Sepsis
Hyperbilirubinemia
Ductal-dependent cardiac anomaly
Renal or intestinal congenital malformation (relative)

forming cyclooxygenase (COX) enzymes. No statistical difference has been demonstrated between ibuprofen and indomethacin in their effectiveness in closing a patent duct. Indomethacin has greater inhibition of COX-1 receptors and consequently greater vasoconstrictive effects. Both drugs have potentially serious adverse effects with indomethacin associated with renal dysfunction, necrotizing enterocolitis, and impairment of cerebral blood flow but potentially protective effect against intraventricular hemorrhage (Table 81.1). Timing of intervention and dosage of pharmacologic treatment also remains a debated topic. The actual trends would support treatment within the first week of life and in symptomatic older infants, but accepting that treatment failure may occur in the older age infants.

A number of safety recommendations should be followed prior to and during the administration of these drugs: (1) check coagulation prior to treatment, (2) control urine output prior and during therapy, (3) check platelet count before and throughout treatment, (4) check renal function prior and throughout treatment, (5) fastening for 48 h, and (6) echocardiographic control prior to and after therapy.

Guidelines for pharmacological treatment are institution dependent. Multiple protocols have been proposed. A common algorithm is as follows: a dose of 0.1–0.2 mg/kg is given intravenously for 3 doses, 12–24 h apart, before the infant is considered for alternative therapies. A scheme of 0.1 mg/kg/day for 6 days may also be used in stable premature patients. Ibuprofen may be administered at 5 mg/kg/day for 5 days.

Nevertheless, the approach to PDA closure in preterm infants continues to be an evolving work in progress since there is not enough accumulated evidence-based data to determine a consistent protocol [16].

Interventional and Surgical Management

PDA closure is indicated for any symptomatic infant, child, or adult, with the exception of patients with high pulmonary vascular resistance. Closure is also indicated in asymptomatic patients with hemodynamically significant left-to-right shunt (LA/Ao ratio >1.5:1).

The issue of closure of small or very small (called "silent duct") PDAs without left atrial enlargement is controversial. The benefit of surgical or transcatheter closure in this setting is uncertain. Currently, the risk of infective endarteritis is quite low in this patient group, and although the risks of the procedure are also low, the cost and risk of the procedure may not be justified in these patients.

The results of PDA closure in adult patients have been good, including those with a left-to-right shunt with mild to moderate pulmonary vascular disease. In those patients with high pulmonary vascular resistance, closure of a PDA would be detrimental. In this clinical setting, it should be necessary to evaluate the response to pulmonary vasodilators and transcatheter duct occlusion tests and then consider closure or pulmonary vasodilator therapy [7].

Interventional Closure

The details of catheter-based interventions to occlude persistent ductus arteriosus can be found in a specific chapter in this textbook.

In preterm infants, transcatheter PDA occlusion is not currently widely developed. Therefore and until further data is available, in these situations, surgical closure is preferred.

For symptomatic infants weighing greater than 5 kg, percutaneous approach can be feasible. However, for infants with an asymptomatic patent arterial duct, it may be better to wait until the child's weight reaches 10–12 kg [13].

Transcatheter PDA occlusion is safe and effective. The success rates have improved over time, owing to the development of new devices and device modifications, evolution of new techniques, and increased operator skill. Available data report complete PDA closure in around 90–95 %. Severe complications related with the procedure are infrequent. Device embolization represents the most common complication. Protruding device, hemolysis by residual shunting, thrombosis related to vascular access, and infection are the other complications [17].

Surgical Closure

Surgical treatment should be considered in three clinical settings:
- Preterm infants
- Term infants and children
- Adults

Indications for Surgery in Infants and Children

The surgical closure of PDA remains the treatment of choice for symptomatic patients weighing less than 5 Kg. Sometimes, the specific ductal anatomy precludes the percutaneous approach (very large, window type, and aneurysmal ducts).

Technical Considerations

Thoracotomy Approach

The standard approach to a PDA is a left posterolateral or anterolateral thoracotomy. The usual technique is through the third or fourth intercostal space. After skin incision, the latissimus dorsi is divided, taken care to preserve the serratus anterior muscle. The scapula is retracted, and the ribs

are counted from the top in order to identify the proper intercostal space. A retractor needs to be gently placed on the lung. The mediastinal pleura is opened over the proximal descending thoracic aorta: pleural traction sutures are pulled to obtain adequate surgical vision. Excessive dissection should be avoided due to the vagus and left recurrent laryngeal nerves and thoracic duct. The ductal tissue is fragile and its dissection should be performed very carefully.

This approach remains appropriate for the preterm infant undergoing surgical ligation of the ductus or for the older infant or child who has a particularly short and wide ductus.

Ligation

The first surgical description was made in 1946 by Alfred Blalock. The operation proceeds as mentioned above. This technique can be performed with a single stitch or a double purse string and transfixion 5-0/6-0 polypropylene suture. In the first situation, a ligature is passed behind and around the PDA using a thick ligature of pleated silk because a finer ligature may cut the ductal tissue causing bleeding. Alternatively, the suture is placed through the ductus and one end is passed beneath it.

Division

Once the PDA is dissected, fine vascular clamps are applied, and the PDA is divided. In order to obtain more length for division, a partial occlusion clamp may be placed at the aortic end of the PDA. Both pulmonary and aortic ends are oversewn, usually with a 5-0/6-0 polypropylene running mattress suture in one layer and then a continuous over-and-over stitch in the second layer [20].

PDA Closure in Adult Patients

In adult patients, the aortic end of the PDA is often calcified and short. Before closure, cardiac catheterization is indicated to assess the hemodynamic situation and pulmonary vascular resistance, and then a transcatheter occlusion test provides important information regarding advisability of closure. Percutaneous closure is recommended as a primary choice for treating adult patients with PDA [18]. When percutaneous closure is not possible, a surgical technique using cardiopulmonary bypass may be required through a median sternotomy, to avoid the risk of tear or even rupture.

Surgical Occlusion in Preterm Infants

Surgical treatment of the PDA in preterm infants is considered in the following situations:
(a) Pharmacological closure failure
(b) Complications of the pharmacological closure
(c) Contraindications for pharmacological closure
   In premature infants, the occlusion of the PDA is suggested with clips because a safe and fast occlusion can be achieved. Once the dissection is deep enough, clips are carefully applied. The first clip is placed close to the pulmonary artery; the second clip is placed on the aortic side of the PDA. The most important advantage of this approach is a limited dissection of a very friable duct, typical of the premature infant; this technique diminishes the chance of bleeding. In the majority of cases, pleural drainage is not necessary.

Closure in Special Situations

Closure from Inside the Pulmonary Artery

This surgical approach must be considered when there are serious adhesions from a previous mediastinal operation. The patient is cooled on CPB, while the PDA is occluded by the surgeon's finger from outside. When the nasopharyngeal temperature reaches 28 °C, the rate of perfusion is temporarily reduced. The pulmonary artery is opened, and the PDA is occluded by the

surgeon's finger or a balloon catheter, and an incision is extended towards the left pulmonary artery, and the orifice of the PDA is identified and oversewn. When the sutures are finished, care must be taken not to occlude a branch of the left pulmonary artery and also to prevent air from entering the aorta.

Closure in the Presence of Acute Endocarditis

Bacterial endarteritis has become extremely uncommon. The prevalence of endocarditis has also declined dramatically because of treatment with antibiotics. If the infection cannot be controlled or if lung embolization occurs, operation during the acute phase of endocarditis may be undertaken on cardiopulmonary bypass.

Video-Assisted Thoracoscopic Surgery (VATS)

VATS approach to PDA ligation was reported by Laborde et al. (1993, 1995) [19]. Three to four small 4–7 mm incisions are made around the tip of the scapula for positioning of a videoscopic camera, one to three lung retractors, an L-shaped diathermy dissector, and the endoscopic clip applicator. No chest wall muscles are cut and the ribs are not retracted.

   The clip applicator with the clip mounted is introduced through the hole. The clip is gently placed with an arm on each side of the PDA. Robotically assisted PDA closure has recently been introduced. It seems to be equally safe but it is more time consuming and expensive.

Surgical Complications

The complications after surgery for PDA closure are very rare. Major bleeding, recurrent laryngeal and phrenic nerve palsy, pneumothorax, and chylothorax have been described in different reports. Treatment of these complications should be using standard procedures.

Outcomes of Surgical Closure

The recurrent ductal patency is very rare, and the literature shows a rate between 0.4 % and 3 % [18, 20].

Postoperative Management

Monitoring of these patients is usually standard. Central and arterial lines are seldom required unless patients have additional risks. Management of fluid should be administered at the physiological rate, except in patients with volume overload and heart failure, particularly premature infants in whom a partial fluid restriction may be indicated.

Thoracotomy is usually painful. Sedation and analgesia combining non-opioid therapy, opioids as required, and low-dose benzodiazepines should be provided in order to keep patients comfortable with spontaneous breathing allowing rapid extubation. In order to optimize respiratory mechanics and pain control, regional blockade and patient-controlled analgesia may be considered. Early extubation usually takes place in the operating room or in the first postoperative hours. Failure of extubation following phrenic or recurrent laryngeal nerve insult is rare, but the former should trigger evaluation to rule out the latter.

References

1. Fransson SG (1999) The botallo mystery (profiles in cardiology). Clin Cardiol 22:434–436
2. Boyer NH (1967) Patent ductus arteriosus. Some historical highlights. Ann Thorac Surg 4:570–573
3. Gross RE, Hubbard JP (1939) Surgical ligation of a patent ductus arteriosus. JAMA 112:729–731
4. Rashkind WJ, Mullins CE, Hellenbrand WE, Tait MA (1987) Nonsurgical closure of patent ductus arteriosus: clinical application of the Rashkind PDA Occluder System. Circulation 75:583–592
5. Benson LN, Cowan KN (2002) The arterial duct: its persistence and its patency. In: Anderson RH, Baker EJ, Macartney FJ, Rigby ML, Shinebourne EA, Tynan M (eds) Paediatric cardiology, 2nd edn. Churchill Livingstone, London, pp 1405–1459
6. Kouchoukos NT, Blackstone EH, Hanley FL, Kirklin JK (2013) Patent ductus arteriosus. In: Kouchoucos NT, Blackstone EH, Hanley FL, Kirklin JK (eds) Cardiac surgery, 4th edn. Elsevier Saunders, Philadelphia, pp 1342–1358
7. Schneider DJ (2012) The patent ductus arteriosus in term infants, children, and adults. Semin Perinatol 36:146–153
8. Emmanoulides GC, Thanopoulos B, Siassi B, Fishbein M (1976) Agenesis of ductus arteriosus associated with the syndrome of tetralogy of Fallot and absent pulmonary valve. Am J Cardiol 37:403–409
9. Schneider DJ, Moore JW (2006) Patent ductus arteriosus. Circulation 114:1873–1882
10. Moore P, Brook MM, Heymann MA (2008) Patent ductus arteriosus. In: Allen HD, Driscoll DJ, Shaddy RE, Feltes TF (eds) Moss and Adams' Heart disease in infants, children and adolescents, 7th edn. Lippincott Williams and Wilkins, Philadelphia, pp 683–702
11. Antonucci R, Bassareo P, Zaffanello M, Pusceddu M, Fanos V (2010) Patent ductus arteriosus in preterm infants: new insights into pathogenesis and clinical management. J Matern Fetal Neonatal Med 23:34–37
12. Krichenko A, Benson LN, Burrows P, Möes CA, McLaughlin P, Freedom RM (1989) Angiographic classification of the isolated persistently patent ductus arteriosus and implications for percutaneous catheter occlusion. Am J Cardiol 63:877–879
13. Lee JH, Shin JH, Park KH, Rhie YJ, Park MS, Choi BM (2013) Can early B-type natriuretic Peptide assays predict symptomatic patent ductus arteriosus in extremely low birth weight infants? Neonatology 103:118–122
14. Giroud JM, Jacobs JP (2007) Evolution of strategies for management of the patent arterial duct. Cardiol Young 17:68–74
15. Habib G et al (2009) Guidelines on the prevention, diagnosis, and treatment of infective endocarditis (new version 2009). The task force on the prevention, diagnosis, and treatment of infective endocarditis of the European Society of Cardiology (ESC). Eur Heart J 30:2369–2413
16. Hammerman C, Bin-Nun A, Kaplan M (2012) Managing the patent ductus arteriosus in the premature neonate: a new look at what we thought we knew. Semin Perinatol 36:130–138
17. Forbes TJ, Turner DR (2012) What is the optimal device for closure of persistently patent ductus arteriosus? Progr Ped Cardiol 33:125–129
18. Wiyono SA, Witsenburg M, De Jaegere PPT, Roos-Hesselink JW (2008) Patent ductus arteriosus in adults. Case report and review illustrating the spectrum of the disease. Neth Heart J 8:225–229
19. Laborde F, Folliguet T, Etienne P, Carbognani D, Batisse A, Petrie J (1997) Video assisted thoracoscopic surgical interruption of PDA. Routine experience in 332 cases. Eur J Cardiothor Surg 11:1052–1055
20. Mavroudis C, Backer CL, Gevitz M (1994) Forty-six years of patent ductus arteriosus division at children's Memorial Hospital of Chicago: standards for comparison. Ann Surg 220:402–410

Atrial Septal Defect

Shellie Kendall, John Karamichalis, Tara Karamlou,
David Teitel, and Gordon Cohen

Abstract

There are commonly three main types of atrial septal defects (ASDs):
ostium secundum (80 %), ostium primum (10 %), and sinus venosus
(10 %). Atrial septal defects were one of the very first congenital cardiac
anomalies to be corrected by operative treatment.

The secundum atrial septal defect (ASD) is the second most common
form of congenital heart disease, representing at least 10 % of all congenital cardiac anomalies. The median incidence of the isolated secundum
atrial septal defect is at least 568 per million live births.

Keywords

Gata4 • Nkx2-5 • Ostium primum ASD • Ostium secundum ASD • Septum
primum • Septum secundum • Sinus venosus ASD • Tbx5

Historical Background

Atrial septal defects were one of the very first congenital cardiac anomalies to be corrected by operative treatment. In fact the diagnosis of ASD holds
a special place in the evolution of cardiac surgery as

S. Kendall (✉) • D. Teitel
Division of Pediatric Cardiology, UCSF School of
Medicine, Benioff Children's Hospital, San Francisco,
CA, USA
e-mail: Shellie.Kendall@ucsf.edu;
David.Teitel@ucsf.edu

J. Karamichalis • T. Karamlou • G. Cohen
Division of Pediatric Cardiac Surgery, UCSF School of
Medicine, Benioff Children's Hospital, San Francisco,
CA, USA
e-mail: John.Karamichalis@ucsfmedctr.org;
tara.karamlou@ucsfmedctr.org; gordon.cohen@ucsf.edu

it was the attempts to surgically close ASDs that
ushered in the contemporary era of cardiac surgery.
For years prior to the advent of cardiopulmonary
bypass, surgeons had tried numerous novel and
creative techniques to close secundum atrial septal
defects. In 1952, Gross introduced the atrial well
technique [1]. The following year (1953), Lewis
and Taufic published their technique of using hypothermia and inflow occlusion to close an ASD [2].
The year after that (1954), Sondergaard published
three cases using a purse-string technique [3]. At
the same time, Dr. John Gibbon was working on the
development of the heart-lung machine, and on
May 6, 1953, Dr. Gibbon successfully closed
an atrial septal defect on an 18-year-old college
student [4]. This operation, for closure of an ASD,
was the beginning of the modern era of cardiac
surgery (Figs. 82.1–82.5).

E.M. da Cruz et al. (eds.), *Pediatric and Congenital Cardiology, Cardiac Surgery and Intensive Care*,
DOI 10.1007/978-1-4471-4619-3_14, © Springer-Verlag London 2014

Introduction

The secundum atrial septal defect (ASD) is the second most common form of congenital heart disease, representing at least 10 % of all congenital cardiac anomalies. The median incidence of the isolated secundum atrial septal defect is at least 568 per million live births [5]. The incidence is likely significantly higher as small defects are often incidentally discovered in adulthood or likely never discovered. Additionally, secundum intra-atrial communications are commonly found in association with other congenital heart defects.

The atrial septum is composed of two structures, the septum primum and the septum secundum. The septum primum is a thin, membranous structure that begins to develop at around 4 weeks' gestation and mostly involutes. Only its inferior portion remains as the valve of the foramen ovale with continuation down to the endocardial cushions that closes the ostium (foramen) primum. The septum secundum is a thick, muscular structure that develops to the right of the septum primum, beginning around 5 weeks' gestation. It is comprised of two rims of tissue – a thin superior component that forms the superior rim of the fossa ovalis and a thicker anterior-inferior rim extending to the atrioventricular valves and the aortic knob. The septum secundum forms from a coalescence of cells with a variety of embryologic origins. Dorsal atrial myocardium folding inward from the roof of the atrium meets an inferior muscular mass called the dorsal mesenchymal protrusion (or vestibular spine) and a region of muscularization of the mesenchymal cap on the leading edge of the primum septum [6, 7]. Our understanding of the septum secundum origins and development continues to evolve, gradually revealing mechanisms by which secundum atrial septal defects could form.

Both hemodynamic and genetic mechanisms for the formation of secundum atrial septal defects have been proposed. Abnormal formation of the atrial septum could be due to increased flow from the IVC across the atrial septum during fetal life, causing a deficient valve of the foramen ovale (septum primum), which then cannot close

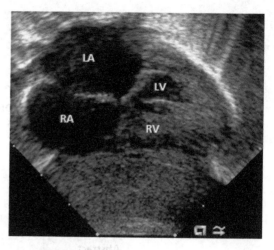

Fig. 82.1 Transthoracic two-dimensional echocardiogram subcostal coronal view of a secundum atrial septal defect. Right atrium (*RA*), right ventricle (*RV*), left atrium (*LA*), left ventricle (*LV*)

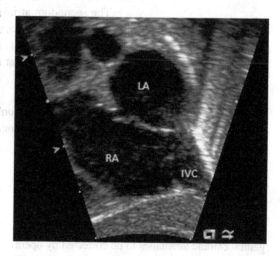

Fig. 82.2 Transthoracic two-dimensional echocardiogram subcostal sagittal view of a secundum atrial septal defect. Left atrium (*LA*), right atrium (*RA*), inferior vena cava (*IVC*)

the foramen ovale at birth. This may be the cause of secundum ASDs seen in association with other congenital heart defects such as tricuspid atresia, but it has not been demonstrated as a cause of isolated ASDs in fetal models [8]. Transcription factors involved in the regulation of atrial septal development in human and murine models include sonic hedgehog (Shh), Gata4, Nkx2-5, and Tbx5; perturbation of these transcription

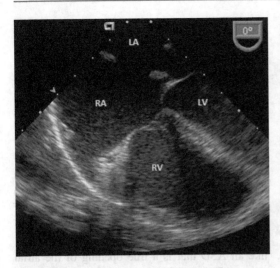

Fig. 82.3 Transesophageal echo view of a secundum atrial septal defect. The transducer is located posterior to the left atrium. Right atrium (*RA*), right ventricle (*RV*), left atrium (*LA*), left ventricle (*LV*)

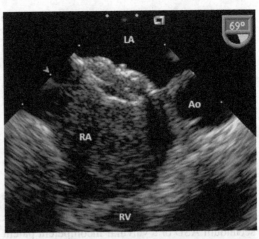

Fig. 82.5 Transesophageal echo view of a secundum atrial septal defect after device occlusion of the atrial septal defect. The transducer is located posterior to the left atrium. Right atrium (*RA*), right ventricle (*RV*), left atrium (*LA*), aortic valve (*Ao*)

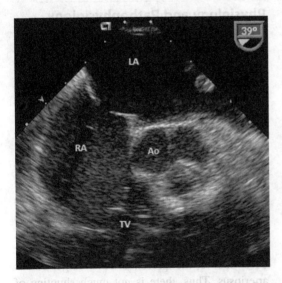

Fig. 82.4 Transesophageal echo view of a secundum atrial septal defect. The transducer is located posterior to the left atrium. Right atrium (*RA*), tricuspid valve (*TV*), left atrium (*LA*), aortic valve (*Ao*)

factors leads to the formation of atrial septal defects [9–11]. Mutations in the gene encoding the Tbx5 transcription factor on human chromosome 12q24.1 have been identified as the cause of both the atrial septal defects and skeletal abnormalities that characterize the autosomal dominantly

inherited Holt-Oram syndrome [11, 12]. Mutations in the gene encoding the Nkx2-5 transcription factor lead to an autosomal dominant disorder characterized by secundum ASDs and progressive atrioventricular block [13]. Emerging research in cardiac development has revealed that pharyngeal mesoderm-derived progenitor cells in the posterior second heart field give rise to atrial septal structures [14]. Progenitor cells in the murine posterior second heart field (SHF) that receive Shh signaling migrate from the posterior SHF to form the primary atrial septum and dorsal mesenchymal protrusion and are necessary for normal septal development [10]. Gata4, Nkx2-5, and Tbx5 are also expressed in the posterior SHF during atrial septal progenitor specification, and Tbx5 expression in the murine posterior SHF is necessary for normal septal development [15]. An understanding of the genetic and molecular mechanisms of normal and abnormal atrial septal development continues to evolve.

Anatomy

There are commonly three main types of atrial septal defects (ASDs): ostium secundum (80 %), ostium primum (10 %), and sinus venosus (10 %).

In the Congenital Heart Surgery Nomenclature and Database Project, [16] three other types of ASD are identified: common atrium, unroofed coronary sinus, and patent foramen ovale.

ASDs are classified according to their location relative to the fossa ovalis and their proposed embryogenesis.

Secundum ASD

Interatrial communications in the region of the fossa ovalis may represent either a true secundum ASD or a valvular incompetent patent or stretched foramen ovale. The limbus of the fossa ovalis are almost always present to some degree. Complete absence of the atrial septum including the fossa ovalis is known as "common atrium" which is generally part of heterotaxy [17, 18].

Primum ASD

An ostium primum defect is anterior to the fossa ovalis, in the inferior portion of the atrial septum immediately adjacent to the atrioventricular valves. It is commonly associated with cleft in the anterior leaflet of mitral valve. These defects constitute part of the spectrum of atrioventricular septal defects or partial or incomplete atrioventricular septal defects, and these are covered in a different chapter [17, 18].

Sinus Venosus ASD

The sinus venosus defects are commonly situated immediately inferior to the junction of the superior vena cava (SVC) and the right atrium, posterior and superior to fossa ovalis. They usually occur in conjunction with anomalous connection of the right upper lobe pulmonary veins. Although the majority of sinus venosus ASDs are close to the SVC/right atrial junction, occasionally they are situated at the inferior vena cava/right atrial junction or directly posteriorly. In these cases there is more likely to be anomalous drainage of the right

lung to the inferior vena cava, e.g., "scimitar" syndrome, rather than abnormal right upper lobe venous drainage [17, 18].

Coronary Sinus ASD

Coronary sinus ASD is the direct communication between the tubelike unroofed coronary sinus and the left atrium. Even though there is no opening in the interatrial septum per se, this results in interatrial communication at the expected site of the coronary sinus ostium, resulting in a left-to-right atrial shunt, acting physiologically just like an ASD that is a true opening of the atrial septum. These defects are often associated with a persistent left superior vena cava draining to the coronary sinus.

Physiology and Pathophysiology

In the absence of other cardiac defects, the magnitude of the left-to-right shunt across the atrial septum depends upon the size of the defect and the relative compliance of the right and left ventricles. The relative compliance of the two ventricles is in turn dependent on the relative resistances of the pulmonary and systemic vascular beds. The higher the resistance that the ventricle sees, the greater its muscle mass and the lesser its compliance. At birth, compliance of the right and left ventricles is similar because pulmonary vascular resistance is high in the fetus, and the two ventricles eject into similar vascular beds due to the presence of a large ductus arteriosus. Thus, there is not much shunting of blood across an ASD at birth, even if the defect is large [8, 19]. Pulmonary vascular resistance decreases and thus right ventricular compliance increases over the next several weeks, during which time left-to-right shunting across the ASD increases substantially.

Once pulmonary vascular resistance is at its minimum, pulmonary blood flow can be three to four times the systemic blood flow in the presence of a large ASD. Normally, this large increase in pulmonary blood flow does not result in a significant increase in pulmonary arterial pressures because the central vessels enlarge and there is recruitment of distal arterioles. Over many years, however, pulmonary arterial pressures may increase in the presence of a large shunt. This is attributed to increasing muscularity of the pulmonary arteries in response to increased pulmonary blood flow [10]. Although significantly elevated pulmonary vascular resistance is exceedingly rare in childhood and young adulthood, resistances as high as 16.5 U x m^2 in a 2-year-old and 15.5 U x m^2 in a 5-year-old have been described [20]. Moreover, many older adults with large shunts throughout their lives have only modest elevations in pulmonary vascular resistance. The pathophysiology of the development of pulmonary vascular disease in the setting of atrial septal defects is an area of ongoing investigation.

Diagnosis

Clinical presentation depends on the magnitude of the left-to-right atrial shunt and the presence of associated problems, particularly pulmonary pathology. Without associated problems, most patients are asymptomatic. Neonates and infants are frequently diagnosed when auscultation of a murmur leads to a cardiac evaluation. With improved imaging via transthoracic echocardiography, very small defects can be appreciated. As a result, the average age at diagnosis has decreased to approximately 6 months of age [19]. If there are associated problems such as chronic lung disease, seen in premature infants, large left-to-right shunts can be associated with failure to thrive, frequent upper respiratory infections, and congestive heart failure. In addition to congestive heart failure, older children, adolescents, and adults may present with exercise intolerance, arrhythmias, and, rarely, symptoms of pulmonary vascular disease or paradoxical embolization (much more common in foramen ovale rather than a large ASD, which causes a large left-to-right shunt due to increased pulmonary blood flow, which prevents right-to-left shunting). Prior to surgical and device closure of large ASDs,

mortality resulted from pneumonia, congestive heart failure, and, less commonly, pulmonary vascular disease. In patients with large defects who survived beyond infancy, the mean age of death was 37.5 ± 4.5 years of age [21]. After the advent of surgical intervention, postoperative survival in patients repaired before 20 years of age parallels survival in the normal population [10]. Patients repaired later have slightly decreased survival with age compared to the normal population. In the current era, the frequency of diagnosis is increasing, while the average age at diagnosis and, with transcatheter approaches, of closure is decreasing. Thus, most patients with isolated ASDs should expect to have a normal life span.

The classic cardiac exam in the setting of a large left-to-right atrial level shunt and normal pulmonary arterial pressures is characterized by the following four features: a hyperdynamic cardiac impulse, a widely split second heart sound, a soft systolic crescendo-decrescendo ejection murmur at the left upper sternal border produced by increased blood flow across the pulmonary valve that radiates along lines of pulmonary blood flow to the axilla bilaterally, and an early to mid-diastolic murmur at the left lower sternal border, reflecting increased blood flow across the tricuspid valve. The second heart sound is widely split because pulmonary valve closure is delayed by two factors – right ventricular volume overload prolongs the right ventricular systolic ejection phase and pulmonary arterial diastolic pressure decreases more slowly in the dilated pulmonary vascular bed. If pulmonary hypertension develops, the left-to-right shunt decreases in volume. As a result, the second heart sound narrows and the pulmonic component is accentuated; the systolic murmur shortens and a diastolic murmur can no longer be auscultated.

Chest X-ray of a patient with a large left-to-right shunt via an ASD reveals an enlarged cardiac silhouette due to right atrial, right ventricular, and main pulmonary arterial dilation, and there are increased pulmonary vascular markings. An electrocardiogram typically demonstrates normal sinus rhythm, right axis deviation with a QRS axis +95– +170 °, PR interval prolongation in older children and adults, and rsR' or RSR' pattern in rV3, eV4, and V1 due to right ventricular dilation. Intermittent or persistent tachycardias such as atrial flutter can be observed with ECG monitoring.

The atrial septum can be best visualized by transthoracic echocardiography (TTE) in infants and children and transesophageal echocardiography (TEE) in adolescents and adults. Subcostal two-dimensional imaging best defines the rims of atrial septal defects of all sizes. Color flow allows visualization of the direction of the shunt across the defect. Doppler investigation determines both shunt direction and quantifies blood flow velocity. Visualization of tiny defects and determination of the magnitude of the shunt can be augmented by saline contrast injection in a peripheral vein during imaging. Doppler evaluation of tricuspid and pulmonary valve insufficiency is used to estimate right ventricular and pulmonary pressures, respectively. The ratio of pulmonary blood flow to systemic outflow (Qp: Qs) can be estimated via echocardiographic evaluation of the tricuspid and mitral inflow velocity or the pulmonary and aortic outflow velocity. TTE, TEE, and intracardiac echocardiography (ICE) are used in older children and adults during transcatheter atrial septal device placement to aid in device positioning and decrease radiation exposure.

Echocardiography in the setting of a large left-to-right atrial shunt demonstrates progressive right ventricular dilation and paradoxical septal motion. Progressive systolic and diastolic right ventricular dysfunction rarely develops. As the right ventricle dilates, the tricuspid annulus dilates as well and tricuspid insufficiency may be observed. Pulmonary valve dilation and insufficiency and main and branch pulmonary dilation also occur in chronic, large left-to-right shunts. Typically, the left atrium and ventricle remain normal in mass and volume, and left ventricular systolic function is normal. If pulmonary arterial hypertension develops, the shunt at the atrial level can become bidirectional or mostly right to left. Right ventricular hypertrophy and/or dilation may progress and failure may occur.

Cardiac magnetic resonance imaging is often performed to evaluate for partial anomalous pulmonary venous return in patients with challenging echocardiography windows. Currently, visualization of the rims of secundum ASD is more difficult with cardiac MRI than with echocardiography.

Today, diagnostic cardiac catheterization is indicated only for the evaluation of secundum ASDs in rare cases where there is a concern for pulmonary arterial hypertension. A hemodynamic evaluation is always performed before and after atrial septal device placement during interventional cardiac catheterization. When a hemodynamic evaluation is performed in the setting of a large secundum ASD with a large left-to-right atrial shunt, no interstitial lung disease, and normal or mildly elevated pulmonary arterial pressures, oxygen saturations are elevated downstream from the SVC and across the right heart due to mixing of highly saturated pulmonary venous blood with systemic venous return at the right atrial level. Systemic saturations are normal. There is equalization of right atrial and left atrial mean pressures across a large defect. Right ventricular systolic and diastolic pressures can be normal or mildly elevated. Due to significantly increased pulmonary blood flow across the fixed diameter of the pulmonary valve, mildly to moderately elevated peak systolic gradients across the pulmonary valve are observed. Pulmonary vascular resistance can be low, normal, or mildly elevated. As described previously, Qp:Qs can be increased to as much as 3–4:1. In the absence of right ventricular failure, systemic blood flow remains normal, so that the elevation in Qp:Qs is due entirely to an increase in pulmonary blood flow [17, 18].

Surgical Decision Making

The decision making surrounding the closure of ASDs has really become very simplified in the current era. Whereas this was the original lesion that surgeons worked to hard to develop techniques to close, now it is a lesion that is rarely closed in an operating room. In the 1990s, ASD closures made up approximately 10 % of open cardiac surgical procedures. However in 2013, ASD closures make up only 1–2 % of the open cardiac surgical volume. The reason for this is the advent of devices that can be placed by interventional cardiologists in the cath lab. Surgeons now only see secundum ASDs that either have failed device closure or were evaluated for device closure and have an absent inferior rim of the defect making device closure not possible. In addition, there are the rare secundum ASDs that are too large for devices.

Sinus venosus ASDs are different in that they cannot be closed in the cath lab and still require open surgical closure. However, sinus venosus ASDs are far less common than secundum ASDs and so they make up a very small volume of a congenital cardiac surgical practice. Because sinus venosus ASDs are often associated with partial anomalous pulmonary venous drainage, they essentially always require closure. Hence, when they are diagnosed and presented to the surgeon, they are usually scheduled for surgery. Typically the biggest decision the surgeon has to make with a sinus venosus ASD is which surgical technique to use. This is discussed in more detail later in this chapter.

Interventional Approach: Decision Making, Postoperative Management, Complications, Controversies, Outcomes and Long-Term Follow-up, and Future Developments

Categorization of ASDs by size varies between publications and institutions. Generally defects less than 3–4 mm in diameter are referred to as patent foramen ovale or tiny ASDs, small ASDs range from 3–4 mm to 6–8 mm, moderate ASDs range from 5–8 mm to 8–12 mm, and large ASDs are greater than 8–12 mm in diameter. ASDs as large as 39 mm have been reported. After more than half a century studying the natural history of isolated secundum ASDs, prediction of which defects will close spontaneously, remain stable in size, or enlarge over time is still challenging. Varying rates of spontaneous closure are reported in the literature, and the differences in reported rates are likely in part attributable to the differences in age of subjects at diagnosis and variation in categorization of ASDs by size between studies [22–26]. We do know, however,

that there is a high incidence of spontaneous closure of defects less than 3 mm diagnosed during infancy. Radzik et al. determined spontaneous rates of isolated secundum ASD closure in 101 asymptomatic infants diagnosed within the first three months of age. All atrial septal defects with a diameter less than 3 mm closed by 18 months of age; 87 % of ASDs with a diameter of 3–5 mm and 80 % with a diameter of 5–8 mm spontaneously closed by 15 months of age [23]. Azari et al. performed a similar analysis on 121 patients more recently and found a similar but less impressive trend, finding that 84 % of small ASDs, 44 % of medium, and 1 % of large defects closed spontaneously, representing 26 % of all patients [24]. Hanslik et al. had very similar findings, with 34 % of 200 patients showing spontaneous closure, but none in patients with ASDs greater than 10 mm [26].

Alternatively, defects larger than 3 mm have the potential to enlarge. In 104 patients diagnosed with small, moderate, and large isolated secundum ASDs, 66 % of ASDs enlarged over time (mean age at diagnosis 4.5 years, range 0.1–71 years). Rate of growth and final size of the defect did not correlate with the initial size of the defect [25].

Despite extensive research into the natural history of isolated secundum ASDs, the need and optimal age for elective closure in the asymptomatic patient is unknown. Elective closure should be delayed until at least three years of age, after which time spontaneous regression is less likely. Closure at this time is frequently performed in asymptomatic young children with moderate-to-large ASDs and signs of right ventricular volume overload, as it is not yet known if the complications of long-term volume overload including arrhythmias and diastolic dysfunction can be alleviated by late closure. Early closure of ASDs in infants with left-to-right shunts of almost any size should be considered if they have bronchopulmonary dysplasia or other causes of chronic lung disease, even in the absence of signs of right ventricular volume overload or pulmonary arterial hypertension, because closure has been associated with improvement in respiratory status [27, 28]. If there is evidence of elevated pulmonary arterial pressure, patients should undergo cardiac catheterization to evaluate pulmonary vascular resistance and its reactivity. Pulmonary vascular resistance greater than 15 Wood Units $X m^2$ is considered an absolute contraindication to closure. In these cases, medical management of pulmonary arterial hypertension should be instituted, then potential for closure reevaluated [29]. Pulmonary vascular resistance from 10 to 15 Wood Units $X m^2$ increases the risk of closure; however, with the appropriate perioperative medical management, successful closure can be achieved.

Indications for transcatheter device closure of secundum ASDs in symptomatic patients include failure to thrive, frequent upper respiratory infections, congestive heart failure, exercise intolerance, and paradoxical embolization (or its risk, in divers). Successful secundum ASD closure leads to improved weight gain in otherwise normal individuals, a decreased frequency of respiratory infections, resolution of congestive heart failure, and improved exercise tolerance and/or removes the risk of paradoxical embolism. Closure of ASDs with large left-to-right shunts decreases the risk for the development of exercise intolerance and congestive heart failure in pregnancy. Although patients consistently report improved exercise tolerance after ASD closure, evaluation of pulmonary and cardiac function during exercise testing has shown that diffusing capacity is still decreased and airway resistance is increased [30, 31]. Patients with cryptogenic strokes are more likely to have a patent foramen ovale [32]. Patients with both a patent foramen ovale and atrial septal aneurysm are at significant risk for stroke [33]. Closure of the patent foramen ovale in patients with cryptogenic stroke to reduce the risk of recurrent stroke is controversial [34–39]. The CLOSURE I trial demonstrated no benefit to patent foramen ovale closure with the STARFlex device and antiplatelet therapy compared to medical management alone in the prevention of recurrent stroke after cryptogenic stroke [35]. As the study did not include patients at high risk for stroke and recurrent strokes attributed to causes other than paradoxical embolism, the scientific community as a whole agrees that further clinical

trials are required to determine whether the risk of recurrent stroke can be decreased by ASD device closure [37, 39].

Evaluation of the morphology of atrial septal defects in heart specimens compared to echocardiography has revealed important anatomical considerations when choosing and sizing ASD devices. Defects are typically oval in shape, fenestrations are a common finding, and the major axis of the defect is variable and best measured using a combination of the apical four chamber, parasternal short axis, and subcostal sagittal views. The anterior-superior rim of the defect is most likely to be the shortest [40]. Residual shunting across the device most often occurs at the anterior and anterior-superior rims [40]. Intracardiac structures that are close to the defects are the aortic mound, coronary sinus, mitral valve, and the right upper pulmonary vein. Real-time three-dimensional echocardiography characterization of PFO and ASD morphology during selection and sizing of ASDs is being explored in hopes of decreasing the frequency of residual shunts, device embolization, and erosion but is not yet widely available [41].

In 1975, Dr. Terry King and Dr. Noel Mills developed the first transcatheter atrial septal defect closure device, the King-Mills Umbrella [42]. It was used successfully to close a large ASD in a 17-year-old girl. There have been a variety of atrial septal devices developed since the King-Mills Umbrella. Historically, widely used devices included the Clamshell Septal Occluder, CardioSEAL, STARFlex, and the Sideris Buttoned Device, but they are no longer available as technology has advanced. Design evolution has been driven by the desire to minimize delivery system size; to facilitate ease of delivery, repositioning, and retrieval; to balance qualities of device flexibility versus metal fatigue resistance; and to minimize risk of embolization, erosion, and thrombus formation. The design feature that has remained constant is double disk design with a left atrial and right atrial disk.

Currently, the two FDA-approved, widely used devices are the Amplatzer Septal Occluder and the HELEX Septal Occluder. The Amplatzer Septal Occluder (ASO) has been in use since

1996 and received FDA approval in 2001. It is composed of a nickel-titanium alloy (Nitinol) mesh filled with polyester fabric and comprised of a larger left atrial disk and smaller right atrial disk joined by central waist. A variation of it, the Cribiform ASO device, has equal-sized disks and a narrower waist to facilitate closure of fenestrated ASDs. The HELEX Septal Occluder consists of a Nitinol wire frame covered with polytetrafluoroethylene that creates a spiral configuration across the ASD when deployed. It was FDA approved in 2006 for use in ASDs up to a 20 mm stretched diameter [43]. The newly developed GORE Septal Occluder has been designed to improve ease of delivery, visibility during and after delivery, and increased durability compared to the HELEX device. Clinical experiences using this device are ongoing [44].

Transcatheter ASD device closure is safe and effective; however, rare major complications can occur including device embolization or malposition requiring interventional or surgical retrieval, retroperitoneal bleeding, vascular injury to the femoral vessels requiring surgical repair, cardiac perforation by the device causing pericardial effusion and/or tamponade, clinically significant arrhythmias, and thromboembolic stroke. There are no randomized controlled trials comparing transcatheter ASD device closure to surgical ASD closure at this time. Butera et al. performed a meta-analysis of nonrandomized studies between 1998 and 2008 comparing short-term complications of transcatheter device closure of ASDs (Amplatzer and HELEX devices) versus surgical ASD closure [45]. Transcatheter device closure had a lower rate of major complications defined as causing hemodynamic instability or needing immediate invasive or surgical treatment when compared to surgery. Surgical risk of major complications was 3.8-fold higher than the risk with transcatheter device closure; however, these results could in selection bias [45]. Transcatheter closure is clearly preferable in elderly patients or patients with other comorbidities that place them at high risk for complications from anesthesia, sternotomy, and cardiac surgery. Additionally, blood transfusion is avoided during transcatheter closure. No significant difference in long-term outcomes of transcatheter device closure compared to surgical closure, such as survival, clinically significant atrial arrhythmias, or stroke, has been demonstrated in patients followed out to 20 years, but further study is needed [46, 47]. Device erosion of the aortic or atrial wall with resultant hemopericardium, tamponade, or aortic to atrial fistula after transcatheter device placement has been reported. The incidence of erosion reported in long-term follow-up varies between institutions, and 73 cases have been reported in the United States to date [40]. The mechanism of device erosion is unknown; however, deficiency of the anterior-superior rim, oversizing of the device, and straddling of the aorta by the device have been proposed as contributing factors; this issue is currently being investigated in a post-market study [48–51]. There have been no HELEX device erosions reported in the literature [48–51].

Worldwide, devices are emerging for use with design modifications made in hopes of reducing cardiac erosion, promoting endothelialization, and decreasing thrombus formation. The most recent evolution of the Atriasept ASD Occluder is a double disk device with no wire arms in the left atrial disk called the Ultrasept ASD Occluder. The bio-absorbable Sideris Patch is now available in an immediate release device. The Occlutech Figulla ASD Occluder and the Cardio-O-Fix ASD Occluder do not have left atrial metal hubs. The PFM NitOcclud ASD-R and CeraFlex have a ceramic coating on their Nitinol frame, and the CeraFlex has no left atrial metal hub. The BioSTAR device is an absorbable acellular porcine intestinal collagen matrix on a nonabsorbable STARFlex frame that has been shown to be feasible, efficacious, and safe in the BioSTAR Evaluation Study (BEST) phase I clinical trial [52, 53]. Despite being 90–95 % absorbable, a case report of frame migration has been published [48]. Since those studies, the BioSTAR device has been discontinued. Other bio-absorbable devices are under development and the future holds a bioengineered tissue membrane that is completely absorbable yet easily deployable.

Surgical Management

Minimally Invasive Techniques for Surgical Closure of ASD

Over the recent years, minimally invasive techniques have been increasingly used to close primarily secundum ASDs. Different approaches have been used though some of them have certain disadvantages which might limit their use [54].

With the *limited anterolateral thoracotomy* technique, significant distortion of breast development can develop, [55] exposure of the aorta can be difficult, and phrenic nerve injury can also occur.

The use of *posterolateral thoracotomy* avoids the problem of breast distortion [56], and the exposure of the aorta is improved; however, scoliosis has been described.

The use of *limited lower sternotomy* is probably the most commonly used minimally invasive technique for ASD closure [57]. This limits the skin incision to approximately 4 cm and still allows passage of all cannulas through the incision itself although different modifications of this technique exist. The incision starts in the midline at the level of the nipples and extends inferiorly for approximately 4 cm. A slightly longer incision may also be employed depending on the comfort and experience of the surgeon.

Standard Surgical Approach

A standard surgical technique for secundum ASD closure is through a median sternotomy approach. This approach also allows repair of other associated intracardiac defects that might be discovered at the time of surgery. Autologous pericardial patch is commonly used for the ASD closure. Alternatively synthetic material can also be used.

Primary or direct suture closure of the ASD is possible for small- to moderate-sized ASDs. Cardiopulmonary bypass is initiated with an aortic cannula and two venous cannulas. The inferior vena cava should be cannulated at the junction

with the right atrium, low enough so that if there is no inferior rim to the ASD, adequate exposure in this area can still be obtained.

After initiation of cardiopulmonary bypass and placement of caval tapes around the SVC and IVC, cardioplegia is administered through the aortic root. The caval tapes are snared and the right atrium is opened.

Ostium Secundum ASD

For ostium secundum defects, an oblique incision is made from the right atrial appendage to in the direction of the inferior vena cava cannula avoiding crossing the crista terminalis to avoid injury to any conduction fibers from the sinoatrial node to the atrioventricular node.

The ostium secundum defect is visualized and closed through the opened right atrium. The left atrium can be vented directly through the ASD. Inspection of the anatomy of the pulmonary veins and their opening in the left atrium is important to avoid missing an anomalous pulmonary venous drainage. The defect can be closed using autologous pericardium in most cases or synthetic patch material or bovine pericardium if autologous pericardium is not available. The patch is sutured around the defect with care taken to avoid the edge of the Eustachian valve being mistaken as the edge of the ASD. Suturing the Eustachian valve to the septum secundum might produce an obligatory shunt of inferior vena cava blood to the left atrium. The patient will then be desaturated after the procedure.

When suturing the patch adjacent to the coronary sinus, care should be taken to avoid taking deep bites to avoid injuring the atrioventricular node. When the suturing is completed all around the defect but before the knot is tied, a Valsalva maneuver is performed to allow de-airing of the left atrium. The right atrial incision is closed and then the cross-clamp is removed.

Air embolism is one of the most feared complications of ASD closure and care should be taken to de-air the left side of the heart before allowing the left ventricle to fully eject. The aortic root can also be vented through a cardioplegia needle connected to suction, and this can be confirmed by using transesophageal echo which is also used to ensure adequate repair and no significant residual defects left behind.

Alternative techniques of closing secundum defects include direct suture closure of the edges of the defect if the defect is of small to moderate size.

Sinus Venosus ASD

A different incision is made for sinus venosus ASD which is carried from the tip of the right atrial appendage in the direction of the superior vena caval – right atrial junction. The incision can be extended across the junction of the superior vena cava and the right atrium along the right lateral margin of the superior vena cava should this be necessary. For sinus venosus defects, the SVC should be cannulated directly high and close to the innominate – SVC junction.

Sinus venosus defects nearly always require closure with a patch because of their location at the junction between the SVC and the right atrium. Direct closure can lead to right superior pulmonary vein or SVC stenosis or both. Transesophageal echocardiography at the conclusion of sinus venosus defect repair can look for residual atrial level shunting, pulmonary vein stenosis, and SVC stenosis. The sinoatrial node is at risk of injury during sinus venosus defects repair. The right phrenic nerve located at the other side of the pericardium immediately adjacent to the right lateral aspect of the SVC is also potentially at risk.

Between 20 % and 40 % of sinus venosus, ASDs can be closed with a simple autologous intracardiac pericardial patch. The suture line is started between the right superior pulmonary vein and the orifice of the SVC. In some cases, the ASD may require enlargement for prevention of right upper pulmonary vein stenosis. At the posterior aspect of the junction with the SVC and the right atrium, suturing should be relatively superficial to avoid injury to the sinoatrial node by deep bites into the atrial septum and junction with the SVC. If the ASD requires enlargement,

this procedure is performed with an incision toward the fossa ovalis and resection of a portion of the limbus of the septum secundum.

Two-Patch Technique

When the anomalous pulmonary veins enter the SVC, the pericardial patch may have to extend up into the SVC itself to partition the left and right sides. Billowing of the patch into the SVC in these patients would cause SVC stenosis. This complication is prevented with a two-patch technique. A second pericardial patch is placed on the SVC. In these cases, the incision across the SVC-right atrial junction should be as lateral as possible to avoid injury to the sinoatrial nodal artery and the sinoatrial node itself.

Warden Procedure

Several other ingenious techniques involving flaps of the atrial appendage or direct anastomosis of the SVC to the right atrial appendage have been used in repair of complex sinus venosus defects to avoid sinoatrial node injury. The Warden procedure was initially described by Warden et al. in 1984 [58]. In the Warden technique, the SVC is transected and oversewn above the entrance site of the right superior pulmonary vein. The SVC is then anastomosed to the right atrial appendage and the ASD is closed with a patch.

Ostium Primum ASD

The management of ostium primum ASD is described in the chapter of atrioventricular septal defects.

Coronary Sinus Septal Defect

The approach for repair of this defect is with standard bicaval cannulation. The coronary sinus ostium is closed with a patch of autologous pericardium. Because of the proximity of the atrioventricular node, fine superficially placed sutures are placed within the ostium avoiding the triangle of Koch and the risk of causing complete heart block. Coronary sinus blood return drains through the unroofed coronary sinus into the left atrium with an acceptable small right-to-left shunt. In the presence of persistent left SVC in continuity with the coronary sinus, it may be necessary to take a different approach.

Technical Pitfalls

A particularly important technical pitfall is the inadvertent suturing of the edge of the ASD to a prominent Eustachian valve mistaken as the edge of the ASD. This can cause an obligatory right-to-left shunt from the inferior vena cava to the left atrium. This shunt will become immediately obvious because of severe oxygen desaturation of the patient. Proper cannulation of the inferior vena cava, adequate-sized atriotomy, and careful placement of the initial sutures in the inferior area where visualization is most critical should prevent these complications.

Sinus venosus ASD repair can result in SVC stenosis and consideration to a two-patch technique or a Warden procedure should be given to avoid such complication.

Postoperative Care

Following ASD closure, many patients can be extubated in the operating room and monitored in the intensive care unit for the first 12–24 h. Systematic monitoring of these patients is routinely done with special focus on postoperative occurrence of arrhythmias, bleeding, and airway problems. Inotropic support is rarely indicated and most patients can be discharged home within 3–4 days. The use of critical pathways can reduce the length of hospitalization [59].

Post-procedure echocardiogram, either in the operating room or prior to discharge, is crucial to document the adequacy of the technical repair and looking for residual lesions.

Surgical Results and Complications

Surgical ASD Closure

Traditional operative strategies, such as pericardial or synthetic patch closure, have been well established, with a low complication rate and a mortality rate of zero among patients without pulmonary hypertension [60–63]. The most frequently reported immediate complicates include post-pericardiotomy syndrome and atrial arrhythmias. Beyond immediate postoperative outcomes, long-term outcomes following surgical closure (up to 20 years) document the low attrition rate and durability of functional status benefit. Importantly, however, atrial arrhythmias are not completely mitigated by closure and can occur in 10–40 % of patients, especially in older patients (>40 years) or those with preexisting arrhythmias [63–66]. Kutty et al. [67] followed 300 patients from their institution, 152 of whom had surgical closure. Late mortality at 10 years was 3 %, and functional health status had declined in only 15 patients during follow-up. Recently, there have been an increasing number of reports regarding the results following surgical closure among elderly patients, over 60 years of age, which demonstrate equivalent survival to younger patients, albeit with slightly higher complication rates [64, 68, 69]. Hanninen and colleagues [64] studied 68 patients between 68 and 86 years at their institution undergoing either surgical ($n = 13$) or device ($n = 54$) closure. Although the 23 % incidence of major complications (including pneumothorax, heart failure, pneumonia) was higher than that recently reported by Mascio et al. [70] using the Society of Thoracic Surgeons' Congenital Database (20 %), or a single-institution review by Hopkins et al. [71], there were no operative deaths among the elderly cohort. Moreover, after ASD closure, echocardiographic indices of right ventricular size and function were significantly improved from preoperative values and functional capacity as measured by standardized survey instruments, were also significantly improved.

New and Future Approaches to Traditional Surgical ASD Closure

Because of the uniformly excellent outcomes with traditional surgery, attention has shifted to improving the cosmetic result and minimizing hospital stay and convalescence. Multiple strategies have been described to achieve these aims, including the right submammary incision with anterior thoracotomy, limited bilateral submammary incision with partial sternal split, and limited midline incision with partial sternal split. Some surgeons use either video-assisted thoracic surgery (VATS), in conjunction with the submammary and transxiphoid approaches to facilitate closure within a constricted operative field, or totally endoscopic repair in selected patients [64, 71–73]. The use of robotics has also been reported in a small series of 12 adult patients by Argenziano and colleagues [73]. The morbidity and mortality of all of these approaches are comparable to those of the traditional median sternotomy; however, each has technical drawbacks. Operative precision must be maintained with limited exposure in any minimally invasive technique. Extended cardiopulmonary bypass and aortic cross-clamp times, coupled with increased cost, may limit the utility of totally endoscopic- or robotic-assisted ASD closure except at limited centers. Certain approaches have a specific patient population in whom they are applicable. For example, the anterolateral thoracotomy should not be employed in prepubescent girls because it will interfere with breast development. Most totally endoscopic approaches are not feasible in very young patients due to the size of the thoracoscopic ports. Despite these potential drawbacks, however, in carefully selected patients, minimally invasive techniques have demonstrated benefits. Luo and associates performed a prospective randomized study comparing ministernotomy (division of the upper sternum for aortic and pulmonary lesions and the lower sternum for septal lesions) to full sternotomy in 100 consecutive patients undergoing repair of septal lesions [74]. The patients in the ministernotomy group had longer procedure times (by 15–20 min), but had less bleeding, and shorter hospital stays. Consistent with these initiatives, conversion of "low-risk" patients undergoing

minimally invasive ASD closure to an ambulatory population (discharge from hospital within 24 h) has recently been described [75].

First performed in 1976, transcatheter closure of ASDs with the use of various occlusion devices is gaining widespread acceptance [76]. Certain types of ASDs, including patent foramen ovale (PFO), secundum defects, and some fenestrated secundum defects, are amenable to device closure, as long as particular anatomic criteria (e.g., an adequate superior and inferior rim for device seating and distance from the atrioventricular valve) are met. Since the introduction of percutaneous closure, there has been a dramatic rise in device closure prevalence to the point where device closure has supplanted surgical therapy as the dominant treatment modality for secundum ASD [77]. A study from Karamlou et al. [77] recently found that ASD and patent foramen ovale closures per capita increased dramatically from 1.08 per 100,000 population in 1988 to 2.59 per 100,000 population in 2005, an increase of 139 %. When analyzed by closure type, surgical closure increased by only 24 % (from 0.86 per 100,000 population in 1988 to 1.07 per 100,000 in 2005), whereas transcatheter closure increased by 3475 % (from 0.04 per 100,000 population in 1988 to 1.43 per 100,000 in 2005). Importantly, this study determined that the paradigm shift favoring transcatheter closure has occurred mainly due to increased prevalence of closure in adults over age 40 years rather than an increase in closure in infants or children.

Despite the simplicity of ASD repair, there are a myriad of options for patients and physicians who care for patients with congenital heart disease. The patient population that might benefit from closure (whether device or surgical) is likely to increase, challenging current ideas and treatment algorithms that optimize outcomes.

References

1. Gross RE, Watkins E Jr, Pomeranz AA, Goldsmith EI (1953) Method for surgical closure of interauricular septal defects. Surg Gynecol Obstet 96L1:1–23
2. Lewis FJ, Taufic M (1953) Closure of atrial septal defect with aid of hypothermia. Surgery 33:52

3. Sondergaard T (1954) Closure of atrial septal defects: report of three cases. Acta Chir Scand 107:492

4. Gibbon JH (1954) Application of a mechanical heart and lung apparatus to cardiac surgery. Minn Med 37:171–185

5. Hoffman JI, Kaplan S (2002) The incidence of congenital heart disease. J Am Coll Cardiol 39(12):1890–1900

6. Briggs LE, Kakarla J, Wessels A (2012) The pathogenesis of atrial and atrioventricular septal defects with special emphasis on the role of the dorsal mesenchymal protrusion. Differentiation 84(1):117–130

7. Anderson RH, Brown NA, Webb S (2002) Development and structure of the atrial septum. Heart 88(1):104–110

8. Rudolph A (2011) Congenital diseases of the heart: clinical-physiological considerations. Wiley, Chichester

9. Lyons I et al (1995) Myogenic and morphogenetic defects in the heart tubes of murine embryos lacking the homeo box gene Nkx2-5. Genes Dev 9(13):1654–1656

10. Hoffmann AD et al (2009) Sonic hedgehog is required in pulmonary endoderm for atrial septation. Development 136(10):1761–1770

11. Basson CT et al (1997) Mutations in human TBX5 [corrected] cause limb and cardiac malformation in Holt-Oram syndrome. Nat Genet 15(1):30–35

12. Vaughan CJ, Basson CT (2000) Molecular determinants of atrial and ventricular septal defects and patent ductus arteriosus. Am J Med Genet 97(4):304–309

13. Schott JJ et al (1998) Congenital heart disease caused by mutations in the transcription factor NKX2-5. Science 281(5373):108–111

14. Kelly RG (2012) The second heart field. Curr Top Dev Biol 100:33–65

15. Xie L et al (2012) Tbx5-hedgehog molecular networks are essential in the second heart field for atrial septation. Dev Cell 23(2):280–291

16. Jacobs JP, Burke RP, Quitessenza JA, Mavroudis C (2000) Atrial septal defect. Ann Thorac Surg 69:S18

17. Mavroudis C, Backer C (2003) Pediatric cardiac surgery, 3rd edn. Futura, Mount Kisco

18. Jonas R (2004) Comprehensive surgical management of congenital heart disease, 1st edn. Arnold, London

19. Hoffman JIE (2009) The natural and unnatural history of congenital heart disease. Wiley, Hoboken

20. Haworth SG (1983) Pulmonary vascular disease in secundum atrial septal defect in childhood. Am J Cardiol 51(2):265–272

21. Campbell M (1970) Natural history of atrial septal defect. Br Heart J 32(6):820–826

22. Brassard M et al (1999) Outcome of children with atrial septal defect considered too small for surgical closure. Am J Cardiol 83(11):1552–1555

23. Radzik D et al (1993) Predictive factors for spontaneous closure of atrial septal defects diagnosed in the first 3 months of life. J Am Coll Cardiol 22(3):851–853

24. Azhari N, Shihata MS, Al-Fatani A (2004) Spontaneous closure of atrial septal defects within the oval fossa. Cardiol Young 14(2):148–155

25. McMahon CJ et al (2002) Natural history of growth of secundum atrial septal defects and implications for transcatheter closure. Heart 87(3):256–259

26. Hanslik A et al (2006) Predictors of spontaneous closure of isolated secundum atrial septal defect in children: a longitudinal study. Pediatrics 118(4):1560–1565

27. Wood AM et al (2011) Transcatheter elimination of left-to-right shunts in infants with bronchopulmonary dysplasia is feasible and safe. Congenit Heart Dis 6(4):330–337

28. Thomas VC et al (2012) Transcatheter closure of secundum atrial septal defect in infants less than 12 months of age improves symptoms of chronic lung disease. Congenit Heart Dis 7(3):204–211

29. Steele PM et al (1987) Isolated atrial septal defect with pulmonary vascular obstructive disease–long-term follow-up and prediction of outcome after surgical correction. Circulation 76(5):1037–1042

30. Weber M et al (2004) Cardiopulmonary exercise capacity increases after interventional ASD-closure. Z Kardiol 93(3):209–215

31. Reybrouck T et al (1991) Cardiorespiratory exercise capacity after surgical closure of atrial septal defect is influenced by the age at surgery. Am Heart J 122 (4 Pt 1):1073–1078

32. Hara H et al (2005) Patent foramen ovale: current pathology, pathophysiology, and clinical status. J Am Coll Cardiol 46(9):1768–1776

33. Mas JL et al (2001) Recurrent cerebrovascular events associated with patent foramen ovale, atrial septal aneurysm, or both. N Engl J Med 345(24):1740–1746

34. Agarwal S et al (2012) Meta-analysis of transcatheter closure versus medical therapy for patent foramen ovale in prevention of recurrent neurological events after presumed paradoxical embolism. JACC Cardiovasc Interv 5(7):777–789

35. Furlan AJ et al (2012) Closure or medical therapy for cryptogenic stroke with patent foramen ovale. N Engl J Med 366(11):991–999

36. Ford MA et al (2009) Percutaneous device closure of patent foramen ovale in patients with presumed cryptogenic stroke or transient ischemic attack: the mayo clinic experience. JACC Cardiovasc Interv 2(5):404–411

37. O'Gara PT et al (2009) Percutaneous device closure of patent foramen ovale for secondary stroke prevention: a call for completion of randomized clinical trials a science advisory from the American Heart Association/American Stroke Association and the American College of Cardiology Foundation the American Academy of Neurology affirms the value of this science advisory. J Am Coll Cardiol 53(21):2014–2018

38. Freund MA et al (2012) Percutaneous device closure of patent foramen ovale for cryptogenic strokes/transient ischemic attacks. JACC Cardiovasc Interv 5(11):1189

39. Kitsios GD et al (2012) Patent foramen ovale closure and medical treatments for secondary stroke prevention: a systematic review of observational and randomized evidence. Stroke 43(2):422–431

40. Momenah TS et al (2000) Transesophageal echocardiographic predictors for successful transcatheter closure of defects within the oval fossa using the CardioSEAL septal occlusion device. Cardiol Young 10(5):510–518

41. Rana BS et al (2010) Three-dimensional imaging of the atrial septum and patent foramen ovale anatomy: defining the morphological phenotypes of patent foramen ovale. Eur J Echocardiogr 11(10):i19–i25

42. King TD, Mills NL (1974) Nonoperative closure of atrial septal defects. Surgery 75:383–388

43. Latson LA et al (2006) Analysis of factors related to successful transcatheter closure of secundum atrial septal defects using the HELEX septal occluder. Am Heart J 151(5):1129.e7–1129.e11

44. Albers E et al (2012) Percutaneous closure of secundum atrial septal defects. Prog Pediat Cardiol 33(2):115–123

45. Butera G et al (2011) Percutaneous versus surgical closure of secundum atrial septal defects: a systematic review and meta-analysis of currently available clinical evidence. Euro Intervention 7(3):377–385

46. Kutty S et al (2012) Long-term (5- to 20-year) outcomes after transcatheter or surgical treatment of hemodynamically significant isolated secundum atrial septal defect. Am J Cardiol 109(9):1348–1352

47. DiBardino DJ et al (2009) Analysis of the US Food and Drug Administration manufacturer and user facility device experience database for adverse events involving amplatzer septal occluder devices and comparison with the society of thoracic surgery congenital cardiac surgery database. J Thorac Cardiovasc Surg 137(6):1334–1341

48. Vottero GV et al (2012) Late migration of percutaneous bio-absorbable devices–a word of caution. J Card Surg 27(2):183–185

49. Masura J, Gavora P, Podnar T (2005) Long-term outcome of transcatheter secundum-type atrial septal defect closure using amplatzer septal occluders. J Am Coll Cardiol 45(4):505–507

50. Diab K, Kenny D, Hijazi ZM (2012) Erosions, erosions, and erosions! Device closure of atrial septal defects: how safe is safe? Catheter Cardiovasc Interv 80(2):168–174

51. Crawford GB et al (2012) Percutaneous atrial septal occluder devices and cardiac erosion: a review of the literature. Catheter Cardiovasc Interv 80(2):157–167

52. Baspinar O et al (2012) Bioabsorbable atrial septal occluder for percutaneous closure of atrial septal defect in children. Tex Heart Inst J 39(2):184–189

53. Mullen MJ et al (2006) BioSTAR evaluation STudy (BEST): a prospective, multicenter, phase I clinical trial to evaluate the feasibility, efficacy, and safety of the BioSTAR bioabsorbable septal repair implant for the closure of atrial-level shunts. Circulation 114(18):1962–1967

54. Bichell DP, Geva T, Bacha EA et al (2000) Minimal access approach for the repair of atrial septal defect: the initial 135 patients. Ann Thorac Surg 70:115

55. Cherup LL, Siewers RD, Futrell JW (1996) Breast and pectoral muscle maldevelopment after anterolateral and posterolateral thoracotomies in children. Ann Thorac Surg 41:492–497

56. Houel L, Petit J, Planche C et al (1999) Right posterolateral thoracotomy for open heart surgery in infants and children. Indications and results. Arch Mal Coeur Vaiss 92:641–646

57. del Nido PJ, Bichell DP (1998) Minimal-access surgery for congenital heart defects. Semin Thorac Cardiovasc Surg 10:75–80

58. Warden HE, Gustafson RA, Tarnay TJ, Neal WA (1984) AN alternative method for repair of partial anomalous pulmonary venous connection to the superior vena cava. Ann Thorac Surg 38:601–605

59. Price MB, Jones A, Hawkins JA et al (1999) Critical pathways for postoperative care after simple congenital heart surgery. Am J Manag Care 5:185

60. Thompson JD, Abuwari EH, Watterson KG et al (2002) Surgical and transcatheter (amplatzer) closure of atrial septal defect: a prospective comparison of results and cost. Heart 87:466–469

61. Du ZD, Hijazi ZM, Kleinman CS et al (2002) Comparison between transcatheter and surgical closure of secundum atrial septal defect in children and adults: results of a multicenter nonrandomized trial. J Am Coll Cardiol 39:1836–1844

62. Highes ML, Maskell G, Goh TH, Wilkinson JL (2002) Prospective comparison of costs and short term health outcomes of surgical versus device closure of atrial septal defect in children. Heart 88:67–70

63. Murphy JG, Gersh BJ, McGoon MD et al (1990) Long-term outcome after surgical repair of isolated atrial septal defect. N Engl J Med 323:1645–1650

64. Hanninen M, Kmet A, Taylor DA et al (2011) Atrial septal defect closure in the elderly is associated with excellent quality of life, functional improvement, and ventricular remodeling. Can J Cardiol 27:698–704

65. Gatzoulis MA, Freeman MA, Siu SD et al (1999) Atrial arrhythmias after surgical closure of atrial septal defects in adults. N Engl J Med 340:839–846

66. Silversides CK, Haberer K, Siu SD et al (2008) Predictors of atrial arrhythmias after device closure of secundum atrial septal defects in adults. Am J Cardiol 101:683–687

67. Kutty S, Hazeem AA, Brown K et al (2012) Long-term (5-to 20-year) outcomes after transcatheter or surgical treatment of hemodynamically significant isolated secundum atrial septal defect. Am J Cardiol 109:1348–1352

68. Jemielity M, Dyszkiewicz W, Paluszkiewicz L et al (2001) Do patients over age 40 years of age benefit from surgical closure of atrial septal defects? Heart 85:300–303

69. Attie F, Rosas M, Granados N et al (2001) Surgical treatment of secundum atrial septal defects in patients > 40 years old. A randomized clinical trial. J Am Coll Cardiol 38:2035–2042

70. Mascio CE, Pasquali SK, Jacobs JP et al (2011) Outcomes in adult congenital heart surgery: analysis of the society of thoracic surgeons (STS) database. J Thorac Cardiovasc Surg 142:1090–1097

71. Hopkins RA, Bert AA, Buchholz B et al (2004) Surgical patch closure of atrial septal defects. Ann Thorac Surg 77:2144–2150

72. Liu G, Qiao Y, Zou C et al (2012) Totally thoracoscopic surgical treatment for atrial septal defect: mid-term follow-up results in 45 consecutive patients. Heart Lung Circ 22:S1443–S9506

73. Argenziano M, Oz M, Kohmoto T et al (2003) Totally endoscopic atrial septal defect repair with robotic assistance. Circulation 108(Suppl II):II-191–II-194

74. Luo W, Chang C, Chen S (2001) Ministernotomy versus full sternotomy in congenital heart defects: a prospective randomized study. Ann Thorac Surg 71:473

75. Srivastava AR, Banerjee A, Tempe DK et al (2008) A comprehensive approach to fast tracking in cardiac surgery: ambulatory low-risk open-heart surgery. Eur J Cardiothorac Surg 33:955–960

76. King TD, Mills NL (1976) Secundum atrial septal defects: nonoperative closure during cardiac catheterization. JAMA 235:2506

77. Karamlou T, Diggs BS, McCrindle BW, Ungerleider RM, Welke KF (2008) The rush to atrial septal defect closure: is the introduction of percutaneous closure driving utilization? Ann Thorac Surg 86:1584–1590

Ventricular Septal Defects

83

Beatrice Bonello, Virginie Fouilloux, Stephane Le Bel,
Alain Fraisse, Bernard Kreitmann, and Dominique Metras

Abstract

The ventricular septal defect is the most common congenital heart defect
and truly represents the success story that is interdisciplinary pediatric
cardiovascular care.

The diagnosis, classification, and management of patients with ventricular septal defect mirror the development and advancement of modern
pediatric cardiology and cardiac surgery. Appropriate medical and surgical
treatment allows severely ill children to have a normal growth and near
normal life expectancy. While the diagnosis and management of patients
with ventricular septal defect is relatively standard and predictable, there
are pitfalls and risks that can account for a complicated perioperative and
critical care course. The progress in the surgical field (cardiopulmonary
bypass, myocardial protection, improved skill, and surgical techniques) and
in the perioperative care has advanced so that standard ventricular septal
defect closure in patients above 2 kg of weight is now obtained with almost
no mortality or major morbidity. The management of ventricular septal

Electronic Supplementary Material: The online version
of this chapter (doi:10.1007/978-1-4471-4619-3_15)
contains supplementary material, which is available to
authorized users.

B. Bonello (✉) • A. Fraisse
Pediatric Cardiology, Children's Hospital La Timone
Aix-Marseille University (France), Marseille, France
e-mail: Beatrice.bonello@ap-hm.fr;
alain.fraisse@ap-hm.fr

V. Fouilloux • B. Kreitmann • D. Metras
Cardiothoracic Surgery, Children's Hospital La Timone
Aix-Marseille University (France), Marseille, France
e-mail: virginie.fouilloux@ap-hm.fr;
bkreitmann@ap-hm.fr; dmetras@apm.fr

S. Le Bel
Pediatric Intensive Care, Children's Hospital La Timone
Aix-Marseille University (France), Marseille, France
e-mail: Stephane.lebel@ap-hm.fr

defect has also been the spark for development of innovative technology and the opportunity for truly interdisciplinary pediatric cardiovascular care.

Keywords

Cardiac catheterization • Cardiac surgery • Cardiopulmonary bypass • Congenital heart defects • Cono-ventricular • Inlet • Interventricular • Muscular • Paramembranous • Perimembranous • Pulmonary hypertension • Supracristal • Vascular resistance • Ventricular septal defect • VSD

Definition

A ventricular septal defect (VSD) is a hole in the interventricular septum. It is one of the most prevalent congenital heart defects (CHD). This chapter will address VSD (single or multiple) as an isolated lesion, with or without associated defects like aortic valve insufficiency or secondary right ventricular outflow stenosis.

A VSD is, however, a frequent and important aspect of a neonatal coarctation syndrome and is very common in many more complex CHD such as tetralogy of Fallot or pulmonary atresia-VSD, double-outlet right ventricle, transposition or malposition of the great arteries, truncus arteriosus, and complete atrioventricular canal defects. When associated with these defects, management of the VSD will be discussed in their respective chapters.

Introduction

Prevalence

The VSD is one of the most prevalent congenital heart defects, accounting for up to 40 % of cardiac anomalies [1]. Frequency of this defect varies according to the age at examination and the mode of diagnosis. Prevalence in neonates has been reported to be as high as 5 % with highly sensitive echocardiography [2], but most studies quote an incidence of 3–3.5 per 1,000 live-born infants [3]. In the adult population, the incidence is lower (0.3 per 1,000). Indeed, many VSDs will close spontaneously or will be repaired in childhood [4].

Genetics

The underlying etiology of VSD is unclear. Nevertheless, there are chromosomal disorders associated with an increased incidence of VSD such as trisomy 21 (Down syndrome), 22q11 deletion (Di George syndrome), and 45X deletion (Turner syndrome). Familial forms of cardiac septation defects have been linked to TBX5, GATA4, and NKX2.5 mutations [5]. Children from an adult with a VSD that is not associated with a genetic disorder may have a risk of VSD as high as 3 % if the father is affected and a 6 % risk if the mother is affected [6].

Historical Background

The VSD was recognized and described by the anatomists and pathologists as far back in time as Vesale (sixteenth century), Morgagni (eighteenth century), and Senac (eighteenth century). However, it was not until Roger (nineteenth century) that the correlation between a cardiac murmur and a hole in the ventricular septum was made. Paradoxically, in France, the term "maladie de Roger" (Roger's disease) is used to describe a very small VSD without any clinical consequence but with a loud murmur, which is in fact probably not a "maladie" at all.

Clinical interest in VSD increased when surgical therapy became possible. Initially, the only possible therapy was to address the consequence of the VSD, namely, excessive pulmonary blood flow via left-to-right shunt, with a palliative surgery to limit pulmonary blood flow by placing a band on the main pulmonary artery (PA), as originally described by Muller and Damman in 1952 [7].

In 1954, Lillehei, Varco, and colleagues at the University of Minnesota were the first to surgically close a VSD with the aid of cross circulation, a technique in which an adult patient, usually a parent, was utilized as a pump and oxygenator to allow cardiotomy [8]. Between 1954 and 1955, 27 patients had a VSD closed this way, with 19 survivors.

Once a usable heart-lung machine was available, a series of 20 patients treated by surgical closure at the Mayo clinic was reported in 1957 [9].

Subsequently, surgical closure of VSD became a worldwide procedure, with progressive reduction of the age of the patients. The technique of deep hypothermia and circulatory arrest that was initially described in 1969 by Okamoto et al. [10], and popularized by Sir B. Barratt-Boyes [11], allowed repair of VSD in small infants. Soon it was shown that, even in small babies, the direct closure of defect was superior to a palliative PA banding.

In the more recent era, two important procedures were added to the armamentarium of the physicians, in a field where interventional cardiologists and surgeons collaborate more and more: first the percutaneous closure of a VSD by a device introduced by catheterization [12] and secondly the intraoperative perventricular closure with a device, without the use of cardiopulmonary bypass [13].

Obviously, these two procedures cannot be used for all VSD closures but are very useful in several situations where conventional surgery on CPB either can be avoided or can be hazardous.

As a result of these technical and strategic developments, the treatment of VSD has led to a real definitive cure and near normal life expectancy.

Anatomy

The morphology of VSDs has been described by various authors using position, embryologic, topographic, or even surgical considerations as the focus. As R.H. Anderson recently wrote [13]: "there is still no consensus concerning the best way to categorize and describe holes between the ventricle." Nevertheless, most surgeons and cardiologists utilize the work of R. Van Praagh [14] and R.H. Anderson [15] as a basis for classification.

The Components of the Interventricular Septum

There are four basic areas of the septum, where a VSD can be found [14]:

1. Atrioventricular or inlet muscular septum (AV) canal (component 1) [15].
2. The muscular or ventricular sinus septum (component 2).
3. The septal band or proximal conal septum (component 3).
4. The parietal band or distal conal septum (component 4). This part is also known as the infundibular septum.

Those four components of the ventricular septum can be seen from the right side of the septum (IA) or the left side (IB).

The nearly transparent fibrous area at the limit of the conal septum and the AV canal septum is also referred to as pars membranacea.

Anatomic Types of VSD

Cono-Ventricular Defects

Cono-ventricular defects are located between the conal septum (component 4) and the ventricular components (2, 3) and at the limit with the AV canal septum (component 1). Many variation and extensions of this type of VSD exist. These VSDs are often beyond the membranous septum and are referred to as perimembranous or paramembranous. When associated with some hypoplasia or displacement of the conal septum, the VSD may be called a "malalignment defect." They can have some extension to the infundibular (outlet) or AV canal (inlet) septum. They are often covered partially with accessory fibrotic tricuspid tissue.

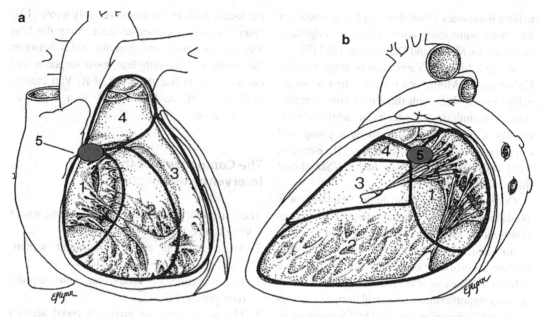

Fig. 83.1 (a) The septum seen from the right side (b) seen from the left side, *Component 1* AV canal septum or inlet septum, *Component 2* muscular septum, *Component* *3* proximal conal septum, *Component 4* distal conal septum or infundibular septum, *Component 5* "pars membranacea" (Figure adapted from Van Praagh et al. [14])

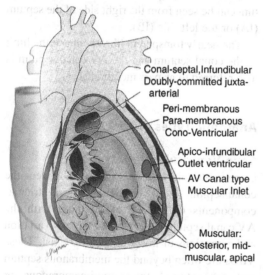

Conal-septal, Infundibular
Doubly-committed juxta-arterial

Peri-membranous
Para-membranous
Cono-Ventricular

Apico-infundibular
Outlet ventricular

AV Canal type
Muscular Inlet

Muscular:
posterior, mid-muscular, apical

Fig. 83.2 VSD classified according to R. Van Praagh [14] and RH Anderson [15] (Drawing adapted from Keane and Fyler [66])

AV Canal or Inlet VSD

Located in the AV canal septum or inlet portion of the interventricular septum, they are very similar to the ventricular component of an atrioventricular septal defect. The cephalad border of these defects is the tricuspid valve annulus; therefore; they have a large part of their edge without muscular tissue.

Both the cono-ventricular and the inlet VSDs can be partially covered by tricuspid chordae and small papillary muscles, seen from the right ventricular side.

Muscular VSD

Muscular VSDs have their entire circumference composed of muscular tissue. They can occur in the mid-muscular, posterior, or apical portion of the interventricular septum. They may be singular or multiple. In some cases there appears to be multiple VSDs from the right ventricular aspect; however, there is often only a singular large defect as viewed from the left ventricular aspect. Multiple defects are sometimes described as "Swiss cheese"-like septum. The anterior area to the septal band is considered by some authors as the apex of the conus and is the location of the apico-infundibular or low outlet ventricular defects. It is not uncommon for muscular defects to coexist with other types of VSD especially cono-ventricular or perimembranous defects.

Conal Septal or Supracristal VSD

These VSDs occur in the infundibular portion of the septum and usually produce near continuity between pulmonary and aortic valves annuli. For this reason, they have also been referred to as doubly committed or juxta-arterial VSDs.

Important Anatomic Relations of VSD

There are clinical and surgically important anatomic relationships of VSDs.

Perimembranous VSDs are closely associated with the aortic valve annulus, and in fact, the aortic valve leaflets may be drawn into the opening of the VSD. Valve leaflets may be injured in the course of a VSD repair. This relationship is one of the major limitations of percutaneous VSD closure with devices.

It is not uncommon for the VSD to be partially obscured by septal leaflet tissue of the tricuspid valve. This may require incision and reconstruction of the tricuspid valve to accomplish VSD closure.

The atrioventricular node and bundle of His are in close proximity to both membranous and inlet-type VSDs. The atrioventricular node of Aschoff-Tawara is located in the upper angle of the triangle of Koch. The bundle of His originates from the node and penetrates the central fibrous body close to the posteroinferior rim of the VSD. From there, the bundle passes in the inferior rim and left ventricular side of the interventricular septum of the perimembranous VSD. During its course, it separates into the left and the right branch, the later has then a course under the right ventricle towards the apex. Conduction tissue is usually remote from muscular or supracristal-type VSDs, although it must be noted that in some large mid-muscular defects, positioned high in the septum and separated from tricuspid annulus only by a small muscular band, the bundle of His course is located at the anterior superior rim of the defect.

Physiology and Pathophysiology

In the heart with normal segmental anatomy and without significant obstruction to pulmonary blood flow or increased pulmonary vascular resistance, a VSD will exhibit significant left-to-right shunt. This increased pulmonary blood flow will manifest as a volume load on the left ventricle. The magnitude of the shunt is determined by the size of the defect, the relative ratio of resistances of pulmonary and systemic vascular beds, and the potential obstruction of either the right or left ventricular outflow tracts.

Small restrictive defects have inherent resistance across the defects and are characterized by limited volume overload and a pulmonary to systemic blood flow ratio lower than 1.5/1 [16]. Small restrictive defects do not have hemodynamic consequences, and 85–95 % will spontaneously close in the first year after birth [17–19].

Moderately sized VSDs, despite some restriction, are usually associated with some increased volume overload. These defects are less likely to close spontaneously and may result in symptoms and require surgical closure.

Large, nonrestrictive VSDs have no restriction to flow across the defect, and hence the degree of shunt is dependent upon relative resistance of pulmonary and systemic vascular beds. This relation varies with the age [20]. In this situation, symptoms are usually present in the absence of increased pulmonary vascular resistance. Those defects are very unlikely to close spontaneously, without treatment, and will result in permanent changes in the pulmonary vasculature or pulmonary vascular occlusive disease with eventual reversal of shunting to right-to-left and Eisenmenger syndrome [21].

Diagnosis

Clinical

VSDs can usually be detected by auscultation; the VSD is characterized by a pansystolic murmur located at the left lower sternal border and radiating across the precordium. The intensity and duration of the murmur depend on the flow velocity across the defect. The smaller the defect is, the louder the murmur. If there is a significant volume load of the left ventricle (moderate size defect or larger and low pulmonary vascular resistance), the precordium impulse may be displaced laterally, and an apical mid-diastolic murmur across the mitral valve and/or a third heart sound can be heard.

In the neonatal period, pulmonary vascular resistance is normally elevated, and consequently, flow across a VSD may be limited, and the newborn is usually asymptomatic. However, as the PVR falls, left-to-right shunt increases and symptoms may be exhibited. These include tachypnea, tachycardia diaphoresis and dyspnea while feeding, poor weight gain, and eventual failure to thrive. After several months or years of significantly increased pulmonary blood flow from a nonrestrictive VSD, reversal of flow across the VSD may occur resulting in no heart failure symptoms but relative desaturation with right-to-left shunt or Eisenmenger syndrome. Occasionally, the usual fall in neonatal pulmonary vascular resistances does not occur. These children may not exhibit signs of heart failure, despite a large VSD.

Electrocardiogram

The electrocardiogram (EKG) is usually normal when the VSD is small. Larger degrees of left-to-right shunt may show sinus tachycardia and evidence of chamber enlargement on EKG. Defects of the inlet septum may show left axis deviation of the frontal plane QRS vector with Q waves in leads I and aVL, as in atrioventricular canal defects, suggesting an abnormal course of the conduction system.

Imaging

Chest X-Ray

Chest X-ray should be normal if the defect is small since birth. In children with moderate or large-sized VSD and low pulmonary resistance, pulmonary vascularity is increased and the pulmonary arteries are dilated. Left atrial and left ventricle may be dilated with cardiomegaly. Lung fields will often demonstrate perihilar edema and enlarged pulmonary arteries.

Echocardiography

Echocardiography is the mainstay of modern diagnosis of VSD. It will demonstrate the number, the size(s) and location(s) of the defect(s), and the anatomical relations to the outflow tracks and the tricuspid valve, and rule out associated cardiac or extracardiac anomalies. Complete imaging of the interventricular septum requires careful assessment and use of multiple echocardiographic views, with and without Doppler color mapping. Parasternal short-axis view, the most important one, scans all the interventricular septum from the conus to the apex. This view allows distinguishing membranous VSD, classically between "9 and 12 h," on a plane through the aortic valve, to infundibular VSD between "12 and 3 h" (Videos 83.1 and 83.2). Parasternal long-axis view will image the conal and muscular septum. Apical 4-chamber view shows the inlet and muscular septum (Figs. 83.1 and 83.2), with a scan up to the outflow tracts to study the conal septum. Subcostal view shows the conal and muscular septum. Tiny defects and small multiple defects in the trabecular muscular septum may be difficult to identify and can sometimes be visualized by Doppler color imaging only (Videos 83.3 and 83.4). In case of a very large unrestrictive defect, color-coded Doppler flow may not easily identify additional VSDs.

The echocardiography will also characterize the cardiac function and the impact of the defect by measuring the left ventricle diameter according to the normal value indexed for the body surface area. Two-dimensional continuous wave Doppler allows reliable estimates of right ventricular pressure. It can be obtained both by measuring the pressure gradient between the right ventricle and the right atrium by the tricuspid regurgitation maximal velocity jet and by

Video 83.1 Apical
4-chamber
echocardiographic view
showing a large mid-
muscular ventricular septal
defect

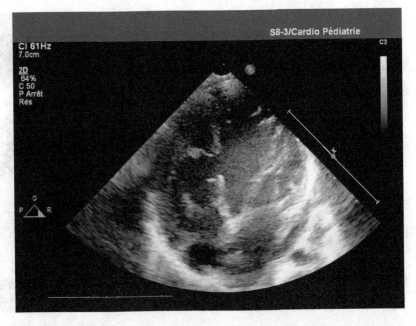

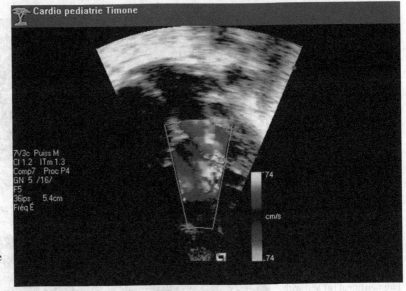

Video 83.2 Apical
4-chamber
echocardiographic view
with color Doppler flow
through a mild to moderate
mid-muscular ventricular
septal defect

measuring the pressure gradient between the left and the right ventricle by the maximal velocity jet trough the defect itself.

Transesophageal echocardiography is rarely used as a diagnostic test but plays a major role in the confirmation of the defects and the effectiveness of surgical closure or percutaneous closure [22, 23].

Three-dimensional echocardiography is becoming widely available and may provide important diagnostic assistance in the case with complex anatomy [24].

Cardiac Catheterization

Cardiac catheterization is only indicated in complicated cases: to assess the pulmonary vascular

Video 83.3 Parasternal short-axis echocardiographic view with color Doppler showing a large membranous ventricular septal defect between "9 and 12 h," on a plane through the aortic valve

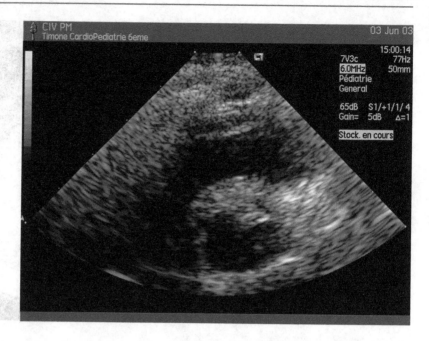

Video 83.4 Parasternal short-axis echocardiographic view showing a mild to moderate infundibular ventricular septal defect between "12 and 3 h" on a plane through the aortic valve, in bidimensional (**a**) and with color Doppler flow (**b**)

resistance in individuals with suspected pulmonary vascular occlusive disease and in suspected multiple VSD or to close the malformation by transcatheter approach. A specific chapter elsewhere in this textbook outlines the details of interventional cardiac catheterization for VSD closure.

Cardiac Magnetic Resonance Imaging

Cardiac magnetic resonance imaging (cMRI) is used increasingly to assess patients with congenital heart disease. In newborn and young children, its indications may be limited due to the sedation often required. cMRI can be used to assess complex anatomy and the VSD impact by measuring the volume overload and the Qp/Qs in patients with poor echocardiographic images [25].

Laboratory Tests

Pre-therapeutic evaluation in symptomatic patients may include standard electrolytes and complete blood count. In patients with significant heart failure symptoms, B-type natriuretic peptide (BNP) has been shown to correlate to clinical heart failure [26]. There is no evidence-based management on BNP level, but it can be helpful in association with other measures of heart failure for the management and follow-up of infants.

Natural History

A large number of VSDs will close spontaneously with time. This is true for cono-ventricular (peri- or paramembranous) and also for many muscular defects. For the former type, closure occurs mainly by proliferation of fibrous tissue, attached to the fibrous edge of the defect and to the ventricular side of the tricuspid adjacent leaflets (often the anteroseptal commissure). It can result in the so-called aneurysm of membranous septum. This can occur until the age of 3 or 4 years, but mainly during the first months of the first year of life, and is more likely to happen in the case of small restrictive defects that usually measure less than 50 % of aortic annulus. Because of this, it is recommended to observe and medically manage small restrictive VSDs until such time that symptoms develop requiring increased medical management, aortic insufficiency develops, evidence of increased PVR develops, or it becomes clear that the defect is moderate to large and is not likely to close.

The AV canal type and supracristal of infundibular VSDs are very unlikely to close spontaneously. These defects generally have a large left-to-right shunt and are more prone to result in complications like development of aortic insufficiency.

The presence of a patent ductus arteriosus or an atrial level shunt will further increase the left-to-right shunt and may increase the necessity of surgical repair.

Increased PVR and the risk for pulmonary vascular occlusive disease increase with age and the degree of left-to-right shunt. This must be evaluated in children with large VSDs after about 1 year of age or 6 months of age for children with Down syndrome. Increased resistance may alter or guide postoperative care or, in some cases, if the resistance is very high, may preclude definitive repair of the VSD. These children may be screened with echocardiography and an estimate of RV and pulmonary artery pressure but may also require direct measurement of the pulmonary artery pressure and calculation of Qp/Qs and resistance indexes by cardiac catheterization. Evidence of a relatively low Qp/Qs (1.3–1.5) in the face of a large defect demonstrates high PVR. In these patients, pulmonary vasodilator testing at the time of catheterization may demonstrate a decrease in resistance in which closure is indicated, or possibly fixed elevated PVR, in which case closure is contraindicated. This situation is unusual in current practice, but is not uncommon in developing countries.

Medical Management

Most children with important VSDs will not exhibit significant signs or symptoms until the PVR begins to fall in the first several weeks of life. The degree of left-to-right shunt will determine the necessity for medical management and eventual surgical repair. Medical management for congestive heart failure (CHF) due to left ventricular volume overload usually begins with the initiation of diuretic therapy. There is increasing use of angiotensin converting enzyme inhibitors as well. Usually, definitive therapy (total repair) is indicated with escalation or failure of medical management. Proper nutritional supplementation is often necessary as caloric requirements are increased in the face of CHF. This may necessitate nasogastric tube feedings. When a patient fails to gain weight despite adequate caloric intake, definitive therapy is indicated. Importantly, prevention of serious viral infections is indicated. Many centers go so far as to recommend repair early in order to avoid the risk of viral infection with a large VSD. Endocarditis prophylaxis was recommended routinely in patients with VSDs to prevent procedure-associated endocarditis. However, this poor evidence-based strategy has resulted in revised guidelines [27]. Patients with uncomplicated VSDs do not need antibiotics when undergoing dental, gastrointestinal, urogenital, and skin and soft tissue procedures, unless there is an established infection. Primary dental prevention is strongly recommended by daily dental hygiene, except for dental procedure requiring manipulation of gingival, periapical region of the teeth or the oral mucosa. Antibiotic prophylaxis is still indicated in high-risk population: patients with previous infective endocarditis, patients with right-to-left shunt, patients with residual shunt after repair, and patients after repair with prosthetic material whether placed by surgery or by percutaneous technique, up to 6 months after the procedure.

Surgical Management

Pulmonary Artery Banding

The pulmonary artery banding historically has been performed in patients with aortic coarctation and ventricular septal defect in order to avoid an open cardiac surgical procedure in early infancy. It is presently rarely done for an isolated VSD unless there is a contraindication to cardiopulmonary bypass and significant CHF that necessitates some intervention. Pulmonary artery banding may also be indicated in particular situations like multiple VSDs and very large apical VSD in small babies.

To perform an adequately positioned and calibrated banding, the best approach is through a median sternotomy, but anterior and posterior thoracotomies have been used. After incision of the pericardium, the main PA (MPA) is cautiously encircled. A band is placed around the MPA. The material used is variable and includes polytetrafluoroethylene (PTFE) strip, Silastic material, and Teflon strip umbilical tape. It is advantageous to use a material that is the least adherent. Once the MPA is encircled with the band, the band is progressively tightened while observing the distal main pulmonary artery pressure and systemic oxygen saturation. This is usually accomplished with titanium clips applied to the band and eventually securing the band to the PA to prevent migration onto the branch PAs. A rough estimate of the band may follow Trusler's rules: length in mm corresponding to the weight in kg of the baby, plus 20 mm. The distal PA pressure should usually be about one half systemic systolic blood pressure so that it is well tolerated hemodynamically, without important cyanosis. End tidal CO_2 measurement is also helpful, since it is almost directly related, in stable operative condition, to pulmonary output.

If the banding is performed through a thoracotomy, with a less easy access to the MPA, it is a good precaution to separate first aorta from PA staying close to the aorta; since the PA is thinner, the right angle dissector can perforate it, and hemostasis might be difficult to obtain. The tape is then passed around the aorta, and by subtraction, through the transverse sinus, it is finally located around the main PA.

Adjustable PA banding is an interesting concept. A specific device, although expensive and rather cumbersome for small babies, does exist and is externally adjustable [28]. This allows for progressive tightening or loosening of the band as necessary. In some cases, construction of the band may be performed so that the band can be disrupted by balloon dilation of the main PA if it is not needed. This is useful in some cases of multiple muscular VSDs or "Swiss cheese" septum. One technique is one in which the PA band in which the circumference was reduced by several staged thin mattress sutures, as 6/0 or 7/0 monofilament. Another is to place only a single clip on the band so that it may be dislodged with balloon dilation.

For debanding of the PA during an intracardiac correction, after some fibrous tissue is dissected on the band, the simple division of

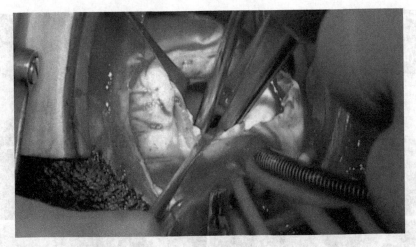

Video 83.5 Closure of VSD by patch through sternotomy (interrupted sutures). After median sternotomy, opening of pericardium, aorta is encircled with tape. Heparin is given, purse-strings are made, and aorta and cavae through right atrium are cannulated. On CPB, cavae are encircled, left venting catheter inserted, and aorta is cross-clamped, then cardioplegia is injected. Cavae are snared and right atrium is opened. The ventricular septum is inspected through the tricuspid. A large paramembranous VSD is exposed. The exposure is improved by a vessel-loop applying a traction on chordae of the septal leaflet and the application of two eyelid retractors in order to expose all the rim of the defect. Alternatively, a pledgeted suture is put from the right atrium through the hinge of septal or commissural leaflet and pulled. A series of pledgeted 5/0 or 6/0 (depending upon the age and size of the child) is placed on the right ventricular aspect of the circumference of the defect. In the area of the septal leaflet, part of the defect, where there is no muscle rim, the pledgeted suture can be put through the hinge of the tricuspid, from the atrium to the ventricular side of the valve. When the rim of the defect is not totally seen properly, a delicate traction on each suture allows to expose the area where the next one has to be placed. The aortic valve is never very far from the VSD! Once all the sutures have been placed, in general at least 8–10, they are inserted on the Dacron patch adequately tailored, the patch is pushed down, and the sutures are tied down. In this video, a second dose of cardioplegia being needed, a right angle is placed in the aorta to start flushing the cardioplegia and thus deairing the ascending aorta. After completion of VSD closure, the right atrium is closed, the aortic clamp is released, and the operation is routinely completed

a PA band allows the band to be removed. But care should be taken as a tear in the PA wall is always possible, and CPB should be immediately available.

When stenosis of the MPA has resulted from the banding, after debanding, it may be necessary to widen it either by simple dilatation, by resection and end-to-end anastomosis, or by patch enlargement. Alternatively, a percutaneous balloon dilatation can be subsequently performed.

Surgical Approach for VSD Closure

Most often, the approach is through a median sternotomy (Video 83.5), on CPB with aortic and bi-caval cannulations, snaring of the cavae, and cardioplegic arrest of the heart. However, the approach (for a membranous defect) through a relatively small right posterolateral thoracotomy is possible mainly after infancy (Video 83.6) [29]. Other approaches include bilateral submammary incisions as well as partial lower sternotomy.

The access of the great majority of VSDs is convenient through a right atriotomy. An angled retractor is placed on the anterior aspect of the tricuspid and pulled. Alternatively, exposure can be obtained by traction sutures on the atrial wall. With a delicate traction on tricuspid septal chordae with an encircling vessel-loop, the vision of almost all of the edges of the defect is possible. At the level of the quadrant where there is tricuspid annulus, a pledgeted suture placed through the annulus from the right atrium allows also gentle traction and provides a good view of the area adjacent to the aortic valve.

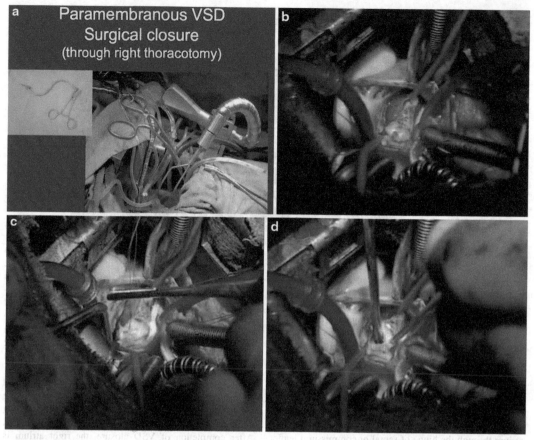

Video 83.6 Closure of VSD through a posterior (cosmetic) thoracotomy. This short video shows the excellent exposure of the paramembranous VSD with fibrous edges, through a posterior thoracotomy, using two perpendicular self-retaining retractors. The first view shows the position of the patient, and the second shows that through this approach all necessary cannulas, the aortic clamp (ideally a flexible arms clamp), and in larger children even an atrial retractor can be put through this approach. Normal CPB, aortic cross-clamping, cardioplegia, deairing are possible. In the video shown, the defect is closed with interrupted pledgeted sutures, but if needed, a patch can be inserted without problem. Infundibular defects have even been closed this way

Occasionally, when chordae and/or papillary muscles crossing the defect impair the vision, the operator can either open perpendicularly the anteroseptal commissural valvular tissue or detach the tricuspid valve at the annulus. In both cases it must be carefully reconstructed with fine sutures. One other option is to detach the base of the small papillary muscle of these chordae, retract it, and reattach it after closure of the VSD, using a small reinforcement pericardial pledget.

The apical and apico-infundibular defects can also be approached through the tricuspid valve. Division of the moderator band in an effort to better visualize the muscular VSD has been recommended but, in general, should be avoided. A better approach for most apical anterior muscular VSDs is through an apical anterior right ventriculotomy close to the interventricular septum [30].

Left ventricular incisions have also been used but should generally be avoided as related LV dysfunction or aneurysms can occur, even years after [31].

Supracristal or infundibular VSDs are best approached through the main pulmonary artery or rarely through an infundibular right ventriculotomy.

VSDs are usually closed with patch material, but occasional small VSDs (usually muscular) may be closed with pledgeted horizontal mattress stitches. Incomplete closure or recurrence may be higher when direct closure is performed in larger defects. The type of patch material used is quite variable. Prosthetic material (PTFE or Dacron) is most often used, but some surgeons prefer either treated bovine pericardium or autologous fixed pericardium. Untreated autologous pericardium should be avoided as it is prone to stretching and aneurysm.

There are basically two techniques of insertion, and the one used is most often determined by surgeons' preference and training. One is using a running continuous monofilament permanent suture. The other is an interrupted technique with pledgeted horizontal mattress sutures. Using braided sutures rather than monofilament facilitates organization of the sutures.

The most commonly used are interrupted 5/0 or 6/0 (in small babies), pledgeted sutures with half-circle, small needles to facilitate the placement. For the cono-ventricular (or perimembranous) defects, care must be taken to avoid conduction tissue by placing the sutures on the right ventricular side, well away from the left side of the interventricular septum (Fig. 83.3). In the anterior superior quadrant of the defect in cono-ventricular defects, care must be taken to avoid deep bites due to the proximity of the aortic valve. In all the quadrant where the tricuspid valve (anteroseptal commissure) is the limit of the VSD and if there is no muscular edge, it is recommended that the sutures be placed through the annulus, with a pledget on the atrial side. This is also valid in the running suture option (Video 83.7), with the suture running through and by the tricuspid annulus, avoiding distortion of the annulus, and in some cases reinforcing this suture line with a small pericardial strip. The aortic leaflet is close and can be better visualized with a short cardioplegia infusion. After completion, the function of the tricuspid valve has to be assessed, and one or two appropriately placed monofilament sutures may be necessary to achieve good competence of the anteroseptal commissure.

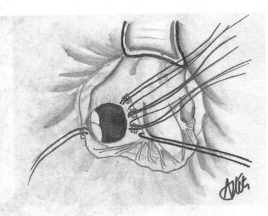

Fig. 83.3 Closure of a cono-ventricular defect (paramembranous, perimembranous). There is an eyelid retractor pulling the anterior leaflet of the tricuspid valve. The VSD area is exposed with a vessel-loop pulling septal leaflet chordae and another eyelid retractor or a pledgeted suture inserted in the tricuspid annulus. Three to four similar sutures will be anchoring the VSD patch in this area. Through the VSD, the aortic leaflets are seen

For the infundibular (or doubly committed) defects, the upper rim is the most critical due to the near continuity of pulmonary and aortic annuli, sometimes separated by only a fine fibrous ridge. When there is not such a ridge, a good option is to use pledgeted interrupted sutures placed through the base of pulmonary leaflets from the pulmonary artery aspect (Fig. 83.4). Using running suture in this situation is difficult and is not recommended.

In some situations, it may be advantageous to partially close a VSD with either a flap-like mechanism or a central fenestration of the patch. This will allow shunting from the right ventricle to the left in the case of elevated right ventricular pressures. This is not infrequently employed when closing a VSD in a patient with severe pulmonary hypertension and increased PVR [32].

VSD with Aortic Insufficiency

Valvular aortic regurgitation (AR) can occur in association with and potentially as a result of a VSD closure. Classically, the regurgitation is due to the lack of support of the aortic leaflet and to the Venturi effect of left-to-right flow across the defect. It has been described mainly in infundibular (or doubly committed) defects but also in

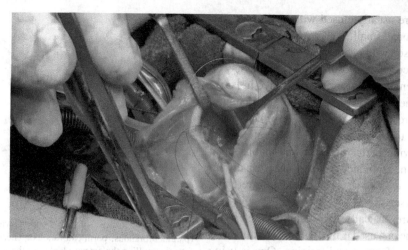

Video 83.7 Closure of VSD by a patch inserted with a continuous suture (through sternotomy). This short video shows the closure of a paramembranous VSD using a running suture. The preferred suture is polypropylene 5/0 or 6/0 according to the age and size of the baby. The first suture, after exposure of the defect, is placed on the anterior aspect of the defect and can be, if the surgeon prefers, reinforced by a small pledget. As for the interrupted suture technique, the stitches are placed on the right ventricular aspect of the defect, at 1–2 mm from the actual rim of the defect. A gentle traction on the running suture allows to expose the next location of stitching if the rim of the defect is not totally seen after usual retraction. The area of tricuspid valve hinge can be continued with a mattress continuous suture, reinforced by a small pericardial band

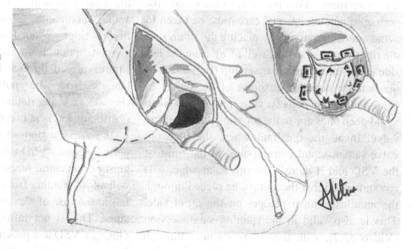

Fig. 83.4 Closure of an infundibular (doubly committed) VSD. The main pulmonary artery is vertically opened. A retractor pulls gently forward the pulmonary valve. The VSD upper rim is represented by the juxtaposed aortic and pulmonary annuli. The pledgeted sutures in this area are taking the pulmonary annulus, being sewn from inside the pulmonary artery

paramembranous (or cono-ventricular) defects [33]. Defects can be large and almost totally occluded by a redundant and prolapsing leaflet producing a small left-to-right shunt. The degree of shunt is often small with the leaflet tissue partially obstructing the VSD. However, the VSD itself is usually quite large.

The potential consequence of this type of situation is enlargement and distortion of the valve leaflet usually by prolapse. Because there is such a strong relationship of aortic valve tissue and potential aortic regurgitation and supracristal-type VSD, there is not much controversy concerning the indication for repair of these defects. Aortic valve repair should also be performed if there is significant regurgitation. In some situations, just closing the defect and removing that Venturi effect is enough to improve aortic valve competence. But if there is significant prolapse of the leaflet, valve repair should be performed. First, the VSD is closed, and then, after aortotomy, the anatomy of the valve is examined. An extremely important maneuver described by R. Frater [34] is done: a thin suture approximates the three nodules of Arantius so that the operator can identify precisely the position and the amount of redundant tissue of the leaflet. Then, a plicature of this excessive amount of tissue is performed with a fine mattress suture between two small pericardial pledgets inside and outside the aorta, as described by Trusler [35] (Fig. 83.5). This shortens the elongated part of the valve and creates a "normal" commissure with resuspension of it. Other procedures like plication [36] or triangular resection [37] of the leaflets may be necessary for more advanced valve disease.

Another concept introduced by Yacoub [38] is based on the fact that the aortic regurgitation is the result of dilation and thinning of the media of the sinus of Valsalva that produces redundancy of tissue and prolapse, separating the solid aortic media from the aortic annulus. Therefore, pledgeted sutures taking the edge of the VSD, the aortic annulus, plicating the thinned portion, and finally taking the true aortic media would treat both the VSD and the AR, without the need to touch the leaflet itself (Fig. 83.6a, b). This type of repair requires significant judgment and experience to know just how much of that sinus of Valsalva to incorporate into the repair.

VSD and Secondary Right Ventricular Outflow Stenosis

It is known that pulmonary stenosis can develop in the natural history of a VSD creating a double-chambered right ventricle. Muscle bundles involving the moderator band and other divisions of distal band may develop and then become covered by fibrous thickening of the endocardium, dividing the right ventricle in two chambers. Often, the VSD gets smaller and even sometimes closes spontaneously so that only the obstruction remains [39]. It is best treated, when necessary, by adequate and extensive fibromuscular resections. This can be done

usually through the tricuspid valve and in case of difficulties through an infundibulotomy. More details about this scenario are described in a chapter specific to right ventricular outflow tract disorders elsewhere in this textbook.

Interventional and Hybrid Management

Transcatheter closure of VSD is an interesting alternative to surgical closure. Since the pioneering work of Lock et al. [40] more than 20 years ago, a variety of devices, originally designed for atrial septal defect or patent ductus arteriosus closure, have been used, mainly for transvascular treatment of *muscular VSDs*. The specifically designed Amplatzer mVSD occluder (AGA Medical Corporation, MN, USA) introduced in 1998 contributed to the widespread use of the technique, with the advantage of smaller delivery systems and self-centering and retrievable device. In the current era, this device is used in the vast majority of the catheter-based closure of muscular VSDs. In properly selected cases, this device is safe and effective. The technique for transcatheter closure is currently well described. The muscular VSD is crossed from the left ventricular side with an exchange soft wire, generally through 4-French Judkins right catheter. The wire is subsequently snared from the pulmonary artery (or inferior or superior vena cavae) and gently pulled out through the vena cavae into the femoral or the jugular catheterized vein to make an arteriovenous loop. A sheath is advanced from the venous access through the VSD, and the appropriate device is implanted thought the defect (Videos 83.8 and 83.9). Importantly, the transcatheter technique for the muscular VSD closure remains challenging, particularly in small patients who may experience more hemodynamic compromise [41] and is generally not recommended for children less than 6–8 kg.

Perimembranous VSD closure has been performed with Amplatzer mVSD occluder. However, such a procedure is relatively contraindicated with this device due to the high frequency of

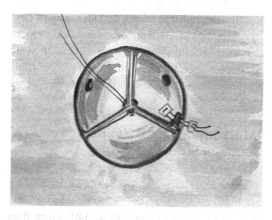

Fig. 83.5 Trusler's technique for associated aortic regurgitation. A fine suture pulling the three Arantius nodules allows to identify the site of excessive tissue and prolapse (Frater). A fine pledgeted suture takes in sandwich the excess valvular tissue and the aortic wall

atrioventricular block [42]. A modification of the device, with an asymmetric left part, designed to decrease risk on the aortic valve, did not offer less risk on the conduction bundle. One of the issues is that sudden AV block has been noted to occur even several days or weeks after the device placement and thus may be life-threatening and difficult to prevent.

In 1998, the closure of VSD, through direct puncture of the right ventricular free wall, without the use of CPB, was performed in an 8-month infant, as a hybrid procedure in the operating room under epicardial echocardiographic guidance. Subsequently, the procedure was applied more widely with an initial report of six patients too small for catheter-based approach and in whom a surgical or catheter-based approach would be difficult or complicated. In this report, the muscular VSDs were limited to large muscular, mid-septal or apical, in a location for which closure of the defect was considered a better option than PA banding [43]. In the majority of cases, perventricular closure is accomplished in a conventional operating room under epicardial and/or transesophageal echocardiographic guidance. In complicated cases with multiple defects, the addition of fluoroscopic guidance has proved to be useful [44]. Done with a close medico-surgical collaboration, these procedures are the essence of good hybrid approach.

Currently, development of hybrid suites is in progress in most of the high activity level centers, and the indications and conducts for hybrid procedures are becoming more refined (Video 83.10).

More recently, important series appeared, particularly coming from China [45], describing perventricular device closure of hundreds of perimembranous VSD, whereas, as stated earlier, this type of defect has been considered as contraindicated to be closed by similar catheter-placed devices, mainly because of the risk of conduction tissue injury. In fact the majority of the perimembranous defects need to be closed in infancy, making the risk of complete heart block even greater.

Critical Care Management

The postoperative course after surgical single VSD repair with CPB is usually uncomplicated. The factors that increase complexity include the presence of multiple VSDs, apical location, presence of aortic regurgitation, straddling of AV valve chordae, and increased PVR. Even though the mortality for closure of most VSDs is less than 1 %, there are significant physiological factors that may increase the risk for an individual patient. The intensivist must be aware of increased PVR, whether the PVR is reactive to pulmonary vasodilator therapy, decreased ventricular function, and presence of additional defects and syndromes. Age and weight must also be considered, as well as past medical history (prematurity, respiratory syncytial virus bronchiolitis). Hyperoxia and hypocapnia should be avoided since both increase pulmonary blood flow and may increase CHF. These issues are usually discussed in regular multidisciplinary meetings, in order to preoperatively identify patients likely to have simple or complicated postoperative courses. A child with a restrictive VSD may benefit from a fast-track strategy, while a 3-month-old infant, with Down syndrome, preoperative signs of heart failure, pulmonary arterial hypertension, and respiratory symptoms, may benefit from a more conservative management. A recent study illustrates the

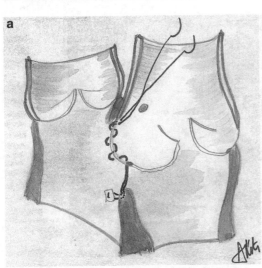
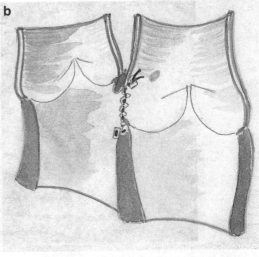

Fig. 83.6 The Yacoub concept and repair. Pledgeted sutures take VSD rim, aortic annulus, dilated thinned Valsalva tissue, and normal thickness aortic wall (**a**). After securing sutures, the structures are approximated; aortic valve leaflet apposition is reestablished (**b**)

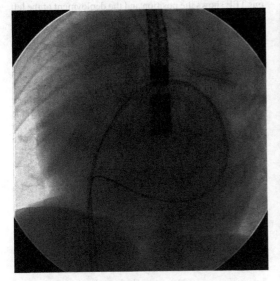
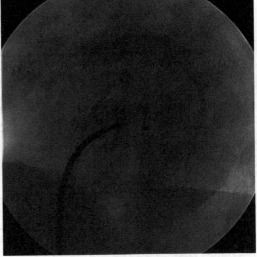

Video 83.8 Transcatheter closure of a large apical muscular VSD in children who previously underwent pulmonary artery banding. In 8, the lateral angiogram demonstrates the large apical VSD that is successfully close in 9 with a 14 mm Amplatzer mVSD device

Video 83.9 Transcatheter closure of a large apical muscular VSD in children who previously underwent pulmonary artery banding. In 8, the lateral angiogram demonstrates the large apical VSD that is successfully close in 9 with a 14 mm Amplatzer mVSD device

difficulties experienced by clinicians to select patients likely to benefit from early extubation [46]. Two hundred and sixty-five children undergoing surgery for CHD with CPB were included in the study. All were planned for early extubation in the operating room, according to local medical procedures. In multivariate analysis, factors associated with delayed weaning from mechanical ventilation were (1) more complex surgeries (RACHS three procedures compared

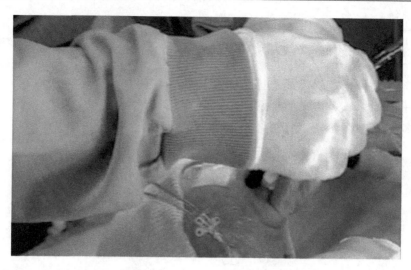

Video 83.10 Closure of a muscular apical VSD by perventricular approach, with a Amplatzer mVSD device. In the operating room, under general anesthesia, a transesophageal echocardiography (*TEE*) confirms the localization, the dimension, and the spatial relationships of the VSD. Surgeon and cardiologist are scrubbed together, while a second cardiologist (*BB*) performs the TEE. Then, median sternotomy and pericardium opening exposes the right ventricle. The point of insertion is exactly defined by a double approach. First, the surgeon depresses the right ventricle free wall with his finger, while the cardiologist locates it by TEE. This helps to define the nearest point to the septal defect. A 5–0 poly-propylene purse-string is placed around this point and a short catheter introduced into the right ventricle. Then, epicardial echography can be used to give the right axis to the guide wire. The guide wire is passed by the surgeon, through the catheter and through the ventricular septal defect under TEE and if necessary epicardial echography guidance. This double echographic approach allows an easy catheterization of each septal defect. The catheter is then removed and a dilatator passed once. Then a sheet is placed and the appropriate device size chosen and inserted in the sheet by the cardiologist, exactly in the same way as it is done for percutaneous procedure. All along, continuous TEE shows the position and the deployment of the left part of the device and the right part, withdrawing the sheet. At each step, additional guidance by epicardial echography is used if necessary. The right ventricular disc is not always perfectly expanded, because of muscular bands. When the summit/outskirts of the disc remain close to the right ventricular free wall, it can be covered with an epicardial running suture. At the end, a complete TEE confirms the right position of the device; exclude significant residual shunting and valvular obstruction or regurgitation, which could have been induced by the procedure

to RACHS2), (2) trisomy 21, and (3) age less than 2 months. In one institution that entered the largest number of patients to the trial, 87 % of VSD cases benefited from a fast-track protocol.

Specific Issues with Postoperative Care

Monitoring in this clinical situation is relatively standard and usually includes EKG monitoring, pulse oximetry, invasive systemic blood pressure, and right atrial pressures associated with end tidal CO_2 [47]. In situations of known increased PVR, placement and monitoring of a PA catheter may be helpful. The goal for all postoperative cardiac patients is to ensure adequate and optimal tissue oxygen delivery and consumption. The use of techniques to continuously or intermittently monitor mixed venous saturations and near-infrared spectroscopy (NIRS) may prove instrumental in anticipating and managing cardiovascular dysfunction with an impact on tissue perfusion. Central venous catheters with optic fibers are available for the pediatric population and allow continuous measurement of central venous oxygen saturation as a surrogate of SvO_2. In a large and heterogeneous population of pediatric patients undergoing congenital heart surgery, Crowley et al. showed that a decrease in central venous saturation below

40 % for more than 18 min was predictive of major adverse events [48]. If inserted as PA line, such a catheter gives oximetric data directly related to mixed SvO_2, given no residual shunt is present. Cerebral oximetry monitored by near-infrared (NIRS) technology has become quite valuable in detection of impaired oxygen delivery. It has been widely adopted by clinicians involved in developing new strategies to reduce neurological morbidity but is also of outmost importance for hemodynamic evaluation and treatment. While there is some discussion about the appropriateness of routine use and adoption of NIRS as a standard of care, objective data is accumulating that supports its use [49, 50]. NIRS technology is also used as a monitor for splanchnic perfusion and oxygen delivery. The renal and abdominal oximetry strongly correlate with gastric tonometry data, venous oxygen saturation, and serum lactate [51]. The use of both cerebral and somatic sensors could provide an elegant solution for noninvasive oximetry monitoring, but the effectiveness of this strategy has yet to be validated [52].

The Low Cardiac Output Syndrome (LCOS)

LCOS is the prerogative of large VSD with pulmonary fluid overload, in children treated for heart failure. There is now evidence that a preventive approach is more appropriate. Early intraoperative milrinone infusion allows a significant reduction of LCOS incidence [53]. Pulmonary vasodilatory properties of milrinone may decrease the risk of postoperative pulmonary hypertension. Low-dose epinephrine is very useful, alone or in combination with other inotropic agents. Very few scientific data are available concerning the calcium channel blocker, levosimendan, in the context of pediatric cardiac surgery. However this therapy, combined with epinephrine, is used by 22 % of medical teams who responded to a survey of European centers concerning management of LCOS with high systemic vascular resistance after pediatric heart surgery [54]. ECMO must be available if needed but is very unlikely to be necessary after "usual" VSD closure.

Residual VSD

In patients with complicated postoperative course, residual VSD must be ruled out. The diagnosis must be established with certainty. This condition should prompt measures appropriate for left-to-right shunt management. In this situation, introduction of a pulmonary vasodilator therapy for pulmonary arterial hypertension may be ineffective or even harmful if there is a significant residual VSD. Postoperative arterial pulmonary hypertension, unexpected elevation of left atrial pressure, postoperative heart failure, and the existence of an increased PA saturation are potential indicators of residual defect. This problem should be relatively rare with the routine use of transesophageal echocardiography in the operating room [55]. Presumably, a significant residual VSD will be addressed before the patient is returned to the ICU. When present, the physiological importance is best approached by estimating the Qp/Qs if there is a PA catheter in place.

Postoperative Pulmonary Hypertensive Crisis (PAH)

PAH secondary to increased PVR is a classical complication after surgical closure of a VSD. A systolic pulmonary artery pressure (PAP) greater than 50 % of systemic systolic blood pressure is considered pathological. Speaking of PAH is addressing (1) the problem of preoperative risk factors identification, (2) the acute PAH onset treatment, and (3) the prevention strategies. Preoperative risk factors associated with pulmonary hypertension occurrence are the existence of long-lasting high pulmonary blood flow, presence of significant pulmonary venous stenosis, associated left heart obstructive lesions with elevated left atrial pressures, and some genetic disorders such as Down syndrome. Occurrence of pulmonary hypertension should prompt echocardiographic investigation for left-to-right residual shunt recognition (see above) as in such a situation pulmonary vasodilator therapy would worsen the shunt. The treatment of an acute PAH crisis combines (1) ventilation with 100 % oxygen, (2) treatment of acidosis either metabolic or respiratory, (3) correction of any hypothermia, (4) deep sedation eventually associated with neuromuscular blockade, (5) inotropic therapy, and (6) pulmonary vasodilator therapy. Vasodilators validated for acute PAH crisis management are inhaled nitric oxide (iNO), prostacyclins, and oral sildenafil. Class 1 level B recommendation supports the use of iNO for treatment of acute postoperative PAH [56]. Weaning is gradual and can be started as soon as the 12th–24th h of treatment. Oral sildenafil has been proved to be effective prevention for rebound effect prevention after iNO withdrawal (Class 1 level B evidence) [57]. Sildenafil is a phosphodiesterase (type 5) inhibitor. Pulmonary vascular relaxation is obtained by inhibiting cGMP breakdown. Although very widely used, enteral administration may be questionable given the reduced bioavailability in the immediate postoperative time [58]. Intravenous sildenafil was tested successfully in the same clinical setting. It is unfortunately not available for daily clinical use [59]. Acute arterial pulmonary hypertensive crisis is a life-threatening condition. Prevention of PAH crisis is the best therapy. ICU nurses, as first-line health-care workers, must be trained to provide appropriate care during at risk procedure such as endotracheal suctioning [60]. Preemptive use of iNO for at risk congenital heart defect (VSD; AVSD) is associated with less occurrence of postoperative arterial pulmonary hypertensive crisis [61].

Postoperative Arrhythmias

Postoperative tachyarrhythmias are unpredictable after surgical closure of VSD. They are almost exclusively of supraventricular origin, most commonly junctional ectopic tachycardia. Treatment is based on rectification of metabolic and electrolytic disturbances, maintenance of normothermia or moderate hypothermia, and decrease of the catecholaminergic stimuli induced by cardiovascular drugs, pacing strategies, and antiarrhythmic drugs. Maintenance of optimal cardiac output is essential. While some inotropic agents are proarrhythmic, cardiac output must be supported to prevent a vicious circle in which arrhythmia precipitates low cardiac output which begets refractory arrhythmia.

Complete atrioventricular block (AVB) after VSD repair is uncommon. It is not infrequent for junctional rhythm or partial atrioventricular block to be present temporarily after surgery. Complete and permanent AVB is estimated between 0.3 % and 0.7 % [62] after perimembranous VSD closure. Most intensivists would prefer placement of both atrial and ventricular temporary pacemaker leads after cardiac surgery. In the presence of AV block, atrioventricular pacing, which is better hemodynamically than ventricular alone, can be initiated. In case of complete heart block, the external pacemaker should be programmed for DDD pacing, ideally with atrial sensing and subsequent ventricular pacing with normal for rate and age AV delay. Careful management of atrial and ventricular sensing and output is warranted to prevent any interruption in pacing therapy. Loss of pacing capability should be considered as a highly emergent surgical indication for new wires (or permanent pace) placement. A complete heart block after the 10th postoperative day, in most cases, reflects high probability of definitive lesion of conduction tissue. Placement of a permanent pacing system is necessary at this stage.

Perioperative Care of Low Birth Weight and Premature Babies

Low weight and prematurity are associated with higher mortality [63]. However, recent data suggest that early surgery on premature infants weighing less than 2.5 kg is possible with an acceptable risk and likely preferable to surgical palliation [64]. Risk seems much higher in neonates less than 2 kg weight and prematurity below 32 weeks of gestational age. There are no available data to say whether or not a strategy promoting growth before surgery is a better option. A recent study suggests that waiting favors morbidity with an associated higher preoperative mortality [65]. Surgery is an option for babies weighing less than 2 kg, in case of severe heart failure precluding any enteral nutritional support. In those cases, a palliative strategy as pulmonary artery banding might be preferable, but this has to be a multidisciplinary team decision adapted to each specific patient.

Outcomes

Operative mortality for isolated VSD repair in most of the developed world is less than 1 %. While each center is different, the routine VSD often has an ICU stay of 2–3 days and hospitalization duration of less than 1 week.

Most VSDs warrant a period of medical management before repair. Indeed some smaller defects will close spontaneously. Surgical therapy is recommended for failure of medical management, presence of supracristal VSD, and in moderate to large VSDs with persistent increased PVR. Surgical therapy is safe and effective. Some VSDs, typically in a mid-muscular position, may be closed by catheter-based therapy or hybrid approaches. In the current era, palliation with a pulmonary artery band is rarely indicated. Due to technical and technological limitation, catheter-based and perventricular VSD closure is rarely indicated in small infants.

In the European Association for Cardio-Thoracic Surgery (EACTS) databank results for VSD patch closure in Europe, about 7,000 procedures have been entered since 1990. The patient's mean weight was 9 kg (from 1.5 to 115 kg). The overall 30-day mortality was 0.89 %.

Conclusion

The diagnosis, classification, and management of patients with VSD mirror the development and advancement of modern pediatric cardiology and cardiac surgery. Appropriately driven medical and surgical treatment allows severely ill children to have a normal growth and near normal life expectancy. Experienced cardiologists can often predict which VSDs will close spontaneously and never need intervention. The progress in the surgical field (CPB, myocardial protection, adequate surgical techniques) and in the perioperative care (with a special mention to PAH treatment) has advanced so that standard VSD closure in patients above 2 kg of weight is now obtained with almost no mortality or major morbidity. The development of interventional catheterization has

dramatically changed the treatment of muscular defects. The "hybrid" approach – presented here as a multidisciplinary approach – offers the capacity to tailor the treatment of complex cases with multiple defects and cardiac insufficiency in infancy. The VSD is the most common congenital heart defect and truly represents the success story that is interdisciplinary pediatric cardiovascular care.

References

1. Hoffman JI (1995) Incidence of congenital heart disease: I – postnatal incidence. Pediatr Cardiol 16:103–113
2. Roguin N, Du ZD, Barak M, Nasser N, Hershkowitz S, Milgram E (1995) High prevalence of muscular ventricular septal defect in neonates. J Am Coll Cardiol 26:1545–1548
3. Hoffman JIE, Kaplan S (2002) The incidence of congenital heart disease. J Am Coll Cardiol 39:1890–1900
4. Hoffman JIE, Kaplan S, Liberthson RR (2004) Prevalence of congenital heart disease. Am Heart J 147:425–439
5. Garg V, Kathiriya IS, Barnes R et al (2003) GATA4 mutations cause human congenital heart defects and reveal an interaction with TBX5. Nature 424:443–447
6. Uebing A, Steer PJ, Yentis SM et al (2006) Pregnancy and congenital heart disease. BMJ 332:401–406
7. Muller WH Jr, Damman JF Jr (1952) The treatment of certain congenital malformations of the heart by the creation of pulmonic stenosis to reduce pulmonary hypertension and excessive pulmonary blood flow: a preliminary report. Surg Gynecol Obstet 95:213
8. Lillehei CW, Cohen M, Warden HE et al (1955) The results of direct vision closure of ventricular septal defects in eight patients by means of controlled cross circulation. Surg Gynecol Obstet 101:446
9. Kirklin JW, Harshbarger HG, Donald DE et al (1957) Surgical correction of ventricular septal defect: anatomic and technical considerations. J Thorac Surg 33:45
10. Okamoto Y (1969) Clinical studies for open-heart surgery in infants with profound hypothermia. Arch Jpn Chir 38:188
11. Barratt-Boyes BG, Simpson M, Neutze JM (1971) Intracardiac surgery in neonates and infants using deep hypothermia with surface cooling and limited cardiopulmonary bypass. Circulation 43(I):25
12. Lock JE, Block PC, MacKay RG et al (1988) Transcatheter closure of ventricular septal defects. Circulation 78:361
13. Amin Z, Berry JM, Foker JE, Rocchini AP, Bass JL (1998) Intraoperative closure of muscular ventricular septal defect in a canine model and application of the technique in a baby. J Thorac Cardiovasc Surg 115:1374–1376

14. Van Praagh R, Geva T, Kreutzer J (1989) Ventricular septal defects: how shall we describe, name and classify them? J Am Coll Cardiol 14:1298

15. Tynan M, Anderson RH (2002) Ventricular septal defect. In: Livingstone C (ed) Paediatric cardiology. Churchill Livingstone, London/New York, pp 983–1015

16. Warnes CA, Williams RG, Bashore TM et al (2008) ACC/AHA 2008 guidelines for the management of adults with congenital heart disease: a report of the American College of Cardiology/American Heart Association Task Forces on Practice Guidelines. Circulation 118:e714–e833

17. Hiraishi S, Agata Y, Nowatari M et al (1992) Incidence and natural course of trabecular ventricular septal defect. J Pediatr 120:409–415

18. Roguin N, Du ZD, Barak M et al (1995) High prevalence of muscular ventricular septal defect in neonates. J Am Coll Cardiol 26:1545–1548

19. Du ZD, Roguin N, Wu XJ (1998) Spontaneous closure of muscular ventricular septal defect identified by echocardiography in neonates. Cardiol Young 8:500–505

20. Rudolph AM (1971) Circulatory adjustments after birth: effects on ventricular septal defect. Br Heart J 33:32–34

21. Hopkins WE, Waggoner AD (2002) Severe pulmonary hypertension without right ventricular failure: the unique hearts of patients with Eisenmenger syndrome. Am J Cardiol 89:34–38

22. Houston AB, Lim MK, Doig WB, Reid JM, Coleman EN (1988) Doppler assessment of the interventricular pressure drop in patients with ventricular septal defects. Br Heart J 60:50–56

23. Bezold LI, Pignatelli R, Altman CA, Feltes TF, Gajarski RJ, Vick GW 3rd, Ayres NA (1996) Intraoperative transesophageal echocardiography in congenital heart surgery. The Texas Children's Hospital experience. Tex Heart Inst J 23(2):108–115

24. Ayres NA, Miller-Hance W, Fyfe DA, Stevenson JG, Sahn DJ, Young LT, Minich LL, Kimball TR, Geva T, Smith FC, Rychik J (2005) Indications and guidelines for performance of transesophageal echocardiography in the patient with pediatric acquired or congenital heart disease: report from the task force of the pediatric council of the American Society of Echocardiography. Pediatric Council of the American Society of the Echocardiography. J Am Soc Echocardiogr 18(1):91–98

25. Bassil R, Acar P, Abadir S, Aggoun Y, Dulac Y, Taktak A, Rumeau P, Paranon S (2006) New approach to perimembranous ventricular septal defect by real-time 3D echocardiography. Arch Mal Coeur Vaiss 99(5):471–476

26. Kilner PJ, Geva T, Kaemmerer H, Trindade PT, Schwitter J, Webb GD (2010) Recommendations for cardiovascular magnetic resonance in adults with congenital heart disease from the respective working groups of the European Society of Cardiology. Eur Heart J 31(7):794–805

27. Habib G, Hoen B, Tornos P, Thuny F, Prendergast B, Vilacosta I, Moreillon P, de Jesus Antunes M, Thilen U, Lekakis J, Lengyel M, Müller L, Naber CK, Nihoyannopoulos P, Moritz A, Zamorano JL, ESC Committee for Practice Guidelines (2009) Guidelines on the prevention, diagnosis, and treatment of infective endocarditis (new version 2009): the task force on the prevention, diagnosis, and treatment of infective endocarditis of the European Society of Cardiology (ESC). Endorsed by the European Society of Clinical Microbiology and Infectious Diseases (ESCMID) and the International Society of Chemotherapy (ISC) for infection and cancer. Eur Heart J 30(19): 2369–2413

28. Bonnet D, Corno AF, Sidi D, Sekarski N, Beghetti M, Schulze-Neick I, Fasnacht M, Le Bret E, Kalangos A, Vouhé PR et al (2004) Early clinical results of the telemetric adjustable pulmonary artery banding FloWatch-PAB. Circulation 110(11): II158–II163

29. Metras D, Kreitmann B (1999) Correction of cardiac defects through a right thoracotomy in children. J Thorac Cardiovasc Surg 117:1040–1041

30. Stellin G, Padalino M, Milanesi O, Rubino M, Casarotto D, Van Praagh R, Van Praagh S (2000) Surgical closure of apical ventricular septal defects through a right ventricular apical infundibulotomy. Ann Thorac Surg 69:597–601

31. Wollenek G, Wyse R, Sullivan I, Elliott M, Deleval M, Stark J (1996) Closure of muscular ventricular septal defects through a left ventriculotomy. Eur J Cardiothorac Surg 10(8):595–598

32. Novick WM, Sandoval N, Lazorhysynets VV, Castillo V, Baskevitch A, Mo X, Reid RW, Marinovic B, Di Sessa TG (2005) Flap valve double patch closure of ventricular septal defects in children with increased pulmonary vascular resistance. Ann Thorac Surg 79(1):21–28; discussion 21–8

33. Praagh RV, Mac Namara JJ (1968) Anatomic types of ventricular septal defect with aortic insufficiency. Diagnostic and surgical consideration. Am Heart J 75:604–619

34. Frater RW (1967) The prolapsing aortic cusp. Ann Thorac Surg 3:63–67

35. Trusler GA, Moes CA, Kidd BS (1973) Repair of ventricular septal defect with aortic insufficiency. J Thorac Cardiovasc Surg 66:394–403

36. Spencer FC, Doyle EF, Danilowicz DA (1973) Long term evaluation of aortic valvuloplasty for aortic insufficiency and ventricular septal defect. J Thorac Cardiovasc Surg 65:15–31

37. Carpentier A (1983) Cardiac valve surgery-the "French correction". J Thorac Cardiovasc Surg 86:323–373

38. Yacoub MH, Khan H, Stavri G (1997) Anatomic correction of the syndrome of prolapsing right coronary cusp, dilatation of the sinus of Valsalva, and ventricular septal defect. J Thorac Cardiovasc Surg 113:253–260

39. Wong PC, Sanders SP, Jonas RA, Colan SD, Parness IA, Geva T, Van Praagh R, Spevak PJ (1991) Pulmonary valve-moderator band distance and association with development of double-chambered right ventricle. Am J Cardiol 68(17):1681–1686

40. Lock JE, Block PC, McKay RG, Baim DS, Keane JF (1988) Transcatheter closure of ventricular septal defects. Circulation 78:361–368

41. Carminati M, Butera G, Chessa M, De Giovanni J, Fisher G, Gewillig M, Peuster M, Piechaud JF, Santoro G, Sievert H, Spadoni I, Walsh K (2007) Investigators of the European VSD registry. Transcatheter closure of congenital ventricular septal defects: results of the European registry. Eur Heart J 28:2361–2368

42. Ovaert C, Dragulescu A, Sluysmans T, Carminati M, Fraisse A (2008) Early surgical removal of membranous ventricular septal device might allow recovery of atrio-ventricular block. Pediatr Cardiol 29(5):971–975

43. Bacha EA, Cao QL, Starr JP, Waight D, Ebeid MR, Hijazi ZM (2003) Perventricular device closure of muscular ventricular septal defects on the beating heart: technique and results. J Thorac Cardiovasc Surg 126:1718–1723

44. Diab KA, Hijazi ZM, Cao QL, Bacha EA (2005) A truly hybrid approach to perventricular closure of multiple muscular ventricular septal defects. J Thorac Cardiovasc Surg 130:892

45. Xing Q, Wu Q, Pan S, Ren Y, Wan H (2011) Transthoracic device closure of VSD without cardiopulmonary bypass: experience in infants weighing less than 8 kg. Eur J Cardiothorac Surg 40(3):591–597

46. Kin N, Weismann C, Srivastava S, Chakravarti S, Bodian C, Hossain S, Krol M, Hollinger I, Nguyen K, Mittnacht AJ (2011) Factors affecting the decision to defer endotracheal extubation after surgery for congenital heart disease: a prospective observational study. Anesth Analg 113(2):329–335

47. Sivarajan VB, Bohn D (2011) Monitoring of standard hemodynamic parameters: heart rate, systemic blood pressure, atrial pressure, pulse oximetry, and end-tidal CO2. Pediatr Crit Care Med 12(4):S2–S11

48. Crowley R, Sanchez E, Ho JK, Lee KJ, Schwarzenberger J, Marijic J, Sopher M, Mahajan A (2011) Prolonged central venous desaturation measured by continuous oximetry is associated with adverse outcomes in pediatric cardiac surgery. Anesthesiology 115(5):1033–1043

49. Kussman BD, Wypij D, Laussen PC, Soul JS, Bellinger DC, DiNardo JA, Robertson R, Pigula FA, Jonas RA, Newburger JW (2010) Relationship of intraoperative cerebral oxygen saturation to neurodevelopmental outcome and brain magnetic resonance imaging at 1 year of age in infants undergoing biventricular repair. Circulation 122(3):245–254

50. Hirsch JC, Charpie JR, Ohye RG, Gurney JG (2009) Near-infrared spectroscopy: what we know and what we need to know – a systematic review of the congenital heart disease literature. J Thorac Cardiovasc Surg 137(1):154–159

51. Kaufman J, Almodovar MC, Zuk J, Friesen RH (2008) Correlation of abdominal site near-infrared spectroscopy with gastric tonometry in infants following surgery for congenital heart disease. Pediatr Crit Care Med 9(1):62–68

52. Ghanayem NS, Wernovsky G, Hoffman GM (2011) Near-infrared spectroscopy as a hemodynamic monitor in critical illness. Pediatr Crit Care Med 12(4): S27–S32

53. Hoffman TM, Wernovsky G, Atz AM, Kulik TJ, Nelson DP, Chang AC, Bailey JM, Akbary A, Kocsis JF, Kaczmarek R, Spray TL, Wessel DL (2003) Efficacy and safety of milrinone in preventing low cardiac output syndrome in infants and children after corrective surgery for congenital heart disease. Circulation 107(7):996–1002

54. Vogt W, Läer S (2011) Treatment for paediatric low cardiac output syndrome: results from the European EuLoCOS-Paed survey. Arch Dis Child 96(12):1180–1186

55. Bettex DA, Schmidlin D, Bernath MA, Prêtre R, Hurni M, Jenni R, Chassot PG, Schmid ER (2003) Intraoperative transesophageal echocardiography in pediatric congenital cardiac surgery: a two-center observational study. Anesth Analg 97(5):1275–1282

56. Barr FE, Macrae D (2010) Inhaled nitric oxide and related therapies. Pediatr Crit Care Med 11(2): S30–S36

57. Namachivayam P, Theilen U, Butt WW, Cooper SM, Penny DJ, Shekerdemian LS (2006) Sildenafil prevents rebound pulmonary hypertension after withdrawal of nitric oxide in children. Am J Respir Crit Care Med 174(9):1042–1047

58. Fraisse A, Wessel DL (2010) Acute pulmonary hypertension in infants and children: cGMP-related drugs. Pediatr Crit Care Med 11(2):S37–S40

59. Fraisse A, Butrous G, Taylor MB, Oakes M, Dilleen M, Wessel DL (2011) Intravenous sildenafil for postoperative pulmonary hypertension in children with congenital heart disease. Intensive Care Med 37(3):502–509

60. Oh H, Seo W (2003) A meta-analysis of the effects of various interventions in preventing endotracheal suction-induced hypoxemia. J Clin Nurs 12(6):912–924

61. Miller OI, Tang SF, Keech A, Pigott NB, Beller E, Celermajer DS (2000) Inhaled nitric oxide and prevention of pulmonary hypertension after congenital heart surgery: a randomised double-blind study. Lancet 356(9240):1464–1469

62. Lin A, Mahle WT, Frias PA, Fischbach PS, Kogon BE, Kanter KR, Kirshbom PM (2010) Early and delayed atrioventricular conduction block after routine surgery for congenital heart disease. J Thorac Cardiovasc Surg 140(1):158–160

63. Ades AM, Dominguez TE, Nicolson SC, Gaynor JW, Spray TL, Wernovsky G, Tabbutt S (2010) Morbidity and mortality after surgery for congenital cardiac disease in the infant born with low weight. Cardiol Young 20(1):8–17

64. Azakie A, Johnson NC, Anagnostopoulos PV, Egrie GD, Lavrsen MJ, Sapru A (2011) Cardiac surgery in low birth weight infants: current outcomes. Interact Cardiovasc Thorac Surg 12(3):409–413

65. Hickey EJ, Nosikova Y, Zhang H, Caldarone CA, Benson L, Redington A, Van Arsdell GS (2012) Very low-birth-weight infants with congenital cardiac lesions: is there merit in delaying intervention to permit growth and maturation? J Thorac Cardiovasc Surg 143(1):126–136

66. Keane JF, Fyler DC (2002) Ventricular septal defect. In: Nadas' pediatric cardiology. Saunders Elsevier Ed, pp 527–558

Atrioventricular Septal Defects

Aditya K. Kaza, L. LuAnn Minich, and Lloyd Y. Tani

Abstract

Atrioventricular septal defects (AVSDs) represent a wide spectrum of defects. Abnormal development of the endocardial cushions can lead to a spectrum of defects that are collectively referred to as AVSD. The presence and size of the ostium primum atrial septal defect (ASD) and inlet ventricular septal defect (VSD) varies and are considered when classifying the AVSD into its four subtypes. One consistent feature among all subtypes is the presence of a common AVV that is always at the same anatomic level within the ventricular mass. The valve may have a single orifice or be divided into two separate orifices by a bridging tongue of tissue. Although the nomenclature varies widely, the underlying anatomy and definitive surgical management of the four basic subtypes of AVSD will be addressed in this chapter.

Introduction

Atrioventricular septal defects (AVSDs) [2, 4] represent a wide spectrum of defects with a common cardiac developmental alteration. During embryogenesis, the atrial and ventricular septa develop in such a way that the endocardial

A.K. Kaza (✉)
Section of Pediatric Cardiothoracic Surgery, Department of Surgery, University of Utah School of Medicine, Salt Lake City, UT, USA
e-mail: ak.kaza@hsc.utah.edu

L.L. Minich • L.Y. Tani
Division of Pediatric Cardiology, Department of Pediatrics, University of Utah School of Medicine, Salt Lake City, UT, USA
e-mail: luann.minich@imail.org; pcltani@ihc.com

cushions orient toward each other to obliterate the interventricular and interatrial pathways. This process also plays an important role in partitioning of the atrioventricular valve (AVV) complex into the right and left components. Abnormal development of these endocardial cushions can lead to a spectrum of defects that are collectively referred to as AVSD. The presence and size of the ostium primum atrial septal defect (ASD) and inlet ventricular septal defect (VSD) vary and are considered when classifying the AVSD into its four subtypes. One consistent feature among all subtypes is the presence of a common AVV that is always at the same anatomic level within the ventricular mass. The valve may have a single orifice or be divided into two separate orifices by a bridging tongue of tissue. Although the nomenclature varies widely, the underlying anatomy and definitive surgical management of the four basic subtypes of AVSD will be addressed in this chapter.

Historical Background

The surgical management of AVSD was first proposed by Dr. Lillehei in 1955. Surgical therapy, at that time, was aimed at the obliteration of the ASD and VSD. As increasing numbers of these children survived surgery, it became apparent that AVV stenosis/regurgitation was complicating their outcomes and focus shifted to repair of the common atrioventricular valve. The improvements in AVSD management over the past few decades have been attributed to a variety of factors, including earlier referral for surgery, avoidance of palliation prior to the complete repair, and techniques to ensure postoperative AVV competency, particularly by closure of the so-called cleft or commissure between the anterior and posterior bridging leaflets. Echocardiographic technology improved over the years and is now the sole imaging modality needed to demonstrate the anatomy of AVSD and the AVV with all surgically relevant details in the vast majority of cases. Because residual AVV insufficiency remains the Achilles heel of AVSD repair, surgeons continue to focus on the development of new and improved techniques for improving its postoperative function and minimizing the need for re-repair or replacement.

Anatomic Subtypes

Partial AVSD

This subtype has also been referred to as a primum ASD. It is characterized by the presence of a large ostium primum ASD (Fig. 84.1). The ventricular component is completely obliterated by chordal and AV valve tissue attached to the ventricular septum and there is no shunt at this level. The common AVV is partitioned into the right and left components that share a common hinge point. The left AVV has a "cleft" along the

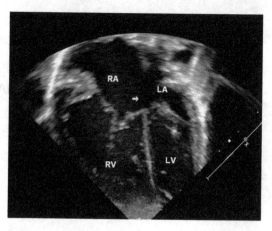

Fig. 84.1 Apical 4-chamber view showing the downwardly displaced AVV with the common hinge point. The *arrow* points to the primum ASD. The leaflets are attached to the ventricular septum and there is no ventricular shunt in this patient with a partial AVSD. *LA* left atrium, *LV* left ventricle, *RA* right atrium, *RV* right ventricle

entire length of the anterior leaflet, and it represents the commissure between the superior and inferior bridging leaflets. Unless there is significant AVV insufficiency, these children are usually asymptomatic until a few years of age and may be diagnosed after a murmur is detected that prompts cardiac evaluation. Traditionally, these children were not referred for repair until 5–10 years of age. Contemporary thinking, however, has led us to believe that they may grow better and/or develop less left AVV regurgitation if referral for surgical repair is earlier or when there is evidence of new onset or progressive AVV insufficiency.

Transitional AVSD

This subtype has also been referred to as intermediate AVSD or incomplete AVSD by some authors. It is characterized by the presence of a large ostium primum ASD and restrictive VSD (Figs. 84.2, 84.3). The ventricular component often consists of multiple small shunts through dense chordal attachments to the crest of the ventricular septum. The common AVV is once again partitioned into the right and left

Fig. 84.2 This apical 4-chamber view from a patient with a transitional AVSD shows the AVV at the same height in the interventricular septum, primum ASD and the dense chordal attachments to the ventricular septum (*arrow*). *LA* left atrium, *RA* right atrium

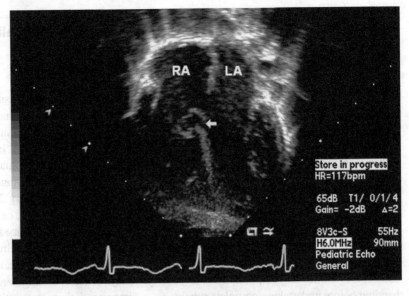

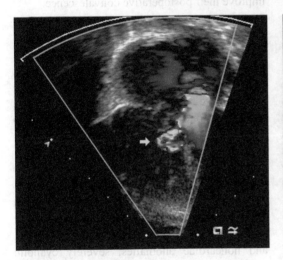

Fig. 84.3 Color Doppler echocardiography shows the dense chordal attachments allow only a small left to right shunt (*arrow*)

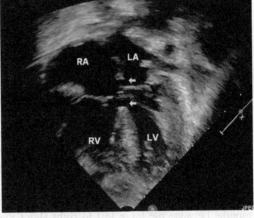

Fig. 84.4 The complete AVSD shown here has a downwardly displaced common AVV and both a primum ASD and inlet VSD (*arrows*). *LA* left atrium, *LV* left ventricle, *RA* right atrium, *RV* right ventricle

components that are at the same level and the left AVV has a cleft along the entire length of the anterior leaflet. Children are typically referred for repair before the age of 1 year.

Complete AVSD

This subtype is characterized by the presence of both a large ostium primum ASD contiguous with a large inlet VSD (Fig. 84.4). The common AVV has a single orifice with a superior and an inferior bridging leaflet. The degree of bridging of these leaflets across the ventricular septum is variable. The Rastelli classification describes the degree of bridging along with the chordal attachments, and has been used to stratify the surgical risk. In Rastelli A, the bridging leaflets are partitioned equally over the right and left ventricle with the chordal attachments from the crest of the ventricular septum to papillary muscles on the appropriate side. In Rastelli B, the left-sided component of the bridging leaflet can have abnormal chordal attachments to the right-sided papillary muscle. In Rastelli C, the superior bridging leaflet is free floating with no chordal attachments to the crest of the ventricular septum. The most common subtype is A, followed by C, with subtype B very rarely occurring. More recently, surgeons rely on a clear echocardiographic description of all components of the valve and supporting structures rather than the Rastelli classification. Currently, infants with complete AVSD are usually referred for repair at 3–6 months of life. Neonatal repair might be necessary if there is evidence of profound and intractable heart failure, frequently associated with AVV regurgitation or additional lesions. Very rarely, neonates with heart failure and significant comorbidities may require pulmonary artery banding before undertaking complete repair.

Canal-Type VSD

This subtype is included in this chapter because of the anatomical and developmental similarities to the other types of AVSD. It is characterized by having a large inlet VSD and no primum ASD. As described with other subtypes, the right and left AVV are at the same level and share the same hinge point and the left AVV has a cleft along the entire length of the anterior leaflet. These children are usually referred for repair at age 3–6 months because the large left to right shunt via the VSD leads to signs and symptoms of uncompensated heart failure.

Conduction Tissue in AVSD

The sinoatrial node is in the usual location at the junction of the right atrium and superior vena cava. The atrioventricular node, which is usually present in the triangle of Koch (bordered by the septal leaflet of the tricuspid valve, tendon of Todaro, and the coronary sinus), is displaced more caudally in hearts with AVSD. Thus, special attention needs to be paid during surgical repair to avoid injury and heart block by placing stitches too close to this area.

Associated Anomalies

Trisomy 21

There is a significant association of AVSD with trisomy 21, predominantly of the complete subtype. Although infants with trisomy 21 are evaluated and treated in a similar fashion to those without this anomaly, they are more likely to have increased pulmonary vascular resistances. Therefore, if a trisomy 21 infant is referred for repair at an older age, careful assessment of pulmonary artery resistance is required to plan a safe operation. In those children with elevated pulmonary vascular resistance, a small atrial level shunt may be left to augment systemic output and improve their postoperative convalescence.

Tetralogy of Fallot Associated with Complete AVSD

This is a rare defect that has components of right ventricular outflow obstruction in addition to complete AVSD. The subpulmonary stenosis is related to the anterior displacement of the infundibular septum with varying degrees of valvar and supravalvar stenosis that is typical of tetralogy of Fallot. These infants may present with cyanosis depending on the severity of pulmonary stenosis. Depending on the size, gestational age, and noncardiac anomalies, severely cyanotic infants may need a palliative aortopulmonary shunt prior to complete repair.

Unbalanced AVSD

This diagnosis implies that the commitment of the AVV over the ventricles is asymmetric and unequal with associated hypoplasia of one of the ventricular chambers. In these cases, careful assessment of the ventricular size and planimetry of the AVV en face using modified subcostal echocardiographic views can help determine if the child is a candidate for high-risk biventricular repair or the single ventricle pathway.

Associated Cardiac Defects

Common associated anomalies include a secundum ASD, patent foramen ovale (PFO) and/or a patent ductus arteriosus (PDA). Other associated cardiac defects that may occur in the AVSD include coarctation of the aorta and heterotaxy syndrome (with abnormal systemic and pulmonary venous drainage, variable outflow tract obstruction, and sometimes transposed or malposed great arteries). When these defects are present, the lesions are usually repaired concomitantly with AVSD repair and a staged approach is required only in select cases.

Diagnosis

Fetal echocardiography is used to diagnose AVSD using the apical 4-chamber view. This view is recommended for all fetuses having obstetrical ultrasounds and may be the reason for referral to the pediatric cardiologist for a fetal echocardiogram. The downwardly displaced AVV is seen with the common hinge point between the right and left AVV leaflets at the same height in the intra-ventricular mass. The primum portion of the atrial septum may reveal a defect and the inlet septum should be inspected for a VSD. Doppler interrogation of the AVVs for insufficiency is routinely performed. The outflow tracts and arch views allow assessment of additional defects. After the infant is born, a complete echocardiogram is obtained to confirm the diagnosis, evaluate valve commitment, and determine the presence of additional lesions.

Clinical Findings

The infant is cared for in a normal fashion except for therapy directed at symptomatic infants. Height and weight are determined and plotted on the appropriate growth charts. Some infants can present with tachypnea, tachycardia, and failure to thrive related to pulmonary over-circulation and/or AVV insufficiency. Infants with significant pulmonary over-circulation

typically have a systolic ejection murmur at the upper left sternal border (related to increase flow across the pulmonary outflow tract); some will have a diastolic flow rumble at the lower sternal border related to increased flow across the common AV valve. Infants with significant AVV insufficiency may have a systolic regurgitant murmur heard between the lower sternal border and apex. A continuous murmur may be audible in those with an associated patent ductus arteriosus.

Chest X-ray

Chest roentgenogram usually demonstrates cardiomegaly with increased pulmonary vascular markings; those with persistently elevated pulmonary resistance with relatively little shunt may show a more normal heart size.

ECG

Electrocardiography usually demonstrates a leftward or superior frontal plane QRS axis. Many have a prolonged PR interval (first degree AV block), atrial enlargement, and changes suggestive of right ventricular hypertrophy. Changes suggestive of left ventricular hypertrophy may also be present.

Diagnostic Imaging

Echocardiography is the most important imaging modality for the evaluation of infants and children with AVSD; angiography is no longer a routine part of the preoperative evaluation. In most cases two-dimensional transthoracic echocardiography demonstrates the AVSD anatomy in excellent detail. A complete systematic exam includes a segmental approach with assessment of chamber sizes and ventricular function. The common AVV leaflets and supporting apparatus are imaged from all possible views with careful attention to the number and location of the papillary muscles and the chordal

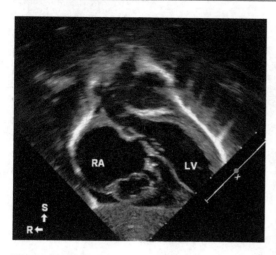

Fig. 84.5 Modified subcostal view of the AVV en face shows the number of orifices and the degree of commitment to each ventricle. This patient has a single orifice with nearly equal commitment of the AVV over each ventricle. *A* anterior, *PA* pulmonary artery, *RV* right ventricle, *S* superior

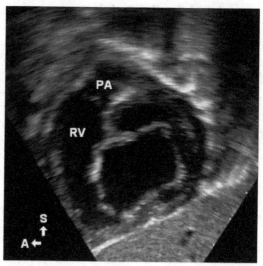

Fig. 84.6 This patient has a 2-orifice AVV with the right AVV slightly larger over the right ventricle. *A* anterior, *PA* pulmonary artery, *RV* right ventricle, *S* superior

attachments of the AVV. En face imaging of the AVV from a modified subcostal view will demonstrate the number of orifices and the degree of commitment of the AVV tissue with relation to the two ventricles. Planimetry of the common AVV should routinely be performed to assess the relative amounts of AVV tissue committed to each ventricular inlet (Figs. 84.5, 84.6). In cases where there is minor discrepancy in the commitment, the valve can be adequately partitioned at the time of surgery.

Investigators have proposed ratios to predict successful biventricular repair but ongoing studies are needed to refine these as surgical repair of the valve evolves. In assessing unbalanced AVSD, Cohen et al. [5] have found that AVVi (AVV index = left/right valve area) >0.67 identified patients with balanced defects. Of those with unbalanced (right dominant) AVSD, an AVVi <0.67 in the presence of a large VSD favored a single ventricle approach, while an AVVi between 0.27 and 0.67 and an intact ventricular septum favored a two-ventricle repair. The Toronto group (Oliveira et al.) [3] looked at the AVVi in LV dominant canals and reported those with AVVi <0.50 required early reoperations due to signs of right ventricular

inadequacy. Overman and colleagues at the Congenital Heart Surgeons Society [6] are currently working on determining more accurate predictors of biventricular versus single ventricular repair based on AVVi in cases of unbalanced AVSD. Standard subcostal long-axis imaging provides insight into the elongated appearance of the left ventricular outflow tract ("goose-neck deformity") and helps identify potential chordae crossing the outflow tract (Fig. 84.7). Multiple views allow assessment of ventricular size and function, inspection of the ventricular septum for an inlet VSD and associated defects in other areas, inspection of the atrial septum for the presence and size of the primum ASD and any additional ASDs, and determination of systemic and pulmonary venous connections. Suprasternal notch imaging allows evaluation of the aortic arch for coarctation and branching of the head and neck vessels and modified high parasternal views will allow visualization of a PDA.

Doppler echocardiography should be routinely performed to assess the degree of AVV regurgitation. Doppler interrogation is not useful for assessment of valve stenosis in the preoperative patient with a primum ASD. Because the left ventricular outflow tract is elongated and narrow

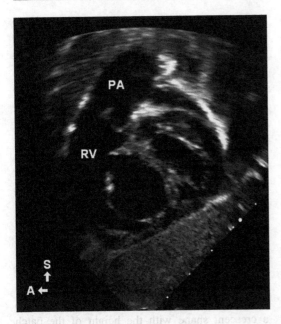

Fig. 84.7 The subcostal view demonstrates the typical elongated and narrow "goose-neck deformity" of the left ventricular outflow tract of the AVSD. *LA* Left ventricle, *RA* right atrium, *R* right, *S* superior

in these infants, they are predisposed to obstruction and this area should be carefully interrogated. The absence of a Doppler gradient may be misleading; however, if there is an inlet VSD, careful measurements of the aortic valve annulus as well as assessment of the arch should be performed if the adequacy of the left ventricular outflow is in question.

Cardiac Catheterization

Cardiac catheterization has no role in the routine evaluation of young infants with AVSD, but may be required in older children with unrepaired AVSD who have a significant ventricular component (to assess pulmonary vascular resistance), in children with tetralogy of Fallot associated with complete AVSD who underwent palliative shunting in infancy, and in those with more complex forms of AVSD. Careful assessment of pulmonary and systemic blood flow and pulmonary vascular resistance should be performed. In addition, the presence of any associated pulmonary venous, systemic venous, or aortopulmonary

collaterals should be assessed and addressed at the time of the catheterization. Other imaging modalities such as cardiac MRI and CT angiography may be of value in evaluating patients with heterotaxy and suspected venous anomalies.

Medical Management

Heart Failure Management

Infants with complete AVSD and inlet VSD usually present with signs and symptoms of heart failure including tachypnea, diaphoresis, and failure to thrive. These infants need to be monitored by a cardiologist. Diuretic therapy including furosemide can be helpful in managing the respiratory symptoms. Digoxin may be helpful in a subset of patients, and angiotensin-converting enzyme inhibition may be of value in some of these patients with significant pulmonary over-circulation. In addition, fortified feeds can be effective in maintaining a positive nitrogen balance in these frail infants. Prior to the dramatic improvements in operative and perioperative management of these infants, medical management was intense and included enteral feeding, often with limited success, and many infants continued to struggle with weight gain. In the current era, these infants undergo definitive surgical therapy, regardless of age, if they fail to gain weight with diuretic therapy and fortified feedings.

Surgery for AVSD

The goal of surgery for AVSD is to eliminate intracardiac shunting and to repair and partition the AVV. The surgical techniques have evolved through the decades with refinements that are highlighted below.

Timing of Surgery

Most children with complete AVSD and inlet VSD require surgery within the first few months of life. This is due to the high degree of shunting leading to pulmonary over-circulation and heart failure that fails to respond to medical management. Our policy has been to perform the complete repair at 3–6 months of age. Rarely, in the setting of significant comorbidities, we have palliated these infants with a pulmonary artery band. In the very rare instance that this is required, the pulmonary artery banding (along with ligation of a patent ductus, if present) can be performed via a left thoracotomy. As with other palliative operations, PA banding has the disadvantages of requiring repeat hospitalization for the definitive surgical correction and the associated morbidity and mortality of this additional procedure.

Surgery for Various Subtypes

The approach to all subtypes of AVSD is via median sternotomy. This can be limited to the lower hemisternum in cases of partial AVSD. Subtotal thymectomy is performed and a generous piece of pericardium is harvested and cross-linked in glutaraldehyde for 10 min. The aorta, superior vena cava and inferior vena cava are all circumferentially dissected. If a PDA is present, this is also circumferentially dissected and ligated using a silk ligature. The child is then heparinized and cannulated with a single aortic cannula in the ascending aorta and two metal right-angled venous cannulae in the superior and inferior vena cavae. A left ventricular vent is placed via the right superior pulmonary vein and a cardioplegia needle is placed in the aortic root. If there is a left superior vena cava present, we either cannulate it directly or put a sump sucker in the coronary sinus once the right atrium is opened. It is important to consult the appropriate charts to know the annular size of the AVV based on the child's body surface area. Aortobicaval bypass is instituted and mild hypothermic full flow cardiopulmonary bypass is utilized for repair. Once the child is on full flow bypass, the ascending aorta is cross-clamped and the heart is arrested by instilling cold blood cardioplegia in the aortic root. Cardioplegia is re-administered at 20–30-min intervals or sooner if necessary. Total bypass is instituted and the right atrium opened

parallel to the atrioventricular groove. Stay stitches are placed to retract the right atrium and expose the AVV. It is paramount to examine the intracardiac anatomy in a systematic fashion. The AVV complex needs to be carefully examined to determine the chordal support and papillary muscles. The degree of chordal bridging and the mobility of the lateral leaflet need to be determined to decide how to partition the common AVV. The borders of the VSD, the extent of the primum ASD, the presence of additional ASDs should also be determined.

There are several techniques used to repair complete AVSDs: single-patch, double-patch, and rarely no-patch or Australian technique. We describe the two-patch technique for repair of complete AVSD where a Dacron patch is utilized for the VSD closure. This patch is cut into a crescent shape with the height of the patch based on static examination of the distance between the nadir of the VSD at the crest of the septum and the level of the AVV at this location. We believe that the height of the patch is important to prevent narrowing the already small left ventricular outflow tract. In cases of associated tetralogy of Fallot, the superior aspect of the patch needs to be more rounded resulting in a comma-shaped patch. A continuous suture of 5-0 polypropylene with a small felt pledget is used to anchor the patch at the nadir of the VSD to the crest of the ventricular septum; the patch is sewn away from the crest of the VSD to avoid injury to the conduction tissue. To avoid trapping any chordal support with the suture, it may be necessary to weave in-and-out to leave the valvar support free of tethering. Once the VSD at the level of the ventricular crest is eliminated, the sutures are brought through the superior and inferior bridging leaflet at the level of the annulus and placed on hemostats.

Attention is then turned to the AVV where the zone of opposition or cleft in the left AVV is delineated by distending the left ventricle using saline solution. Interrupted or figure-of-eight 5-0 or 6-0 polypropylene sutures are used to close the cleft along its entire length. It is important to use "kissing" type suture where the already opposed edges of the valve leaflet are sutured together instead of suturing the free edges of the leaflet. This is a more durable technique that can help prevent unnecessary distortion of the valve. A running mattress suture combined with an over-and-over suture is another technique for closing the cleft. Proponents of this technique believe that the closure is more secure with little distortion of the valve and even distribution of the tension along the suture line. The cleft needs to be closed along its entire length in the vast majority of patients. The exception to this rule is the presence of a single or closely related/fused papillary muscle(s) on the left side. In these rare cases, we elect to leave the cleft partially open to avoid postoperative LAVV stenosis. Once the cleft has been repaired, we test the competency of the AVV by instilling saline in the left ventricle. If there is any leakage noted on passive testing, this is addressed by additional maneuvers. If there is significant annular dilatation, we perform a posterior annuloplasty using absorbable suture (5-0 or 6-0 polydiaxone). The annulus is cinched down to a z-score of 0 to -1. It is important to ensure that the valve is competent on passive testing before proceeding.

We then turn our attention to the primum ASD and an appropriate sized patch of treated pericardium is shaped. We use interrupted mattress sutures at the level of the AVV to close the VSD and to anchor the ASD patch. Suture are passed from the right ventricular aspect through the Dacron VSD patch and then though the AVV at the imaginary line of partitioning and finally through the pericardial patch. These interrupted sutures are all tied down to close the VSD at the level of the ventricular septum. The suture arms from the VSD closure brought out at the level of the AVV annulus are used to anchor the remainder of the ASD patch. At the level of the coronary sinus, we orient the ASD patch and suture line close to the left AVV annulus to avoid injury to the conduction system. Alternatively, the ASD patch can be shaped with a flange and sutured widely away from the coronary sinus, thus leaving this structure on the left atrial side, and avoiding injury to the conduction system. Additional ASDs are addressed at this point and the atriotomy closed. After adequate de-airing

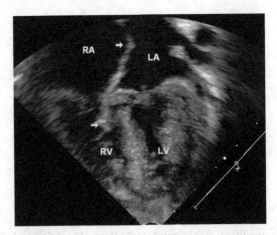

Fig. 84.8 This patient has undergone closure of the primum ASD and inlet VSD with a single-patch technique (*arrows*). *LA* left atrium, *LV* left ventricle, *RA* right atrium, *RV* right ventricle

maneuvers, the cross-clamp is released and the child rewarmed and weaned off cardiopulmonary bypass. We use left atrial and pulmonary artery pressure lines selectively. Epicardial pacing wires are placed and postoperative transesophageal echocardiogram (TEE) performed. The TEE assessment is performed to look for residual lesions and evaluate the function of the AVV (Fig. 84.8). If there are significant intracardiac shunts or AVV insufficiency, these need to be addressed by going back on cardiopulmonary bypass. After heparin reversal and hemostasis, the chest is widely drained and closed.

Although the operative plan may vary depending on the particular subtype of AVSD, the fundamental sequence of the operation remains constant. In cases of canal-type VSD, it may be necessary to incise the interatrial septum at the level of the oval fossa to access and repair the cleft in the left AVV. In children with associated tetralogy of Fallot, it is necessary to relieve the pulmonary stenosis either through the right atrium, pulmonary artery, and/or an infundibular incision. In cases of severe pulmonary valvar hypoplasia, a trans-annular repair may be required, with or without the placement of a monocusp valve. Although studies show no long-term benefits of the monocusp valve, we routinely use it if a trans-annular reconstruction is necessary to facilitate a smoother immediate postoperative course. Gore-tex patch which is 0.1-mm thick is used to make the monocusp valve and either 0.4-mm thick Gore-tex or treated pericardium is used for the trans-annular patch. In this subset of patients, subsequent surgery is usually required for the placement of a competent valve in the pulmonary position. With the availability of percutaneous pulmonary valves, the need for future surgery may be avoided in select cases.

Other techniques that can be utilized for the repair of complete AVSD include the no-patch technique, the single-patch technique, and the modified single-patch technique. The utility of the no-patch technique is mostly limited to patients with a very shallow VSD and small primum ASD (the Lillehei repair, also referred to as the Australian repair). It should be avoided in the majority of complete AVSD patients who have a deep VSD to prevent distortion of the AVV and to avoid creating a potential substrate for the development of left ventricular outflow tract obstruction in the future. Proponents of this technique highlight the speed and ease of repair and the avoidance of prosthetic material inside the heart. The long-term fate of the AVV is yet to be determined with this particular technique.

The one-patch technique involves the division of the superior and inferior bridging leaflet at the proposed site of partition into right and left components. A single patch of pericardium is used to close the VSD and the divided AVV leaflets are reattached to the pericardial patch to close the VSD at the level of the valve and the remainder of the patch is used to close the atrial level shunt. This is a technique that is used widely with results comparable to the two-patch technique. The modified single-patch technique is used to describe AVSD repair where the VSD is closed primarily and a patch used for ASD closure.

There is a small risk of heart block or other conduction abnormalities after AVSD repair. Younger patients require the placement of epicardial pacemaker system. The need for single or double chamber pacing system is based on the individual patient. Although a transvenous system is an option in older patients, we still tend to favor the epicardial system to avoid having leads

crossing the right-sided AVV in the immediate postoperative period.

In cases of unbalanced AVSD with associated ventricular hypoplasia or where there are extensive chordal attachments to the crest of the ventricular septum and the AVV is not amenable to partitioning, the child may need to be palliated down the single ventricle pathway. These children usually require palliation with banding of the main pulmonary artery during infancy to protect the pulmonary vasculature from excessive flow and to maintain low pulmonary vascular resistance. Cardiac catheterization is needed to calculate pulmonary vascular resistance and to measure pulmonary pressures prior to the cavopulmonary shunts. Superior cavopulmonary anastomosis is performed at around 4–6 months of age. The antegrade pulmonary blood flow can be either interrupted at this stage or at the time of the completion of the Fontan. We usually transect and oversew the pulmonary valve to avoid any dead space that can act as a nidus for thrombus formation. The Fontan operation is performed at the age of 2–5 years. Interval development of AVV insufficiency needs to be addressed at the time of these operations or independently if cardiac output is impaired.

Postoperative Care

Postoperative care in the cardiac intensive care unit is aimed at proper sedation, airway control, and maintenance of good hemodynamics. We strive to keep the systemic blood pressure well controlled to reduce any increased afterload on the repaired AVV. Children with Down syndrome are at increased risk of pulmonary hypertensive episodes after surgery. Avoidance of pain, respiratory or metabolic acidosis, alveolar hypoxia, atelectasis, and low cardiac output are important principles in the avoidance and management of pulmonary hypertension. Pulmonary hypertensive episodes may be initiated with suctioning and may be diminished with pretreatment with increased oxygen delivery, adequate/additional analgesia, and use of intratracheal lidocaine. In the presence of pulmonary hypertensive episodes, and after standard principles in the avoidance and treatment of pulmonary hypertension are implemented, inhaled nitric oxide may be very beneficial. Failure to respond to inhaled nitric oxide should warrant further investigation of residual lesions, inadequate lung recruitment, severe plexiform arteriopathy, or associated lung hypoplasia or parenchymal lung disease. Intravenous sildenafil has been used in the setting of pulmonary hypertension that is not completely ameliorated by inhaled nitric oxide and also in the withdrawal of inhaled nitric oxide. Although we have not systematically studied this, we believe that adequate blood pressure control in the immediate postoperative period is paramount to preserve long-term AVV competency. We always obtain an echocardiogram prior to hospital discharge to document the function of the AVV, assess for residual shunts, and to rule out pericardial effusion.

Reoperations After AVSD Repair

The most common reason for reoperation after AVSD repair is the development or persistence of AVV insufficiency. In the recent report from the Pediatric Heart Network (PHN) [1, 7, 8], the risk of moderate to severe LAVV insufficiency at 6 months postoperatively ranged from 22 % to 33 % depending on the type of AVSD. Predictors of LAVV insufficiency after surgery included the presence of LAVV insufficiency prior to surgery and later age at time of surgery. Development of signs and/or symptoms of heart failure (tachypnea, dyspnea on exertion), pulmonary hypertension, arrhythmias, or marked chamber enlargement is usually used to determine the need for reoperative surgery. Once the diagnosis, progression, and mechanism of AVV insufficiency are established, these patients are referred for reoperation. In most cases, the AVV insufficiency is through a residual cleft, but it can also occur centrally through a dilated annulus. The geometry of the annulus is one of the fundamental differences between the AVV in AVSD and normal hearts. In normal hearts, the AVV annulus

is usually oval shaped; however, in AVSD, the AVV annulus is more oblong with an increase in annular height. Thus, traditional annuloplasty rings are not well suited for the repair of these valves. Suture annuloplasty with buttress of pericardium or felt usually has good results. The bioabsorbable annuloplasty ring (Bioring®), which is flexible, would theoretically be an excellent choice for repair of the AVV. The surgeon should make every attempt to repair these valves, but in some instances, repair is not achievable and replacement may be necessary. Any additional residual lesions such as shunts need to be addressed at the time of reoperation.

In cases of uneven AVV commitment, patients can be left with AVV stenosis. Reoperation may be needed if the stenosis is moderate to severe as this is poorly tolerated in infants and small children who have faster heart rates. Techniques to open the valvar orifice by the use of a combination of commissurotomy, division of secondary chordae, and rarely division of a fused papillary muscle may relieve the stenosis. Once again, if a good repair is not achievable, valve replacement may be necessary. The type of prosthetic valve used varies and is beyond the scope of this monograph.

Development of left ventricular outflow tract obstruction is a less frequent complication of AVSD repair. It tends to develop with time and may not require reoperation for years after the initial repair. The narrow, elongated, "gooseneck" outflow tract and the presence of chordae crossing the outflow tract predispose these patients to the development of obstruction. Left ventricular outflow tract obstruction is more common with patient with a partial AVSD; however, it can be seen with the other subtypes as well. Patients whose outflow tract obstruction that has progressed to $\geq$ moderate or those who develop aortic insufficiency are referred to surgery. The goal of surgery is to remove obstruction regardless of its cause. This may require removal of any discreet subaortic membrane, removal of any aberrant chordae that are not providing support to the AVV, septal myomectomy, and/or removal of any membrane on the underside of the aortic valve leaflets to improve their mobility. In rare instances, a modified Konno procedure with incision of the old VSD patch and re-patching may be necessary to adequately relieve the obstruction.

Our policy is to utilize transesophageal echocardiography (TEE) to assess the repair in the operating room. TEE to determine residual lesions should be a standard part of operative repair of these complex defects. The postoperative TEE should include a two-dimensional and Doppler assessment of the left ventricular outflow for residual obstruction and evaluation of valve competency and ventricular function. In instances where there is a significant residual left ventricular outflow obstruction or significant aortic regurgitation, we elect to go back on bypass to address the residual lesion.

A baseline postoperative transthoracic echocardiogram is obtained when the child is ready to leave the hospital, and this is used as a reference point for subsequent serial studies. AVV dysfunction and left ventricular outflow tract obstruction may develop and progress over time, so children with AVSD must undergo routine serial exams even after initial successful repair. These infants and children require a lifetime of follow-up and it is important to reinforce this with the parents.

Contemporary Benchmarking For AVSD Repair

The PHN reported the 6-month follow-up of AVSD repair in 215 children from seven centers [1, 7, 8]. There were 120 infants in the complete AVSD group, 60 in the partial AVSD group, 27 in the transitional AVSD group, and 8 patients in the canal-type VSD group. Trisomy 21 was present in 80 % of complete, 44 % of transitional, and 28 % of partial AVSD patients. The median age at surgery repair was 4 months for the complete AVSD group, 5 months for the canal-type VSD group, 8 months for the transitional AVSD group, and 3.1 years for the partial AVSD group. Operative mortality for the entire cohort was 3 %. Cardiopulmonary bypass times and cross-clamp times were significantly higher for the complete

AVSD group when compared to the other subtypes. Similarly, the complete AVSD cohort had significantly higher resource utilization as shown by their longer ICU and total hospital stays. One of the more important conclusions of the paper relates to the timing of surgery and left AVV insufficiency. In the partial AVSD group, there was a significant association between surgery performed after age 4 years and subsequent $\geq$ moderate left AVV insufficiency. In the other groups, there was a linear association between older age at surgery and postoperative left AVV insufficiency. The only statistically significant predictors of at least moderate AVV regurgitation at 6-months after surgery were older age at repair and the presence of at least moderate left AVV insufficiency on the one-month postoperative echocardiogram. Finally, the study also showed that infants and children with AVSD who undergo earlier repair have significantly better weight gain after surgery.

Conclusion

Contemporary results of AVSD repair are excellent. Recurrent AVV insufficiency remains the Achilles heel of AVSD repair. We have learned valuable lessons from the past and now perform total cleft closure in nearly everyone. Despite our best efforts, however, there remains a certain cohort of patients who develop recurrent AVV insufficiency. As we have learned from the PHN study, early referral for surgery seems to impact the long-term function of the AVV. In addition, if there is significant AVV insufficiency before surgery, careful assessment with preoperative transthoracic echocardiography and intraoperative echocardiography can help identify the precise mechanism of insufficiency and allow appropriate planning for valve repair. Additional maneuvers such as commissuroplasty and annuloplasty at the time of complete repair can help improve the function of the AVV. The development of novel techniques of valve repair may be needed to improve the outcomes of infants and children undergoing repair of AVSD.

References

1. Kaza AK, Colan SD, Jaggers JG et al (2011) Surgical interventions for atrioventricular septal defect subtypes: the pediatric heart network experience. Ann Thorac Surg 92(4):1468–1475

2. Cetta F, Minich L, Williams E, Dearani J, Puga F. Atrioventricular septal defecs. In: Allen H, Driscoll D, Shaddy R, Feltes T (eds) Moss and Adam's heart disease in infants, children, and adolescents including the fetus and young adult, 7th edn. Lippincott Williams and Wilkins, Philadelphia, PA

3. Oliveira NC, Sittiwangkul R, McCrindle BW et al (2005) Biventricular repair in children with atrioventricular septal defects and a small right ventricle: anatomic and surgical considerations. J Thorac Cardiovasc Surg 130:250–257

4. Kaza AK, del Nido P (2010) Atrioventricular septal defects. In: Selke F, Swanson S, del Nido P (eds) Sabiston and spencer's surgery of the chest, 8th edn. Elsevier

5. Cohen MS, Jacobs JL, Weinberg PM, Rychik J (1996) Morphometric analysis of unbalanced atrioventricular canal using two-dimensional echocardiography. J Am Coll Cardiol 28(4):1017–1023

6. Jegatheeswaran A, Pizarro C, Caldarone CA et al (2010) Echocardiographic definition and surgical decision-making in unbalanced atrioventricular septal defect: a congenital heart surgeons' society multiinstitutional study. Circulation 122(11 Suppl): S209–S215

7. Minich LL, Atz AM, Colan SD et al (2010) Partial and transitional atrioventricular septal defect outcomes. Ann Thorac Surg 89(2):530–536

8. Atz AM, Hawkins JA, Lu M et al (2011) Surgical management of complete atrioventricular septal defect: associations with surgical technique, age, and trisomy 21. J Thorac Cardiovasc Surg 141(6): 1371–1379

Aortopulmonary Window

Moritz C. Wyler von Ballmoos, Michael Barnes,
Stuart Berger, Michael E. Mitchell, and James S. Tweddell

Abstract

Aortopulmonary window is a rare defect caused by failure of fusion of the two opposing conotruncal ridges that are responsible for separating the truncus arteriosus into the aorta and pulmonary artery. Aortopulmonary window may occur as an isolated lesion, or it can be associated with other cardiac abnormalities in a third to one-half of cases. The most common associated lesions are arch abnormalities including interrupted aortic arch and coarctation of the aorta. Other less common associated lesions may also occur. Antenatal diagnosis is rare. In the current era, early mortality following repair of simple aortopulmonary window approaches zero percent and depends on the presence of associated lesions especially

M.C. Wyler von Ballmoos (✉)
Division of Cardiothoracic Surgery, Department of
Surgery, Medical College of Wisconsin, Wauwatosa,
WI, USA
e-mail: mcwyler@mcw.edu

M. Barnes
Cardiothoracic Surgery Department, Children's Hospital
of Wisconsin, Milwaukee, WI, USA
e-mail: MBarnes@chw.org

S. Berger
Department of Pediatrics, Division of Pediatric
Cardiology, The Herma Heart Center The Medical
College of Wisconsin, Children's Hospital of Wisconsin,
Milwaukee, WI, USA
e-mail: sberger@chw.org

M.E. Mitchell
Department of Cardiothoracic Surgery, Children's
Hospital of Wisconsin, Milwaukee, WI, USA
e-mail: mmitchell@chw.org

J.S. Tweddell
Department of Pediatrics and Surgery (Cardiothoracic),
Medical College of Wisconsin and Herma Heart Center at
Children's Hospital of Wisconsin, Milwaukee, WI, USA
e-mail: jtweddell@chw.org

interrupted aortic arch. Long-term outcome should be excellent. Early morbidity includes pulmonary artery stenosis and residual aortopulmonary septal defects. Long-term follow-up is indicated to look for recurrent lesions such as the development of branch pulmonary artery stenosis and arch obstruction.

Keywords

Acyanotic • Anterior sandwich patch technique • Aortic • Aortopulmonary septal defect • Aortopulmonary window • Cardiac development • Cardiac surgery • Cardiopulmonary bypass • Congenital • Congestive • Echocardiography • Heart defects • Heart failure • Hypertension • Interrupted aortic arch • Murmur • Pulmonary

Introduction

Aortopulmonary window is a rare lesion, with a prevalence among patients with congenital heart disease of only 0.1–0.2 % [1–3]. Aortopulmonary window may occur as an isolated lesion, or it can be associated with other cardiac abnormalities in a third to one-half of cases. Simple aortopulmonary window is often not identified by fetal echocardiography, and only recently has antenatal diagnosis of aortopulmonary window with interrupted aortic arch been reported. Presentation of the defect will differ depending on the size of the window and other associated defects. But generally, patients present in the first few weeks of life with symptoms consistent with a left-to-right shunt and heart failure. With early surgical intervention in the modern era, patients with aortopulmonary window have an early mortality that approaches zero percent. Long-term follow-up is required to monitor for branch pulmonary stenosis or coarctation of the aorta in the case of repaired aortopulmonary window with interrupted aortic arch.

Epidemiology, Embryology, and Anatomy

Aortopulmonary window is a rare defect and accounts for about 0.1–0.2 % of all structural congenital cardiac defects [1–3]. Major academic centers could anticipate taking care of 1 or 2 infants with aortopulmonary window per year.

Antenatal diagnosis of aortopulmonary window is challenging, and delayed diagnosis may occur; the actual prevalence at birth is hence more difficult to estimate.

Aortopulmonary window is caused by failure of fusion of the two opposing conotruncal ridges that are responsible for separating the truncus arteriosus into the aorta and pulmonary artery. The aortopulmonary window therefore occurs between the two structures that normally result from septation of the truncus arteriosus, namely, the ascending aorta and the main pulmonary artery. Normal anatomy of the aortic and pulmonary valves separates this defect from the persistent truncus arteriosus. The similarity among conotruncal defects raises the question of a common underlying pathogenesis, but anatomic studies suggest it develops by a different mechanism than truncus arteriosus [1, 4]. Furthermore, to date, no genetic association or environmental risk factors have been linked to aortopulmonary window.

A classification of aortopulmonary window based on location has been proposed by Mori, dividing aortopulmonary window into three types: proximal (type I), distal (type II), and total (type III) [5]. The classification introduced by the Society of Thoracic Surgeon adds a fourth, "intermediate" category accounting for the fact that this defect likely has a continuum of morphologies. For patients with aortopulmonary window without additional lesions, it is the size rather than the location of defect that impacts management or outcome (Fig. 85.1) [6].

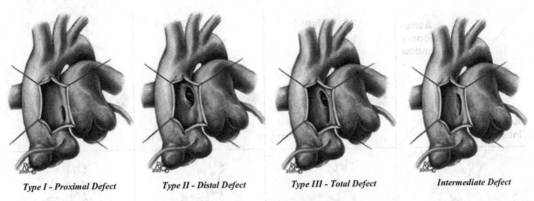

Type I - Proximal Defect   Type II - Distal Defect   Type III - Total Defect   Intermediate Defect

Fig. 85.1 The Society of Thoracic Surgeons classification of aortopulmonary window (Reproduced from reference [9] with permission)

Origin of the right pulmonary artery from the ascending aorta and arch hypoplasia with interruption or coarctation are additional anomalies occurring with large aortopulmonary windows. With increasing size of the aortopulmonary window, aberrations in flow result in abnormal incorporation of the right sixth arch, destined to become the right pulmonary artery, such that the right pulmonary artery arises from the rightward aspect of the ascending aorta [7]. Similarly, with large aortopulmonary windows, flow patterns can be disturbed such that there is preferential flow through the ductus arteriosus and diminished flow in the developing aortic arch, resulting in distal arch hypoplasia including coarctation or interrupted aortic arch. It has been suggested that when associated with interrupted aortic arch, aortopulmonary windows are larger with greater distal extension [7]. The Congenital Heart Surgeons' Society multi-institutional study of aortopulmonary window with interrupted aortic arch found that all types of aortopulmonary window were more or less equally represented among patients with interrupted aortic arch (Fig. 85.2) [8]. Aortopulmonary window is not associated with DiGeorge syndrome, suggesting that aortopulmonary window is a distinct malformation not related to abnormalities of the conal septum, such as interrupted aortic arch with ventricular septal defect (VSD), tetralogy of Fallot, and persistent truncus arteriosus.

In reports based on the cumulative experience at high-volume centers, aortopulmonary window was associated with other defects in 58 % of cases, the most common being ventricular and atrial septal defect, interrupted aortic arch or coarctation of the aorta, tetralogy of Fallot, and transposition of the great arteries [9–15]. Abnormal origin of the coronary arteries is also commonly associated with aortopulmonary window. The coronary arteries may arise from the edge of the defect, or the origin may occur just on the pulmonary artery side of the defect.

Presentation, Diagnostic Considerations, and Indications for Surgery

Antenatal diagnosis of aortopulmonary window was first reported in 2002 [16]. Simple aortopulmonary window may not be identified by fetal echocardiography because equal pressure in the ascending aorta and pulmonary root in the fetus results in minimal detectable flow through the defect. Interrupted aortic arch associated with aortopulmonary window lacks the characteristic posterior deviation of the infundibular septum that may prompt further interrogation of the aortic arch. As a consequence, antenatal diagnosis of aortopulmonary window with interrupted aortic arch has only recently been reported [17].

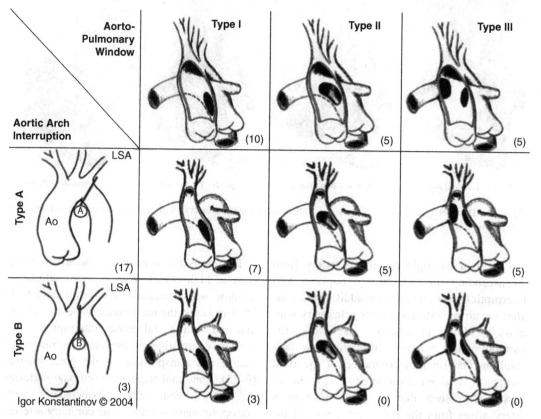

Fig. 85.2 The observed morphologies of aortopulmonary window with interrupted aortic arch. Type A interrupted arch predominated, but the position of aortopulmonary window was essentially evenly divided between proximal and distal (Reproduced from reference [8] with permission)

The presentation of patients with aortopulmonary window is similar to that of other patients with left-to-right shunts, such as patent ductus arteriosus or VSD. Although small, restrictive aortopulmonary windows do occur; generally, the communication is large, and patients present in the first weeks of life when pulmonary vascular resistance drops and increased pulmonary blood flow with congestive heart failure develops. Tachypnea, diaphoresis, poor feeding, and inadequate weight gain are common. In early infancy, cyanosis is usually not a prominent feature, but with large defects, bidirectional shunting can produce systemic desaturation [18, 19].

Physical examination demonstrates a tachypneic infant with accessory respiratory muscle use. Cardiac examination reveals an enlarged heart, and similar to patients with patent ductus arteriosus, the pulses are bounding. A systolic murmur can be heard along the left sternal border; however, unlike patients with a patent ductus arteriosus, a diastolic component to the murmur is rare. Chest X-ray films reveal cardiomegaly and increased pulmonary vascular markings consistent with increased pulmonary blood flow. Patients with associated arch abnormalities frequently present with pulmonary edema, low cardiac output, and metabolic acidosis coinciding with closing of the ductus arteriosus [18, 19].

The diagnosis is routinely made with echocardiography. The location and size of the communication as well as associated anomalies are carefully identified. Echocardiography as the sole imaging modality has been shown to be accurate and sufficient for preoperative evaluation of even complex congenital defects including aortopulmonary windows with or without associated defects [20]. Cardiac catheterization is rarely indicated and reserved for the patient who presents after early infancy and therefore is at risk for elevated pulmonary vascular resistance or any patient in whom the anatomy cannot be adequately defined by echocardiography. Although using cardiac catheterization to assess the origin of the coronary arteries is theoretically appealing, the large defect occurring just above the sinuses of Valsalva combined with the tremendous pulmonary flow makes assessment of coronary artery anatomy with catheterization impractical. Those patients who are found to have an elevated pulmonary vascular resistance should undergo testing with pulmonary vasodilators to determine if the pulmonary vascular resistance can be reduced. Presence of an aortopulmonary window is an indication for surgery because untreated infants die of intractable heart failure or rapidly develop pulmonary vascular obstructive disease [18, 19].

Preoperative Management

Because aortopulmonary window is rarely diagnosed antenatally, preoperative stabilization is still required with some regularity. For the patient with a large aortopulmonary window presenting in shock, initial resuscitative efforts are aimed at improving systemic output by limiting excessive pulmonary blood flow and are similar to those used in the patient with single ventricle anatomy and unobstructed pulmonary blood flow, or patients with truncus arteriosus. Measures may include intubation and mechanical ventilation as well as sedation and on occasion neuromuscular blockade. The use of hypercapnea will increase the pulmonary vascular resistance, decrease left-to-right shunting, and improve systemic oxygen delivery. Inotropic and vasodilator support may be required. Prostaglandin infusion is necessary to maintain ductal patency in patients with aortopulmonary window and interrupted aortic arch or coarctation. These measures should be successful in restoring systemic output, and the patient should go to surgery without a metabolic acidosis [18, 19].

Operative Technique

Simple Aortopulmonary Window

A median sternotomy incision is used for aortopulmonary window regardless of associated abnormalities. Once the pericardium is opened, the anatomy should be carefully assessed (Fig. 85.3). External inspection can reveal the extent of the aortopulmonary window and provides clues to abnormal origins of the coronary arteries. Coronary arteries involved in the defect can be seen arising from the area of the communication and coursing down the proximal aorta before reaching the myocardium. The position of the right pulmonary artery should be noted.

The right and left pulmonary arteries should be loosely encircled with snares so that once cardiopulmonary bypass is established, pulmonary flow can be controlled. The aorta should be dissected nearly circumferentially distal to the extent of the aortopulmonary window to allow for subsequent placement of the cross-clamp. After the administration of heparin, the aortic cannula is placed in the ascending aorta near the origin of the innominate artery (Fig. 85.4). If there is an associated atrial septal defect or VSD, bicaval cannulation should be undertaken; otherwise, a single venous cannula can be used. Cardiopulmonary bypass is begun, and simultaneously the branch pulmonary arteries are snared. A cardioplegia cannula is placed in the ascending aorta. For simple aortopulmonary window, repair can be completed with normothermic cardiopulmonary bypass or moderate hypothermia (32 °C). The aorta is cross-clamped distal to the communication. Cardioplegic solution is infused while the pulmonary arteries are snared. The defect can be repaired via an incision in the window itself, through the aorta, or through the pulmonary artery (Fig. 85.5). An approach through the window is preferable because the origin of the coronary arteries can be easily assessed and the patch placed such that an abnormal coronary ostial origin is incorporated into the aorta. In addition, there is less potential for compromise of either of the great vessels or injury of the semilunar valves.

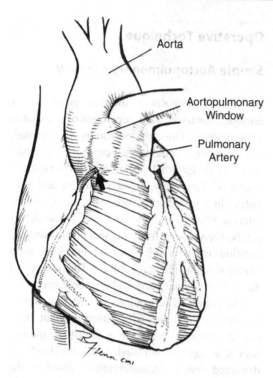

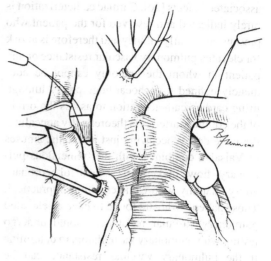

Fig. 85.4 Preliminary steps in repair of simple aortopulmonary window. The left and right branch pulmonary arteries are loosely encircled. The aorta is cannulated beyond the distal extent of the aortopulmonary window so that there is adequate room for a cross-clamp. Generally, a single venous cannula placed through the right atrial appendage is used for venous drainage. After cardiopulmonary bypass has begun, the branch pulmonary artery snares are tightened (Reproduced from reference [19] with permission)

Fig. 85.3 External view of aortopulmonary window. The area of communication between the great vessels can be easily identified. The extent of the defect and the origins of the right pulmonary artery and right coronary artery should be identified. As in this figure, the right coronary artery (*arrow*) can be sometimes seen originating near the inferior margin of the defect and coursing proximally on the aorta before taking its normal position in the atrioventricular groove. This finding should prompt careful internal inspection for abnormal origin of the coronary artery from the inferior ridge of the defect or the pulmonary artery (Reproduced from reference [19] with permission)

The incision is initiated in the anterior-superior portion of the window, and, after the origin of the right coronary artery is identified, the incision is extended proximally, transecting the anterior half of the window. After the origins of the coronary arteries and the right pulmonary artery are identified, an appropriately sized patch of polytetrafluoroethylene (PTFE), autologous glutaraldehyde-fixed pericardium, or homograft is secured to the posterior wall of the defect using continuous suture (Fig. 85.6a). The anterior incision in the window is then closed, incorporating the patch into the suture line (Fig. 85.6b). Rewarming to normothermia is begun as the window is closed. The aortic root is de-aired, and the

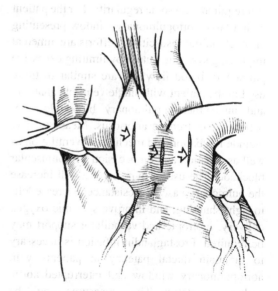

Fig. 85.5 Aortopulmonary window can be repaired via an incision in the window itself, through the aorta, or through the pulmonary artery (Reproduced from reference [19] with permission)

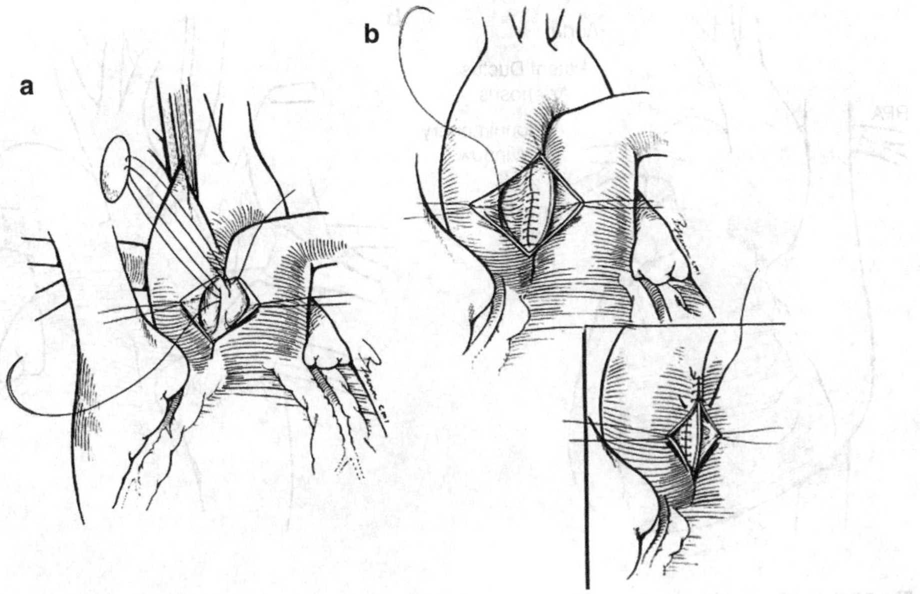

Fig. 85.6 (a) Approach through the aortopulmonary window. An incision is initiated in the anterior-superior portion of the window, and after the origin of the right coronary artery is identified, the incision is extended proximally, transecting the anterior half of the window. After the origins of the coronary arteries and the right pulmonary artery are identified, an appropriately sized patch of PTFE or pericardium is secured to the posterior rim of the defect. (b) The patch is secured to the posterior margin of the aortopulmonary window using a continuous suture technique. Anteriorly, closer of the arteriotomy in the aortopulmonary window incorporates the patch (Reproduced from reference [19] with permission)

cross-clamp is removed. Inotropic support may be necessary, and milrinone should be considered as this provides both inotropy and pulmonary vasodilatation. Additional pulmonary vasodilators such as inhaled nitric oxide should be available especially in the older infant.

Aortopulmonary Window with Interrupted Aortic Arch

Aortopulmonary window with interrupted aortic arch is usually a large defect and can be associated with abnormal origin of the right pulmonary artery (Fig. 85.7a). A median sternotomy incision is used. Initial preparation is the same as for simple aortopulmonary window; again, the branch pulmonary arteries are loosely encircled with snares. Because of the large aortopulmonary communication, a single arterial cannula can be used. This is placed in the ascending aorta (Fig. 85.7b). Flow to the distal half of the body will be through the aortopulmonary window and then via the ductus arteriosus.

After cardiopulmonary bypass is established, the branch pulmonary arteries are snared. The patient is cooled over a period of at least 30 min to a bladder temperature of 18 °C. During the cooling period, the aortic arch, head vessels, ductus arteriosus, and proximal descending thoracic aorta are mobilized. After reaching the target temperature, circulatory arrest is established, the head vessels are snared, a C-shaped vascular clamp is placed across the descending thoracic aorta at least 1 cm distal to the insertion of the ductus arteriosus, and cardioplegic solution is infused via the arterial cannula. With the branch pulmonary arteries, descending thoracic aorta, and head vessels occluded, cardioplegic solution will be directed into the coronary arteries. The entire procedure can be performed using deep hypothermic circulatory arrest, or alternatively continuous cerebral perfusion can be used. The ductus arteriosus is ligated near the pulmonary artery, and all ductal tissue is excised from the descending thoracic aorta. An incision is made

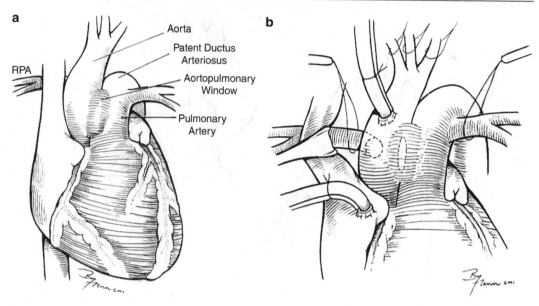

Fig. 85.7 (a) External appearance of the aortopulmonary window and interrupted aortic arch (RPA = right pulmonary artery). (b) Cannulation for repair of aortopulmonary window and interrupted aortic arch. The right and left branch pulmonary arteries are loosely encircled with snares. Unlike interrupted aortic arch with ventricular septal defect, a single aorta cannula is satisfactory because distal perfusion can be carried via the aortopulmonary window and a ductus arteriosus to the lower half of the body. Aortopulmonary window and interrupted aortic arch are rarely associated with ventricular septal defect, and a single venous cannula is usually all that is required. After establishment of cardiopulmonary bypass, the branch pulmonary artery snares are tightened. During the period of cooling, the brachiocephalic vessels are mobilized and loosely encircled with snares (Reproduced from reference [19] with permission)

from the base of the left subclavian artery and extended proximally into the aortopulmonary window (Fig. 85.8). The posterior edge of the descending thoracic aorta is then joined to the posterior edge of the distal arch in order to achieve as much tissue-to-tissue continuity as possible (Fig. 85.9). A single patch of pulmonary homograft is then used to augment the arch and septate the window taking care to prevent compromise of the proximal right pulmonary artery (Fig. 85.10).

Catheter-Based Approaches

The utility of transcatheter closure is limited by the large size of the defect, small size of patients with correspondingly small femoral vessels, and the potential for complications related to anomalous origin of the coronary arteries that are hard to define prior to intervention. Nevertheless, device closure of aortopulmonary window may be suitable for small defects in which the risk of anomalous origin of the coronary arteries is low, specifically those with a more distal location.

Postoperative Care

For simple aortopulmonary window and even aortopulmonary window with interrupted aortic arch, postoperative inotropic support should be minimal. Like other patients with large left-to-right shunts, there is potential for acute elevation of pulmonary vascular resistance with the development of critically low cardiac output following repair. Patients operated on in the first 2 weeks of life should be at low risk for pulmonary vascular resistance elevation and may be candidates for early extubation. Older patients may require sedation and neuromuscular blockade for the first 12–24 h. In higher-risk patients, pulmonary artery pressure should be continuously monitored until extubation. If pulmonary hypertension develops,

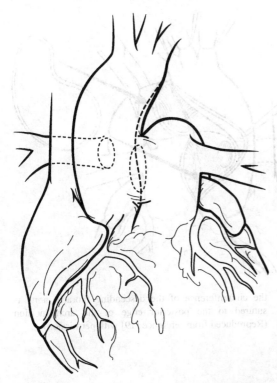

Fig. 85.8 A patch (either pulmonary homograft or pericardium) is fashioned as shown in the illustration. The dashed line indicates the initial suture line. Reconstruction begins by suturing the patch to the anterior one-half of the proximal descending thoracic aorta and then transitioning the suture line to the posterior wall of the ascending aorta such that the abnormally positioned right pulmonary artery is placed on the left side of the patch. The suture line then continues to the bottom of the aortopulmonary window (Reproduced from reference [19] with permission)

pulmonary vasodilators (inhaled nitric oxide) should be started promptly. In addition to routine hemodynamic monitoring, the adequacy of systemic oxygen delivery might be assessed by sampling of mixed venous blood from the pulmonary artery or with near-infrared spectroscopic (NIRS) monitoring the cardiac intensive care unit.

Results of Surgery

As with other defects, the trend towards early repair along with the advances in diagnosis and perioperative management has substantially improved outcomes over the last decades. In the current era, early mortality following repair of uncomplicated

aortopulmonary window approaches zero, and long-term outcome should be excellent. Early morbidity includes pulmonary artery stenosis and residual aortopulmonary septal defects.

In a pooled analysis of 370 patients, from 22 reports over six decades, the median age at surgery was 3 months (ranging from neonate to 27-year-old adults), and 58 % of the patients had associated defects [9–15, 21–35]. There was one reported death during surgery in all patients with isolated aortopulmonary window (128 patients). No late death was reported for this group, but some of the patients needed re-intervention for residual shunting or pulmonary artery stenosis in older series and in cases where simple ligation of the aortopulmonary window was performed. In the group with associated defects, 35 patients (17 %) died during or immediately after surgery. Seven additional patients (3.4 %) died during follow-up that varied in length but were greater than 2.5 years in all reports (median follow-up 6.5 years). Importantly, these estimates include the experience from six decades; in more recent series, the mortality approaches zero percent, even for cases of aortopulmonary window with associated defects. In three studies reporting long-term outcomes, actuarial survival was between 84 % and 90 % at 10 years, and freedom from re-intervention was 43 %–70 % at 5–10 years after the initial procedure, including patients with associated defects. Among these studies, associations with higher morbidity and mortality were found for combination of aortopulmonary window with another defect, for simple ligation of the window, and for the transpulmonary repair technique.

Between 1983 and 2009, 25 patients with aortopulmonary window and associated lesions have undergone repair at our institution. Patients were divided into two categories based on the presence of important additional lesions. Simple aortopulmonary window (n = 12) included those patients with an isolated aortopulmonary window with or without an atrial level communication. Complex aortopulmonary window (n = 13) included those patients with important additional lesions including interrupted aortic arch or coarctation of the aorta (n = 8), ventricular septal

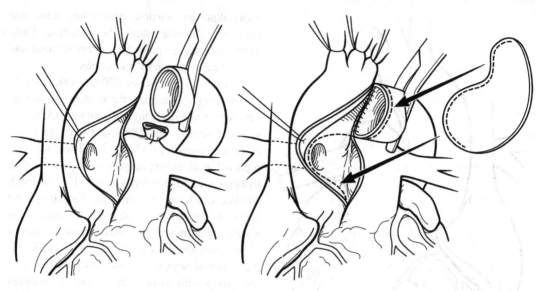

Fig. 85.9 (a) An incision is made from the base of the left subclavian artery and extended proximally into the aortopulmonary window. (b) The posterior one-half of the circumference of the descending thoracic aorta is sutured to the posterior edge of the arch incision (Reproduced from reference [19] with permission)

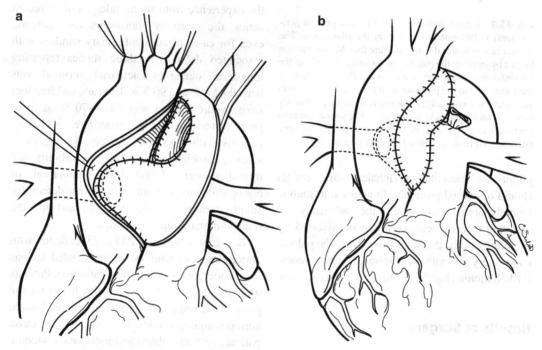

Fig. 85.10 (a) The posterior suture line is in place. The anterior edge of the patch will now be secured to the edge of the ascending aorta. (b) Completion of the repair. The pulmonary artery edge of the aortopulmonary window is sutured to the centerline of the patch to complete closure of the main pulmonary artery. In this way, the patch augments both ascending aorta and main pulmonary artery and minimizes the potential for compromise of the caliber of either of these vessels or the right pulmonary artery. In addition, the patch allows augmentation of the arch reconstruction (Reproduced from reference [19] with permission)

defect (n = 1), pulmonary atresia with ventricular septal defect and anomalous origin of the right coronary artery (n = 1), pulmonary atresia with intact ventricular septum and partial anomalous pulmonary venous return (n = 1), aortopulmonary window with d-malposed great vessels (n = 1), and congenital absence of the left pulmonary artery with pulmonary artery hypertension (n = 1). There were no deaths early or late in the simple aortopulmonary window group. In the complex aortopulmonary window group, there was one early death in the patient with aortopulmonary window, pulmonary atresia, and intact ventricular septum. There was one late death following lung transplantation in the patient with aortopulmonary window, absent left pulmonary artery, and pulmonary hypertension.

In the current era, early mortality following repair of simple aortopulmonary window approaches zero percent, and long-term outcome should be excellent. Early morbidity includes pulmonary artery stenosis and residual aortopulmonary septal defects. Long-term follow-up is indicated to observe for the development of branch pulmonary artery stenosis. For patients with aortopulmonary window and interrupted aortic arch, the outcome should also be good with low operative mortality. Long-term observation for recurrent coarctation and pulmonary artery stenosis is indicated.

References

1. Kutsche LM, Van Mierop LH (1987) Anatomy and pathogenesis of aorticopulmonary septal defect. Am J Cardiol 59(5):443–447
2. Talner CN (1980) Report of the New England Regional Infant Cardiac Program, by Donald C. Fyler, MD. Pediatrics 65(suppl):375–461, (1998) Pediatrics 102(1 Pt 2): 258–259
3. Samanek M, Voriskova M (1999) Congenital heart disease among 815,569 children born between 1980 and 1990 and their 15-year survival: a prospective Bohemia survival study. Pediatr Cardiol 20(6):411–417
4. Van Praagh R (1987) Truncus arteriosus: what is it really and how should it be classified? Eur J Cardiothorac Surg 1(2):65–70
5. Mori K, Ando M, Takao A, Ishikawa S, Imai Y (1978) Distal type of aortopulmonary window. Report of 4 cases. Br Heart J 40(6):681–689
6. Jacobs JP, Quintessenza JA, Gaynor JW, Burke RP, Mavroudis C (2000) Congenital heart surgery Nomenclature and database project: aortopulmonary window. Ann Thorac Surg 69(4 Suppl):S44–S49
7. Berry TE, Bharati S, Muster AJ et al (1982) Distal aortopulmonary septal defect, aortic origin of the right pulmonary artery, intact ventricular septum, patent ductus arteriosus and hypoplasia of the aortic isthmus: a newly recognized syndrome. Am J Cardiol 49(1):108–116
8. Konstantinov IE, Karamlou T, Williams WG et al (2006) Surgical management of aortopulmonary window associated with interrupted aortic arch: a Congenital Heart Surgeons Society study. J Thorac Cardiovasc Surg 131(5):1136–1141, e1132
9. Backer CL, Mavroudis C (2002) Surgical management of aortopulmonary window: a 40-year experience. Eur J Cardiothorac Surg 21(5):773–779
10. Hew CC, Bacha EA, Zurakowski D, del Nido PJ Jr, Jonas RA (2001) Optimal surgical approach for repair of aortopulmonary window. Cardiol Young 11(4):385–390
11. Tanoue Y, Sese A, Ueno Y, Joh K (2000) Surgical management of aortopulmonary window. Jpn J Thoracic Cardiovasc Surg 48(9):557–561, Official publication of the Japanese Association for Thoracic Surgery = Nihon Kyobu Geka Gakkai zasshi
12. Soares AM, Atik E, Cortez TM et al (1999) Aortopulmonary window. Clinical and surgical assessment of 18 cases. Arq Bras Cardiol 73(1):59–74
13. Tkebuchava T, von Segesser LK, Vogt PR et al (1997) Congenital aortopulmonary window: diagnosis, surgical technique and long-term results. Eur J Cardiothorac Surg 11(2):293–297
14. Bertolini A, Dalmonte P, Bava GL, Moretti R, Cervo G, Marasini M (1994) Aortopulmonary septal defects. A review of the literature and report of ten cases. J Cardiovasc Surg (Torino) 35(3):207–213
15. van Son JA, Puga FJ, Danielson GK et al (1993) Aortopulmonary window: factors associated with early and late success after surgical treatment. Mayo Clin Proc 68(2):128–133, Mayo Clinic
16. Collinet P, Chatelet-Cheront C, Houze de l'Aulnoit D, Rey C (2002) Prenatal diagnosis of an aortopulmonary window by fetal echocardiography. Fetal Diagn Ther 17(5):302–307
17. Hayashi G, Inamura N, Kayatani F, Kawazu Y, Hamamichi Y (2010) Prenatal diagnosis of aortopulmonary window with interrupted aortic arch by fetal echocardiography. Fetal Diagn Ther 27(2):97–100
18. Qureshi SA (2010) R. Arterio-venous Fistulas and Related Conditions. In: Anderson RH, Baker EJ, Redington A, Rigby ML, Penny DJ, Wernovsky G (eds) Paediatric cardiology, 3rd edn. Churchill Livingston, Philadelphia
19. Tweddell J (2006) Aortopulmonary window. In: Kaiser LR KI, Spray TL (eds) Mastery of cardiothoracic surgery, 2nd edn. Lippincott, Williams and Wilkins, Philadelphia

20. Tworetzky W, McElhinney DB, Brook MM, Reddy VM, Hanley FL, Silverman NH (1999) Echocardiographic diagnosis alone for the complete repair of major congenital heart defects. J Am Coll Cardiol 33(1):228–233

21. Barnes ME, Mitchell ME, Tweddell JS (2011) Aortopulmonary window. Semin Thorac Cardiovasc Surg Pediatr Card Surg Annu 14(1):67–74

22. Freitas I, Parames F, Rebelo M, Martins JD, Pinto MF, Kaku S (2008) Aortopulmonary window. Experience of eleven cases. Rev Port Cardiol 27(12):1597–1603, Orgao oficial da Sociedade Portuguesa de Cardiologia = Portuguese journal of cardiology: an official journal of the Portuguese Society of Cardiology

23. Santos W, Rossi R, Abecasis M et al (2008) Aortopulmonary window–a review of nine cases. Rev Port Cardiol 27(11):1453–1462, Orgao oficial da Sociedade Portuguesa de Cardiologia = Portuguese journal of cardiology: an official journal of the Portuguese Society of Cardiology

24. Bhan A, Gupta M, Abraham S, Sharma R, Kothari SS, Juneja R (2007) Surgical experience of aortopulmonary window repair in infants. Int Cardiovas Thoracic Surg 6(2):200–203

25. Chen CA, Chiu SN, Wu ET et al (2006) Surgical outcome of aortopulmonary window repair in early infancy. J Formos Med Assoc 105((10):813–820, Taiwan yi zhi

26. Jansen C, Hruda J, Rammeloo L, Ottenkamp J, Hazekamp MG (2006) Surgical repair of aortopulmonary window: thirty-seven years of experience. Pediatr Cardiol 27(5):552–556

27. Mert M, Paker T, Akcevin A et al (2004) Diagnosis, management, and results of treatment for aortopulmonary window. Cardiol Young 14(5):506–511

28. Bagtharia R, Trivedi KR, Burkhart HM et al (2004) Outcomes for patients with an aortopulmonary window, and the impact of associated cardiovascular lesions. Cardiol Young 14(5):473–480

29. Erez E, Dagan O, Georghiou GP, Gelber O, Vidne BA, Birk E (2004) Surgical management of aortopulmonary window and associated lesions. Ann Thorac Surg 77(2):484–487

30. Di Bella I, Gladstone DJ (1998) Surgical management of aortopulmonary window. Ann Thorac Surg 65(3):768–770

31. McElhinney DB, Reddy VM, Tworetzky W, Silverman NH, Hanley FL (1998) Early and late results after repair of aortopulmonary septal defect and associated anomalies in infants <6 months of age. Am J Cardiol 81(2):195–201

32. Prasad TR, Valiathan MS, Shyamakrishnan KG, Venkitachalam CG (1989) Surgical management of aortopulmonary septal defect. Ann Thorac Surg 47(6):877–879

33. Ravikumar E, Whight CM, Hawker RE, Celermajer JM, Nunn G, Cartmill TB (1988) The surgical management of aortopulmonary window using the anterior sandwich patch closure technique. J Cardiovasc Surg (Torino) 29(6):629–632

34. Tiraboschi R, Salomone G, Crupi G et al (1988) Aortopulmonary window in the first year of life: report on 11 surgical cases. Ann Thorac Surg 46(4):438–441

35. Ventemiglia RA, Oglietti J, Izquierdo J, Muasher I, Frazier OH, Cooley DA (1983) The surgical treatment of aortopulmonary window. Tex Heart Inst J 10(1):31–37, from the Texas Heart Institute of St. Luke's Episcopal Hospital, Texas Children's Hospital

Tetralogy of Fallot

86

Jennifer S. Nelson, Edward L. Bove, and Jennifer C. Hirsch-Romano

Abstract

Tetralogy of Fallot is one of the most common congenital cardiac malformations and consists of (1) ventricular septal defect, (2) right ventricular outflow tract obstruction, (3) aortic override, and (4) right ventricular hypertrophy. The initial presentation of the patient with Tetralogy of Fallot is variable and dependent on the degree of right ventricular outflow tract obstruction. Initial medical management of Tetralogy of Fallot is aimed at monitoring and managing hypoxemia and preventing hypercyanotic spells. A small percentage of patients will present with significant cyanosis in the neonatal period. The majority, however, will have stable pulmonary artery blood flow and require no immediate treatment. Cyanosis gradually progresses as pulmonary blood flow is limited by increasing right ventricular outflow tract obstruction. Diagnosis is usually established with transthoracic echocardiography. Further anatomic detail and some functional data may also be garnered with cardiac MRI or cardiac catheterization, which may help define and characterize additional sources of pulmonary blood flow or abnormalities of systemic venous return.

Indications for surgical intervention are symptoms of hypercyanotic episodes or the presence of oxygen saturations that are persistently below 75–80 %. In most children with Tetralogy of Fallot, elective complete repair is recommended by 1 year of age with most centers recommending elective repair in the first 3–6 months of life. While palliative procedures can be performed to delay the need for definitive complete repair, most centers favor early complete repair, reserving palliative procedures for those patients that have contraindications to open cardiac surgery. In the current era, outcomes for complete repair are excellent, even when definitive repair is required in the neonatal period.

J.S. Nelson (✉) • E.L. Bove • J.C. Hirsch-Romano
Department of Cardiac Surgery, University of Michigan
Medical School, Ann Arbor, MI, USA
e-mail: jensnels@med.umich.edu; elbove@umich.edu;
jhirsch@umich.edu

E.M. da Cruz et al. (eds.), *Pediatric and Congenital Cardiology, Cardiac Surgery and Intensive Care*,
DOI 10.1007/978-1-4471-4619-3_18, © Springer-Verlag London 2014

Morphology and associated defects in tetralogy of Fallot may include tetralogy of Fallot with absent pulmonary valve, tetralogy of Fallot with complete atrioventricular septal defect, and tetralogy of Fallot with pulmonary atresia and multiple aortopulmonary collaterals. These entities may behave differently, and strategy and timing for surgical repair are often more complicated than for simple tetralogy of Fallot. Following repair of tetralogy of Fallot, lifelong follow-up is usually indicated in order to monitor for recurrent or persistent pathology of the right ventricular outflow tract and for appropriate intervention if indicated.

Keywords

Absent pulmonary valve • Complete atrioventricular septal defect • Hypercyanotic spells • Junctional ectopic tachycardia (JET) • Low cardiac output syndrome • Multiple aortopulmonary collateral arteries (MAPCAs) • Pulmonary atresia • Pulmonary blood flow • Pulmonary stenosis • Pulmonary valve replacement • Right ventricular outflow tract obstruction • Surgical palliation • Surgical repair • Tetralogy of Fallot

Introduction

Tetralogy of Fallot (TOF) is the most common complex congenital heart defect, with an estimated incidence of 3.3 per 10,000 live births [1, 2]. The first complete description of TOF was published in 1888 by the French physician Etienne-Louis Arthur Fallot [3]. It was not until 1945, however, that the first surgical treatment for TOF was performed by Alfred Blalock at Johns Hopkins University [4]. This landmark operation ushered in the era of surgery for congenital heart defects. A number of innovative systemic-to-pulmonary artery shunt procedures were soon described [5, 6] followed by the first successful intracardiac repair using human cross-circulation by Lillehei and Varco at the University of Minnesota in 1954 [7]. The first successful repair using a pump oxygenator was performed by Kirklin at the Mayo Clinic 1 year later [8]. Numerous contributions have been made in the management of TOF since these initial pioneering efforts, which have led to a long-term survival rate approaching 90 % [9, 10]. Now, with increasing duration of follow-up, adult patients with repaired TOF are presenting new medical and surgical challenges. The latter will be further discussed in a specific chapter elsewhere in this textbook.

Anatomy and Associated Defects

The classic components of the "tetrad" that comprise this defect are malalignment ventricular septal defect (VSD), right ventricular outflow tract obstruction (RVOTO), aortic override, and right ventricular hypertrophy (RVH) (Fig. 86.1a, b). The subpulmonary infundibulum in TOF is characterized by a smaller volume, shorter and thicker infundibular septum, and anterosuperior deviation of the infundibular septum [11]. The VSD in TOF is a large, nonrestrictive defect that results from malalignment of the leftward or septal extent of the infundibular septum with the septal band [12]. The bundle of His penetrates at the posteroinferior edge of the defect [13, 14]. Although the VSD is generally subaortic in position, it may extend to the subpulmonary region when the infundibular septum is absent or deficient [15, 16]. Additional ventricular septal defects may exist in approximately 5 % of patients and generally occur in the muscular septum.

The anterior and superior displacement of the infundibular septum also results in RVOTO from hypoplasia of the right ventricular infundibulum. The pulmonary valve (PV) is nearly always involved in the obstruction. The leaflets may be thickened and tethered to the pulmonary artery

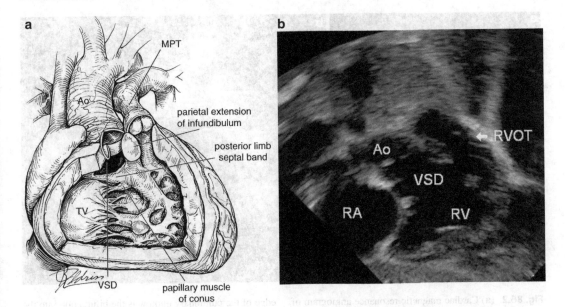

Fig. 86.1 (**a**) Artist's rendering and (**b**) transthoracic echocardiography highlighting the pathologic anatomy of TOF. Images demonstrate a nonrestrictive malalignment VSD with aortic override, the papillary muscle of the conus along with the hypertrophied parietal and septal bands (**a**) which result in RVOTO, an infundibular "chamber," and a stenotic, hypoplastic main pulmonary trunk and valve (From Hirsch and Bove [89])

wall. The PV is bicuspid in 58 % of patients, but it is the narrowest part of the outflow tract in a small minority of patients [17, 18]. The "annulus" of the PV, although not a true fibrous structure, is usually hypoplastic.

Important degrees of obstruction may also occur at the level of the right and left branch pulmonary arteries. Hypoplasia of one or both branches may be seen. Uncommonly, the left pulmonary artery may take origin from the ductus arteriosus, and its intrapericardial portion may be completely absent. More commonly, localized narrowing of the origin of the right or left pulmonary arteries will be present. The ductus may also insert into the proximal left pulmonary artery and may result in localized stenosis at this level. In extreme cases of anterior displacement of the infundibular septum, complete atresia of the distal right ventricular infundibulum and main pulmonary artery trunk may result.

Pulmonary atresia (PA) is present in approximately 7 % of patients with TOF [19]. Multiple major aortopulmonary collateral arteries (MAPCAs) are usually found in those patients without an associated patent ductus arteriosus (PDA) and provide a variable degree of the pulmonary blood flow. Additionally, these systemically perfused lung segments often demonstrate aberrant arborization of the pulmonary vasculature that can result in further flow derangements. Unlike patients without PA who possess centrally located areas of discrete pulmonary arterial stenoses, those with PA and MAPCAs are more likely to have peripheral pulmonary stenoses.

Approximately 5 % of patients with TOF will have complete absence of the pulmonary valve leaflets [20]. Severe pulmonary regurgitation is generally present with RVOTO at the level of the hypoplastic annulus. Aneurysmal dilatation of the main pulmonary artery and the right and left branch pulmonary arteries occurs and may result in compression of the distal tracheobronchial tree [21].

Aortic override is caused by dextroposition of the aortic root and results in a biventricular origin of the aorta. Continuity between the aortic and mitral valves is present by definition, even in extreme degrees of override. Double outlet right

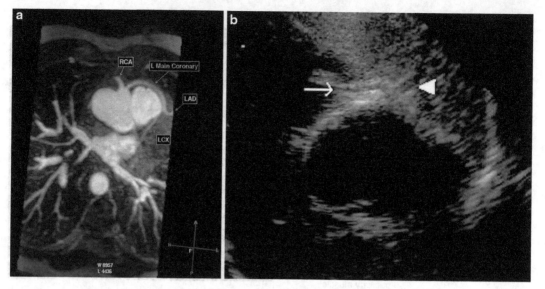

Fig. 86.2 (a) Cardiac magnetic resonance angiogram of a patient with TOF and a single coronary artery from the right facing sinus. This transverse oblique maximum intensity projection shows the single coronary artery with the right and left main coronary arteries traveling anterior to the pulmonary outflow tract. At the leftward edge of the pulmonary outflow is the bifurcation into the LAD and the circumflex which then courses posteriorly. (b) Transthoracic echocardiogram subcostal view of a TOF patient with LMCA (*arrowhead*) originating from the RCA (*arrow*) and crossing the RVOT

ventricle (DORV) is considered to exist with TOF when the right ventricle supports 90 % or more of the aorta or in the case of aortic and mitral discontinuity.

The origin of the left anterior descending (LAD) coronary artery from the right coronary artery (RCA) occurs in approximately 3–5 % of patients with TOF [22]. The LAD will cross the RVOT a short distance below the PV annulus to reach the anterior interventricular septum and is susceptible to injury from an incision in this area. Other important coronary artery patterns include a dual LAD distribution with the lower half of the septum supplied from the RCA and the upper half from the left coronary artery along with the presence of large right ventricular conal branches. Rarely, a single RCA gives rise to the left main coronary artery (LMCA), which then crosses the RVOT (Fig. 86.2a, b).

Major associated cardiac defects are relatively uncommon in TOF. The most frequently associated lesions are atrial septal defect (ASD), PDA, complete atrioventricular septal defect, and multiple ventricular septal defects. Other less common defects include persistent left superior vena cava, anomalous aortic origin of the coronary artery, and aberrant origin of the right or left pulmonary artery.

Genetics

The genetics of TOF are incompletely understood. The heritability of TOF is thought to be about 54 % according to a large study by Boon et al. [23]. This study also suggested that if one sibling has TOF, there is a 1 % risk of a second sibling having TOF. Other early research was able to show an association of TOF with DiGeorge syndrome, Alagille syndrome, and trisomies 21, 18, and 13 [24]. More recently, specific mutations have been correlated with TOF including a microdeletion in chromosome 22q11 (found in 15 % of TOF patients and in up to 40 % of those with TOF/PA), a mutation in Jagger-1 (JAG-1) (found in 1–2 %), a mutation in NKX2.5 (found in 4 %), and a mutation in zinc-finger protein, multi-type 2 (ZFPM2, found in 4 %) [24, 25].

Important transcription factors such as TBX1, TBX5, and GATA4 have also been implicated in the pathogenesis [24].

Pathophysiology

The initial presentation of the patient with TOF is dependent on the degree of RVOTO. Most commonly, cyanosis is mild at birth and gradually progresses with age as the obstruction increases due to increasing hypertrophy of the right ventricular infundibulum and failure of growth of the hypoplastic pulmonary valve. Initially, the predominant shunt across the VSD may even be left to right in patients with mild obstruction (pink TOF), and the clinical picture is one of congestive heart failure. Cyanosis tends to become significant within the first 6–12 months of life in these patients. In such situations, the obstruction is entirely or predominantly at the infundibular level. The pulmonary valve annulus and the branch pulmonary arteries are usually of good size.

Some patients may develop characteristic hypercyanotic or "tet spells," which are periods of profound systemic hypoxemia typically occurring in the context of crying, eating, or defecation. Rarely, these hypercyanotic spells can lead to loss of consciousness, neurologic injury, or death. These spells are characterized by a marked decrease in pulmonary blood flow and an increase in the right-to-left shunt across the VSD into the left ventricle and out the aorta. The precise pathophysiology of these spells is uncertain but may involve alterations in systemic vascular resistance.

A smaller percentage of patients will present with significant cyanosis at or shortly after birth. In this group, the outflow tract obstruction is nearly always due to a hypoplastic pulmonary valve annulus with or without severe right ventricular infundibular obstruction or hypoplasia. Although the peripheral pulmonary arteries may appear hypoplastic, they are generally adequate in size when there is TOF with pulmonary stenosis. The small appearance is due to reduced pressure and flow [26]. Cyanosis is constant in these patients due to the fixed nature of the obstruction to pulmonary blood flow. Patients with atresia of the PV and main pulmonary trunk will be dependent on a PDA or systemic aortopulmonary collateral arteries for pulmonary blood flow. In the latter situation, the collateral arteries may be such that pulmonary overcirculation exists and congestive heart failure (CHF) is present [27, 28]. Older patients with untreated TOF and long-standing cyanosis will develop clubbing of the fingers and toes, dyspnea, exercise intolerance, brain abscesses, and polycythemia with pulmonary and cerebral thromboses.

Diagnosis

Physical Examination

Cyanosis is the main physical finding. The first heart sound is normal, but the second sound is often single due to an inaudible pulmonary component resulting from the low pulmonary artery pressure and the location of the aorta which may obscure the soft pulmonary closure sound. The characteristic systolic murmur results from the RVOTO and is usually moderate in intensity. Typically, the murmur disappears in the presence of a "tet" spell. A thrill is uncommon. Continuous murmurs, best heard over the back, will be heard with significant systemic aortopulmonary collateral artery flow. Patients with absent pulmonary valve syndrome will often exhibit signs of respiratory distress and a diastolic murmur from the pulmonary regurgitation. In older children and adults, clubbing of the fingers and toes occurs. Clubbing usually develops after 6 months of age and persists until after operative correction.

Electrocardiogram

The characteristic electrocardiographic finding is that of RVH from pressure overload of the right ventricle. This finding is consistent with normal RVH in the neonatal period and may not clearly represent an abnormality before 3 or 4 months

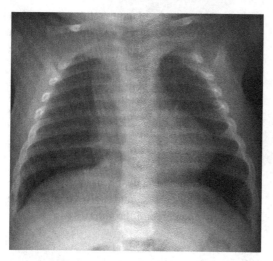

Fig. 86.3 Typical chest radiograph of the "coeur en sabot" (*boot-shaped* heart) in a patient with TOF and right-sided aortic arch. The image demonstrates the displacement of the cardiac apex upward and toward the right. This appearance results from right ventricular hypertrophy and hypoplasia of the main pulmonary artery (Image courtesy of Dr. Michael Di Pietro)

of age. Right axis deviation will also be found. Left ventricular hypertrophy (LVH) may be seen in those patients with increased pulmonary blood flow from large shunts or collaterals. Other abnormal findings are rare.

Chest Radiography

The heart size is generally normal, and the pulmonary artery segment may be small. The characteristic "boot-shaped" heart results from elevation of the cardiac apex from the hypertrophied right ventricle and a concave upper left heart border caused by a narrow main pulmonary artery (Fig. 86.3). This is most commonly observed in older infants and children. When pulmonary blood flow is derived from aortopulmonary collateral arterial supply, the peripheral markings often appear disorganized and irregular. Rib notching may even result from increased collateral flow in these circumstances. Asymmetry in the pulmonary blood flow pattern may result from branch pulmonary artery

stenoses or non-confluent pulmonary arteries. The aortic arch is right-sided in approximately 25 % of patients.

Echocardiography

The diagnosis is generally easily established by echocardiography [29]. The typical malalignment VSD with aortic override and RVOTO is well visualized (Fig. 86.1b). Often, the location of the LAD can be determined by transthoracic echo by following the left main coronary artery until it bifurcates. If an anomalous origin of the LAD from the right coronary is suspected, this should be defined by another imaging study. The anomalous LAD may be confused for a large conus branch of the right coronary artery. If the anatomy of the peripheral pulmonary arteries is not well seen, cardiac MRI or catheterization can be useful for clarification.

Cardiac Catheterization

In the majority of patients, diagnostic cardiac catheterization is not necessary. Catheterization is more commonly used for interventional procedures before and after TOF repair to address branch pulmonary artery stenoses. In the rare instance when the coronary artery anatomy is not well delineated by echocardiography, cardiac catheterization may be of benefit. In TOF with pulmonary atresia and MAPCAs, catheterization is essential for delineating the pulmonary artery and aortopulmonary collateral anatomy for surgical planning. Adult patients with repaired TOF may require cardiac catheterization if there is concern for coronary artery disease or prior to pulmonary valve replacement.

Cardiac MRI

Cardiac MRI (cMRI) provides an accurate noninvasive modality for assessing anatomic and physiologic features of TOF. It provides excellent detail and specific flow data and can quantify

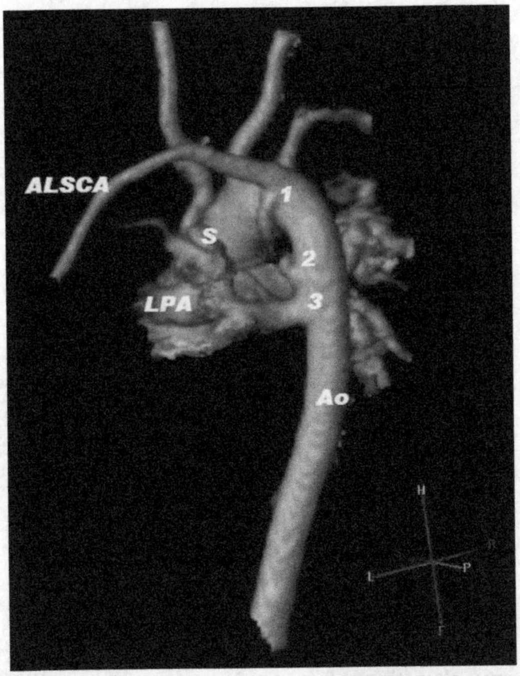

Fig. 86.4 Three-dimensional reconstruction from a gadolinium-enhanced magnetic resonance angiogram in a 2-month-old with TOF/PA status post modified Blalock-Taussig (BT) shunt. This image is viewed from posterior and leftward. It shows the shunt from the left common carotid artery to the pulmonary arteries (S) and three major collaterals *1* from just inferior to the anomalous left subclavian artery, which travels inferior to the arch and rightward; *2* from the leftward aspect of the descending aorta, traveling to the right; and *3* just inferior to 2, traveling to the left (and joining with the left pulmonary artery)

myocardial function and percentage of pulmonary valve regurgitation [30, 31]. It does not expose the patient to ionizing radiation or iodinated contrast, which is important in pediatric patients who may need multiple exams over their lifetime. Most commonly, cMRI is used in TOF to provide follow-up imaging after repair. However, gadolinium-enhanced MR angiography is becoming a critical adjunct to the preoperative workup of TOF patients specifically with branch pulmonary artery anomalies or aortopulmonary collaterals and can function as a 3D "road map" for surgical planning (Fig. 86.4). Because cMRI requires patient cooperation (breath-holding and lying still), pediatric patients often require general anesthesia.

Therapy

Medical Management

Initial medical management is aimed at monitoring and managing hypoxemia and preventing hypercyanotic spells until such time that definitive repair can be performed. A progressive decrease in systemic arterial saturation is usually associated with fixed RVOTO and will not respond to medical intervention. Hypercyanotic spells result from transient reductions in pulmonary blood flow due to a sudden increase in RVOTO and/or a decrease in systemic vascular resistance (SVR). Conditions that predispose to hypercyanotic spells include dehydration, anemia, increased catecholamine levels, acidosis, fever, or anything else that can decrease systemic vascular resistance. In the acute setting, therapy is directed at (1) increasing the total cardiac output by increasing blood volume with fluid administration or blood transfusion administration, (2) treating acidosis with sodium bicarbonate and supplemental oxygen, (3) decreasing the cardiac hyperdynamic state with sedation and intravenous beta-blockers, and (4) increasing systemic vascular resistance with postural changes or intravenous α-agonists (phenylephrine) administration. In rare refractory cases, mechanical ventilation followed by emergent cardiopulmonary bypass and surgical intervention may be required. In patients in whom it is desirable to delay definitive repair, oral beta blockade may be used to decrease myocardial contractility and decrease the dynamic infundibular obstruction. However, clinical response has been variable, and once hypercyanotic spell occur, plan for surgical repair should be made [32].

In neonates with TOF/PA, in which the pulmonary blood flow is dependent upon a patent ductus, ductal patency should be maintained with Prostaglandin E_1, (PGE$_1$) until either complete repair is performed or until a stable source of pulmonary blood flow is established. Patients with TOF/PA often do not have a patent ductus, and the pulmonary blood flow is dependent upon MAPCAS, and PGE$_1$ is not necessary.

Indications for and Timing of Operation

At birth, most patients with TOF have satisfactory systemic arterial oxygen saturation and require no specific intervention. Progression of hypoxemia will ultimately occur, and when the oxygen saturation falls below 75–80 %, operative intervention is recommended. The occurrence of hypoxemic spells is also generally an indication for operation, although in select cases, medical management with propranolol may be used to delay surgery. In patients not meeting specific indications, elective complete repair is generally recommended by 1 year of age and in most centers by 3–6 months of age [33, 34]. Single-stage complete repair can be safely performed and is preferred [35, 36]. However, some surgeons prefer an initial palliative systemic-to-pulmonary artery shunt if the patient becomes cyanotic in early infancy, in order to defer definitive repair until the child is older, usually 6–12 months [37]. A modified Blalock-Taussig (BT) shunt may also be indicated in patients that are cyanotic or are having hypercyanotic episodes but also have concomitant conditions, like intracranial hemorrhage or severe sepsis that contraindicate the use of CPB. Also, the presence of PA, significant branch pulmonary artery hypoplasia, or severe associated noncardiac anomalies has been reported as indication for an initial palliative shunt rather than primary repair. The need for a transannular patch because of significant hypoplasia of the pulmonary valve annulus was formerly considered a contraindication to complete repair in the neonate, but this risk has now been neutralized [38–41].

In the rare case of a symptomatic infant with TOF whose RVOTO is predominantly due to valvular pulmonary stenosis, and a larger operation is contraindicated (e.g., recent intracranial hemorrhage, comorbidities, prematurity), ductal stenting and catheter-based balloon pulmonary valvuloplasty are temporary palliative options [42]. While some have advocated stenting of the right ventricular outflow tract, this maneuver will destroy any possibility of a valve sparing procedure and may complicate the subsequent definitive surgical procedure and should therefore be avoided if possible.

Preoperative Care

Standard cardiac anesthesia practices are generally followed. However, a few important points specific to the care of the patient with TOF should be mentioned. Preoperatively, dehydration should be avoided. NPO status should be minimized as much as possible or the child admitted the night prior to surgery for intravenous hydration if they have a history of significant hypercyanotic spells. It is not uncommon for TOF patients to experience hypercyanotic episodes after induction of anesthesia because of the decrease in SVR associated with anesthetic agents. The patient is also at risk with any alteration of systemic venous return like when the pericardium is tented up to cradle the heart. This risk can be ameliorated with anesthetic choices that maintain SVR and proper intravenous hydration after induction. Should important hypoxemia persist, α-agonist drugs are recommended to increase SVR and minimize the right-to-left shunt. In the rare case of a refractory spell, emergent sternotomy and initiation of cardiopulmonary bypass (CBP) may be required.

Monitoring and Vascular Access

Monitoring lines including arterial and central venous catheters are placed. In patients with TOF/PA and MAPCAs, femoral access should be minimized given their expected future need for repeat groin access for percutaneous interventions. Additional peripheral intravenous lines and a bladder catheter are placed. Nasopharyngeal, cutaneous, and rectal temperature probes are utilized. A transesophageal echocardiogram (TEE) probe is placed after anesthesia is induced. Additional intracardiac lines may be placed at the termination of the procedure as indicated.

Surgical Management

Systemic-to-Pulmonary Shunt Procedures

When an initial systemic-to-pulmonary shunt procedure is chosen as part of a staged repair, the classic or modified form of the BT shunt is most commonly selected [34]. The classic BT shunt is performed on the side opposite the aortic arch (ipsilateral to the innominate artery) in order to allow the most favorable angle for the subclavian artery to reach the pulmonary artery without kinking. In the modified procedure, an interposition polytetrafluoroethylene (PTFE) conduit is placed between the subclavian or innominate and pulmonary arteries [43]. A 3.5 or 4 mm graft is generally preferred because early complete repair may be performed and larger shunts may result in CHF. This procedure is now most often performed through a median sternotomy approach with or without CPB. The results achieved by this procedure have been excellent with an extremely low shunt failure rate and an acceptable duration of palliation [44, 45]. This shunt has the advantage of being able to be performed on either side without regard to anomalies of the aortic arch vessels. However, a right-sided shunt is preferred because of the ease of takedown at the time of complete repair. Takedown of either the modified or the classic form of BT shunt is generally uncomplicated, and pulmonary artery distortion, CHF, and pulmonary artery hypertension are rare with properly performed shunts. In patients with non-confluent branch pulmonary arteries, initial unifocalization procedures may be required, either in combination with palliative shunts or in conjunction with complete repair.

Technique of Complete Repair

Understanding the relevant anatomic details is essential for successful complete repair. Because RVOTO in TOF may be present at multiple levels, a surgical strategy to accurately address

these must be planned. Important factors include size and distribution of the branch pulmonary arteries, the nature and size of the PV annulus (junction between the right ventricle and main pulmonary trunk), extent of the infundibular obstruction, coronary artery distribution, anatomy of the VSD, and the presence of any associated defects. A midline sternotomy incision is performed. The precise location of the coronary artery branches is confirmed, and preparation is made for cardiopulmonary bypass (CPB). Little manipulation of the heart is done in order to avoid precipitating a hypoxemic spell. Existing systemic-to-pulmonary artery shunts are exposed for subsequent takedown. After administration of heparin, the patient is cannulated for CPB. Standard bicaval cannulation is employed for all repairs with mild-to-moderate hypothermia (28–32 °C). The left ventricle is vented through the right superior pulmonary vein.

All shunts are ligated and/or divided, the main pulmonary trunk and bifurcation (if branch stenoses are present) are mobilized, and the PDA is ligated if present. After the aortic cross-clamp is applied and the cardioplegic solution is administered, a right atriotomy is made to assess the anatomy. If an atrial septal defect or patent foramen ovale is present, it is closed at this time. In neonates with a patent foramen ovale only, it is often left open to allow for a limited degree of right-to-left shunting in case right heart pressure is significantly elevated that cardiac output is limited. This may help to maintain the systemic output early after repair, although at the expense of mild systemic desaturation. The anatomy of the VSD and RVOTO is viewed from the tricuspid valve (Fig. 86.5a–e). A retractor placed anteriorly through the tricuspid valve aids in the exposure of the distal outflow tract. When the repair is accomplished entirely through the right atrial approach, the outflow tract obstruction is approached first. Traction sutures placed in the anterior and septal leaflets of the tricuspid valve facilitate exposure of the VSD and distal infundibulum. The position of the anterior margin of the VSD and the aortic valve leaflets are noted, and the parietal extent of the anterosuperiorly

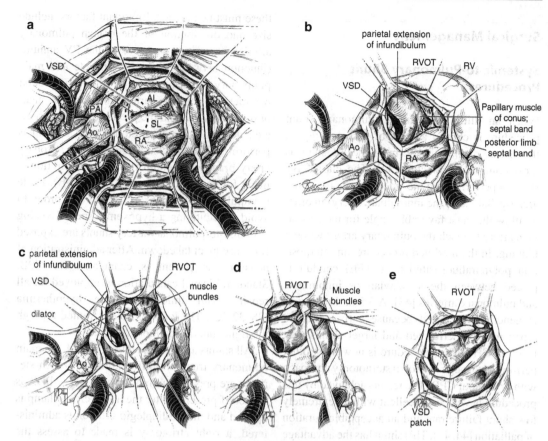

Fig. 86.5 The surgical anatomy as viewed through a right atriotomy. The free edge of the atrial wall is retracted with stay sutures. The location of the VSD is denoted by the dashed line. (**a**) Stay sutures are placed in the septal and anterior leaflets of the TV for retraction. (**b**) The TV leaflets have been retracted and a single valve retractor is placed to aid exposure. The inferior margin of the VSD can be seen superior to the posterior limb of the septal band. (**c**) A dilator placed through the pulmonary annulus delineates the course of the RVOT. The parietal extension of the infundibulum is visible at the tip of the dilator. The parietal extension can be resected at its origin from the infundibular septum, dissected up toward the free wall, and amputated at the free wall. Note: removal of this portion of the outflow tract is not performed routinely. (**d**) Division of the obstructing muscle bundles along the anterior limb of the septal band. Division of these muscle bundles is usually sufficient to relieve the outflow tract obstruction when repair is performed in infancy (see text for details). (**e**) View through the right atriotomy and TV following patch closure of the VSD. The ends of the divided muscle bundles can be visualized. *AL, SL* anterior leaflet, septal leaflet of TV, *TV* tricuspid valve, *Ao* aorta, *PA* pulmonary artery, *RA* right atrium, *RV* right ventricle, *RVOT* right ventricular outflow tract (From Hirsch and Bove [89])

malpositioned infundibular septum is visualized [46–49]. Invaginating the right ventricular free wall with a finger placed from outside the heart facilitates this exposure. Muscle trabeculations along the anterior limb of the septal band are divided down to the level of the moderator band if necessary. The moderator band should be spared regardless of the approach. When repair is performed in infancy, excision of the parietal extent of the infundibular septum is almost never necessary and simple division of the obstructing muscle bundles is all that is required. A pulmonary valvotomy can now be performed through the right atrial approach. If exposure is not adequate, a vertical incision is made in the main pulmonary artery through which a pulmonary valvotomy may be performed [50, 51]. Valve leaflets may be mobilized and

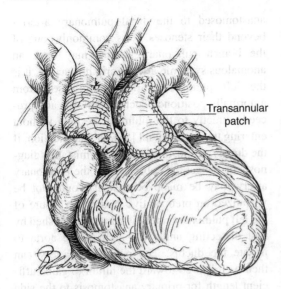

Transannular patch

Fig. 86.6 The appearance of a transannular patch used to enlarge a hypoplastic PV annulus and main pulmonary trunk. The patch extends onto the origin of the left pulmonary artery as well. The proximal extent of the patch on the RVOT should be kept to as short as possible (From Hirschand Bove [89])

fused commissures divided all the way to the pulmonary artery wall. At this time, an assessment of the diameter of the PV annulus is made by inserting calibrated dilators across the PV. In select patients (no unicusp valve, PV z-score > -3), a valve-preserving technique is an option. PV commissurotomy may be followed by high-pressure balloon dilation of the pulmonary valve annulus after complete relief of RVOTO. Early results are encouraging [52].

The decision to place a transannular patch is made if the estimated post-repair RV/LV pressure ratio is predicted to exceed 0.7 [53–55]. In this situation, the main pulmonary artery incision is extended onto the RVOT across the PV annulus (Fig. 86.6). It can be kept quite short, extending only a few millimeters proximal to the annulus, as the infundibular obstruction has been adequately relieved transatrially. Whenever possible, this incision is placed directly through the anterior commissure of the valve to allow the pulmonary valve leaflets to remain functional and decrease the amount of pulmonary regurgitation. It is often possible to limit the incision such that it remains superior to an anomalous LAD when a transatrial repair is done.

Closure of the VSD is accomplished from the transatrial approach regardless of whether or not a transannular patch is needed, as that allows the ventricular extent of the incision to be minimized to the length necessary only for relief of obstruction, not for VSD exposure [56]. Visualization of the VSD is generally adequate through the tricuspid valve and is facilitated by dividing the obstructing right ventricular muscle bundles first. A patch of PTFE is cut to the appropriate size and sutured to the right side of the septum utilizing a continuous-suture technique. Suturing is commenced at the angle between the anterior and posterior limbs of the septal band, directly opposite the perimembranous rim, and begun superiorly over the infundibular septum and aortic valve. The sutures are kept close to the aortic valve annulus itself to avoid residual defects in muscle trabeculations. This initial arm of the suture is brought into the right atrium by passing the needle through the annulus of the tricuspid valve at its junction with the ventriculo-infundibular fold. The other needle is then brought inferiorly, past the medial papillary muscle, and under any chordae tendineae from the septal leaflet, until the posteroinferior rim of the defect is reached. At this point, suturing is done approximately 5 mm away from the crest of the VSD itself and only on the right ventricular side in order to avoid the A-V node or bundle of His which penetrate the floor of the atrial septum in the apex of the triangle of Koch and pass adjacent to this margin of the VSD. Attaching the patch to the base of the septal leaflet of the tricuspid valve over the penetrating bundle completes suturing.

After the operation is complete and the patient is separated from CPB, transesophageal echocardiography is performed to identify residual defects and adequacy of repair. The peak RV/LV pressure ratio is measured to ensure that significant residual RVOTO does not persist. If the post-repair RV/LV pressure is in excess of 0.7 and a transannular patch has not been placed, bypass is resumed and a patch is inserted across the PV annulus. If a transannular patch has been placed, other causes of persistent elevation of right ventricular pressure must be considered, including branch pulmonary artery stenosis, hypoplastic peripheral pulmonary arteries, residual VSD, or residual infundibular obstruction. Often, this elevation in right ventricular pressure can result from dynamic RVOTO, particularly when an outflow patch is avoided, as in the case of a transatrial repair. Administration of an ultrashort-acting beta-blocking agent such as esmolol can help to differentiate dynamic versus fixed residual right ventricular outflow tract obstruction intraoperatively.

Special Circumstances: Pulmonary Artery Abnormalities

Stenosis of the origin of the left and/or right pulmonary arteries is frequently encountered in patients with TOF, and additional imaging may be necessary to detect its presence if not otherwise visualized by echocardiography. Left pulmonary artery stenosis is best augmented with placement of a separate patch. Simple extension of the RVOT patch onto the left pulmonary artery can cause flow disturbances as well as distortion of the left pulmonary artery takeoff due to the acute posterior course of the vessel [41]. Stenosis at the origin of the right pulmonary artery is more difficult to repair because of the right angle that this vessel takes from the main pulmonary artery and the more difficult exposure resulting from the overlying ascending aorta. Although transection of the aorta can be done to improve exposure, mobilization alone is generally adequate. In this situation, a separate patch may be necessary to enlarge the proximal right pulmonary artery. Alternatively, resection of the stenotic area, if it is relatively localized, with end-to-end anastomosis may also provide good results. This technique may also be used for the left pulmonary artery. Bifurcation stenoses involving both pulmonary artery origins may be repaired with a resection and end-to-end anastomoses of both pulmonary arteries. Alternatively, each branch of a bifurcated pulmonary artery allograft may be anastomosed to the distal pulmonary arteries beyond their stenoses. Less commonly, one of the branch pulmonary arteries may have an anomalous systemic arterial origin. Usually, it is the left pulmonary artery that arises from a normally positioned ductus arteriosus and proceeds directly to the hilum of the lung without entering the pericardium [57]. In this situation, if the ductus arteriosus has closed, a mistaken diagnosis of congenital "absence" of the pulmonary artery may be made because it would not be visualized on preoperative studies. Exposure of the left pulmonary artery is best accomplished by first dissecting under the arch of the aorta to isolate the ductus. The pulmonary artery can then be followed toward the hilum to gain sufficient length for primary anastomosis to the side of the main pulmonary artery trunk. When the right pulmonary artery is not in continuity with the left, it is likely to originate from a right-sided ductus off the innominate artery. Rarely, it may take origin from the descending aorta. When the branch pulmonary arteries are non-confluent, or confluent but with a significant stenosis centrally (usually at the insertion of the ductus itself), reconstruction of the central pulmonary artery bifurcation is required, using one or more of the techniques outlined is preferred in order to provide symmetric pulmonary blood flow. This is best combined with complete intracardiac repair, although placing a shunt to the reconstructed pulmonary arteries may also be done [57].

Hypoplastic Pulmonary Arteries

Significant pulmonary artery hypoplasia occurs uncommonly in patients with TOF and pulmonary stenosis [58]. It may be considered to be present when the McGoon ratio (the diameter of the right pulmonary artery plus that of the left divided by the diameter of the descending aorta at the level of the diaphragm) is below 1.2 [26]. This corresponds to a Nakata index of approximately 70 [59]. However, hypoplasia in this setting is most likely to be a result of underperfusion of the pulmonary arteries, and prompt enlargement can be expected when pressure and flow are restored [60].

This may not be the situation with TOF/PA, in which case the hypoplasia is more likely to be due to fixed peripheral arterial stenoses and/or arborization anomalies, and may not respond to the usual palliative or reparative procedures [28]. If after correction of TOF in the setting of hypoplastic pulmonary arteries the intraoperative right ventricular pressure equals or exceeds that of the left ventricle, CPB should be resumed and a large, nonrestrictive perforation should be created in the VSD patch. Closure of this residual defect may then be considered at a later date, particularly if sufficient pulmonary artery growth occurs as indicated by the development of a net left-to-right shunt.

Pulmonary Atresia with Multiple Aortopulmonary Collateral Arteries

Patients with pulmonary atresia and diminutive main pulmonary arteries with or without multiple aortopulmonary collateral arteries (MAPCAs) are a heterogeneous and difficult operative challenge. These patients often have peripheral pulmonary artery stenoses and abnormal pulmonary vascular arborization which further complicate operative planning. The potential for complete repair and long-term survival is dependent upon the size and distribution of the pulmonary arteries [25, 61]. Overall, the operative mortality is greater in this population as a result of the complexity. In addition, many of these patients require palliative procedures either prior to or *in lieu* of repair. The goal is to provide physiologic flow (volume and pressure) to the greatest number of pulmonary segments to maximize normal development of the peripheral vasculature along with minimal pressure overload. The management of this problem continues to be debated. Initial therapy can be provided with a systemic-to-pulmonary artery shunt with delayed repair, placement of a right ventricle to pulmonary artery conduit to increase flow to the main pulmonary arteries with delayed complete repair, or unifocalization of MAPCAs to the central pulmonary vasculature with simultaneous complete repair. All of these have unique positive and negative aspects depending on the individual patient's anatomy. Placement of a right ventricle to pulmonary artery transannular patch or conduit when central pulmonary arteries are present, even if extremely diminutive in size, by 3–6 months of age aims to increase pulmonary blood flow and stimulate growth of the central pulmonary arteries. Alternatively, a systemic-to-pulmonary shunt may be utilized. Unifocalization is delayed unless MAPCAs are clearly demonstrated to provide the sole blood supply to major areas of the lung and are severely stenotic and at risk of thrombosis. Establishing antegrade pulmonary blood flow with a transannular patch or conduit will allow better evaluation of dual blood supply from MAPCAs at subsequent catheterization and may minimize or eliminate the need for unifocalization in some patients. The use of a non-valved conduit with the resultant pulmonary regurgitation can be of benefit by stimulating pulmonary artery growth from the increased stroke volume. The frequent presence of peripheral pulmonary artery stenoses protects the distal vasculature from high pressures, but this must be carefully evaluated in each patient as some segments may be free of obstruction and would then be at risk of developing pulmonary vascular obstructive disease. Complete repair then follows with coil occlusion or incorporation of MAPCAs as appropriate. A pulmonary or aortic allograft or valved xenograft (Contegra®, Medtronics, Minneapolis, MN) generally is preferred to porcine heterografts in view of their improved handling characteristics, lower transvalvular gradients, and greater longevity [62]. However, if postoperative pulmonary artery pressure is predicted to be significantly elevated, a porcine valved heterograft is preferred to ensure a competent pulmonary valve after repair.

Tetralogy of Fallot with Absent Pulmonary Valve

In this condition, which occurs in approximately 5 % of patients with TOF, the pulmonary valve leaflets are absent, resulting in pulmonary regurgitation [21]. A ductus arteriosus is most often absent. In approximately one half of the patients

Fig. 86.7 Axial oblique minimum intensity projection from turbo spin echo black blood imaging MRI of a 5-year-old boy with TOF-absent PV s/p repair with RV-PA conduit. Shown are severely dilated branch PAs and narrowed left mainstem bronchus (LMS)

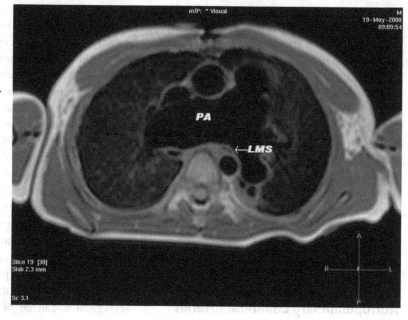

born with this condition, the pulmonary regurgitation results in aneurysmal dilatation of the central pulmonary arteries and obstruction of the tracheobronchial tree (Fig. 86.7). These infants may present with severe respiratory insufficiency from airway compression [20]. Many of these infants require preoperative mechanical ventilation, often in the prone position, and occasionally extracorporeal membrane oxygenation (ECMO). Urgent operative intervention is often required. Although a variety of techniques have been proposed over the years, most centers prefer complete intracardiac repair with the insertion of a valved conduit to restore pulmonary valve competence [63]. The aneurysmal right and left pulmonary arteries are plicated to reduce their diameter and relieve compression of the distal trachea, right and left mainstem bronchi. Alternatively, after intracardiac repair, the pulmonary arteries may be translocated anterior to the aorta in order to reduce compression on the trachea and bronchi. In this technique, a transverse aortotomy is performed above the commissures and a short segment of aorta resected to bring the aorta down and to the left. The PA is transected above the annulus and brought anterior to the aorta. End-to-end

anastomosis of the aorta is followed by direct anastomosis of the PA to the RVOT. Plication of the PA is done as necessary [64, 65].

For those patients not presenting with severe respiratory compromise early in infancy, elective repair can be accomplished by 6 months of age. The insertion of a competent pulmonary valve may not be necessary in this group but is still preferred by some. The mortality for surgical repair of this lesion remains significant primarily due to airway issues. Spray et al. reported an early mortality rate of 21.4 %, with a 1-year survival of 77 % and 10-year survival of 71 %. Preoperative mechanical ventilation was associated with a significantly poorer outcome [66].

Tetralogy of Fallot with Complete Atrioventricular Septal Defect

Complete atrioventricular septal defect (CAVSD) occurs in approximately 2 % of patients with TOF and is more common in patients with Down syndrome. The anatomy is that of the typical AVSD although the left anterior bridging leaflet is always undivided and unattached to the crest of the ventricular septum (Rastelli type "C"). There is anterosuperior displacement of the infundibular septum such that the VSD has a large outlet component in addition to the inlet portion associated with the CAVSD. The aortic valve overrides the outlet component of the VSD. The RVOTO is the same as that for isolated TOF. The repair is complicated by the increased difficulty of placing an intraventricular patch without causing left ventricular outflow tract obstruction or atrioventricular valve regurgitation. Marked overriding of the aortic valve makes this more difficult as exposure is not easily obtained via the atrial approach. Although some authors have advocated a combined atrial and right ventricular approach, this is unnecessary except in rare circumstances [67, 68].

Postoperative and Critical Care

Routine Postoperative Management

A typical postoperative course for neonates and infants undergoing repair of TOF is uneventful. Careful monitoring of tissue perfusion, gas exchange, and urine output may be facilitated by measurement of mixed venous oxygen saturation, serum lactate levels, and near infrared spectroscopy (NIRS). Using these data, inotropic, lusitropic, and vasodilator therapy can be titrated in patients who require it postoperatively. Unless there is significant cardiac dysfunction or arrhythmia postoperatively, the majority of children undergoing complete TOF repair are extubated within 24 h of surgery.

Management of Postoperative Complications: Low Cardiac Output Syndrome

Although most children undergoing TOF repair have a short ICU stay including early extubation, some patients will experience low cardiac output syndrome (LCOS) and may require prolonged inotropic support. Seen in approximately 25 % of infants with congenital heart disease who have any type of cardiac surgery, LCOS is characterized by signs of decreased systemic perfusion and

is a risk factor for increased length of stay and postoperative morbidity and mortality [69–71]. Typically, LCOS presents as tachycardia, oliguria, and metabolic acidosis. Among patients undergoing repair of TOF, approximately 1/3 will experience LCOS due to RV diastolic dysfunction or "restrictive RV physiology" [70]. Preoperative RV hypertrophy, myocardial injury, and edema after right ventriculotomy all decrease right ventricular compliance and result in diastolic dysfunction. Arrhythmias, residual anatomic lesions such as VSD, RVOTO, tricuspid regurgitation, and pulmonary insufficiency (PI) may also add to the cardiopulmonary dysfunction. In postoperative patients with LCOS, repeat bedside echocardiography is useful to rule out clinically significant residual anatomic lesions. Children with RV diastolic dysfunction require elevated RA pressures for adequate RV filling in diastole. Without an atrial-level communication, this situation leads to high central venous pressure, which can cause hepatic congestion, oliguria, ascites, and pleural effusions [70]. Decreased RV filling leads to decreased LV preload and resultant low cardiac output. An atrial fenestration can decompress the right atrium via a right-to-left shunt, which can help augment cardiac output, albeit at the expense of lower oxygen saturation.

Cullen et al. [70] showed that in patients with RV diastolic dysfunction, the noncompliant RV acts more like a passive conduit than a compliant chamber and results in antegrade diastolic flow into the pulmonary arteries during atrial systole. This flow pattern, though abnormal, is an important contributor to cardiac output in these patients. They also note that cardiac output is adversely affected by both the loss of sinus rhythm and the inspiratory phase of mechanical ventilation [70]. These findings have important implications for postoperative management. In particular, maintenance of low mean airway pressures and early (within 24 h of ICU admission) extubation should be goals. Use of temporary pacing is recommended if there is a loss of AV synchrony. The management of LCOS may also require inotropic support with dopamine, epinephrine, and milrinone infusions and sedation and neuromuscular blockade in refractory cases. In patients with severe right-sided failure, mechanical ventilation strategies to maintain a slightly alkalotic pH and the use of pulmonary vasodilators may prove beneficial in selected cases by relieving the dysfunctional RV afterload and by optimizing filling of the left ventricle and therefore systemic stroke volume.

Junctional Ectopic Tachycardia

Junctional ectopic tachycardia (JET) is a rapid, catecholamine-sensitive, and self-limited arrhythmia that occurs in 4–22 % of patients following TOF repair [72, 73]. The onset is typically within the first 24 h postoperatively. The management of JET includes correction of electrolyte derangements, sedation, limiting catecholaminergic drugs and endogenous catecholamines, systemic cooling to 34–35 °C, and amiodarone infusion with temporary epicardial pacing as necessary. In a randomized clinical trial, intravenous magnesium given on cardiopulmonary bypass during rewarming decreased the incidence of postoperative JET compared to placebo in congenital heart surgery patients, including those with TOF [74].

Outcomes

The early (hospital) mortality after repair of TOF is currently between 1 % and 5 % in most reported series [26, 75, 76]. Results of repair of TOF in neonates have improved dramatically over time. A review of TOF repair from 1973 to 1988 showed an early mortality rate of 18.5 % [35]. A 26-year retrospective review demonstrated a decrease in mortality following primary repair of TOF across all age groups from 11.1 % before 1990 to 2.1 % after 1990 [77]. A more recent review of neonates and infants undergoing complete repair from 1993 to 2010 demonstrated a very low early mortality of 4.3 % [75]. These data suggest that early repair has no increased operative mortality in the modern era.

Reoperation

For patients undergoing complete repair in the first month of life, 1-month, 1-year, and 5-year freedom from reoperation was 100 %, 89 %, and 58 %, respectively [75]. Most common indications for reoperation are residual or recurrent VSD, recurrent RVOT obstruction or aneurysm formation, conduit failure, and severe PI or PS [68, 75, 78, 79].

In the case of residual VSD, even relatively small residual defects are poorly tolerated after TOF repair, and reoperation is recommended when the pulmonary-to-systemic flow ratio exceeds 1.5. The most common location for a residual VSD is at the posteroinferior margin of the patch, presumably because suturing in this area is done superficially to avoid heart block. Other sites of residual VSD are at the superior aspect where the ventricular infundibular fold can sometimes be mistaken for the superior aspect of the VSD.

The exact amount of residual RV outflow tract obstruction required for reoperation is controversial, but an immediate post-op RV/LV pressure ratio of 0.75 is an independent risk factor for reoperation [41]. In this situation, either incision or resection of additional muscle bundles or placement of a transannular patch repair is indicated. Overall survival and functional status following reoperation is very good with a 10-year actuarial survival of 92 % with 93 % of these patients in a New York Heart Association classification of I or II [68]. The incidence of complete heart block following TOF repair requiring permanent pacemaker is less than 1 %.

Effect of Pulmonary Insufficiency

Long-standing PI is associated with significant complications after the second postoperative decade. These include exercise intolerance, right heart failure, arrhythmia, and sudden death [80, 81]. Two recent large studies of patients 30 years after TOF repair revealed that the annualized risk of death more than triples during the third postoperative decade (increasing from .27 % to .95 %) [78, 79]. The observation that pulmonary valve replacement (PVR) in symptomatic patients late after TOF repair did not necessarily lead to functional recovery has supported replacement of the pulmonary valve before the onset of symptoms in many cases [82].

Timing of Reoperation for Pulmonary Valve Replacement

The indications for pulmonary valve replacement in the absence of symptoms of exercise intolerance or congestive heart failure are not well defined, but this procedure should be considered in the presence of right ventricular systolic dysfunction, tricuspid insufficiency, and progressive right ventricular dilatation. Early reoperation for asymptomatic RV dysfunction improves the chance of full recovery of ventricular function, increases submaximal exercise capacity, as well as decreases the prevalence of ventricular arrhythmias [83, 84]. A review of patients undergoing elective PVR has demonstrated that the operative risk was low (1.1 %) and functional status was NYHA I for 90 % of patients following repair with a 10-year survival of 95 % [85]. Advances in cardiac imaging have demonstrated the deleterious effects of RV remodeling secondary to PI, and cMRI is now the standard modality for assessing RV size and function. High-risk cMRI parameters include a preoperative RVEDV z-score >7 (=172 mL/m^2 in women and 185 mL/m^2 in men), RVEF <45 %, and LVEF <55 % [86]. It should be noted that most of the echo- and CMR-derived indicators for reintervention have been in adult-sized patients. There are not universally agreed indications derived imaging studies from growing children.

Indications for pulmonary valve replacement continue to evolve. Generally agreed upon indications are shown in Table 86.1. The timing of pulmonary valve replacement must weigh the risk of operating too early which may subject the patient to repeat interventions versus the risk of waiting too long to offload a failing right ventricle. At most major institutions, cMRI in

Table 86.1 Indications for pulmonary valve replacement after TOF repair

Attributable symptoms or signs:
Exertional dyspnea
Exercise intolerance
Heart failure
Syncope
Symptomatic or sustained arrhythmias related to right heart enlargement and severe PR
Asymptomatic patients with:
Decline in functional aerobic capacity (maximum VO2) on exercise testing to <70 % of gender-age predicted or a decline >20 % compared with serial testing
Progressive RV enlargement and/or dysfunction noted on serial imaging studies:
Cardiothoracic ratio on CXR
Echocardiogram
Cardiac MRI (CMR)
RV EF < 40 %
Moderate or severe TR related to long-standing PR
TOF patients with moderate or severe PR (regurgitation fraction ≥25 % measured by CMR) and coexisting cardiac lesions requiring surgical intervention such as:
Significant residual ASD or VSD
Severe aortic regurgitation
RVOT obstruction (RVSP ≥ 2/3 systemic)
Ventricular arrhythmia prevention
QRS ≥ 180 ms
QRS prolongation > 3.5 ms/y
RV volume criteria
RV end diastolic volume index between 150 mL/m^2 and 170 mL/m^2
RV end systolic volume index ≥ 85 mL/m^2
Moderate to severe PR and 2 or more of
RVEDV index ≥ 160 mL/m^2 (z-score > 5)
RVESV index ≥ 70 mL/m^2
LVEDV index ≤ 65 mL/m^2
RVEF < 40 %
RVOT aneurysm

Adapted from Geva [90] and [91]

conjunction with echocardiography are the standard surveillance imaging modalities in patients with repaired TOF. Cardiac MRI provides accurate data regarding biventricular size and function as well as flow measurements and practical quantification of pulmonary regurgitation volume (Fig. 86.8a, b). Not dependent on acoustic windows, cMRI gives detailed anatomic information without the use of ionizing radiation.

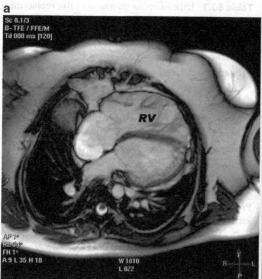
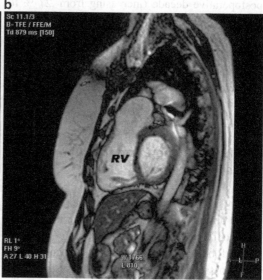

Fig. 86.8 (a) Axial cMRI image of a 36-year-old woman with repaired TOF with a transannular patch. RV is severely dilated (RVEDV 180 ml/m², z-score +7.6), with low-normal to mildly depressed systolic function (RVEF 50 %). The LV is mildly depressed with an EF of 52 %. (b) Sagittal cMRI image of the same patient. The RVOT is dilated, with free PI, which was severe by volume (regurgitant fraction 50 %)

Role of Percutaneous Pulmonary Valve Insertion

Percutaneous PVR now offers patients with repaired TOF a low-risk alternative to open PVR in patients that have had a RV-PA conduit placed either at the initial TOF repair or at subsequent reoperation. The currently available devices have been approved only for such patients in whom the conduit measured between 14 and 22 mm at the time of implant [87] (Fig. 86.9a, b). In patients that have either their native outflow tract or have had a transannular patch, surgically placed valve is indicated.

Mortality for the transcatheter valve implant is reported as less than 0.3 % in recent studies [87]. Early freedom from reintervention is also favorable at 95.4 % at 1 year and 87.6 % at 2 years [88]. As with surgical intervention, early results show a decrease in RVEDV, improved effective RV and LV stroke volume, as well as improvement in New York Heart Association class [87, 88]. Long-term outcome on biventricular function remains to be seen. Typically, PI is resolved after percutaneous PVR. However, there are

risks associated with the procedure including stent fracture, conduit rupture, and coronary artery compression. Stent fracture and recurrent or residual RVOTO are among the most common reasons for reintervention [87, 88]. When choosing a valve in the operating room during initial TOF repair or subsequent PVR, consideration should be given to the possibility of future catheter-based PVR. Further details about this technique are exhaustively discussed in a specific chapter elsewhere in this textbook.

Conclusion

Tetralogy of Fallot is one of the most common congenital heart lesions. Early surgical efforts with this defect are the foundation of the entire field of congenital cardiac surgery. Most programs have adopted early primary repair for TOF, and the outcomes are excellent. The management of the freshly repaired TOF patient has many nuances, but convalescence is generally predictable. While initially it was believed that complete repair for this defect was curative, it is

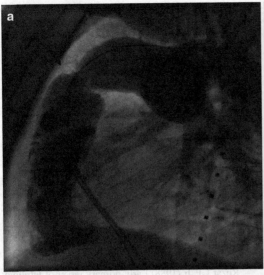 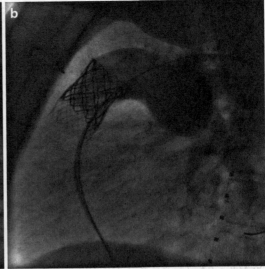

Fig. 86.9 (a) Lateral angiogram injecting contrast into the pulmonary homograft conduit. The conduit valve appears mildly stenotic, and the branch pulmonary arteries are dilated. (b) Lateral angiogram after placement of Melody® transcatheter pulmonary valve (TPV) injecting contrast into the MPA showing a widely patent Melody® TPV and trivial insufficiency with stiff wire and catheter across the valve

now known that many patients will require additional surgical and medical management within their lifetimes.

References

1. Eldadah ZA, Hamosh A, Biery NJ, Montgomery RA, Duke M, Elkins R, Dietz HC (2001) Familial tetralogy of Fallot caused by mutation in the jagged1 gene. Hum Mol Genet 10:163–169
2. Goldmuntz E, Geiger E, Benson DW (2001) NKX2.5 mutations in patients with tetralogy of Fallot. Circulation 104:2565–2568
3. Fallot ÉLA (1988) Contribution à l'anatomie pathologique de la maladie bleue (cyanose cardiaque). n.p.
4. Blalock A, Taussig HB (1945) The surgical treatment of malformation of the heart in which there is pulmonary stenosis or pulmonary atresia. JAMA 128:189
5. Potts WJ, Smith S, Gibson S (1946) Anastomosis of the aorta to a pulmonary artery; certain types in congenital heart disease. J Am Med Assoc 132:627–631
6. Waterston DJ (1962) Treatment of Fallot's tetralogy in children under 1 year of age. Rozhl Chir 41:181–183
7. Lillehei CW, Cohen M, Warden HE, Read RC, Aust JB, Dewall RA, Varco RL (1955) Direct vision intracardiac surgical correction of the tetralogy of Fallot, pentalogy of Fallot, and pulmonary atresia defects; report of first ten cases. Ann Surg 142:418–442
8. Kirklin JW, Dushane JW, Patrick RT, Donald DE, Hetzel PS, Harshbarger HG, Wood EH (1955) Intracardiac surgery with the aid of a mechanical pump-oxygenator system (gibbon type): report of eight cases. Proc Staff Meet Mayo Clin 30:201–206
9. Bacha EA, Scheule AM, Zurakowski D, Erickson LC, Hung J, Lang P, Mayer JE Jr, del Nido PJ, Jonas RA (2001) Long-term results after early primary repair of tetralogy of Fallot. J Thorac Cardiovasc Surg 122:154–161
10. Lindberg HL, Saatvedt K, Seem E, Hoel T, Birkeland S (2011) Single-center 50 years' experience with surgical management of tetralogy of Fallot. Eur J Cardiothorac Surg 40:538–542
11. Van Praagh R, Van Praagh S, Nebesar RA, Muster AJ, Sinha SN, Paul MH (1970) Tetralogy of Fallot: underdevelopment of the pulmonary infundibulum and its sequelae. Am J Cardiol 26:25–33
12. Suzuki A, Ho SY, Anderson RH, Deanfield JE (1990) Further morphologic studies on tetralogy of Fallot, with particular emphasis on the prevalence and structure of the membranous flap. J Thorac Cardiovasc Surg 99:528–535
13. Dickinson DF, Wilkinson JL, Smith A, Hamilton DI, Anderson RH (1982) Variations in the morphology of the ventricular septal defect and disposition of the atrioventricular conduction tissues in tetralogy of Fallot. Thorac Cardiovasc Surg 30:243–249
14. Kurosawa H, Imai Y (1988) Surgical anatomy of the atrioventricular conduction bundle in tetralogy of Fallot. New findings relevant to the position of the sutures. J Thorac Cardiovasc Surg 95:586–591

15. Anderson RH, Allwork SP, Ho SY, Lenox CC, Zuberbuhler JR (1981) Surgical anatomy of tetralogy of Fallot. J Thorac Cardiovasc Surg 81:887–896

16. Vargas FJ, Kreutzer GO, Pedrini M, Capelli H, Rodriguez CA (1986) Tetralogy of Fallot with subarterial ventricular septal defect. Diagnostic and surgical considerations. J Thorac Cardiovasc Surg 92:908–912

17. Altrichter PM, Olson LJ, Edwards WD, Puga FJ, Danielson GK (1989) Surgical pathology of the pulmonary valve: a study of 116 cases spanning 15 years. Mayo Clin Proc 64:1352–1360

18. Shimazaki Y, Blackstone EH, Kirklin JW (1984) The natural history of isolated congenital pulmonary valve incompetence: surgical implications. Thorac Cardiovasc Surg 32:257–259

19. Chiariello L, Meyer J, Wukasch DC, Hallman GL, Cooley DA (1975) Intracardiac repair of tetralogy of Fallot. Five-year review of 403 patients. J Thorac Cardiovasc Surg 70:529–535

20. Miller RA, Lev M, Paul MH (1962) Congenital absence of the pulmonary valve. The clinical syndrome of tetralogy of Fallot with pulmonary regurgitation. Circulation 26:266–278

21. Bove EL, Shaher RM, Alley R, McKneally M (1972) Tetralogy of Fallot with absent pulmonary valve and aneurysm of the pulmonary artery: report of two cases presenting as obstructive lung disease. J Pediatr 81:339–343

22. Humes RA, Driscoll DJ, Danielson GK, Puga FJ (1987) Tetralogy of Fallot with anomalous origin of left anterior descending coronary artery. Surgical options. J Thorac Cardiovasc Surg 94:784–787

23. Boon AR, Farmer MB, Roberts DF (1972) A family study of Fallot's tetralogy. J Med Genet 9:179–192

24. Di Felice V, Zummo G (2009) Tetralogy of Fallot as a model to study cardiac progenitor cell migration and differentiation during heart development. Trends Cardiovasc Med 19:130–135

25. Kirklin JW, Barratt-Boyes BG (1993) Cardiac surgery: morphology, diagnostic criteria, natural history, techniques, results, and indications. Churchill Livingstone, New York

26. Groh MA, Meliones JN, Bove EL, Kirklin JW, Blackstone EH, Lupinetti FM, Snider AR, Rosenthal A (1991) Repair of tetralogy of Fallot in infancy. Effect of pulmonary artery size on outcome. Circulation 84: III206–III212

27. Ramsay JM, Macartney FJ, Haworth SG (1985) Tetralogy of Fallot with major aortopulmonary collateral arteries. Br Heart J 53:167–172

28. Shimazaki Y, Maehara T, Blackstone EH, Kirklin JW, Bargeron LM Jr (1988) The structure of the pulmonary circulation in tetralogy of Fallot with pulmonary atresia. A quantitative cineangiographic study. J Thorac Cardiovasc Surg 95:1048–1058

29. McConnell ME (1990) Echocardiography in classical tetralogy of Fallot. Semin Thorac Cardiovasc Surg 2:2–11

30. Norton KI, Tong C, Glass RB, Nielsen JC (2006) Cardiac MR imaging assessment following tetralogy of Fallot repair. Radiographics 26:197–211

31. Chung T (2000) Assessment of cardiovascular anatomy in patients with congenital heart disease by magnetic resonance imaging. Pediatr Cardiol 21:18–26

32. Garson A Jr, Gillette PC, McNamara DG (1981) Propranolol: the preferred palliation for tetralogy of Fallot. Am J Cardiol 47:1098–1104

33. Castaneda AR, Freed MD, Williams RG, Norwood WI (1977) Repair of tetralogy of Fallot in infancy. Early and late results. J Thorac Cardiovasc Surg 74:372–381

34. Castaneda AR (1990) Classical repair of tetralogy of Fallot: timing, technique, and results. Semin Thorac Cardiovasc Surg 2:70–75

35. Di Donato RM, Jonas RA, Lang P, Rome JJ, Mayer JE Jr, Castaneda AR (1991) Neonatal repair of tetralogy of Fallot with and without pulmonary atresia. J Thorac Cardiovasc Surg 101:126–137

36. Gustafson RA, Murray GF, Warden HE, Hill RC, Rozar GE Jr (1988) Early primary repair of tetralogy of Fallot. Ann Thorac Surg 45:235–241

37. Karl TR, Sano S, Pornviliwan S, Mee RB (1992) Tetralogy of Fallot: favorable outcome of nonneonatal transatrial, transpulmonary repair. Ann Thorac Surg 54:903–907

38. Kirklin JK, Kirklin JW, Blackstone EH, Milano A, Pacifico AD (1989) Effect of transannular patching on outcome after repair of tetralogy of Fallot. Ann Thorac Surg 48:783–791

39. Kirklin JW, Blackstone EH, Jonas RA, Shimazaki Y, Kirklin JK, Mayer JE Jr, Pacifico AD, Castaneda AR (1992) Morphologic and surgical determinants of outcome events after repair of tetralogy of Fallot and pulmonary stenosis. A two-institution study. J Thorac Cardiovasc Surg 103:706–723

40. Kirklin JW, Blackstone EH, Kirklin JK, Pacifico AD, Aramendi J, Bargeron LM Jr (1983) Surgical results and protocols in the spectrum of tetralogy of Fallot. Ann Surg 198:251–265

41. Hennein HA, Mosca RS, Urcelay G, Crowley DC, Bove EL (1995) Intermediate results after complete repair of tetralogy of Fallot in neonates. J Thorac Cardiovasc Surg 109:332–342, 344, discussion 342–333

42. Remadevi KS, Vaidyanathan B, Francis E, Kannan BR, Kumar RK (2008) Balloon pulmonary valvotomy as interim palliation for symptomatic young infants with tetralogy of Fallot. Ann Pediatr Cardiol 1:2–7

43. Di Benedetto G, Tiraboschi R, Vanini V, Annecchino P, Aiazzi L, Caprioli C, Parenzan L (1981) Systemic-pulmonary artery shunt using PTFE prosthesis (Gore-Tex). Early results and long-term follow-up on 105 consecutive cases. Thorac Cardiovasc Surg 29:143–147

44. Bove EL, Kohman L, Sereika S, Byrum CJ, Kavey RE, Blackman MS, Sondheimer HM, Rosenthal A (1987) The modified Blalock-Taussig shunt: analysis of adequacy and duration of palliation. Circulation 76: III19–III23

45. McKay R, de Leval MR, Rees P, Taylor JF, Macartney FJ, Stark J (1980) Postoperative angiographic assessment of modified Blalock-Taussig shunts using expanded polytetrafluoroethylene (Gore-Tex). Ann Thorac Surg 30:137–145

46. Pacifico AD, Sand ME, Bargeron LM Jr, Colvin EC (1987) Transatrial-transpulmonary repair of tetralogy of Fallot. J Thorac Cardiovasc Surg 93:919–924

47. Binet JP (1988) Correction of tetralogy of Fallot with combined transatrial and pulmonary approach: experience with 184 consecutive cases. J Card Surg 3:97–102

48. Edmunds LH Jr, Saxena NC, Friedman S, Rashkind WJ, Dodd PF (1976) Transatrial repair of tetralogy of Fallot. Surgery 80:681–688

49. Dietl CA, Torres AR, Cazzaniga ME, Favaloro RG (1989) Right atrial approach for surgical correction of tetralogy of Fallot. Ann Thorac Surg 47:546–551; discussion 551–542

50. Pacifico AD, Kirklin JK, Colvin EV, McConnell ME, Kirklin JW (1990) Transatrial-transpulmonary repair of tetralogy of Fallot. Semin Thorac Cardiovasc Surg 2:76–82

51. Coles JG, Kirklin JW, Pacifico AD, Kirklin JK, Blackstone EH (1988) The relief of pulmonary stenosis by a transatrial versus a transventricular approach to the repair of tetralogy of Fallot. Ann Thorac Surg 45:7–10

52. Vida VL, Padalino MA, Maschietto N, Biffanti R, Anderson RH, Milanesi O, Stellin G (2012) The balloon dilation of the pulmonary valve during early repair of tetralogy of Fallot. Catheter Cardiovasc Interv 80:915–921

53. Blackstone EH, Kirklin JW, Pacifico AD (1979) Decision-making in repair of tetralogy of Fallot based on intraoperative measurements of pulmonary arterial outflow tract. J Thorac Cardiovasc Surg 77:526–532

54. Naito Y, Fujita T, Manabe H, Kawashima Y (1980) The criteria for reconstruction of right ventricular outflow tract in total correction of tetralogy of Fallot. J Thorac Cardiovasc Surg 80:574–581

55. Pacifico AD, Kirklin JW, Blackstone EH (1977) Surgical management of pulmonary stenosis in tetralogy of Fallot. J Thorac Cardiovasc Surg 74:382–395

56. Kavey RE, Bove EL, Byrum CJ, Blackman MS, Sondheimer HM (1987) Postoperative functional assessment of a modified surgical approach to repair of tetralogy of Fallot. J Thorac Cardiovasc Surg 93:533–538

57. Shanley CJ, Lupinetti FM, Shah NL, Beekman RH 3rd, Crowley DC, Bove EL (1993) Primary unifocalization for the absence of intrapericardial pulmonary arteries in the neonate. J Thorac Cardiovasc Surg 106:237–247

58. Shimazaki Y, Blackstone EH, Kirklin JW, Jonas RA, Mandell V, Colvin EV (1992) The dimensions of the right ventricular outflow tract and pulmonary arteries in tetralogy of Fallot and pulmonary stenosis. J Thorac Cardiovasc Surg 103:692–705

59. Nakata S, Imai Y, Takanashi Y, Kurosawa H, Tezuka K, Nakazawa M, Ando M, Takao A (1984) A new method for the quantitative standardization of cross-sectional areas of the pulmonary arteries in congenital heart diseases with decreased pulmonary blood flow. J Thorac Cardiovasc Surg 88:610–619

60. Pagani FD, Cheatham JP, Beekman RH 3rd, Lloyd TR, Mosca RS, Bove EL (1995) The management of tetralogy of Fallot with pulmonary atresia and diminutive pulmonary arteries. J Thorac Cardiovasc Surg 110:1521–1532; discussion 1532–1523

61. Kirklin JW, Blackstone EH, Shimazaki Y, Maehara T, Pacifico AD, Kirklin JK, Bargeron LM Jr (1988) Survival, functional status, and reoperations after repair of tetralogy of Fallot with pulmonary atresia. J Thorac Cardiovasc Surg 96:102–116

62. Clarke DR, Campbell DN, Pappas G (1989) Pulmonary allograft conduit repair of tetralogy of Fallot. An alternative to transannular patch repair. J Thorac Cardiovasc Surg 98:730–736; discussion 736–737

63. Snir E, de Leval MR, Elliott MJ, Stark J (1991) Current surgical technique to repair Fallot's tetralogy with absent pulmonary valve syndrome. Ann Thorac Surg 51:979–982

64. Hraska V (2005) Repair of tetralogy of Fallot with absent pulmonary valve using a new approach. Semin Thorac Cardiovasc Surg Pediatr Card Surg Annu 8:132–134

65. Hraska V, Kantorova A, Kunovsky P, Haviar D (2002) Intermediate results with correction of tetralogy of Fallot with absent pulmonary valve using a new approach. Eur J Cardiothorac Surg 21:711–714; discussion 714–715

66. McDonnell BE, Raff GW, Gaynor JW, Rychik J, Godinez RI, DeCampli WM, Spray TL (1999) Outcome after repair of tetralogy of Fallot with absent pulmonary valve. Ann Thorac Surg 67:1391–1395; discussion 1395–1396

67. Ilbawi M, Cua C, DeLeon S, Muster A, Paul M, Cutilletta A, Arcilla R, Idriss F (1990) Repair of complete atrioventricular septal defect with tetralogy of Fallot. Ann Thorac Surg 50:407–412

68. Oechslin EN, Harrison DA, Harris L, Downar E, Webb GD, Siu SS, Williams WG (1999) Reoperation in adults with repair of tetralogy of Fallot: indications and outcomes. J Thorac Cardiovasc Surg 118:245–251

69. Hoffman TM, Wernovsky G, Atz AM, Kulik TJ, Nelson DP, Chang AC, Bailey JM, Akbary A, Kocsis JF, Kaczmarek R, Spray TL, Wessel DL (2003) Efficacy and safety of milrinone in preventing low cardiac output syndrome in infants and children after corrective surgery for congenital heart disease. Circulation 107:996–1002

70. Cullen S, Shore D, Redington A (1995) Characterization of right ventricular diastolic performance after complete repair of tetralogy of Fallot. Restrictive physiology predicts slow postoperative recovery. Circulation 91:1782–1789

71. Rajagopal SK, Thiagarajan RR (2011) Perioperative care of children with tetralogy of Fallot. Curr Treat Options Cardiovasc Med 13:464–474

72. Plumpton K, Justo R, Haas N (2005) Amiodarone for post-operative junctional ectopic tachycardia. Cardiol Young 15:13–18

73. Hoffman TM, Bush DM, Wernovsky G, Cohen MI, Wieand TS, Gaynor JW, Spray TL, Rhodes LA (2002) Postoperative junctional ectopic tachycardia in children: incidence, risk factors, and treatment. Ann Thorac Surg 74:1607–1611

74. Manrique AM, Arroyo M, Lin Y, El Khoudary SR, Colvin E, Lichtenstein S, Chrysostomou C, Orr R, Jooste E, Davis P, Wearden P, Morell V, Munoz R (2010) Magnesium supplementation during cardiopulmonary bypass to prevent junctional ectopic tachycardia after pediatric cardiac surgery: a randomized controlled study. J Thorac Cardiovasc Surg 139:162–169 e162

75. Hirsch JC, Mosca RS, Bove EL (2000) Complete repair of tetralogy of Fallot in the neonate: results in the modern era. Ann Surg 232:508–514

76. Park CS, Lee JR, Lim HG, Kim WH, Kim YJ (2010) The long-term result of total repair for tetralogy of Fallot. Eur J Cardiothorac Surg 38:311–317

77. Knott-Craig CJ, Elkins RC, Lane MM, Holz J, McCue C, Ward KE (1998) A 26-year experience with surgical management of tetralogy of Fallot: risk analysis for mortality or late reintervention. Ann Thorac Surg 66:506–511

78. Murphy JG, Gersh BJ, Mair DD, Fuster V, McGoon MD, Ilstrup DM, McGoon DC, Kirklin JW, Danielson GK (1993) Long-term outcome in patients undergoing surgical repair of tetralogy of Fallot. N Engl J Med 329:593–599

79. Nollert G, Fischlein T, Bouterwek S, Bohmer C, Klinner W, Reichart B (1997) Long-term survival in patients with repair of tetralogy of Fallot: 36-year follow-up of 490 survivors of the first year after surgical repair. J Am Coll Cardiol 30:1374–1383

80. Bove EL, Byrum CJ, Thomas FD, Kavey RE, Sondheimer HM, Blackman MS, Parker FB Jr (1983) The influence of pulmonary insufficiency on ventricular function following repair of tetralogy of Fallot. Evaluation using radionuclide ventriculography. J Thorac Cardiovasc Surg 85:691–696

81. Burchill LJ, Wald RM, Harris L, Colman JM, Silversides CK (2011) Pulmonary valve replacement in adults with repaired tetralogy of Fallot. Semin Thorac Cardiovasc Surg Pediatr Card Surg Annu 14:92–97

82. Therrien J, Siu SC, McLaughlin PR, Liu PP, Williams WG, Webb GD (2000) Pulmonary valve replacement in adults late after repair of tetralogy of Fallot: are we operating too late? J Am Coll Cardiol 36:1670–1675

83. Frigiola A, Tsang V, Bull C, Coats L, Khambadkone S, Derrick G, Mist B, Walker F, van Doorn C, Bonhoeffer P, Taylor AM (2008) Biventricular response after pulmonary valve replacement for right ventricular outflow tract dysfunction: is age a predictor of outcome? Circulation 118:S182–S190

84. Ilbawi MN, Idriss FS, DeLeon SY, Muster AJ, Gidding SS, Berry TE, Paul MH (1987) Factors that exaggerate the deleterious effects of pulmonary insufficiency on the right ventricle after tetralogy repair. Surgical implications. J Thorac Cardiovasc Surg 93:36–44

85. Yemets IM, Williams WG, Webb GD, Harrison DA, McLaughlin PR, Trusler GA, Coles JG, Rebeyka IM, Freedom RM (1997) Pulmonary valve replacement late after repair of tetralogy of Fallot. Ann Thorac Surg 64:526–530

86. Knauth AL, Gauvreau K, Powell AJ, Landzberg MJ, Walsh EP, Lock JE, del Nido PJ, Geva T (2008) Ventricular size and function assessed by cardiac MRI predict major adverse clinical outcomes late after tetralogy of Fallot repair. Heart 94:211–216

87. Lurz P, Bonhoeffer P, Taylor AM (2009) Percutaneous pulmonary valve implantation: an update. Expert Rev Cardiovasc Ther 7:823–833

88. McElhinney DB, Hellenbrand WE, Zahn EM, Jones TK, Cheatham JP, Lock JE, Vincent JA (2010) Short- and medium-term outcomes after transcatheter pulmonary valve placement in the expanded multicenter us melody valve trial. Circulation 122:507–516

89. Hirsch JC, Bove EL (2003) Tetralogy of Fallot. In: Mavroudis C, Backer CL (eds) Pediatric cardiac surgery, 3rd edn. Mosby, Philadelphia

90. Geva T (2011) Repaired tetralogy of Fallot: the roles of cardiovascular magnetic resonance in evaluating pathophysiology and for pulmonary replacement decision support. J Cardiov Magn Reson 13(9)

91. Ammash NM, Dearani JA, Burkhart HM et al. (2007) Pulmonary regurgitation after tetralogy of Fallot repair: clinical features, sequelae, and timing of pulmonary valve replacement. Congenital Heart Dis 2(6):386–403

Pulmonary Atresia with Ventricular Septal Defect

87

Asad A. Shah, John F. Rhodes, Jr., and Robert D. B. Jaquiss

Abstract

The management of patients with pulmonary atresia with ventricular septal defect is complex, in correspondence with the array of anatomic subtypes, and within subtypes there is substantial controversy about the optimal management strategy. In this chapter an overview of the most commonly encountered subtypes of PA-VSD will be presented, along with a review of the pathophysiology and presentation of the these subtypes, a description of the options for management, and a brief review of the outcomes for the variety of treatments which have been proposed.

Keywords

Central shunt • Coil occlusion of aortopulmonary collaterals • Congenital heart disease • Cutting balloon angioplasty • DiGeorge syndrome • Major aortopulmonary collateral arteries • Nakata index • Neonatal heart surgery • Percutaneous pulmonary valve replacement • Pulmonary artery stenosis • Pulmonary artery stent • Pulmonary atresia • Right ventricle-to-pulmonary artery conduit • Systemic shunt • Tetralogy of Fallot • Unifocalization • Velo-cardio-facial syndrome • Ventricular septal defect

A.A. Shah (✉)
Duke University Medical Center, Durham, NC, USA
e-mail: asad.shah@duke.edu

J.F. Rhodes, Jr.
The Heart Program at Miami Children's Hospital, Miami, FL, USA
e-mail: jfrhodes47@gmail.com

R.D.B. Jaquiss
Section of Pediatric Cardiac Surgery, Duke Children's Hospital & Duke University School of Medicine, Durham, NC, USA
e-mail: Robert.jaquiss@duke.edu

Introduction

The term PA-VSD, standing for pulmonary atresia with ventricular septal defect, is commonly used to describe a heterogeneous group of congenital cardiac malformations, which share the features of absence of luminal continuity between the pulmonary arteries and the "pulmonary ventricle" as well as a nonrestrictive interventricular defect. A comprehensive description of this group of malformations was recently presented by Tchervenkov and Roy and emphasized the wide spectrum of anatomic subtypes comprised in this diagnosis, including all types of ventricular morphology, ventricular septal defect (VSD) location, ventricular looping, and sources of pulmonary blood flow [1]. As a practical matter, the vast majority of such patients have a consistent cardiac morphology, similar to that seen in tetralogy of Fallot. Inter-patient variability occurs most importantly in the sources and morphology of pulmonary blood flow, with consistency found only in the absence of a patent connection between the pulmonary ventricle and the native pulmonary arteries (NPRs).

Embryology

The malformation of PA-VSD is most consistently believed to be characterized by absence of septation and poor development of the subpulmonary myocardium. Many believe that the anatomical finding that often distinguishes PA-VSD from other conotruncal abnormalities is echocardiographic evidence of a pulmonary valve remnant. However, this remains controversial as Kirby emphasized that if the pulmonary atresia develops embryonically before a pulmonary valve is formed, then this criterion would not distinguish conotruncal abnormalities [2]. Also, The´veniau-Ruissy and colleagues reported recent data suggesting that if the subpulmonary myocardium is absent from the right ventricular outflow tract from the beginning, then this tissue would not have a chance to form the pulmonary trunk [3]. Since septation of the great arteries requires a neural crest cell-driven developmental process and junction of the subpulmonary and subaortic myocardium, it is possible that septation is present for patients with PA-VSD, but abnormal, because of the deficient subpulmonary myocardium.

Anatomy

Intracardiac and Valvar Anatomy

The least variable component of the constellation of lesions constituting PA-VSD is the interventricular communication (VSD). This defect is commonly referred to as a "tetralogy-type VSD" and is a type of perimembranous defect with outlet extension, sometimes termed an anterior malalignment defect. As with tetralogy of Fallot and often truncus arteriosus, the aorta may be described as overriding the VSD. The conduction system is in the usual location and should not be at particular risk during closure of the VSD, although injury to the right bundle branch is not uncommon. Additional muscular VSDs as well as coronary artery fistulae [4] may be present with PA-VSD, although these are both unusual.

Another consistent, and defining, feature of PA-VSD is absence of a patent pulmonary

Fig. 87.1 Native central pulmonary arteries supplied by a ductus arteriosus. This angiogram demonstrates well-developed central pulmonary arteries with a catheter in the takeoff of the ductus from the aorta in the AP projection (**a**), and the lateral projection (**b**)

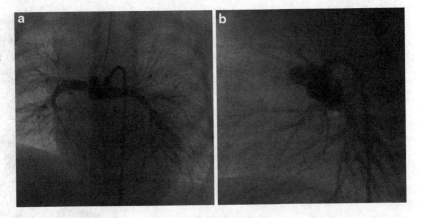

valve. At one end of the spectrum of severity, there may be a valve annulus present with a plate of fibrous tissue instead of mobile valve leaflets. The inference often drawn from this finding is that the atresia occurred relatively late in cardiac development. Typically in such cases, there is a patent main pulmonary artery (MPA) segment with a lumen extending all the way to the valve plate. At the other end of the spectrum, there may be complete absence of valve tissue and valve annulus, with no true pulmonary artery present at all. Occasionally, a fibrous remnant or cord may mark the location where the pulmonary valve and MPA would or should have been. When there is no pulmonary valve or pulmonary artery present at all, it may be speculated that the arrest in development occurred earlier in fetal cardiogenesis.

Sources of Pulmonary Blood Flow

In PA-VSD, pulmonary blood flow must, by definition, arise from a systemic artery [5]. The most favorable circumstance is that in which native pulmonary arteries (NPAs), often with a reasonably well-developed MPA segment, are supplied by a ductus arteriosus (Fig. 87.1). More commonly, pulmonary blood supply is provided by both small NPAs, which may be supplied by a patent ductus or by intraparenchymal collateral-to-pulmonary artery connections, and major (or multiple) aortopulmonary collateral arteries (MAPCAs). In such cases, individual pulmonary

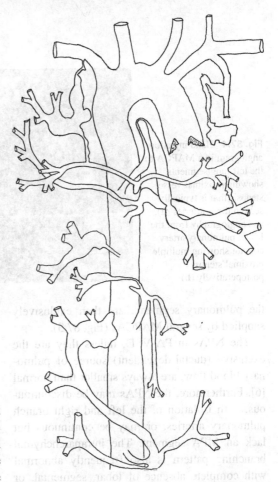

Fig. 87.2 Schematic of MAPCAs and central pulmonary arteries

segments may be supplied by NPAs, by MAPCAs, or by both (dual supply) (Fig. 87.2). Alternatively, there may be no NPAs present and

Fig. 87.3 Schematic of MAPCAs without central pulmonary arteries in (**a**) and a descending aorta angiogram showing MAPCAs without central pulmonary arteries in (**b**)

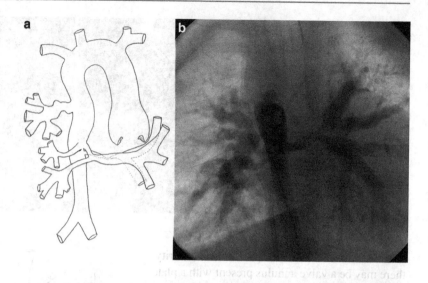

Fig. 87.4 Hand injection angiogram in a MAPCA to the left lung segments showing proximal vessel stenosis that is typically seen in these arteries (**a**), and angiography from the RV to pulmonary artery conduit showing multiple proximal stenoses postoperatively (**b**)

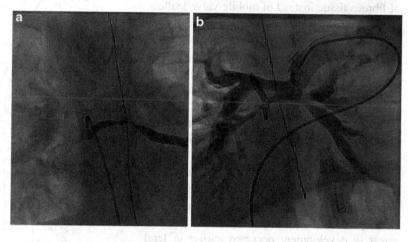

the pulmonary segments are then exclusively supplied by several MAPCAs (Fig. 87.3).

The NPAs in PA-VSD, unless they are the exclusive (ductal-dependent) source of pulmonary blood flow, are always smaller than normal [6]. Furthermore, the NPAs may be discontinuous, with isolation of the left and right branch pulmonary arteries, or may be continuous but lack an MPA segment. The intraparenchymal branching pattern is also frequently abnormal with complete absence of lobar, segmental, or subsegmental arteries.

The MAPCAs seen in PA-VSD are even more variable than NPAs and may arise directly from the aorta (most commonly the anterior-lateral descending aorta near the level of the tracheal carina) or from one or several of its major branches. Although it has been suggested that MAPCAs simply represent massively enlarged bronchial arteries [7], this seems unlikely as their courses are not typical for those of bronchial arteries [8] (although true bronchial arteries may provide significant amount of pulmonary blood flow). It is more likely, as outlined by Rabinovitch and colleagues [9], that most clinically relevant MAPCAs represent segmental branches of the descending aorta or indirect branches arising from aortic arch vessels. Regardless of their embryologic origin, MAPCAs are notoriously prone to the sometimes-rapid early development of proximal stenosis. These stenoses may occur initially in the NPAs (Fig. 87.4a) or after surgical reconstruction with an RV to pulmonary artery conduit (Fig. 87.4b).

Fig. 87.5 Schematic of a MAPCA with dual supply (**a**), of the right lung segments from the MAPCA and the native central pulmonary arteries and a hand injection angiogram in the same anatomy (**b**)

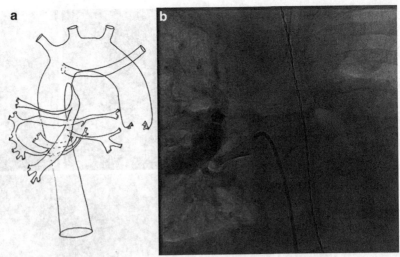

In many patients with PA-VSD, the blood flow to a particular pulmonary segment may appear to have dual supply, with angiographic opacification of vascular inflow and outflow seen on injection of either NPA or MAPCA (Fig. 87.5). Whether this represents actual parallel inflow all the way to the pulmonary acinar unit or simply intraparenchymal communication between the two alternative systems may be impossible to discern angiographically.

Clinical Presentation, Pathophysiology, and Natural History

With the increasing use of fetal echocardiography, it is possible to make the diagnosis of PA-VSD in utero [10]. More commonly, however, the diagnosis is made after birth. The typical presentation is that of cyanosis, in approximately 50 % of patients, [11] seen most dramatically with ductal closure in patients with ductal-dependent pulmonary blood flow. Other patients, without ductal dependence, may also present with cyanosis if the total pulmonary blood flow (Qp) is inadequate. In some cases, the development of clinically apparent cyanosis is subtler and delayed, reflecting the development of important stenoses in the MAPCAs responsible for pulmonary blood flow. In some patients, perhaps 25 %, the total Qp may actually be excessive, resulting to volume overload and tachypnea [11]. In extremely unusual circumstances, untreated patients may actually live for decades, naturally "palliated" with just the right amount of pulmonary blood flow [12].

In considering how and when to intervene in patients with PA-VSD, it is helpful to consider the natural history of patients with the disease [13]. For those patients with ductal-dependent pulmonary blood flow, death is nearly certain with ductal involution. For children without ductal dependence, the prognosis is far less clear. For example, Bull and colleagues described a cohort of 43 patients with PA-VSD who did not undergo surgery [11]. At last follow-up (duration unfortunately not specified) 30 were alive, and 10 were more than 20 years old. In this report, the period of greatest attrition was the first year of life, with a much slower rate of patient attrition thereafter. Because of the widely variable natural history, it is therefore not surprising that there remains some controversy about the optimal timing of intervention in patients with PA-VSD [14].

Diagnostic Evaluation

The initial diagnosis of PA-VSD is made echocardiographically in virtually all cases in the present day. With the diagnosis established, the first question to be answered is whether

Fig. 87.6 Multiple selective angiograms to map out the MAPCA anatomy prior to surgical intervention: (**a**) is a selective angiogram of a MAPCA to the right lung segments, (**b**) is a selective angiogram of a MAPCA to the left lung segments for the same patient, and (**c**) is a selective hand injection angiogram in a MAPCA filling the central native pulmonary arteries retrograde

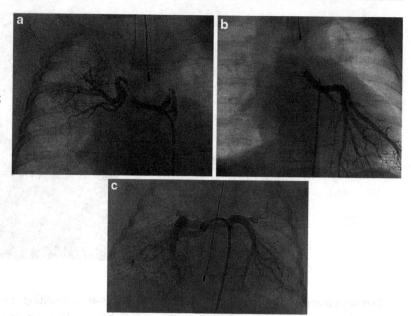

pulmonary blood flow is truly ductal dependent, with obvious implications for the need for prostaglandin infusion. In some cases, it may be extremely difficult to determine whether a ductus is actually present because of the frequent presence of MAPCAs near the usual location of a ductus. Often neither the echocardiographic appearance of the blood flow pattern nor the morphology of the putative ductus is determinant, and either a trial of prostaglandin or cardiac catheterization is required.

Regardless of the presence or absence of a ductus, cardiac catheterization with angiography is eventually necessary in essentially all cases. The purpose of catheterization (beside definition of ductal presence) is to outline as completely as possible all sources of pulmonary blood flow. Because of the possibility of dual supply, and the notorious variability and multiplicity of MAPCAs, numerous aortic and selective MAPCA injections (Fig. 87.6a, b) are typically required to provide all desired information [15]. The most important angiographic assessment is to determine the presence of continuous (Fig. 87.6c) or discontinuous central NPAs. Although distal hand injection angiograms in the MAPCAs most often demonstrate this central NPA anatomy, occasionally

pulmonary venous wedge injections may also be helpful to identify diminutive central NPAs.

If NPAs are present, their size and extent should be quantified as objectively as possible. The number of pulmonary segments supplied by NPAs should be counted. In order to define the size of NPAs, the Nakata index may be calculated [16] as the sum of the areas (in mm^2) of the right and left branch NPAs, indexed to body surface area.

The angiography of the MAPCAs must also include a diligent search for multiple levels of stenoses in these vessels both proximally and distally (Fig. 87.7). Many times MAPCAs may have an early branching pattern with a bifurcation into branches that provide flow to both lungs. Particular attention should be paid to the possibility of "dual" supply of a pulmonary segment or lobe by both MAPCA and NPA.

The roles of newer imaging modalities such as cardiac magnetic resonance imaging (CMR) [17–19] and computed tomographic angiography (CTA) [20–23] continue to evolve. These techniques may supplant traditional angiography in initial or subsequent diagnostic evaluations or serve to target angiography [18]. However, because of the frequent need for catheter-based intervention in patients with

Fig. 87.7 Hand injection angiogram in a stenotic MAPCA to the right lung segments showing multiple levels of stenoses proximally and distally (**a**), and an angiogram in the RV to pulmonary artery conduit showing multiple levels of stenoses proximally and distally (**b**)

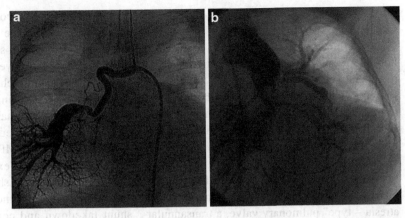

PA-VSD, it is likely that all of these imaging modalities will continue to play important and complementary roles in the management of these patients. In the consideration of which of the imaging modalities to employ, the issue of "invasiveness" is particularly important in this group of patients because of the frequent need for vascular access to permit repeated transcatheter rehabilitation [24] of the pulmonary arterial tree and, more recently, percutaneous pulmonary valve replacement. Preservation of vascular access via one or both femoral veins is therefore of paramount importance in this patient population.

Associated Lesions

An important part of the evaluation of children with PA-VSD includes genetic testing to determine whether there is a deletion of chromosome 22q11.2. This deletion has several genetic presentations such as DiGeorge syndrome and velo-cardio-facial syndrome that may be present in as many as 30–40 % of patients with PA-VSD [25]. The presence of 22q11.2 deletion in PA-VSD patients is thought to portend a particularly poor outcome [26]. Furthermore, both DiGeorge syndrome and velo-cardio-facial syndrome have important multisystem prognostic implications, which were recently reviewed [27]. The salient features of this deletion can be summarized using the mnemonic CATCH-22 where "C" is for cardiac abnormality, "A" is

for abnormal facies, "T" is for thymic aplasia, "C" is for cleft palate, and "H" is for hypocalcemia/hypoparathyroidism. PA-VSD is also associated with Alagille syndrome, related to a mutation on the JAG1 gene [28], and outcomes for PA-VSD with Alagille syndrome may also be worse than for non-syndromic patients [28, 29].

Treatment

Once the diagnosis has been established and the sources of pulmonary blood flow have been completely defined, a treatment plan can be established. The complexity of the plan is related directly to the complexity of the sources of pulmonary blood flow, which may be conveniently organized into three groups as proposed by Tchervenkov [1]:

Group A: Ductal dependent, with well-developed NPA (Fig. 87.1)

Group B: Blood supply by both NPAs and MAPCAs (Fig. 87.2)

Group C: Absent NPA, with all pulmonary blood flow provided by MAPCAs (Fig. 87.3)

As a practical matter, patients in group B may behave either similar to group A or group C, depending on the size and confluence of the NPAs as well as the number of pulmonary segment subtended by the dual pulmonary blood flow sources. The following section will detail the anatomy-driven algorithms for the various subtypes of PA-VSD.

Group A

For the group A patients, there are two alternative treatment plans which are commonly followed, with the choice based on both institutional preference and patient factors (Fig. 87.8a). The more aggressive and increasingly more common approach is to proceed to neonatal complete repair. In extremely favorable anatomy, with a well-developed main pulmonary artery and "membranous atresia – type" pulmonary valve, a transannular patch may be constructed [30], with or without the use of a monocusp neo-pulmonary valve [31]. In essence, this patient population is very similar to tetralogy of Fallot patients. More frequently, transannular patching may not be feasible and establishment of right ventricle-to-pulmonary artery continuity requires implantation of a tubular connection, typically with an

allograft or xenograft conduit. In neonatal complete repair cases, the atrial septal defect is often only partially closed, and delayed sternal closure may be employed.

A different approach to group A patients is to proceed with initial palliation with a systemic-to-pulmonary shunt. This technique has been utilized with a central "Melbourne" shunt [32] (MPA stump to ascending aorta), central Gore-Tex shunt [33, 34], modified Blalock-Taussig shunt, or by creation of an aortopulmonary window [35, 36]. Elective shunt takedown and complete repair are then performed several months later [37]. This staged approach has been employed successfully for many years and may be used, even in centers that prefer neonatal complete repair, if the patient is judged to have coexistent factors that would significantly increase the risk of cardiopulmonary bypass such as prematurity, small size, or intracranial hemorrhage.

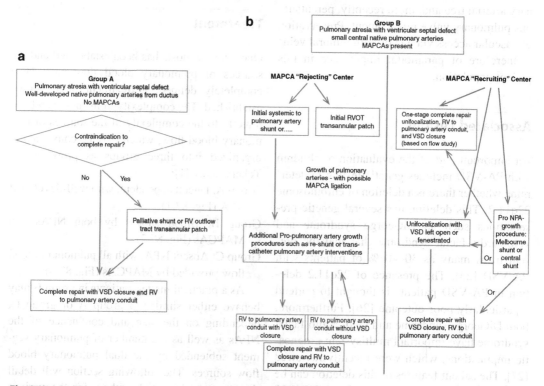

Fig. 87.8 (a) Algorithm for surgical treatment of PA-VSD patients in group A, and (b) algorithm for surgical treatment of PA-VSD patients in group B

No randomized trial comparing one-stage versus two-stage repair has been undertaken, and, for reasons of institutional preference as well as patient comorbidities, it is likely that both one- and two-stage approaches will retain a place in the care of PA-IVS patients.

Group B

Patients with both MAPCAs and NPAs represent a controversial subgroup (Fig. 87.8b). In some centers, management is directed at preservation and amalgamation of virtually all sources of pulmonary blood flow [38–40]. In other centers [41], the MAPCA vessels are not felt helpful, and surgical strategies are directed at maximizing growth of NPAs in a staged sequence, leading to complete repair utilizing only NPAs. Advocates of this latter approach suggest that MAPCAs are derived from bronchial arteries and are therefore inappropriate for use as pulmonary arteries [7], although this viewpoint has been carefully rebutted [8, 42, 43].

Another area that remains unsettled is the optimal timing of intervention, which is in turn related to whether inclusion of MAPCAs is planned. For protocols that focus on optimizing NPA growth without planned MAPCA inclusion, intervention in early infancy or the neonatal period is the rule. Advocates of this approach assert that most discontinuity of the NPAs is an acquired abnormality, which can be averted by neonatal intervention [44]. The initial intervention may be the construction of a central Melbourne shunt [32, 37], whereby the diminutive MPA stump is anastomosed to the lateral wall of the ascending aorta, insertion of a central prosthetic shunt to the diminutive MPA stump [33, 34, 45], or placement of a "transannular patch" [30, 46].

For protocols which seek inclusion of all possible sources of pulmonary blood flow, early intervention is also planned, with establishment of RV to pulmonary artery continuity to the unifocalized neo-pulmonary circulation by age 3–6 months or 5 kg [37, 47, 48]. If possible, based on intraoperative flow study as described subsequently, closure of the VSD is accomplished at the same step (one-stage repair) [49].

Group C

At the other end of the spectrum of complexity are those patients, group C, in whom there are no NPAs (Fig. 87.9). In these patients, the treatment strategy is directed towards the amalgamation of all MAPCAs into a single neo-pulmonary artery, a process known as unifocalization [37–52]. Under ideal circumstances, placement of a valved conduit between the RV and the neo-pulmonary artery and VSD closure would also be accomplished. The three components of complete repair – unifocalization, conduit placement, and VSD closure – may be accomplished simultaneously or in multiple stages, depending on the pulmonary artery anatomy. The choice of approach may be dictated by protocol or by institutional preference, and there are advocates for, and reports of, success with each strategy [37–52]. An additional variation is to accomplish partial closure of the VSD using a patch with a calibrated hole in its center, a so-called fenestrated VSD patch, [48] which would permit later closure by transcatheter placement of an occluder device. As an alternative, the residual VSD could be closed surgically at the time of an elective conduit change.

In the event that a staged approach is elected, the first step is typically the amalgamation of the sources of pulmonary blood flow. As part of the operative goals for this procedure, the elimination MAPCAs that are redundant (provide dual supply) is undertaken to prevent over circulation of one or several pulmonary segments. Care must obviously be taken to determine that true redundancy is actually present to avoid sacrifice of the unique source of blood supply to a parenchymal unit. Once the neo-pulmonary artery has been constructed or "unifocalized," inflow to the amalgamation may be provided by a systemic-to-neo-pulmonary artery shunt or by placement of a conduit between the RV and the vessel. The advantage of the latter method is to allow antegrade (transvenous as opposed to

Fig. 87.9 Algorithm for surgical treatment of PA-VSD patients in group C

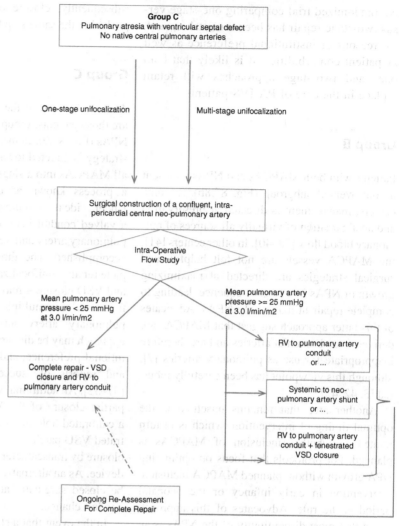

trans-arterial) access to the neo-pulmonary circulation for interventional catheterization procedures such as balloon angioplasty or stent placement. For patients with PA-VSD, such procedures are often necessary multiple times.

The unifocalization procedure itself may be performed in stages, using a thoracotomy approach and a systemic-to-pulmonary shunt. More commonly, a single-stage unifocalization is elected, via sternotomy, typically with support using cardiopulmonary bypass. For midline unifocalization, in the vast majority of circumstance, the source of pulmonary blood flow would be a conduit between the RV and the

neo-pulmonary artery. A nontraditional approach was described by Levi and colleagues in 2006 for RV outflow track transannular patch repair without cardiopulmonary bypass [30].

Complete Surgical Repair

With unifocalization accomplished and continuity established between the RV and the neo-pulmonary artery, all that remains to achieve a "complete" repair is to accomplish closure of the ventricular septal defect. The step is accomplished while the heart is arrested to allow for a right ventriculotomy and proximal conduit anastomosis. The VSD, if it is to be closed, is approached through the same ventriculotomy.

For complete closure of the VSD is to be tolerated, without RV failure, the post-closure RV systolic pressure must be acceptably low. Definition of "acceptably low" may be inferred by analogy to long-established standard employed in repair of tetralogy of Fallot, i.e., RV systolic pressure < 2/3 systemic [51]. To achieve this favorable hemodynamic circumstance, the cross-sectional area of the pulmonary arterial bed must be maximized during the unifocalization procedure(s), and residual focal stenosis in the reconstructed neo-pulmonary arterial tree must be eliminated as completely as possible.

A means of prediction of an acceptably low postoperative RV pressure is obviously desirable. A method for assessing whether the VSD may be closed with a tolerably low postoperative RV pressure has been proposed by Reddy and colleagues [47]. By this technique, a flow study is performed after the pulmonary unifocalization has been completed and the distal anastomosis of the conduit accomplished. Using blood from the cardiopulmonary bypass circuit and an accessory pump on the bypass apparatus flow is sequentially increased via the conduit into the neo-pulmonary circulation while monitoring the pressure in the neo-pulmonary artery. In the original description of the technique, a mean pulmonary artery pressure below 30 mmHg, with a flow rate of 2.5 L/min/m^2, was advocated as predictive of acceptably low pulmonary artery pressures with closure of the VSD [47], and this has been confirmed by others [38, 52]. More recently the original proponents for the flow study have adopted a more stringent threshold and now propose a mean pulmonary artery pressure below 25 mmHg at flow rates of 3.0 L/min/m^2 [52].

If the flow study suggests that the neo-pulmonary vascular bed cannot be perfused with a normal cardiac output at acceptably low pressures, the VSD may simply be left open. Alternatively, the VSD may be closed with a fenestrated patch [48]. A fenestration in the patch has the advantage of potentially permitting subsequent transcatheter device closure, in the event that the distal pulmonary artery resistance falls to an acceptable degree. If the fenestration is "appropriately restrictive," pulmonary blood flow will at least theoretically be encouraged. This favorable circumstance may require direct catheter intervention with balloon angioplasty, often employing cutting balloons, as well as stent implantation [53–57]. With enhanced forward flow, favorable remodeling of the more distal resistance vessels may occur. In either case, the evolution of the pulmonary vascular bed may be crudely indicated by changing arterial oxygen saturation and more precisely estimated by detailed echocardiographic examination of direction of flow across the residual VSD or fenestration. Quantification of RV pressure may also be accomplished by means of Doppler interrogation of trans-VSD gradients and tricuspid valve regurgitant flow jets. A formal assessment of whether the fenestration can be closed can be made in the catheterization laboratory with a test occlusion using a standard balloon and simultaneous RV and pulmonary artery pressure measurement.

Postoperative Management

The postoperative management after total repair of patients with PA-VSD with confluent pulmonary arteries of a reasonable diameter resembles to the relatively straightforward principles followed with tetralogy of Fallot and pulmonary stenosis patients. On the other end of the spectrum, with complex anatomic forms of PA-VSD with MAPCAs, postoperative management may be complex. The main potential complications that may arise are related to postoperative bleeding, low cardiac output, residual stenosis of the newly created "neo-pulmonary artery network" (after unifocalization), and diastolic dysfunction, particularly but not exclusively of the right ventricle.

These patients require comprehensive monitoring with indwelling arterial and central venous lines, a left atrial line (upon institutional preference), continuous ECG, oximetry, and ideally monitoring of mixed venous saturations and near-infrared spectroscopy (NIRS).

Cardiovascular support concentrates on the use of inotropic and lusitropic drugs, associated with systemic vasodilators. In some circumstances, adding iNO may help relieve the afterload of a dysfunctional right ventricle and also may optimize the perfusion of the better-ventilated lung areas. This resource is all the more important that some patients may develop pulmonary hypertensive crisis due to "reactive" pulmonary vasculature or "stiff" neo-pulmonary arteries.

Mechanical ventilation remains a mainstay of therapy and must take into consideration cardiopulmonary interactions. The main target is to promote reduction of right ventricular afterload while recruiting lung parenchyma. The latter involves a significant investment in anticipating, preventing, and intensively managing atelectasis, lung hemorrhage, and pleural effusions. Ventilator strategies should avoid reaching high "plateau" pressures and reducing functional residual capacity. An important detail regards extubation and the need for close evaluation of laryngopharyngeal pathology (i.e., incoordination, vocal cord dysfunction, or primary airway obstruction) or diaphragmatic palsy, mostly in those who fail extubation.

Patients may remain with a significant intracardiac right-to-left shunt, mostly after the preemptive creation of "pop-offs" at the atrial or ventricular levels. This cyanosis is usually secondary to poor right ventricular compliance allied to poorly compliant pulmonary vessels. Caregivers should therefore be permissive with regard to hemodynamically well-tolerated cyanosis that might persist for weeks.

Deep sedation, analgesia, and paralysis, as required, should be utilized until stabilization. Multiple combinations of drugs, targeting minimal efficient doses, may be used depending on institutional preferences. The most common combinations include opioids and benzodiazepines. Dexmedetomidine is also a very attractive alternative, in that it maintains sedation without compromising respiratory drive.

Nutritional support is another important pillar of success after intervention. Enteral feeding should be resumed as soon as safe and possible; if not, parenteral support ought to be initiated as early as possible.

Subsequent Interventions

After complete repair has been accomplished, with unifocalization, conduit implantation, and VSD closure, essentially all patients will require subsequent re-intervention. In the best of cases, those with well-developed distal pulmonary vascular beds, subsequent re-interventions will be needed to replace RV to pulmonary artery conduits, or at least valves in those conduits, typically for stenosis related to patient somatic growth, conduit insufficiency, or both. With the availability of percutaneous pulmonary valve replacement for patients of an appropriate size, initial management strategies must be directed to permit such procedures [58, 59]. In all cases, this mandates zealous attention to the preservation of femoral vein patency. Furthermore, this consideration may influence the choice of conduit sizing or even which type of pulmonary valve is implanted. For example, a stented bioprosthesis may be providing a better "landing site" for a percutaneous pulmonary valve (Fig. 87.10) than an allograft or stentless heterograft conduit [60]. Close consultation with interventional cardiology colleagues is an absolutely mandatory part of both individual operative planning and developing an overall strategy for each patient.

Another important consideration in approaching the revision or replacement of an RV to pulmonary artery conduit is the status of the distal vascular bed. If the resistance is particularly elevated, with associated proximal pulmonary artery hypertension, the stresses on the valve in the pulmonary position will be predictably higher than if the pulmonary resistance is lower. This circumstance may be associated with a shorter longevity of an allograft valve as opposed to a stented bioprosthesis valve. Furthermore, the proximal pulmonary arterial tree may require address at the time of RV to pulmonary

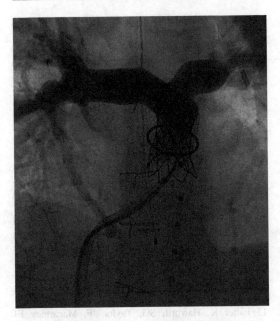

Fig. 87.10 Percutaneous pulmonary valve-in-valve replacement using a Melody valve in a previously placed bioprosthetic valve for a patient with PA-VSD

artery conduit revision, either by surgical patch angioplasty or, when the stenosis is more peripherally located, by intraoperative balloon angioplasty and stenting [61].

Beyond the need to revise or replace RV to pulmonary artery conduits, it may be anticipated, particularly in group C patients, that multiple catheter-based interventions on the pulmonary arterial tree will be necessary. MAPCA-derived pulmonary vessels are notoriously prone to the development of stenoses. In the most favorable circumstance, this may be managed by balloon dilatation alone, with or without stent placement [53, 54]. In other, more fibrotic stenoses, ultimate success may require the use of cutting balloon angioplasty [55–57] or a combination of cutting balloons and stents.

Besides intervention on the RV outflow tract (pulmonary valve) and peripheral pulmonary arteries, transcatheter manipulation may also be helpful to coil-occlude residual (and redundant) MAPCAs [62]. The closure of the fenestration in a ventricular septal defect patch may also be conveniently accomplished in the catheterization laboratory in some cases [63].

Outcomes

To evaluate the outcomes of various alternative management for children with a diagnosis as complex as PA-VSD, the extreme heterogeneity of the patient population must be borne carefully in mind. For example, a comparison of children who have group A PA-VSD who undergo complete repair in the neonatal period to children with group C who require multiple staging procedures is of relatively little value. Furthermore, many published clinical series represent selected subpopulations, and management strategies described in such reports may not be generalizable. With these caveats in mind, it is clear that various currently employed management strategies represent a significant improvement over the natural history of PA-VSD whereby the mortality rate reported in 1994 was at least 40 % by 1 year of age [11].

For patients with group A PA-VSD, outcomes can be expected to be excellent, whether patients undergo neonatal complete repair or initial palliative shunt followed by repair in a few months. For all PA-VSD patients, the reported natural history for patients prior to the mid-1990s was that 65 % of patients survived to 1 year of age and slightly more than 50 % survived to 2 years of age even with surgical interventions. Reddy and colleagues reported in 2000 regarding 85 patients with PA-VSD operated on between 1992 and 2000, demonstrating that early-staged unifocalization was performed successfully in more than 90 % of patients and the intermediate outcome for actuarial survival at 3 years was 80 % [50].

Among the less favorable patients, those in whom some or all pulmonary blood flow is supplied by MAPCAs at the time of presentation, early mortality rates as low as 2–12 % have been reported for "definitive" procedures in recent series from large centers who have included MAPCAs in the ultimate reconstruction [38–40]. A variety of risk factors for mortality have been identified including the presence of a genetic syndrome, young age, and the ability to close the ventricular septal defect at the time of conduit implantation [38–40]. Interesting, in some series, there has been minimal difference in mortality risk for patients who have discontinuous NPAs (all supply from MAPCAs) as compared to those who have continuous NPAs [37].

Similarly excellent results have been reported in smaller from centers whose strategy does not include the inclusion of MAPCAs in the final reconstruction [44]. In these centers, the initial operation is directed at promotion of NPA growth either by placement of a central shunt or with a transannular patch. It must be pointed out that these series do not include patients who only have MAPCAs, and they could not be entered into such a protocol. Nonetheless, for selected patients in centers experienced with an NPA-only strategy, good outcomes are possible.

References

1. Tchervenkov CI, Roy N (2000) Congenital heart surgery nomenclature and database project: pulmonary atresia – ventricular septal defect. Ann Thorac Surg 69(4):S97–S105
2. Kirby ML (2008) Pulmonary atresia or persistent truncus arteriosus: is it important to make the distinction and how do we do it? Circ Res 103:337–339
3. The'veniau-Ruissy M, Dandonneau M, Mesbah K et al (2008) The del22q11.2 candidate gene Tbx1 controls regional outflow tract identity and coronary artery patterning. Circ Res 103:142–148
4. Collison SP, Dagar KS, Kaushal SK et al (2008) Coronary artery fistulas in pulmonary atresia and ventricular septal defect. Asian Cardiovasc Thorac Ann 16(1):29–32
5. Macartney F, Deverall P, Scott O (1973) Hemodynamic characteristics of systemic arterial blood supply to the lungs. Br Heart J 35(1):28–37
6. Rome JJ, Mayer JE, Castaneda AR, Lock JE (1993) Tetralogy of Fallot with pulmonary atresia. Rehabilitation of diminutive pulmonary arteries. Circulation 88:1691–1698
7. Nørgaard MA, Alphonso N, Cochrane AD et al (2006) Major aorto-pulmonary collateral arteries of patients with pulmonary atresia and ventricular septal defect are dilated bronchial arteries. Eur J Card Thor Surg 29(5):653–658
8. Hanley FL (2006) MAPCAs, bronchials, monkeys, and men. Eur J Cardiothorac Surg 29(5):643–644
9. Rabinovitch M, Herrera-deLeon V, Castaneda AR, Reid L (1981) Growth and development of the pulmonary vascular bed in patients with tetralogy of Fallot with or without pulmonary atresia. Circulation 64(6):1234–1249
10. Vesel S, Rollings S, Jones A et al (2006) Prenatally diagnosed pulmonary atresia with ventricular septal defect: echocardiography, genetics, associated anomalies and outcome. Heart 92(10):1501–1505
11. Bull K, Somerville J, Ty E, Spiegelhalter D (1995) Presentation and attrition in complex pulmonary atresia. J Am Coll Card 25(2):491–499
12. Fukui D, Kai H, Takeuchi T et al (2011) Longest survivor of pulmonary atresia with ventricular septal defect: well-developed major aortopulmonary collateral arteries demonstrated by multi-detector computed tomography. Circulation 124(19):2155–2157
13. Warnes CA, Williams RG, Bashore TM et al (2008) ACC/AHA 2008 guidelines for management of adults with congenital heart disease. Circulation 118:e117–e833
14. Leonard H, Derrick G, O'Sullivan J et al (2000) Natural and unnatural history of pulmonary atresia. Heart 84(5):499–503
15. Fäller K, Haworth SG, Taylor JF, Macartney FJ (1981) Duplicate sources of pulmonary blood supply in pulmonary atresia with ventricular septal defect. Br Heart J 46(3):263–268
16. Nakata S, Imai Y, Takanashi Y et al (1984) A new method for the quantitative standardization of cross-sectional areas of the pulmonary arteries in congenital heart diseases with decreased pulmonary blood flow. J Thorac Cardiovasc Surg 88:610–619
17. Boechat MI, Ratib O, Williams PL et al (2005) Cardiac MR imaging and MR angiography for assessment of complex tetralogy of Fallot and pulmonary atresia. Radiographics 25(6):1535–1546
18. Srinivas B, Patnaik AN, Rao DS (2011) Gadolinium-enhanced three-dimensional magnetic resonance angiographic assessment of the pulmonary artery anatomy in cyanotic congenital heart disease with pulmonary stenosis or atresia: comparison with cineangiography. Pediatr Cardiol 32(6):737–742
19. Romeih S, Al-Sheshtawy F, Salama M et al (2012) Comparison of contrast enhanced magnetic resonance angiography with invasive cardiac catheterization for evaluation of children with pulmonary atresia. Heart Int 7(2):e9
20. Westra SJ, Hurteau J, Galindo A et al (1999) Cardiac electron-beam CT in children undergoing surgical repair for pulmonary atresia. Radiology 213(2):502–512
21. Lin MT, Wang JK, Chen YS et al (2012) Detection of pulmonary arterial morphology in tetralogy of Fallot with pulmonary atresia by computed tomography: 12 years of experience. Eur J Pediatr 171(3):579–586
22. Yin L, Lu B, Han L et al (2011) Quantitative analysis of pulmonary artery and pulmonary collaterals in pre-operative patients with pulmonary artery atresia using dual-source computed tomography. Eur J Radiol 79(3):480–485

23. Rajeshkannan R, Moorthy S, Sreekumar KP et al (2009) Role of 64-MDCT in evaluation of pulmonary atresia with ventricular septal defect. Am J Roentgenol 194(1):110–118

24. Kreutzer J, Perry SB, Jonas RA et al (1996) Tetralogy of Fallot with diminutive pulmonary arteries: preoperative pulmonary valve dilation and transcatheter rehabilitation of pulmonary arteries. JACC 27(7):1741–1747

25. Anaclerio S, Marino B, Carotti A et al (2001) Pulmonary atresia with ventricular septal defect: prevalence of deletion 22q11 in the different anatomic patterns. Italian Heart J 2(5):384–387

26. Mahle WT, Crisalli J, Coleman K et al (2003) Deletion of chromosome 22q11.2 and outcome in patients with pulmonary atresia and ventricular septal defect. Ann Thorac Surg 76(2):567–571

27. Kobrynski LJ, Sullivan KE (2007) Velocardiofacial syndrome, DiGeorge syndrome: the chromosome 22q11.2 deletion syndromes. Lancet 370(9596): 1443–1452

28. Mainwaring RD, Sheikh AY, Punn R et al (2012) Surgical outcomes for patients with pulmonary atresia / major aortopulmonary collaterals and Alagille syndrome. Eur J Cardiothorac Surg 42(2):235–241

29. Blue GM, Mah JM, Cole AD et al (2007) The negative impact of Alagille syndrome on survival of infants with pulmonary atresia. J Thorac Cardiovasc Surg 133(4):1094–1096

30. Levi DS, Glotzbach JP, Williams RJ et al (2006) Right ventricular outflow tract transannular patch placement without cardiopulmonary bypass. Pediatr Cardiol 27(1):149–155

31. Turrentine MW, McCarthy RP, Vijay P et al (2002) PTFE monocusp valve reconstruction of the right ventricular outflow tract. Ann Thorac Surg 73:871–880

32. Mumtaz MA, Rosenthal G, Qureshi A et al (2008) Melbourne shunt promotes growth of diminutive central pulmonary arteries in patients with pulmonary atresia, ventricular septal defect, and systemic-to-pulmonary collateral arteries. Ann Thorac Surg 85(6):2079–2083, discussion 2083–2084

33. Gates RN, Laks H, Johnson K (1998) Side-to-side aorto-Gore-Tex central shunt. Ann Thorac Surg 65(2):515–516

34. Barozzi L, Brizard CP, Galati JC et al (2011) Side-to-side aorto-GoreTex central shunt warrants central shunt patency and pulmonary arteries growth. Ann Thorac Surg 92(4):1476–1482

35. Rodefeld MD, Reddy VM, Thompson LD et al (2002) Surgical creation of aortopulmonary window in selected patients with pulmonary atresia with poorly developed aortopulmonary collaterals and hypoplastic pulmonary arteries. J Thorac Cardiovasc Surg 123(6):1147–1754

36. Mainwaring RD, Reddy VM, Perry SB et al (2012) Late outcomes in patients undergoing aortopulmonary window for pulmonary atresia/stenosis and major aortopulmonary collaterals. Ann Thorac Surg 94(3):842–848

37. Duncan BW, Mee RB, Prieto LR et al (2003) Staged repair of tetralogy of Fallot with pulmonary atresia and major aortopulmonary collateral arteries. J Throacic Cardiovasc Surg 126:694–702

38. Carotti A, Albanese SB, Filippelli S et al (2010) Determinants of outcome after surgical treatment of pulmonary atresia with ventricular septal defect and major aortopulmonary collateral arteries. J Thorac Cardiovasc Surg 140(5):1092–1103

39. Malhotra SP, Hanley FL (2009) Surgical management of pulmonary atresia with ventricular septal defect and major aortopulmonary collaterals: a protocol-based approach. Semin Thorac Cardiovasc Surg Pediatr Card Surg Annu 12(1):145–151

40. Davies B, Mussa S, Davies P et al (2009) Unifocalization of major aortopulmonary collateral arteries in pulmonary atresia with ventricular septal defect is essential to achieve excellent outcomes irrespective of native pulmonary artery morphology. J Thorac Cardiovasc Surg 138(6):1269–1275

41. d'Udekem Y, Alphonso N, Norgaard MA et al (2005) Pulmonary atresia with ventricular septal defects and major aortopulmonary collateral arteries: unifocalization brings no long-term benefits. J Thorac Cardiovasc Surg 130(6):1496–1502

42. Rabinovitch M, Herrera-deLeon V, Castaneda AR et al (1981) Growth and development of the pulmonary vascular bed in patients with tetralogy of Fallot with or without pulmonary atresia. Circulation 64(6):1234–1249

43. Anderson RH, Devine WA, Del Nido P (1991) The surgical anatomy of tetralogy of Fallot with pulmonary atresia rather than pulmonary stenosis. J Card Surg 61:41–58

44. Liava'a M, Brizard CP, Konstantinov IE et al (2012) Pulmonary atresia, ventricular septal defect, and major aortopulmonary collaterals: neonatal pulmonary artery rehabilitation without unifocalization. Ann Thorac Surg 93(1):185–191

45. Watterson KG, Wilkinson JL, Karl TR, Mee RBB (1991) Very small pulmonary arteries: central end-to-side shunt. Ann Thorac Surg 52(5):1132–1137

46. Metras D, Chetaille P, Kreitmann B et al (2001) Pulmonary atresia with ventricular septal defect, extremely hypoplastic pulmonary arteries, major aorto-pulmonary collaterals. European Journal of Cardio Thoracic Surgery 20(3):590–596, discussion 596–597

47. Reddy VM, Petrossian E, McElhinney DB et al (1997) One-stage complete unifocalization in infants: when should the ventricular septal defect be closed? J Thorac Cardiovasc Surg 113(5):858–866, discussion 866–868

48. Marshall AC, Love BA, Lang P et al (2003) Staged repair of tetralogy of Fallot and diminutive pulmonary arteries with a fenestrated ventricular septal defect patch. J Thorac Cardiovasc Surg 126(5):1427–1433

49. Tchervenkov CI, Salasidis G, Cecere R et al (1997) One-stage midline unifocalization and complete repair in infancy versus multiple-staged unifocalization followed by repair for complex heart disease with major aortopulmonary collaterals. J Thorac Cardiovasc Surg 114(5):727–735

50. Reddy VM, McElhinney DB, Amin Z et al (2000) Early and intermediate outcomes after repair of pulmonary atresia with ventricular septal defect and major aortopulmonary collateral arteries: experience with 85 patients. Circulation 101:1826–1832

51. Dragulescu A, Kammache I, Fouilloux V et al (2011) Long-term results of pulmonary artery rehabilitation in patients with pulmonary atresia, ventricular septal defect, pulmonary artery hypoplasia, and major aortopulmonary collaterals. J Thorac Cardiovasc Surg 142:1374–1380

52. Honjo O, Al-Radi OO, MacDonald C et al (2009) The functional intraoperative pulmonary blood flow study is a more sensitive predictor than preoperative anatomy for right ventricular pressure and physiologic tolerance of ventricular septal defect closure after complete unifocalization in patients with pulmonary atresia, ventricular septal defect, and major aortopulmonary collaterals. Circulation 120(11):S46–S52

53. Bergersen L, Lock JE (2006) What is the current option of first choice for treatment of pulmonary arterial stenosis? Cardiol Young 16:329–338

54. El-Said HG, Clapp S, Fagan TE et al (2000) Stenting of stenosed aortopulmonary collaterals and shunts for palliation of pulmonary atresia/ventricular septal defect. Catheter Cardiovasc Interv 49(4):430–436

55. Mertens L, Dens J, Gewillig M (2001) Use of a cutting balloon catheter to dilate resistant stenoses in major aortic-to-pulmonary collateral arteries. Cardiol Young 11(5):574–577

56. Rhodes JF, Lane GK, Mesia IG et al (2002) Cutting balloon angioplasty for children with small-vessel pulmonary artery stenoses. Catheter Cardiovasc Interv 55(1):73–77

57. Bergersen L, Gauvreau K, Justino H et al (2011) Randomized trial of cutting balloon compared with high-pressure angioplasty for the treatment of resistant pulmonary artery stenosis. Circulation 124:2388–2396

58. Zahn EM, Hellenbrand WE, Lock JE, McElhinney DB (2009) Implantation of the Melody transcatheter pulmonary valve in patients with a dysfunctional right ventricular outflow tract conduit early results from the U.S. clinical trial. JACC 54:1722–1729

59. Kenny D, Hijazi ZM, Kar S et al (2011) Percutaneous implantation of the Edwards SAPIEN transcatheter heart valve for conduit failure in the pulmonary position. Early phase 1 results from an international multicenter clinical trial. J Am Coll Cardiol 58(21):2248–2256

60. Gillespie MJ, Rome JJ, Levi DS et al (2012) Melody valve implant within failed bioprosthetic valves in the pulmonary position: a multicenter experience. Circ Cardiovasc Interv 5:862–870

61. Angtuaco MJ, Sachdeva R, Jaquiss RD et al (2010) Long-term outcomes of intraoperative pulmonary artery stent placement for congenital heart disease. Catheter Cardiovasc Interv 77(3):395–399

62. Hornung TS, Benson LN, McLaughlin PR (2002) Catheter interventions in adult patients with congenital heart disease. Curr Cardiol Rep 4:54–62

63. Knauth AL, Lock JE, Perry SB et al (2004) Transcatheter device closure of congenital and postoperative residual ventricular septal defects. Circulation 110:501–507

Pulmonary Atresia with Intact Ventricular Septum

88

Mark G. Hazekamp, Adriaan W. Schneider and Nico A. Blom

Abstract

Pulmonary atresia with intact ventricular septum is a rare congenital cardiac malformation characterized by underdevelopment of the right ventricle. Pulmonary atresia with intact ventricular septum can be difficult to manage due its wide variety spectrum of anatomic variations. Pulmonary atresia can be muscular or membranous, and right ventricular size in these patients can range from normal to severely hypoplastic. The tricuspid valve is often affected as well. Type of management is based on individual patient characteristics and is typically staged. Interventions can be percutaneous, surgical, or a combination of both. End goal of treatment may be biventricular repair, univentricular palliation, or one and a half ventricle repair. The appropriate treatment strategy depends mainly on right ventricle and tricuspid valve morphology. Definitive repair should be aimed for at an age of 4–5 years. Late re-interventions are sometimes necessary and include pulmonary valve replacement, tricuspid valve repair, and ablation procedures to treat arrhythmias. Although results of treatment have improved over the last decades due to better patient-treatment matching and improved surgical and interventional techniques, management of patients with pulmonary atresia with intact ventricular septum remains challenging.

M.G. Hazekamp (✉)
Leiden University Medical Center, Leiden,
The Netherlands

Department of Cardiothoracic Surgery, Leiden University
Medical Center, Leiden and Academic Medical Center,
Amsterdam, The Netherlands
e-mail: m.g.hazekamp@lumc.nl

A.W. Schneider • N.A. Blom
Department of Cardiothoracic Surgery, Leiden University
Medical Center, Leiden and Academic Medical Center,
Amsterdam, The Netherlands

E.M. da Cruz et al. (eds.), *Pediatric and Congenital Cardiology, Cardiac Surgery and Intensive Care*,
DOI 10.1007/978-1-4471-4619-3_20, © Springer-Verlag London 2014

Keywords

Aortopulmonary shunt • Atrial septostomy • Cardiac catheterization • Congenital heart disease • Glenn • Hypoplastic right heart syndrome • Intact ventricular septum • One and a half ventricle repair • Pulmonary atresia • Valvuloplasty • Fontan

Introduction

Pulmonary atresia with intact ventricular septum (PA/IVS) is a rare congenital cardiac malformation that is characterized by underdevelopment of the right ventricle (RV). PA/IVS has to be distinguished from pulmonary atresia with VSD (PA/VSD) where the RV is normally developed.

Morphology

PA/IVS comprises a spectrum of morphological varieties. At one end of the spectrum, severe RV cavity hypoplasia with RV hypertrophy is found, while at the other end, the RV is only mildly hypoplastic. The degree of RV underdevelopment is typically associated with the degree of tricuspid valve (TV) hypoplasia.

To categorize PA/IVS, it is practical to divide the RV into three components: an inflow part, a trabecular or apical part, and an outflow tract (RVOT) or infundibular portion. When the trabecular part is missing or diminutive, the RV is "bipartite." Absence of severe hypoplasia of both trabecular and outflow components makes the RV "unipartite," while a "tripartite" RV will have three reasonably developed components. It is usually the inlet portion that is present as long as there is a patent tricuspid valve.

The pulmonary valve (PV) may be present but in an imperforated form. This membranous atresia may or may not be accompanied by some degree of annular hypoplasia. When the atresia is muscular, the distance between the chamber of the RV and pulmonary artery is considerably bigger than in the valvar form of atresia. Underdevelopment of the RVOT is typically related to the type of atresia: In valvar atresia, the RVOT is open but may be hypoplastic, while in muscular

atresia, the RVOT is diminutive or absent. In critical pulmonary stenosis, the pulmonary valve is severely stenotic, but with a small central opening. This is frequently associated with RV hypertrophy and some (usually mild) degree of RV cavity underdevelopment. These patients will present and behave similar to PA/IVS.

The severity of RV hypoplasia is clearly associated with the degree of tricuspid valve hypoplasia. In addition to annular hypoplasia, the TV leaflets can be thickened and dysplastic. The tendinous chords are often shorter than normal and may be positioned differently. This may result in variable severity of TV regurgitation. Unusually, a severely insufficient TV, with or without Ebstein-like features, is associated with a dilated and thin-walled RV. This separate entity stands somewhat apart from the rest of the PA/IVS spectrum (Fig. 88.1).

Sinusoidal connections between RV cavity and coronary arteries are frequently observed in PA/IVS. The presence of these sinusoids is related to the severity of RV hypoplasia. In some patients with sinusoids, there are fistulous communications from the RV to the epicardial coronary arteries. Sometimes the coronary arteries develop stenosis or atresia of the proximal coronary artery. In this situation, coronary artery flow is dependent upon flow from the cavity of the right ventricle through these fistulous communications. This is referred to as right ventricular-dependent coronary circulation (RVDCC) [1]. Anything that decreases the pressure in the RV cavity and thus the flow through these fistulae will result in decreased coronary flow and potential ischemia.

Pulmonary arteries (PA) are normally developed in PA/IVS, although PA branch hypoplasia and distal stenosis have been reported [2].

Pulmonary artery circulation is dependent on the patency of the ductus arteriosus. Anomalous

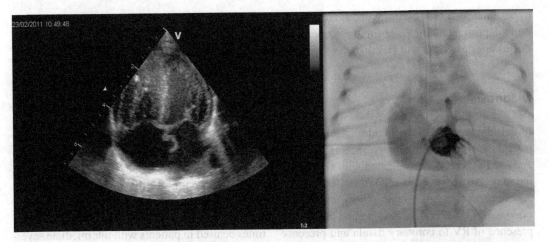

Fig. 88.1 *Left*: Echocardiographic apical four-chamber view of an 11-day-old male infant with PA/IVS at presentation. Note the small RV cavity compared to the LV. *Right*: RV angiography in the same patient

systemic-to-pulmonary collateral arteries have been very rarely observed in PA/IVS and may be associated with the absence of a patent ductus.

A patent foramen ovale (PFO) or atrial septal defect (ASD) is usually present and allows systemic venous return to shunt to the left side of the heart.

The left ventricle (LV) is morphologically normal in PA/IVS, but LV function may be impaired because of suprasystemic RV pressure. In patients with RVDCC, LV function may also be impaired secondary to ischemia.

Embryology

The pathophysiology of PA/IVS is not exactly known, although different studies have shed more light on the mechanisms that may play a role. As there is no VSD present, the changes that lead to maldevelopment of the RV together with pulmonary atresia must occur after the process of ventricular septation has been completed. It is generally accepted that PA/IVS develops relatively late in gestation. Earlier theories had pointed to the importance of pulmonary atresia as being the principal factor being responsible for hypertrophy and luminal underdevelopment of the RV. Sinusoids and RV to coronary artery fistulae could be explained by the excess of pressure in the RV due to the atretic pulmonary valve,

but this is now disputed to be the solitary mechanism [3, 4]. Nowadays, hypotheses have changed, and it is postulated that primarily there is a disturbance of RV development. This is supported by several observations by fetal echocardiography that mild pulmonary stenosis can progress to full-blown pulmonary atresia with subsequent RV luminal hypoplasia. Among others, the group of Gittenberger de Groot has reported that deficient ingrowth of epicardial coronary arteries may be involved. Specimens show a marked disarray of capillaries that was closely interrelated to disarray of cardiomyocytes. There appears to be a relation between the severity of capillary and myocardial disarray and the grade of PA/IVS: More disarray gives a more severe form of PA/IVS [1, 5, 6].

Pathophysiology

Systemic venous blood mixes through an interatrial communication with pulmonary venous blood in the left atrium and will be ejected into the systemic circulation. In PA/IVS, the interatrial communication is usually nonrestrictive. Systemic arterial saturation is dependent on pulmonary blood flow through a patent ductus arteriosus. Pulmonary blood flow will decrease completely when the arterial duct closes postnatally. This will result in a rapid onset of arterial hypoxemia and acidosis. Intravenous administration of prostaglandin E_1 normally reopens the ductus arteriosus and will stabilize the neonate.

Diagnosis

Initial diagnosis can be made in almost all patients by echocardiography. Sizing the RV and the TV is best accomplished with echocardiography. Angiography is recommended if there are concerns about pulmonary artery anatomy or presence of collateral vessels and to clarify the presence of RV to coronary fistula and presence of RVDCC, which may determine initial management strategy and long-term prognosis. The electrocardiogram is usually notable as the typical neonatal signs of RV dominance are decreased or absent. A bigger P wave is related to enlargement of the right atrium, and P waves will be especially high when PA/IVS is associated with severe tricuspid insufficiency. The chest X-ray only shows an enlarged cardiac silhouette when the right atrium is large as a consequence of important tricuspid valve regurgitation.

Management

As PA/IVS may present in many different forms, there is no uniform management strategy. At first presentation, an attempt must be made to define the optimal goal that can be obtained in each patient.

Treatment of PA/IVS is virtually always staged. One-stage neonatal repair has been reported but should be regarded with suspicion [7].

Surgical therapy can be variable, with some patients achieving two-ventricle repair and others requiring a single-ventricle palliation. Some patients with intermediate severity of disease may be managed with the so-called one and a half ventricle repair. When biventricular repair is pursued in the presence of an unfavorable anatomy, this is termed overtreatment, which may result in considerable morbidity and mortality. On the other hand, suboptimal treatment results when univentricular management is chosen when the anatomy would support either biventricular repair or one and a half ventricle palliation and may deprive some patients of the presumed benefits of a two-ventricle and separated circulation.

Individual planning of the optimal treatment strategy has greatly improved outcomes in patients with PA/IVS. At both ends of the spectrum, decision making is fairly easy: A severely hypoplastic and unipartite RV can only be palliated by univentricular management, while valvar atresia with a mildly hypoplastic tripartite RV can nearly always be managed with biventricular repair. One and a half ventricle repair may sometimes be used in patients with intermediate severity of RV and TV hypoplasia. Fenestrating the ASD patch has been reported in biventricular and one and a half repair, in order to decompress the right side of the heart. The biggest challenge presents in the middle "gray" zone of the spectrum where it may be difficult to know and decide upon the best treatment.

Management goals, regardless of the individual morphology, should be to separate the systemic and pulmonary circulation while avoiding venous congestion and decompression of the RV, promoting antegrade pulmonary blood flow whenever possible. It is important to define the management strategy early in the patients' course. Several groups have extensively reported on management algorithms for PA/IVS. Optimal management depends upon morphological characteristics and comparing them to outcomes of treatment [8–13].

One practical management algorithm would be to divide PA/IVS in three groups based on RV anatomy and TV sizes: mildly hypoplastic, moderately hypoplastic, and severely hypoplastic. Mild hypoplasia means that actual RV size is more than two thirds of normal, moderate hypoplasia is an actual RV size in between one third and two thirds of normal, while severe hypoplasia is characterized by an RV size that is less than one third of normal [12]. Mild RV hypoplasia correlates with tripartite RV, and a severely hypoplastic RV is usually unipartite with only an inflow compartment. Moderate RV hypoplasia is typically associated with a bipartite RV where the trabecular component is lacking.

Quantitative RV measurements have been proposed. These include RV inlet length Z-score and RV area Z-score as measured in the echocardiographic four-chamber view. RV inlet Z-score quantifies the distance from TV annulus to RV apex. More sophisticated indices have been reported such as RVDI (RV Development Index) that may be of help in indeterminate cases [13]. Generally speaking, however, qualitative or semiquantitative measurements of the RV are sufficient to decide upon the strategy that has to be followed.

There is a good correlation between RV size and TV annulus Z-score. In general, TV annulus Z-scores greater than −2 correlate with an RV chamber size that allows for biventricular repair, while Z-scores lower than −4 uniformly predict the need for univentricular palliation. TV Z-scores between −2 and −4 indicate an RV of intermediate anatomy that may be amenable to one and a half ventricle repair, assuming the remainder of the right heart anatomy is favorable. In general, TV annulus diameters are measured by echocardiography, and it should be stressed that Z-scores may vary between reported lists of normal values. Z-scores reported in studies from Zilberman et al. or Pettersen et al. are preferred because in neonates and infants, the TV annulus Z-scores reported in these studies are comparable to observed surgical Z-scores [14, 15].

TV Z-scores should be used together with the above-mentioned qualitative or semiquantitative estimates of RV size [2, 12]. It is almost never necessary to require more complex measurements to help predict the adequacy of the RV. Structural anomalies of the TV and TV insufficiency should be taken into account when making treatment decisions. More than moderate regurgitation from a structurally abnormal TV is unfavorable for biventricular repair, even when annular size is sufficiently large.

RV to coronary fistula is associated with severe RV hypoplasia but does not uniformly exclude biventricular or one and a half ventricle repair. However, the presence of RVDCC mandates univentricular palliation.

Heart transplantation in PA/IVS is normally not considered to be a primary therapeutic modality. As both interventional and surgical tools have become much more refined in the last decades, transplantation has now a secondary role and is used as salvage therapy for older infants and children who have severe cardiac dysfunction during the staging course or who have a failing Fontan circulation. Ischemic LV damage in PA/IVS with right ventricular-dependent coronary circulation (RVDCC) may in some institutions form a rare exception to the above mentioned [16].

Fetal Management

There have been an increasing number of reports regarding fetal diagnosis of PA/IVS and prognosis dependent upon in utero morphological parameters [17, 18]. PA/IVS can be reliably diagnosed in the second trimester of gestation. Fetal diagnosis will be earlier and easier in the more severe forms of PA/IVS. Recognition of PA/IVS at an early stage may have several consequences. It may be that for the more severe cases, the rate of pregnancy termination will be higher, but exact data are not available. There is a tendency of progressive hypoplasia of the right side of the heart [17, 18]. This observation may have consequences for prenatal counseling. Fetal tricuspid Z-scores and rate of TV growth predict postnatal outcome [17]. Furthermore, the observation that RV hypoplasia is progressive in the fetus has led to efforts to open the PV by fetal intervention. This has been described by the Boston group in 2009. They performed fetal balloon dilatation of the PV and showed that RV growth and postnatal outcomes may be promoted. However, currently, it still has to be determined whether fetal intervention on the PV will reliably result in significant and predictable growth of RV and TV. To be successful, the PV must be identifiable or membranous, the ventricular septum must be intact, and TV Z-scores must be less than −2 in the presence of a small but identifiable RV. Access to the pulmonary valve for balloon valvuloplasty is via trans uterine, direct puncture of the right ventricle in mid-gestation [19, 20].

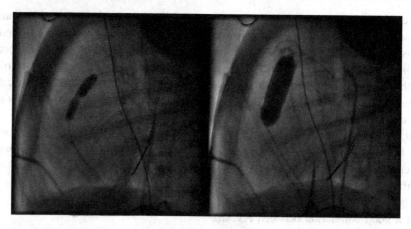

Fig. 88.2 Angiography of balloon dilatation of the PV in the same patient as Fig. 88.1. *Left*: A tight waist is visible during the initial dilatation with a 4 mm coronary balloon. *Right*: After the second balloon dilatation (8 mm), the waist has disappeared indicating that the atretic valve is fully patent. Patient needed subsequent balloon atrioseptostomy and placement of an aortopulmonary shunt due to inadequate pulmonary blood flow from the RV

Neonatal Management

In the great majority of neonates with PA/IVS, some intervention will be necessary in the neonatal period as pulmonary flow depends on ductal patency. The duct must be kept patent by intravenous administration of prostaglandin E1. Thereafter, semi-elective interventions are aimed at maintaining pulmonary blood flow from the aorta or antegrade from the RV. When the interatrial connection is restricted, a Rashkind balloon atrial septostomy may be necessary but is rarely necessary. Pulmonary blood flow may be established by construction of an aortopulmonary shunt or by stent placement in the arterial duct. An aortopulmonary shunt in the neonatal phase is typically a right-sided modified Blalock-Taussig shunt (MBTS) using a 3.5 or 4.0 mm thin-walled PTFE vascular prosthesis. Patency of the MBTS may be 1–2 years, but sometimes longer. An alternative for surgical shunt placement may be stent placement in the ductus arteriosus by percutaneous catheter-based intervention. This method is sometimes difficult in patients with PA/IVS as the ductus can have a long tortuous course and difficult angles of origin and insertion. It is also important to rule out the need for pulmonary arterioplasty before placing a ductal stent. Ductal stent patency may be less durable than surgically created shunts because of neointimal formation. For the moment, discussion remains whether a ductal stent is to be preferred over a surgical aortopulmonary shunt [21–23].

Decompression of RV is indicated for two reasons: to guarantee pulmonary blood flow and to promote growth of an underdeveloped RV. Leaving the RV disconnected to the PAs is thought to induce more hypertrophy that will obliterate the RV cavity even further and will result in more diastolic dysfunction of the RV. Opening the RVOT will decompress the RV and potentially allow for regression of hypertrophy. RV decompression can be performed both surgically and by percutaneous intervention. The percutaneous approach is preferred when atresia is valvular (Fig. 88.2). The imperforate valve is opened by radiofrequency (RF) perforation, followed by balloon dilatation. This is especially useful when the RV infundibulum is sufficiently patent. In the presence of a narrow infundibulum, opening of the valve will not result in adequate forward flow to the PAs. When atresia is muscular or when the PV annulus is hypoplastic, surgical transannular patch augmentation is preferred. Even after adequate opening of the RVOT, either by surgical or percutaneous procedure, forward flow may be insufficient secondary to persistence of severe hypertrophy of the RV and associated poor compliance. Longer administration of prostaglandin or surgical shunt placement may then be needed, even in the presence of a reasonably developed RV until the right ventricular compliance improves.

PA/IVS with severe RV hypoplasia and RVDCC can only be managed by univentricular strategy. Decompression of the right ventricle is contraindicated in this situation, and placement of a MBTS or ductal stent is sufficient for the neonatal period.

When TV regurgitation is important or does not decrease after decompression of the RV, open TV repair should be taken into consideration in all forms of PA/IVS.

The small subgroup of patients with Ebstein malformation of the TV and PA/IVS is very challenging to manage. In the absence of RVDCC, the patient with PA/IVS and "Ebsteinoid" TV valve should undergo decompression of the RV in the neonatal period. This may have to be accompanied by establishment of an alternative source of pulmonary blood flow. While TV repair may be helpful in some of these patients, many times the TV cannot be repaired and severe insufficiency remains. (Fenestrated) patch closure of the TV in association with aortopulmonary shunt placement may be required. Alternatively, the pulmonary artery can be disarticulated from the RV, and atrial septectomy and a BT shunt can be performed. Most patients with Ebstein malformation of the TV and PA/IVS will have inadequate RV function and usually require univentricular palliation [10, 24, 25].

Right ventricular "overhaul" is the term for enlargement of the RV cavity by resecting excessive muscular hypertrophy and trabeculations. This may be helpful in augmenting the RV infundibulum and may prevent persistence or recurrence of subvalvular obstruction. RV overhaul may then be combined with transannular patch augmentation. Enlarging the trabecular part of the RV by extensive muscle resection may result in a larger cavity but has not been demonstrated to promote RV growth. While several authors have reported in favor of extensive muscle resection procedures, the Melbourne group has recommended against aggressive RV overhaul techniques. In their opinion, these procedures did not improve outcomes and must be regarded in the light of earlier philosophies of achieving biventricular repair whenever possible [7, 11, 12].

Several authors have described RV exclusion techniques, but the efficacy of the procedure is difficult to discern. LV dysfunction may result secondary to excessive leftward bulging of the septum by suprasystemic RV pressure which eventually may result in obstruction of the LV outflow tract. If RV decompression is not possible and LV function is impaired by a suprasystemic pressurized and bulging RV, then an RV exclusion procedure may pose a solution [26–31]. The procedure consists of filling the RV lumen with coils or with absorbable gelatin surgical sponge material and subsequently direct or patch closure of the TV. RVDCC is a contraindication for RV exclusion, as acute myocardial ischemia would develop. However, in the absence of proximal coronary artery obstruction, RV exclusion may prevent progression of RV to coronary fistula and associated competitive flow.

Numerous authors have recently reported hybrid management strategies that may have advantages over conventional treatment in selected patients. Although treatment of PA/IVS is already one of the most "hybrid" in the field of congenital heart disease as interventions are both by pediatric cardiologists and surgeons, here "hybrid" refers to a combined intervention and open chest procedure. In one such scenario, following a median sternotomy, the RVOT is opened by guiding a wire (inserted via the RV) through the PV that is subsequently balloon dilated under echocardiographic control. During the same procedure, a MBTS can be placed if saturations drop following ductal ligation. Balloon atrial septostomy is performed when deemed necessary. The procedure should probably be selected only for those patients that will need a MBTS combined with RV decompression. Some patients may be treated with a RF ablation and balloon dilation and continuation of PGE until the compliance of the right ventricle improves to allow adequate antegrade pulmonary blood flow and systemic-to-pulmonary blood flow source is avoided. Other advantages of this type of hybrid approach are that damage to the femoral vessels will be less and that PV opening is possibly safer in a surgical setting [32, 33].

Management After the Neonatal Period

In those patients with severe RV hypoplasia, management in infancy is clear: The patient needs to be staged toward total cavopulmonary connection (TCPC). Thus, the next step after initial neonatal treatment will be to convert the MBTS to a bidirectional cavopulmonary anastomosis (BCPA) where the superior vena cava (SVC) is connected end-to-side to the right PA. In our practice, this is done at the age of 6–8 months. If there are bilateral SVCs, the left SVC is also connected to the left PA. As SVCs are smaller when they present bilaterally, it may be preferable to perform the bilateral BCPA later at the age of 10–12 months.

BCPA may be accompanied with an atrial septectomy in patients for whom TCPC is planned. In some patients for whom a one and a half ventricle repair is performed, the atrial septum may be closed completely or partially at the time of the BCPA to allow inferior vena caval blood to travel to the pulmonary arteries through the TV and patent right ventricle.

At this author's institution, the optimal age for TCPC is considered to be 3–4 years with a minimal weight of 12–15 kg, to accommodate an 18 mm PTFE extracardiac conduit from the inferior vena cava (IVC) to the right PA. A 4 mm fenestration from the conduit to the adjacent right atrium is added when deemed necessary. Some centers may prefer the hemifontan procedure and a lateral tunnel TCPC.

Management after the neonatal phase of patients with mild or moderate RV hypoplasia is less obvious. When RVOT stenosis recurs or persists after initial RF perforation and balloon dilatation, this should be addressed by surgical opening of the RVOT, resection of obstructive and hypertrophic muscle tissue, and a

transannular patch augmentation. The ASD may be closed at the same time but only when the RV is able to accommodate full cardiac output. In practice, this will be feasible only in PA/IVS with mild RV hypoplasia and a reasonable TV. If RV hypoplasia is moderate, a BCPA may be added to surgical opening of the RVOT. The ASD is then left open in hope of further growth of the RV after which closure of the interatrial communication may be carried out. This may take several years, and the final decision to close the ASD may sometimes be difficult. If closure is considered to be possible, this is normally done by percutaneous device placement. For that reason, the surgeon should leave a sufficiently large border of the atrial septum when performing an atrial septectomy.

In patients with a good TV, mild RV hypoplasia, and unobstructed RVOT, the ASD can be closed with catheter-based device, usually at 2–4 years of age. The decision to close the ASD and occlude a patent systemic-to-pulmonary shunt is usually made in the catheterization laboratory after temporary occlusion of the shunt and ASD is performed and cardiac output is measured. If cardiac output does not decrease significantly and right atrial pressures are not too elevated, then it is safe to close the shunt and ASD.

When RV hypoplasia is moderate and TV and RVOT are sufficiently developed, construction of a BCPA may be postponed for some years to allow the RV to grow. If growth of the RV is inadequate and cyanosis persists, a one and a half ventricle repair may be preferred. When RV development appears to be adequate, the ASD may be closed (Fig. 88.3).

Management in Adulthood

Patients with PA/IVS repaired or palliated at pediatric age will need continued management by cardiologists well versed in congenital heart disease. This is true for both patients with cavopulmonary connections and for patients who have a biventricular circulation.

Univentricular palliations will need to be followed in centers with expertise and experience in the care for adults with congenital heart

Fig. 88.3 Same patient at age 7 months. The RV has grown more compared to the LV. Although the RV has grown, growth was insufficient and 1.5 ventricle repair seems to be necessary for this patient

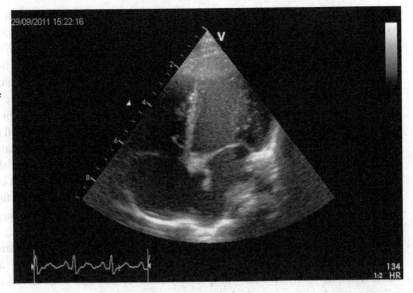

disease. A majority of these patients may suffer from supraventricular arrhythmias that may need medication and interventional ablation procedures. Total or partial cavopulmonary connections may be in need of revision, especially with older style Fontan operations such as atriopulmonary connections with or without the use of (valved) conduits. Revision will be necessary when patients present with a greatly enlarged right atrium, lower extremity edema, hepatomegaly, cirrhosis, or refractory atrial arrhythmias. The surgical procedure will then consist of revision of the original Fontan connection to an extracardiac TCPC and atrial septectomy. These Fontan revisions are usually combined with right atrial or biatrial MAZE procedures to prevent or mitigate later arrhythmias. Permanent epicardial pacemaker electrodes and devices are recommended.

Older patients with PA/IVS and biventricular repair also suffer arrhythmias, most commonly supraventricular tachyarrhythmia. Obstruction and insufficiency of the right-sided heart valves will need constant attention as the tricuspid and pulmonary valve in PA/IVS are abnormal both intrinsically and following previous interventions in childhood.

All previous interventions aimed at opening the pulmonary valve and RVOT will lead to some degree of pulmonary insufficiency (PI). Residual or recurrent pulmonary stenosis is not uncommon. In PA/IVS, the RV is typically hypertrophic and with decreased compliance and therefore PI should be tolerated fairly well for many years. However, adult PA/IVS patients who need PV replacement because of RV dilatation as a consequence of serious PI are now regularly seen. This population is expected to increase as survivorship of early repair increases.

Tricuspid valve in PA/IVS is usually smaller than normal, and a substantial amount of TV is structurally abnormal with thickened and dysplastic leaflets. For that reason, it is to be expected that TV repair or replacement may occur in adulthood. This is consistent with observations of different institutions [34–37].

Postoperative Intensive Care

Following initial neonatal palliation by aortopulmonary stent placement with or without opening the RVOT, it is important to manage pulmonary artery flow carefully. Both pulmonary underflow and overflow must be avoided. Typically, an arterial oxygen saturation around 80 % should be aimed for. Too much pulmonary flow may result in systemic hypoperfusion, while an inadequate pulmonary blood flow will lead to hypoxemia. Systemic hypoperfusion results in lactate acidosis and severe hypoxemia as a consequence of pulmonary hypoperfusion. Low oxygen saturations should prompt an echo-cardiographic study to determine adequate shunt patency. Shunt thrombosis can usually be suc-cessfully managed by thrombolysis and subse-quent heparinization. It is not uncommon that in the immediate period following neonatal pallia-tion O_2 saturations are lower than desirable. Ade-quate ventilation and nitric oxide may be useful in these instances. Furthermore, it is of importance to obtain an adequate mean arterial pressure to provide sufficient flow across the aortopulmonary shunt. Using combinations of vasoconstrictors (noradrenaline, phenylephrine, vasopressin) and milrinone can help fine-tune the balance between systemic and pulmonary circulations. Milrinone is preferred over dopamine or dobutamine [38]. After RVOT decompression (surgically or percu-taneously), RV function, both systolic and diastolic, may take days to some weeks to improve. Upon RV recovery, this will typically lead to an increase of pulmonary flow and improvement of arterial oxygen saturations.

Pulmonary artery growth is usually not a problem after palliation of PA/IVS and therefore the postoperative course following a bidirectional cavopulmonary anastomosis is normally unevent-ful. It may be considered to leave some antegrade pulmonary flow: Flow through a stenotic RVOT is usually well tolerated after BCPA and helps to keep oxygen saturations at an adequate level. Azygos veins should always be closed. Moderate or severe tricuspid insufficiency should be dealt with by repairing the tricuspid valve during the same procedure. The patency of the interatrial communication ought to be verified preopera-tively and optimized if considered insufficient. Again, if inotropic support is needed, a combina-tion of milrinone and vasoconstrictors is the opti-mal choice. Nitric oxide is rarely necessary in these patients. Following BCPA, the upper body segment should be raised to promote pulmonary flow and to prevent venous congestion of head and arms. Ventilation should be as non-aggressive as possible avoiding high pressures at all times.

Spontaneous ventilation should be permitted as soon as possible to permit an optimal flow through to the Glenn shunt. When oxygen saturations remain low following BCPA, the threshold for catheterization and angiography should be low. Catheterization can demonstrate an obstruction at the anastomosis between superior vena cava and pulmonary artery as well as obstructions between right and left pulmonary artery. Furthermore, veno-venous collaterals should be sought for and closed as they can result in considerable cyanosis. Finally, a depressed LV function should be treated aggressively as this may also impair the flow through the BCPA because of elevated atrial pres-sures and thus a higher trans-pulmonary gradient.

Completion toward a total cavopulmonary connection (TCPC) is typically performed at a body weight of approximately 12–15 kg. Again, all remaining or recurrent cardiovascular defects should have been diagnosed preopera-tively and when present dealt with during the TCPC procedure. Following TCPC, a similar intensive care policy should be followed as after a bidirectional Glenn shunt [39].

When biventricular or 1.5 ventricle repair is considered, preoperative evaluation should have confirmed adequate volume and function of the RV as well as an absence of important RVOT obstruction. Nevertheless, when 1.5 ventricle repair or biventricular repair of PA/IVS has been performed, diastolic dysfunction of the RV may sometimes cause venous congestion (only in the lower body half after 1.5 ventricle repair) as there is no longer an interatrial communication. This pathophysiology should preferably be con-firmed by catheterization before recurring to fenestrating an ASD patch or take down of a 1.5 ventricle repair.

Results

PA/IVS remains a heterogeneous anomaly with different treatment strategies. The more severe forms of PA/IVS may be difficult to manage, and high mortality rates persist even today. Evidence-based treatment algorithms have led to a more balanced and consistent approach to

PA/IVS and much better overall outcomes. A UK ongoing collaborative multicenter study reports 1 and 5 years survival rates of 70.8 % and 63.8 % in 183 patients with PA/IVS born from 1991 through 1995. Low birth weight, unipartite RV morphology, and a dilated RV were risk factors for mortality. No more than 29 % reached to a biventricular circulation in this study [10].

Outcomes of 81 patients operated in Melbourne between 1990 and 2006 were better, with 80 % 10 years survival rate. Risk factors for mortality were RVDCC and lower TV Z-scores. Only 38 % of their patients reached to biventricular repair [11].

A multicenter report that was published in 2004 and contained 408 patients revealed survival rates of 68 %, 60 %, and 58 % at 1, 5, and 15 years, respectively. Biventricular repair was obtained in 33 %. The study concluded that in the current era, 85 % of PA/IVS should survive with 50 % having a biventricular repair [9].

Another group has described 86 patients operated between 1974 and 2003 with a mortality rate of 31 %. Sixty-five percent reached biventricular repair. Predictors for biventricular repair were a tripartite RV morphology, RV decompression (with or without systemic-to-pulmonary artery shunt) as initial procedure, and the absence of coronary fistulae [40].

Others report better results, but populations are usually smaller than in the above-mentioned studies. One study reports an overall survival rate of 91.7 % with 10 of 24 patients reaching biventricular state. Patients were operated from 1996 to 2007 [41].

Mortality rates may be decreased when a more balanced approach is taken in choosing the appropriate treatment strategy for each patient. Fetal diagnosis and possibly fetal intervention may also result in earlier treatment with consequently lower mortality rates and a higher incidence of patients that will finally obtain a biventricular circulation.

Preferential use of univentricular management will obviously result in lower mortality rates but may deny some patients with more favorable anatomy the advantages of two-ventricle circulation. In general, it is assumed that cardiac function

and functional results after biventricular repair are more favorable than after univentricular repair. However, data do not necessarily support this bias. Sanghavi et al. showed that peak exercise capacity varied widely in both groups with a significant overlap. In this study, many patients had abnormal peak VO2, and there was a trend toward impaired exercise performance in older patients with PA/IVS irrespective of the type of operation [42]. In contrast, other studies including those from Romeih et al. demonstrate that pediatric PA/IVS patients after biventricular repair have a better exercise capacity and cardiac reserve as compared to the univentricular group [43, 44].

However, concern still remains whether the relatively small and hypertrophied RV in PA/IVS is capable of supporting adequate cardiac output especially with exercise. Studies showed that following a biventricular repair, PA/IVS patients still have abnormal RV diastolic function and atrial dilatation, which may eventually negatively influence clinical outcome [36, 45]. A study in PA/IVS patients following biventricular repair showed that the presence of RV myocardial fibrosis, detected with delayed contrast enhancement MRI, was correlated with both the occurrence of late pulmonary diastolic forward flow and reduced myocardial tissue velocities, indicating impairment of RV diastolic function [46].

In asymptomatic PA/IVS patients using dobutamine stress MRI and bicycle ergonometry, Romeih et al. showed that both exercise capacity and biventricular stroke volume response decreased with age. RV diastolic function decreased in older PA/IVS patients and was correlated with impaired RV-stroke volume response to pharmacological stress [47].

Whether the one and a half ventricle repair gives a better long-term clinical outcome than univentricular repair still remains unclear and study data are limited. During long-term follow-up, there appears to be no major difference in exercise capacity and cardiac reserve between these groups of patients, although in the 1.5 ventricle repair group, a better chronotropic response is maintained [44, 48, 49].

Conclusions

Pulmonary atresia with intact ventricular septum (PA/IVS) is an uncommon congenital heart disease (CHD) with variable severity right ventricular (RV) hypoplasia and tricuspid valve (TV) abnormalities. Due to the wide spectrum of anatomic variations, the management of PA/IVS remains challenging and is based on detailed measurements of the RV and tricuspid valve. Long-term studies into adulthood are necessary to determine whether biventricular repair, using the currently accepted selection criteria, is always preferable to a univentricular or a one and a half ventricle repair. A balanced approach based on RV size, TV Z-scores, and presence of RVDCC will provide optimal outcomes in this difficult defect.

References

1. Gittenberger-de Groot AC, Sauer U, Bindl L et al (1988) Competition of coronary arteries and ventriculo-coronary arterial communications in pulmonary atresia with intact ventricular septum. Int J Cardiol 18:243–258
2. Hanley FL, Sade RM, Freedom RM et al (1993) Outcomes in critically ill neonates with pulmonary stenosis and intact ventricular septum: a multiinstitutional study. Congenital Heart Surgeons Society. J Am Coll Cardiol 22:183–192
3. Allan LD, Crawford DC, Tynan MJ (1986) Pulmonary atresia in prenatal life. J Am Coll Cardiol 8:1131–1136
4. Bonnet D, Gaultier-Lhermitte I, Bonhoeffer P et al (1998) RV myocardial sinusoidal coronary artery connections in critical pulmonary valve stenosis. Pediatr Cardiol 19:269–271
5. Gittenberger-de Groot AC, Eralp I, Lie-Venema H et al (2004) Development of coronary vasculature and its implications for coronary abnormalities in general and specifically in pulmonary atresia without ventricular septal defect. Acta Paediatr Suppl 93:13–19
6. Oosthoek P, Moorman AF, Sauer U et al (1995) Capillary distribution in the ventricles of hearts with pulmonary atresia and intact ventricular septum. Circulation 91:1790–1798
7. Shinkawa T, Yamagishi M, Shuntoh K et al (2005) One-stage definitive repair of pulmonary atresia with intact ventricular septum and hypoplastic right ventricle. J Thorac Cardiovasc Surg 130:1207–1208
8. Alwi M (2006) Management algorithm in pulmonary atresia with intact ventricular septum. Catheter Cardiovasc Interv 67:679–686
9. Ashburn DA, Blackstone EH, Wells WJ et al (2004) Determinants of mortality and type of repair in neonates with pulmonary atresia and intact ventricular septum. J Thorac Cardiovasc Surg 127:1000–1007
10. Daubeney PE, Wang D, Delany DJ et al (2005) Pulmonary atresia with intact ventricular septum: predictors of early and medium-term outcome in a population-based study. J Thorac Cardiovasc Surg 130:1071
11. Liava'a M, Brooks P, Konstantinov I et al (2011) Changing trends in the management of pulmonary atresia with intact ventricular septum: the Melbourne experience. Eur J Cardiothorac Surg 40:1406–1411
12. Odim J, Laks H, Plunkett MD et al (2006) Successful management of patients with pulmonary atresia with intact ventricular septum using a three tier grading system for right ventricular hypoplasia. Ann Thorac Surg 81:678–684
13. Yoshimura N, Yamaguchi M, Ohashi H et al (2003) Pulmonary atresia with intact ventricular septum: strategy based on right ventricular morphology. J Thorac Cardiovasc Surg 126:1417–1426
14. Pettersen MD, Du W, Skeens ME et al (2008) Regression equations for calculation of z scores of cardiac structures in a large cohort of healthy infants, children, and adolescents: an echocardiographic study. J Am Soc Echocardiogr 21:922–934
15. Zilberman MV, Khoury PR, Kimball RT (2005) Two-dimensional echocardiographic valve measurements in healthy children: gender-specific differences. Pediatr Cardiol 26:356–360
16. Chinnock RE, Bailey LL (2011) Heart transplantation for congenital heart disease in the first year of life. Curr Cardiol Rev 7:72–84
17. Salvin JW, McElhinney DB, Colan SD et al (2006) Fetal tricuspid valve size and growth as predictors of outcome in pulmonary atresia with intact ventricular septum. Pediatrics 118:e415–e420
18. Tuo G, Volpe P, Bondanza S et al. (2012) Impact of prenatal diagnosis on outcome of pulmonary atresia and intact ventricular septum. J Matern Fetal Neonatal Med 25:669–674
19. Tworetzky W, McElhinney DB, Marx GR et al (2009) In utero valvuloplasty for pulmonary atresia with hypoplastic right ventricle: techniques and outcomes. Pediatrics 124:e510–e518
20. McElhinney DB, Tworetzky W, Lock JE (2010) Current status of fetal cardiac intervention. Circulation 121:1256–1263
21. Alwi M (2008) Stenting the ductus arteriosus: case selection, technique and possible complications. Ann Pediatr Cardiol 1:38–45
22. Gibbs JL, Uzun O, Blackburn ME et al (1999) Fate of the stented arterial duct. Circulation 99:2621–2625

23. Santoro G, Gaio G, Palladino MT et al (2008) Stenting of the arterial duct in newborns with duct-dependent pulmonary circulation. Heart 94:925–929

24. Coles JG, Freedom RM, Lightfoot NE et al (1989) Long-term results in neonates with pulmonary atresia and intact ventricular septum. Ann Thorac Surg 47:213–217

25. Starnes VA, Pitlick PT, Bernstein D et al (1991) Ebstein's anomaly appearing in the neonate. A new surgical approach. J Thorac Cardiovasc Surg 101:1082–1087

26. Akagi T, Benson LN, Williams WG et al (1993) Ventriculo-coronary arterial connections in pulmonary atresia with intact ventricular septum, and their influences on ventricular performance and clinical course. Am J Cardiol 72:586–590

27. Akiba T, Becker AE (1994) Disease of the left ventricle in pulmonary atresia with intact ventricular septum. The limiting factor for long-lasting successful surgical intervention? J Thorac Cardiovasc Surg 108:1–8

28. Amin P, Levi DS, Likes M et al (2009) Pulmonary atresia with intact ventricular septum causing severe left ventricular outflow tract obstruction. Pediatr Cardiol 30:851–854

29. Waldman JD, Karp RB, Lamberti JJ et al (1995) Tricuspid valve closure in pulmonary atresia and important RV-to-coronary artery connections. Ann Thorac Surg 59:933–940, discussion 940–931

30. Williams WG, Burrows P, Freedom RM et al (1991) Thromboexclusion of the right ventricle in children with pulmonary atresia and intact ventricular septum. J Thorac Cardiovasc Surg 101:222–229

31. Yang JH, Jun TG, Park PW et al (2008) Exclusion of the non-functioning right ventricle in children with pulmonary atresia and intact ventricular septum. Eur J Cardiothorac Surg 33:251–256

32. Burke RP, Hannan RL, Zabinsky JA et al (2009) Hybrid ventricular decompression in pulmonary atresia with intact septum. Ann Thorac Surg 88:688–689

33. Li S, Chen W, Zhang Y et al (2011) Hybrid therapy for pulmonary atresia with intact ventricular septum. Ann Thorac Surg 91:1467–1471

34. Ekman Joelsson BM, Sunnegardh J, Hanseus K et al (2001) The outcome of children born with pulmonary atresia and intact ventricular septum in Sweden from 1980 to 1999. Scand Cardiovasc J 35:192–198

35. John AS, Warnes CA (2012) Clinical outcomes of adult survivors of pulmonary atresia with intact ventricular septum. Int J Cardiol 161:13–17

36. Mishima A, Asano M, Sasaki S et al (2000) Long-term outcome for right heart function after biventricular repair of pulmonary atresia and intact ventricular septum. Jpn J Thorac Cardiovasc Surg 48:145–152

37. van der Velde ET, Vriend JW, Mannens MM et al (2005) CONCOR, an initiative towards a national registry and DNA-bank of patients with congenital heart disease in the Netherlands: rationale, design, and first results. Eur J Epidemiol 20:549–557

38. Hoffman TM, Wernovsky G, Atz AM et al (2003) Efficacy and safety of milrinone in preventing low cardiac output syndrome in infants and children after corrective surgery for congenital heart disease. Circulation 107:996–1002

39. Bronicki RA, Chang AC (2011) Management of the postoperative pediatric cardiac surgical patient. Crit Care Med 39:1974–1984

40. Cleuziou J, Schreiber C, Eicken A et al (2010) Predictors for biventricular repair in pulmonary atresia with intact ventricular septum. Thorac Cardiovasc Surg 58:339–344

41. Hannan RL, Zabinsky JA, Stanfill RM et al (2009) Midterm results for collaborative treatment of pulmonary atresia with intact ventricular septum. Ann Thorac Surg 87:1227–1233

42. Sanghavi DM, Flanagan M, Powell AJ et al (2006) Determinants of exercise function following univentricular versus biventricular repair for pulmonary atresia/intact ventricular septum. Am J Cardiol 97:1638–1643

43. Ekman-Joelsson BM, Gustafsson PM, Sunnegardh J (2009) Exercise performance after surgery for pulmonary atresia and intact ventricular septum. Pediatr Cardiol 30:752–762

44. Romeih S, Groenink M, Roest AA et al (2012) Exercise capacity and cardiac reserve in children and adolescents with corrected pulmonary atresia with intact ventricular septum after univentricular palliation and biventricular repair. J Thorac Cardiovasc Surg 143:569–575

45. Mi YP, Cheung YF (2006) Assessment of right and left ventricular function by tissue Doppler echocardiography in patients after biventricular repair of pulmonary atresia with intact ventricular septum. Int J Cardiol 109:329–334

46. Liang XC, Lam WW, Cheung EW et al (2010) Restrictive right ventricular physiology and right ventricular fibrosis as assessed by cardiac magnetic resonance and exercise capacity after biventricular repair of pulmonary atresia and intact ventricular septum. Clin Cardiol 33:104–110

47. Romeih S, Groenink M, van der Plas MN et al (2012) Effect of age on exercise capacity and cardiac reserve in patients with pulmonary atresia with intact ventricular septum after biventricular repair. Eur J Cardiothorac Surg 42:50–55

48. Kreutzer C, Mayorquim RC, Kreutzer GO et al (1999) Experience with one and a half ventricle repair. J Thorac Cardiovasc Surg 117:662–668

49. Numata S, Uemura H, Yagihara T et al (2003) Long-term functional results of the one and one half ventricular repair for the spectrum of patients with pulmonary atresia/stenosis with intact ventricular septum. Eur J Cardiothorac Surg 24:516–520

Pulmonary Stenosis and Insufficiency

James Jaggers, Cindy Barrett, and Bruce Landeck

Abstract

Pulmonary stenosis refers to either fixed or dynamic obstruction to blood flow from the pulmonary ventricle to the pulmonary arterial vasculature. The most common form of this is pulmonary valvar stenosis, which often presents in infancy but may present throughout life. *Subvalvar stenosis* may be in two forms, either infundibular stenosis or double-chambered right ventricle. *Supravalvar stenosis* may be isolated but often occurs in association with other defects like tetralogy of Fallot. Supravalvar stenosis may be associated with genetic syndromes like Williams syndrome. In the broad sense, pulmonary stenosis is present either in isolation or associated with 20–30 % of all congenital heart defects. Pulmonary valvar stenosis is most often treated with catheter-based therapy with good results. Supravalvar and subvalvar defects most commonly require surgical therapy; other lesions are more often treated surgically. In this chapter, management of these defects in the intensive care unit has some common principles that will be discussed along with the morphology and current therapy and outcomes.

Electronic Supplementary Material: The online version of this chapter (doi:10.1007/978-1-4471-4619-3_21) contains supplementary material, which is available to authorized users.

J. Jaggers (✉)
The Heart Institute, Department of Pediatrics, Children's Hospital Colorado, University of Colorado School of Medicine, Denver, Aurora, CO, USA

Cardiothoracic Surgery, University of Colorado School of Medicine The Children's Hospital Pediatrics, Aurora, CO, USA
e-mail: James.Jaggers@childrenscolorado.org

C. Barrett • B. Landeck
Division of Pediatric Cardiology, Department of Pediatrics, Childrens Hospital of Colorado, University of Colorado School of Medicine, Aurora, CO, USA
e-mail: cindy.barrett@childrenscolorado.org;
bruce.landeck@childrenscolorado.org

Keywords

Double-chambered right ventricle • Noonan syndrome • Pulmonary insufficiency • Pulmonary stenosis • Valvotomy • Williams syndrome

Introduction

Obstruction of blood flow from the right ventricle to the pulmonary artery may occur at various levels. Pulmonic stenosis (PS) refers to a dynamic or fixed anatomic obstruction to flow from the right ventricle (RV) to the pulmonary arterial vasculature. In the broadest sense, it is associated with 20–30 % of all forms of congenital heart disease. In this chapter, the discussion will be limited to defects with primary pulmonary stenosis at either the subvalvar, valvar, or supravalvar level.

Embryology

The pulmonic valve develops between the 6th and 9th week of gestation. Normally, the pulmonic valve is formed from three swellings of subendocardial tissue called the semilunar valves. These tubercles develop around the orifice of the pulmonary tree. The swellings are normally hollowed out and reshaped to form the three thin-walled cusps of the pulmonary valve. In Noonan syndrome, tissue pad overgrowth within the sinuses interferes with the normal mobility and function of the valve.

The myocardial cushion begins as a matrix of endothelial cells and an outer mitochondrial layer separated by cardiac jelly. After endocardial cushion formation, the endothelial mesenchymal transformation (EMT), which is specified endothelial cells, differentiates and migrates into the cardiac jelly. Through a poorly understood process, the cardiac jelly goes through local expansion and bolus swelling, and cardiac valves are formed. The aortic and pulmonic valves develop from the outflow tract of the endocardial cushion and are also believed to involve neural crest cell migration from the brachial crest during development [1].

The process of endothelial–mesenchymal transformation is integral to the development of heart valves. Several factors play a role in this process and include vascular endothelial cell growth factor (VEGF), which is important in endothelial cell proliferation during valve development. In utero, hypoxia and hyperglycemia may affect VEGF and prevent endothelial cell proliferation and thus inhibit valve development. Infants born to hyperglycemic mothers have a threefold increase in cardiovascular abnormalities. There has been correlation between intrapartum hypoxic events and valvular disease. Other research suggests that the numerous signaling pathways have been implicated in development of valvar lesions including the NFAT family of proteins, connexins, and NOTCH family proteins [1].

Anatomy

Valvar Pulmonic Stenosis

The pulmonary valve is normally made up of three thin semilunar leaflets attached to a circular fibrous annulus. Congenital heart lesions of the pulmonary valve can range from abnormalities in the size of the annulus to discrepancies in the thickness of leaflets, to abnormal number of leaflets to fusion of the leaflets, or to any combination thereof. In most patients, the valve commissures are partially fused and the three leaflets are thin and pliable, resulting in a conical or dome-shaped structure with a narrowed central orifice. This classic form of pulmonary valve stenosis comprises about 12 % of congenital heart disease [2]. Post-stenotic pulmonary artery dilation may occur owing to "jet-effect" hemodynamics. In approximately 10–15 % of individuals with valvar PS, the pulmonary valve is dysplastic. These valves have irregularly shaped, thickened leaflets,

Fig. 89.1 Critical PS still – "In this parasternal short-axis image, one can see the aortic valve in cross section, with the valve open in systole. In contrast the pulmonary valve (1 o'clock in relation to the aortic valve) does not open very much. Also note the right ventricular hypertrophy"

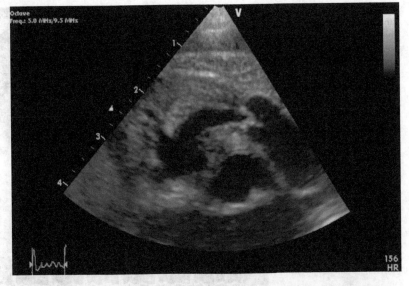

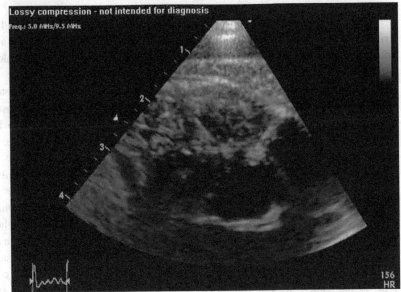

Fig. 89.2 Critical PS MPG – "In this parasternal short-axis loop, one can see the aortic valve opening and closing normally, while the pulmonary valve (1 o'clock in relation to the aortic valve) does not open much. Note the right ventricular hypertrophy"

with minimal commissural fusion, and reduced mobility (Figs. 89.1 and 89.2). The leaflets are composed of myxomatous tissue, which may extend to the vessel wall. The valve annulus and the supravalvular area of the pulmonary trunk is usually hypoplastic. Post-stenotic dilation of the pulmonary artery is uncommon. Approximately two thirds of patients with Noonan syndrome have PS due to dysplastic valves. A bicuspid valve is found in as many as 90 % of patients with tetralogy of Fallot, whereas it is rare in

individuals with isolated valvar PS. Isolated hypoplasia of the pulmonary valve annulus with a normal appearing leaflets can occur but is rare.

With severe valvular PS, subvalvular right ventricular hypertrophy can result in secondary infundibular narrowing and contribute to the right ventricular outflow obstruction. This often regresses after relief of valvular stenosis.

Associated defects like patent foramen ovale or atrial septal (ASD) are not uncommon, and when present in a patient with severe PS and

Fig. 89.3 Infundibular stenosis from still 2 – "In this subcostal image, 2D imaging on left shows a muscle bundle underneath the pulmonary valve, which is shown on the color Doppler image on the right to cause acceleration of blood flow"

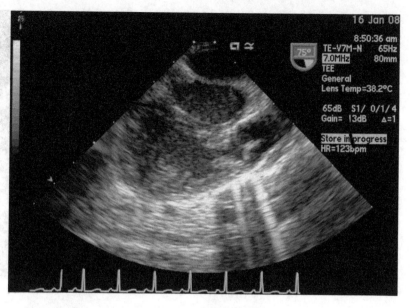

decreased right ventricular chamber compliance, cyanosis can result secondary to right-to-left shunting across the atrial level communication.

Subvalvar Pulmonic Stenosis

Subpulmonary stenosis has two forms: double-chambered right ventricle (DCRV) and primary infundibular stenosis. In DCRV, stenosis of the proximal portion of the infundibulum is due to a fibrous or muscle band at the junction of the main cavity of the RV and the infundibulum. The end result is separation of the right ventricle into a proximal high-pressure chamber and a distal low-pressure chamber. Importantly this lesion does not involve the moderator band. The second type is associated with a thickened muscular infundibulum that forms a narrow outlet to the RV. The infundibulum appears shrunken. In this second type, the narrowed area may be short or long and may be located immediately below the pulmonary valve or lower into the outflow tract but above the moderator band (Figs. 89.3–89.5).

Supravalvar Pulmonic Stenosis

Obstruction of the right ventricular outflow tract above the pulmonary valve will be considered supravalvar stenosis in this chapter. Prevalence is estimated at 2–3 % of all congenital heart defects, and it is associated with another dominant congenital heart defect like tetralogy of Fallot in two thirds of patients. In some patients with isolated supravalvar pulmonary stenosis, the cause may be related to in utero exposure to congenital rubella syndrome or related to inherited conditions like cutaneous laxa, Alagille, Noonan, Ehlers–Danlos, and Williams syndromes. The level of obstruction may be in the main pulmonary artery or in the branches, well into the lung parenchyma. The inheritance pattern of pulmonic valvular stenosis is poorly understood, although Noonan and Leopard syndromes display an autosomal dominant pattern. Rarely, pulmonic stenosis is associated with recessively transmitted conditions such as in the Laurence–Moon–Biedl syndrome. Mutations in germ lines PTPN1 and RAF1 have been associated with these valvular abnormalities [3, 4].

Pathophysiology

Much of what is known about the natural history and pathophysiology of pulmonic valvular stenosis comes from the natural history study of congenital heart defects and the second natural history study of congenital heart defects. The natural history study of congenital heart defects

Fig. 89.4 Infundibular
stenosis MPG – "In this
subcostal loop, one can see
the 2D imaging on the left
showing a muscle bundle
underneath the pulmonary
valve, which is shown on
the color Doppler image on
the right to cause
acceleration of blood flow"

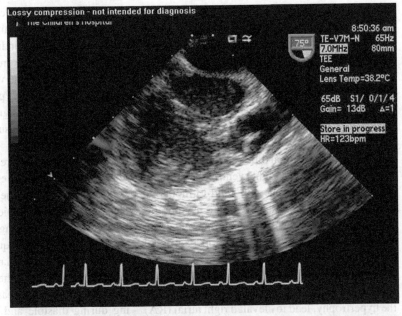

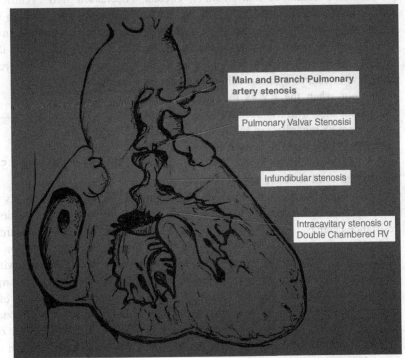

Fig. 89.5 Anatomic
positions of various types
of right ventricular outflow
tract obstruction: main and
branch PS, valvar PS,
infundibular PS, and
intracavitary stenosis or
double-chambered RV

included an initial cardiac catheterization and
then follow-up for events over an 8-year period.
The Second Natural History Study of Congenital
Heart Defects reported on 16–27 years of follow-
up from the same cohort [5].

Common to all three forms of right ventricle
outflow tract obstruction (RVOTO) is the hemodynamic consequence of the obstruction with
elevated pressure within the RV cavity.
The degree of elevation depends on the severity

of obstruction. When severe, the resulting RV systolic pressure may exceed that of the left ventricle (supra-systemic). In the absence of multilevel obstruction, lower or even normal pressures are present beyond the obstruction site. This rise in right ventricular pressure leads to compensatory RV myocardial hypertrophy. If this hypertrophy is severe, impaired subendocardial coronary blood flow may result in ischemia and eventual dilation or fibrosis of the RV with subsequent right ventricular failure. Although most children with mild-to-moderate pulmonary valve stenosis (PVS) are asymptomatic, there are reported cases of patients with moderate-to-severe PS who develop exertional angina, syncope, and even sudden death [6]. Elevation of RV end-diastolic pressure and decreased compliance of the RV, consequent to the hypertrophy, lead to elevated right atrial (RA) pressure and dilation of that chamber. Greater right atrial pressures is required to fill the ventricle, and relative right and left atrial pressures may be reversed, favoring persistent patency of the foramen ovale and right-to-left shunting. This gives rise to central cyanosis. This phenomenon may occur when the RV is hypoplastic, even when associated with less severe PS. In neonates with severe PS regardless of location, the pulmonary blood flow depends on the patency of the ductus arteriosus. Prostaglandin therapy must be maintained until a stable source of pulmonary blood flow can be obtained and/or until the right ventricular compliance and pulmonary vascular resistance decrease.

In patients with severe PS and intact ventricular septum (IVS), the presentation and pathophysiology are very similar to pulmonary atresia with intact ventricular septum (PAIVS). However, unlike PAIVS, it is very uncommon for patients with PS instead of pulmonary atresia to have a significant degree of right ventricular hypoplasia.

Deformity and malfunctioning of the left ventricle (LV) occur in proportion to RV hypertension and can be demonstrated using sophisticated techniques. These alterations in LV mechanics are readily reversible with the relief of the RVOTO and decompression of the right ventricle.

Patients with isolated valvar PS may have subsequent infundibular hypertrophy that could elicit a reactive infundibular obstruction especially in the face of exercise or inotropic therapy. Following relief of the valvar PS, the infundibular hypertrophy may persist for an extended period but generally regresses over time.

Pulmonary valve insufficiency is a risk factor for development of late, right ventricular dysfunction and failure, secondary to chronic ventricular volume overload [7]. As the right ventricle enlarges, the ventricular geometry changes. The tricuspid valve annulus may become dilated, leading to poor coaptation of valve leaflets and subsequent regurgitation. Additionally, right ventricular dilation and increased diastolic volume shift the interventricular toward the left ventricle, decreasing left ventricular filling during diastole and ultimately may lead to decreased left ventricular function [8, 9]. The conduction system is also affected by right ventricular enlargement. The QRS becomes prolonged, increasing the vulnerability of the RV to ventricular tachycardia and the patient to sudden death [10].

Diagnosis

Clinical Pulmonary Stenosis

The majority of patients with right ventricle outflow tract (RVOT) lesions, if not diagnosed in utero by fetal echocardiography, will present with heart murmur on physical examination. Most RVOT lesions with stenosis will have a harsh systolic ejection murmur which will vary in intensity by severity of the stenosis. Additionally, those with pulmonary valve stenosis may have an audible click corresponding with the valve snapping open in early systole. The murmur from RVOT or pulmonary valve stenosis may be heard throughout the precordium but will be loudest at the left upper sternal border. Branch pulmonary artery stenosis will have a murmur audible at the same place but will have pronounced radiation to the axillae of the affected artery. The presence of a prominent second heart sound may indicate main or branch PS. Moderate or severe pulmonary valve insufficiency will also have a diastolic decrescendo murmur. With subvalvar stenosis, a loud, long, systolic crescendo–decrescendo murmur (ejection type), with its maximal intensity at mid-systole or later (indistinguishable from that of isolated pulmonary valvar stenosis), is heard at the left sternal border and is well conducted to the precordium, neck, and back. The later the peak intensity of the murmur occurs, the greater the obstruction. Patients with dysplastic valves may not have a systolic ejection click. If the valve is pliable, a systolic ejection click is often heard.

Although murmur loudness does not necessarily increase with severity, murmurs of less than grade 3/6 usually occur with mild stenosis. With moderate-to-severe stenosis, murmurs are usually systolic and grade 4/6 or louder. The length of the murmur depends on duration of RV systole that, in turn, depends on severity of the stenosis. Thus, mild stenosis is associated with a short murmur, with its peak earlier than mid-systole. In moderate stenosis, the murmur ends at or slightly after the aortic component of the second heart sound, which remains audible. With marked-to-severe obstruction, the murmur extends beyond the aortic component, which may be obscured [4].

Severe pulmonic valvular stenosis and resultant right ventricular dysfunction may be associated with tricuspid insufficiency, elevated central venous pressure, hepatosplenomegaly, a pulsatile liver, jugular venous pulsations, and hepatojugular reflux. Significant pulmonic stenosis is characterized by a prominent jugular venous *a* wave and a right ventricular lift. Cyanosis may occur with right-to-left shunting at the atrial level as with a patent foramen ovale (PFO) or septal defect. If the right ventricle becomes significantly hypertrophied due to increased afterload, arrhythmias can present.

Pulmonary Insufficiency

Pulmonary valve insufficiency usually exists as a primary defect in combination with pulmonary valve stenosis or as a secondary defect resulting from undesired sequelae of catheter-based or surgical intervention on the pulmonary valve. It is usually well tolerated at least initially, however, if severe, may cause severe right heart enlargement, tricuspid valve insufficiency, exercise intolerance, and atrial and ventricular arrhythmias due to the volume load placed on the right ventricle. Clinical exam findings of pulmonary insufficiency are typically limited to diastolic murmur but may include hepatomegaly if tricuspid valve insufficiency develops as the right ventricle begins to fail. The diastolic murmur is best located at the left upper sternal border and is described as a decrescendo murmur, graded from I to IV based on loudness of the murmur.

Diagnosis

Electrocardiogram

The electrocardiogram (ECG) can be normal in patients with mild stenotic lesions, but more severe lesions can demonstrate right axis deviation, right atrial enlargement, and right ventricular hypertrophy. ECG is also helpful to rule out associated arrhythmias and electrical signs associated with the risks of sudden cardiac death, particularly in older patients with chronically hypertrophied or dilated RV and pulmonary regurgitation.

Radiography

Although not commonly employed as a diagnostic method of detecting RVOT lesions, some patients who have chest X-rays for other reasons may have RVOT lesions discovered incidentally. Findings on CXR may be cardiomegaly, due to right ventricular enlargement, or hypertrophy or pulmonary artery enlargement due to post-stenotic dilation.

Echocardiography

Echocardiogram is the most commonly used tool for diagnosis and follow-up evaluation of RVOT lesions. In subvalvar stenotic lesions, 2D imaging will show the hypertrophied muscle bands of double-chambered right ventricle (DCRV) or the abnormal thickening of primary infundibular stenosis. 2D imaging of the pulmonary valve will show its anatomy and function, including a measurement of the annulus diameter, number of leaflets, and size and morphology of the leaflet tissue. Doming of the valve can be seen. 2D imaging of the main pulmonary artery and proximal branches will show discrete stenotic lesions or post-stenotic dilation. Color Doppler provides a visualization of relative flow velocity, size of the effective orifice in valvar stenosis, and will show the presence of valvar insufficiency. Spectral Doppler will provide velocity of flow information, allowing for the calculation of pressure gradients. Clinical practice guidelines for estimation of valve stenosis severity exist [7].

Pulmonary valve insufficiency is readily detected on echocardiogram. It is seen in multiple views, including parasternal long- and short-axis, apical, and subcostal views. The insufficiency is seen in diastole, and severity is typically categorized as trivial, mild, moderate, or severe. Trivial insufficiency may be a normal finding. The narrowest width of the insufficient jet (called the vena contracta) can be compared to the valve annulus diameter to help in grading insufficiency. Typically, severe insufficiency will show echo findings of a wide vena contracta, flow reversal in the branch pulmonary arteries, longer jet length, and right ventricular dilation (due to volume overload). Pressure half-time, the time it takes for the pressure gradient between the pulmonary artery and right ventricle at end-systole to decrease by half, can be measured on the spectral Doppler tracing of the pulmonary insufficiency jet and is typically shorter in more severe insufficiency. Pressure half-time, however, is heart rate dependent and is likely more helpful in older patients with a slower heart rate [11].

Cardiac Catheterization

Cardiac catheterization is commonly used for interventional purposes after echo diagnosis but can also be an excellent tool for evaluating the severity of main and branch pulmonary artery stenosis. Catheter pullbacks provide directly measured pressure gradients, and angiography allows for precise measurements and definition of the stenotic area. Further details related to diagnostic

and interventional cardiac catheterization of these patients can be found in other chapters in this textbook. Cardiac catheterization is generally not required for diagnosis of pulmonary insufficiency but may be indicated to document the condition of the branch pulmonary arteries, pulmonary vascular resistance, and atrial and ventricular pressures and potentially for electrophysiologic study to rule out or document atrial and ventricular arrhythmia.

Other Imaging Studies

Computed tomography (CT) and cardiac MRI (cMRI) are typically reserved for cases in which the anatomy is complex or whenever necessary to evaluate the ventricular volume and mass indexes or the proximal and distal pulmonary branch anatomical details. End-systolic and end-diastolic volumes are readily available with cMRI along with accurate ejection fraction. Along with this, the cMRI can accurately quantify the differential blood flow to each lung in the case of branch pulmonary stenosis. MRI has also become very useful for quantification of regurgitant fraction in pulmonary insufficiency. These tests provide excellent visualization of anatomy, especially of the main and branch pulmonary arteries. CT scan can be performed in a fraction of the time it takes to do cMRI but comes at the risk of radiation exposure. CT gives very accurate information about intraluminal abnormalities of the PAs and very good definition of the pulmonary veins. However, cMRI usually requires sedation in children younger than 7–8 years of age.

Indications for Intervention and Decision-Making

Children with mild pulmonary valve stenosis (RVOT gradient <40 mmHg) do not require intervention, either surgical or catheter-based. These children can be followed at regular but infrequent intervals with periodic electrocardiogram and echocardiogram. There is no limitation on activity and subacute bacterial endocarditis prophylaxis is recommended.

In patients with moderate pulmonary stenosis (RVOT gradient of 40–50 mmHg), therapy is certainly indicated if symptoms are present. In the asymptomatic patient, controversy exists about the necessity of intervention. Certainly, cardiologists have been increasingly willing to subject patients to catheter-based procedures as opposed to surgical procedures for the asymptomatic patient. The long-term efficacy of this course is unclear, although most feel that potential prevention of right ventricular hypertrophy may be beneficial in the long term.

Patients with severe pulmonary stenosis (RVOT gradient >50 mmHg) usually present as neonates or in early infancy and should have an intervention. The usual approach is a diagnostic cardiac catheterization, with the intention for balloon valvotomy. In the neonatal patient, safety of this procedure is guaranteed by a ductus arteriosus and maintained patent with a prostaglandin (PGE_1) infusion. If there is inadequate pulmonary blood flow after the intervention, PGE_1 therapy is continued to the intensive care unit. Over the following days, it is expected that the right ventricular compliance will improve and forward flow into the lungs will increase. Prostaglandin medication is then stopped to allow ductal closure. If this is successful, cardiac output and oxygenation are maintained. If, however, there is continued severe and poorly tolerated cyanosis with the ductus closed, an alternative source of pulmonary blood flow is indicated.

Surgical or Interventional Management

Critical Pulmonary Stenosis of the Neonate

Neonates with severe pulmonary stenosis present in the early after delivery with cyanosis and usually ductal-dependent pulmonary blood flow. Differential diagnosis includes severe TOF or pulmonary atresia with intact ventricular septum. Most often the obstruction is isolated to the valve. The valve is typically a tricuspid pulmonary

valve with a relatively preserved annulus size. Because in utero flow through the right ventricle is limited, there may be variable degrees of right ventricular hypertrophy and infundibular hypertrophy. There may also be associated tricuspid valve hypoplasia. In contrast to pulmonary atresia with intact septum, the right ventricular hypoplasia is rarely severe and RV to coronary artery fistulae is also rare.

Most neonates with critical RVOTO have excess right-to-left shunting across an interatrial communication (patent foramen ovale or ASD), and pulmonary blood flow is dependent on a patent ductus arteriosus (PDA). Because of increased afterload, the hypertrophied right ventricle may develop decreased function, and increased pulmonary blood flow via the PDA can result in left ventricular volume overload and congestive heart failure. If undetected and ductal patency is not preserved, the patient will develop low cardiac output and hypoxemia and eventually succumb.

Therapy is directed at relief of right ventricular outflow tract obstruction. In the current era, this is most often accomplished with catheter-based intervention and balloon valvotomy with surgical valvotomy or transannular incision reserved for patients with inadequate relief of stenosis and persistent requirement for ductal pulmonary blood flow. Details of interventional catheterization are further discussed in a specific chapter in this book. The success of balloon valvotomy has been very good, and with proper management, the need for surgical intervention in patients with critical pulmonary stenosis presenting as neonates is relatively uncommon. These are often patients with multiple levels of severe RVOTO or significant right ventricular and tricuspid valve hypoplasia. Regardless of whether the balloon valvotomy or surgical valvuloplasty is performed, the results are very good. Freedom of re-intervention on the pulmonary valve after surgery was 98.4 %, 93.5 %, 87.7 %, 70.9 %, and 55.7 % at 5, 10, 20, 30, and 40 years postoperatively. Freedom of re-intervention in the patients undergoing primary balloon valvotomy was 95.1 %, 87.5 %, and 84.4 % at 5, 10, and 20 years post-procedure.

Fig. 89.6 Typical pulmonary valvar stenosis with doming and thickened valve exposed via main pulmonary artery incision

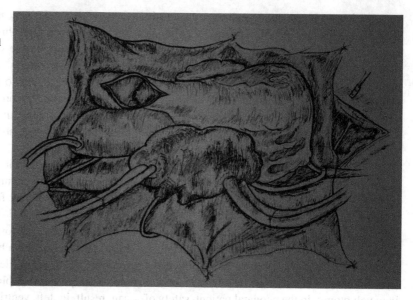

The most common indication for re-intervention in the surgical group was for pulmonary insufficiency while in the balloon valvotomy group was for residual or recurrent stenosis [12].

Surgical Therapy for Pulmonary Valvotomy

Surgical intervention is recommended in symptomatic patients, those with associated defects that require intervention, patients with a significant left-to-right shunt and those with a high RV–PA gradient or a progressively increased gradient. In many patients with pulmonary valvar stenosis, catheter-based balloon valvotomy is the first-line therapy, with surgery being reserved for failures or need for additional source of pulmonary blood flow like a modified Blalock–Tausig shunt. Certainly, when patients present at older ages, catheter-based therapy may be more successful and durable. It is not uncommon for there to be mild residual pulmonary stenosis, but this is usually well tolerated and may be advantageous in that the pulmonary insufficiency may be limited by the mild right ventricular hypertrophy.

Surgical valvotomy is performed via median sternotomy. While this procedure can be performed with inflow occlusion techniques, it is currently most commonly performed with cardiopulmonary bypass (CPB) at normothermic or mildly hypothermic temperatures. After CPB is established, the PDA is occluded with a tourniquet. If a systemic-to-pulmonary shunt is also necessary, this is easily performed with this approach. If an inter-atrial level communication exists, it is often left patent if poor right ventricular compliance and consequently elevated right atrial pressure is anticipated. The communication will allow some degree of right to left shunting and a subsequent decrease in right atrial pressure. The PDA may be left patent if there is any concern about the ability of the right ventricle to provide adequate pulmonary blood flow. The PDA is most often ligated in patients with reasonable antegrade pulmonary blood flow and a systemic-to-pulmonary shunt in order to avoid competitive pulmonary blood flow.

The pulmonary valvotomy is performed by making a longitudinal incision in the main pulmonary artery down to the level of the pulmonary valve annulus (Fig. 89.6). In most cases the main pulmonary artery is normal to mildly dilated in caliber. The pulmonary valve is most often tricommissural, and valvotomy of each commissure is carried out with a scalpel from the luminal aspect to the annulus. The free edges of the valve leaflets may be mildly thickened but usually do not require debridement of fibrotic tissue. The pulmonary valvotomy is usually closed primarily but can be patched if the main pulmonary artery is small. The goal of the valvotomy should be complete relief of the obstruction and preservation of valve function.

It is rare that the annulus of the PV is hypoplastic enough to require transannular incision for relief of obstruction. If necessary, it should be extended through the annulus onto the RV only far enough to relieve annular obstruction. Occasionally, infundibular muscle bundles may be resected through this incision if necessary. The transannular incision is patched with any patch material, like native pericardium or bovine pericardium.

Alternative Source of Pulmonary Blood Flow

In patients in whom there is inadequate antegrade pulmonary blood flow despite an adequate pulmonary valvotomy, an alternative source of pulmonary blood flow may be necessary in order to alleviate the need for PGE$_1$ therapy and eventual discharge. As many as 17–21 % of neonates that undergo a balloon pulmonary valvotomy will require prostaglandin infusion to maintain ductal patency and pulmonary blood flow for 3–21 days after balloon valvotomy [13, 14]. In the congenital heart surgeon society study of critical pulmonary stenosis, Hanley found that regardless of the whether a balloon pulmonary valvotomy or a surgical valvotomy is performed, 25 % required re-intervention for the right ventricular outflow tract and 10 % will require additional source of pulmonary blood flow [15]. This may be accomplished with interventional ductal stent placement or with systemic-to-pulmonary shunt, most commonly a modified Blalock–Taussig (BT) shunt. While there is growing enthusiasm for catheter-based ductal stenting, the successful placement of these stents is limited to experienced centers and operators as well as specific ductal anatomy without risk of pulmonary artery coarctation from

ductal tissue. The efficacy, safety, and outcomes of this technique have yet to be established.

The modified BT shunt can be performed via either lateral thoracotomy or via median sternotomy. Many groups advocate for BT shunt construction via median sternotomy due to the ease of access to the vessels, the flexibility of choice for placement of the shunt, and avoidance of two incisions on the child, and because conversion to the use of CPB is readily available via median sternotomy. If a pulmonary valvotomy is not necessary, the BT shunt is usually performed without the aid of CPB; however, CPB should be utilized if hemodynamic instability or hypoxia ensues during the procedure or if there is necessity of pulmonary arterioplasty. The modified BT shunt is usually between the innominate artery and the right pulmonary artery, although patients in whom there is a right aortic arch, it may be easier to perform on whichever side the innominate artery travels and to the ipsilateral pulmonary artery. In a normal-sized neonate, usually a 3.5–4 mm polytetrafluoroethylene tube graft is used, as this will prevent excessive pulmonary blood flow and CHF. The proximal anastomosis is carried out with an end graft to side innominate artery and 7–0 Prolene suture with slight bevel to allow smooth takeoff from the vessel. The distal anastomosis is an end graft to the right pulmonary artery. It is important that the graft not be excessively short so as to distort the right PA and, as the patient grows, not too long so as to increase potential for kinking and resistance and hence potential for thrombosis. Occasionally there may be some potential for left pulmonary artery stenosis at the insertion of the PDA into the pulmonary artery. In this case, CPB may be necessary to perform a left pulmonary arterioplasty as well as the BT shunt.

Valvar Stenosis in Older Children

The presentation of valvar pulmonary stenosis in older children is due to either delayed diagnosis or progression of the stenosis over time to the point of detection. In some patients, the pulmonary valve annulus fails to grow with somatic growth and the relative stenosis increases due to this mismatch. In other patients, the increased stenosis may be due to the progression of right ventricular hypertrophy due to the valvar obstruction. In these patients, interventional catheter balloon valvotomy is the procedure of choice in the absence of other defects that require surgical intervention like a VSD or severe infundibular stenosis. The only exception to the latter scenario may be the patient with a secundum ASD and pulmonary stenosis, for which catheter-based therapy both have good results. Surgical therapy is indicated for patients with failed catheter balloon valvotomy or multilevel obstruction. Surgical valvotomy is accomplished in the same way as in the neonate, except that the valve leaflets and the annulus are often significantly dysplastic and the need for a transannular patch (TAP) is increased. Some surgeons might place a monocusp valve at the time if a TAP is necessary.

Direct comparison of outcomes for catheter-based therapy and open surgical therapy has limitations because surgical accuracy and technical advances have made historical series of surgical therapy outcomes obsolete. In general, caregivers could expect greater reduction of the gradient is observed after surgery, but, at least historically, the degree and frequency of pulmonary insufficiency may be higher after surgery than after balloon therapy [12, 16].

Supravalvar Stenosis

Supravalvar stenosis of the main pulmonary artery (MPA) is relatively rare in the absence of tetralogy of Fallot. Two thirds of patients with supravalvar PS also have additional congenital heart defects. If present, MPA stenosis may be associated with Noonan or Williams syndromes. Williams syndrome and Alagille's syndrome are most often associated with main and branch pulmonary artery stenosis. Patients with Noonan syndrome will often have proximal main pulmonary artery stenosis in addition to dysplastic valvar stenosis. Surgical therapy is accomplished with the aid of cardiopulmonary bypass. Complete relief of obstruction is the goal; however, with stenosis associated with Williams or

Alagille's syndrome, this is usually not possible and future catheter-based therapy can be anticipated. Usually patch pulmonary arterioplasty is required and these patches may extend well into the hilum of the lung. The best opportunity for surgical success is with the first operation. The choice of patch material varies, but most surgeons choose either minimally fixed or unfixed native pericardium; however, allograft material is acceptable. Newer materials, like extracellular matrix, have been used, but long-term outcome data is pending.

Subvalvar Stenosis

Isolated subvalvar stenosis accounts for a small minority of isolated RVOTO. Indications for repair are similar to those for valvar stenosis. Sometimes the subvalvar or muscular stenosis will regress after treatment of an associated valvar stenosis. The only effective and durable therapy for subvalvar or infundibular stenosis is surgical. Two types of subvalvar stenosis exist: one in which there is infundibular fibromuscular stenosis immediately below the pulmonary valve that does not involve the septal or parietal muscle bands and another that is primary hypertrophy of the septal and parietal muscle at the junction of the body of the right ventricle and the infundibular or outlet chamber of the RV. This type of obstruction is sometimes referred to as "double-chambered RV" (DCRV) and will be further discussed below. In the case of the true infundibular stenosis, infundibular incision up to, but not into, the pulmonary valve, with outflow tract gusset of prosthetic or treated autologous pericardium, is the preferred approach. While techniques have been described to accomplish this without cardiopulmonary bypass, these authors recommend its use to accomplish an accurate and safe approach.

DCRV is a heart defect in which the right ventricular chamber is separated into two chambers by thick hypertrophied muscle bundles. In the usual situation, the septal and parietal bands hypertrophy to the point of creating an opening between the hypertrophied hypertensive

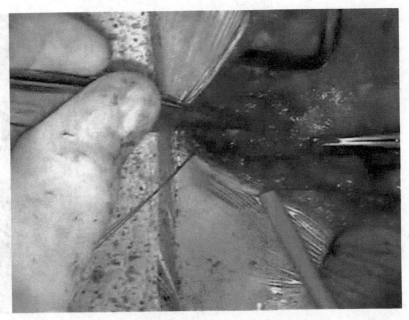

Video 89.1 A 17-year-old male with history of VASD repair at age 4. Developed severe subvalvar RVOTO with decreased exercise tolerance and occasional chest pain. Operation consisted of division and resection of large muscle bundles in mid-cavity of the RV. RVOT gusset placed

proximal inlet and trabecular right ventricle and a low-pressure infundibular or outlet chamber. While this defect is most often diagnosed in the pediatric patient, it can present later in adult life. In a report of 26 surgical cases, the anomalous obstructive muscular lesion identified was, in the majority, a muscular shelf originating from the body of the septomarginal trabeculation and extending toward the ventricular apex. In nine of these patients, the obstructive muscular shelf was positioned low and diagonally across the apical component. In the other 11 patients, the obstructive shelf was high and horizontal. The important distinction in this study was that, irrespective of its location, the two parts of the right ventricle to either side of the shelf each possessed part of the apical ventricular component, with the trabeculated proximal chamber in continuity with the ventricular inlet, and the distal chamber, with its own coarse trabeculations, supporting the subpulmonary infundibulum [17].

DCRV is associated with a ventricular septal defect in 60–90 % of the cases [17]. The VSD is usually perimembranous and localized between the hypertensive proximal RV chamber and the LV. Therefore, left-to-right shunt is usually limited. In this situation, the presentation is often

similar to tetralogy of Fallot with limitation of pulmonary blood flood predominating. However, the VSD can be in any portion of the septum, and when it is associated with the lower-pressure infundibular chamber, the presentation is more often like a large VSD with nonrestrictive left-to-right shunt. DCRV is usually a primary defect but may be acquired in some patients with VSD and pulmonary stenosis or TOF after repair. In this situation, previously unrecognized or recurrent hypertrophied muscle bundles can result in DCRV [18] (Video 89.1).

Repair consists of relief of the mid-cavitary muscular obstruction and repair of intracardiac shunts. Defects, including cor triatriatum, ASD, DORV, subaortic stenosis, and Ebstein's malformation, may coexist. These are most often repaired at the same operation. The cavitary RV obstruction may be surgically relieved from either a right atrial or right ventricular incision. It is important to resect muscle to relieve the obstruction completely in order to prevent recurrence. Most often this is best accomplished via a ventriculotomy with an outflow tract gusset of prosthetic material or pericardium. The VSD is most often approached from a right atrial approach but may be closed through the right ventriculotomy or pulmonary

Video 89.2 Surgical video of pulmonary valve replacement in a 7-year-old patient with a previous RV–PA conduit. This technique allows placement of an over sized (adult-sized) bioprosthetic valve in very small patients (in the author's experience (2–3 years of age)). The technique is equally applicable for mechanical or bioprosthetic valve insertion

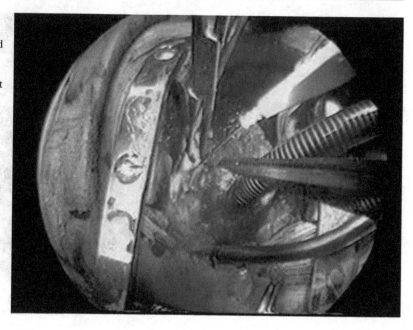

artery if the VSD is associated with the distal aspect of the RV cavity. Surgical repair outcomes are quite gratifying with very low mortality and durable relief of symptoms and recurrence of obstruction [19, 20].

For all patients with various forms of pulmonary stenosis, the prospect of total catheter-based therapy may be on the horizon. Currently, any intervention on the pulmonary valve, either surgical or catheter-based, is imperfect, and a significant number of patients will be left with either residual stenosis or valvar insufficiency or both. In this population catheter-based stent and valve therapy may be possible as newer generations of percutaneous valves are developed. Nonetheless, there will continue to be an important and necessary role for open surgical therapy in many patients.

Surgical therapy for pulmonary insufficiency is primarily relegated to replacement of the pulmonary valve. Attempts at repair of the pulmonary valve are usually unsuccessful. One can reconstruct leaflets of the pulmonary valve, but an important difference between the pulmonary valve and the aortic valve is that the pulmonary valve annulus is supported only by the very pliable, not rigid infundibulum of the right

ventricular outflow tract. Unless the pulmonary insufficiency is associated with previous balloon or surgical valvotomy or tetralogy repair, there is usually coexistent pulmonary stenosis, making repair attempt unlikely to be successful and durable. Therefore, pulmonary valve replacement is most often indicated for severe pulmonary insufficiency. Replacement can be accomplished by open cardiac surgical techniques or by catheter-based techniques. Catheter-based techniques are currently limited to patients that have had a previous RV–PA conduit or to patient that have had a stented bioprosthetic pulmonary valve replacement. Valves placed surgically fall in into three categories: (1) valved conduits (human allografts, bovine jugular venous valved conduits, xenograft stentless valved conduit or Dacron tube valved conduit), (2) prosthetic xenograft valves, or (3) prosthetic mechanical valves. Stented valves include either porcine pulmonary valve or pericardial valves. Mechanical valves have been used in the pulmonary position with generally good results but generally limited to patients that require anticoagulation for another reason or those that have very high risk for redo sternotomy [21] (Video 89.2).

Critical Care Management

Pre-intervention Phase

Pre-intervention management of RVOT obstruction in the intensive care environment is almost exclusive to the neonate with critical PS, with or without ductal and therefore PGE_1 dependency. The latter is determined by the degree of cyanosis upon ductal closure or restrictive pattern. Alternatively, and for the safety reasons mentioned above, PGE_1 infusion may be arbitrarily pursued throughout the peri-interventional phase. Patients in this condition require a comprehensive cardiovascular assessment (chest X-ray, ECH, echocardiography) and noninvasive monitoring, namely, a continuous ECG, serial noninvasive blood pressure measurement, continuous oximetry, and eventually near-infrared spectroscopy (NIRS); some patients diagnosed perinatally may have a venous or arterial umbilical catheter that caregivers should strive to remove as soon as deemed safe. Otherwise, a safe and reliable intravenous line (two if peripherally inserted, one if indwelling) should be kept at all times, mostly in PGE_1-dependent patients. Very seldom do neonates with critical PS require mechanical ventilation although this may be necessary for transport between institutions or in patients with high risk for central apnea. In patients in whom the RVOT obstruction is multistaged or not deemed adequate for interventional cardiac catheterization, the surgical indication is clear. These patients shall remain on a PGE_1 infusion until operated upon. While awaiting for interventional catheterization or surgery, caution is required concerning the risks of over-circulating and mismatch of systemic and pulmonary circulation with tissue perfusion compromise (unlikely but possible), proper nutritional support, evaluation and management of comorbidities, and noninvasive or invasive respiratory support in case of apnea.

Post-interventional Phase

Establishing a post-intervention baseline is important. Patients should be monitored with continuous telemetry to recognize and assess changes in heart rate and rhythm. Continuous pulse oximetry monitoring allows continuous monitoring of oxygen saturation.

Invasive blood pressure monitoring via a peripheral arterial line is helpful as it allows continuous monitoring of blood pressure as well as arterial access for monitoring of arterial blood gases to ensure adequate oxygenation and ventilation. Even if the patient has an arterial line, it is advised to obtaining intermittent noninvasive blood pressure measurement to establish a baseline.

Cardiac assessment post-intervention should also include obtaining an ECG in the immediate post-intervention to evaluate for any arrhythmias and to use as a baseline to compare against if further rhythm issues should arise.

For those patients who have undergone surgical correction of their right ventricular outflow tract obstruction, presence of a central venous line located the right atrium SVC junction or at the RA–IVC junction is helpful for obtaining an accurate central venous pressure (CVP) and systemic venous saturation. Central venous pressure monitoring allows the caregiver to establish a baseline CVP and allows easier diagnosis of atrial and ventricular dyssynchrony (via monitoring atrial and ventricular wave characteristics) and right ventricular response to volume changes and/or use of inotropes. It is also helpful to have real-time SVO_2 with oximetric catheter technology for early detection of low cardiac output. Near-infrared spectroscopy (NIRS) monitoring is used in many centers to evaluate the trends in cerebral and/or renal venous saturations in the post-intervention period. Cerebral NIRS is most similar to and may be a surrogate of SVO_2 and may be a helpful adjunctive way to trend SVO_2 particularly in patients who do not have a central venous access to monitor SVO_2 via venous blood. Alternatively, in patient with a well-positioned peripherally inserted central catheter (PICC), serial SVO_2 may be checked. Renal or flank NIRS may allow a more sensitive way to monitor changes in renal blood flow which often precede changes in cerebral blood flow.

A chest radiograph should be obtained post-intervention to evaluate for endotracheal tube and/or central line position, as well as establishing a baseline view of the patient's cardiac silhouette and lung parenchyma.

An echocardiogram is useful to establish a baseline cardiac function as well as diagnose any potential residual disease and to grade and trend any residual obstructive gradient and the potential for de novo regurgitation. Optimal oxygen delivery may be monitored with laboratory testing including arterial blood gas measurements, serum lactate, systemic venous saturation, hemoglobin and hematocrit, as well as blood chemistries for evaluation of renal function. For patients where there are ongoing concerns of right ventricular dysfunction, blood natriuretic peptide levels can be informative.

Therapy

Cardiac

Management of children with obstruction from the RV to the pulmonary arteries varies with the type of intervention required for relief of the obstruction. Additionally it is not unusual for patients to have potential residual obstruction or new valvar insufficiency after intervention.

To ensure optimum cardiac output, adequate preload needs to be maintained to allow right ventricular filling. Right ventricular systolic dysfunction may be impaired especially after intervention but is unusual. Use of inotropes helps improve RV contractility; however, inotropic agents like dopamine and epinephrine may also increase the incidence of arrhythmia and may actually increase dynamic obstruction of the RVOT if there is residual muscular subvalvar pulmonary obstruction. Right ventricular diastolic function may also be impaired following intervention. Measurement and monitoring of the right atrial pressure and waveform may be very helpful in diagnosis and management of right ventricular diastolic dysfunction. Use of phosphodiesterase inhibitors such as milrinone may improve diastolic function and may also decrease the pulmonary vascular resistance. Levosimendan, a calcium-sensitizing agent more commonly used and available only in Europe, is also used in children with low cardiac output and may have improved efficacy compared to milrinone.

Coronary artery flow to the right ventricle occurs primarily in systole, and flow depends on the pressure difference between the aorta and the right ventricle intracavitary pressure. In a right ventricle that is hypertrophied and hypertensive, the difference between the RV pressure and the aortic pressure is decreased. This issue may be further exacerbated if right ventricular afterload is increased via increased ventilator pressure. Thus, the endocardium is at risk of becoming ischemic, and adequate aortic diastolic pressure needs to be maintained to ensure effective coronary artery filling. Lower dose vasopressin has been particularly useful in this situation.

Maintaining normothermia in the post-intervention period is important as hyperthermia increases myocardial oxygen consumption increased heart rate and decreased ventricular filling time. The incidence of arrhythmia, particularly ectopic junctional tachycardia, may also be increased with hyperthermia. Low cardiac output may result in central hyperthermia. It is important to topically cool the patient to normothermia. This, along with other measures like treating acidosis and inotropic support, will improve cardiac output. Cooling the patient beyond normothermia will likely result in increased SVR and further deterioration of cardiac output.

Tachycardia should be avoided and aggressively managed since it may impact the filling of a poorly compliant and "stiff" right ventricle. Some patients, particularly neonates after balloon valvotomy, maintain a significant functional or reactive subvalvar gradient and may benefit from the use of beta-blockers. In the latter case, an infusion of esmolol, which has a short half-life and can be titrated to effect, is a reasonable choice. After the critical phase, the patient may be transitioned to oral beta-blockers if necessary.

Ventilator Support

If the patient is receiving positive pressure mechanical ventilation, mean airway pressure should remain as low as possible to maintain functional residual capacity yet allow appropriate gas exchange. Close monitoring of the patient's arterial blood gas parameters with a goal of maintaining a normal pH and CO_2 will help ensure lower pulmonary vascular resistance. Discontinuation of positive pressure ventilation is ideal as spontaneous respiration decreases intrathoracic pressure and subsequently improves right atrial filling. If pulmonary vascular resistance is high, then initiation of inhaled nitric oxide may be indicated.

Fluid Management

Optimization of right ventricular function and cardiac output may necessitate supplemental fluid administration to maintain adequate filling pressure in the face of a hypertrophied, noncompliant right ventricle. Central venous monitoring is strongly advised. If the patient has had a procedure, communication with the anesthesiologist as to the optimal filling pressure is beneficial to guide postoperative management. As for the pre-intervention phase, resuming nutritional support, enteral or parenteral, may significantly impact patient progression.

Complications

Residual Obstruction

Obstruction to right ventricular outflow may persist after intervention. This is often seen in patients who undergo catheterization intervention using balloon dilation of their pulmonary valve obstruction to find later that they also have significant subpulmonic obstruction. As previously described, dosing with beta-blockers can decrease the heart rate and decrease the dP/dT and may decrease the muscular or dynamic subvalvar obstruction. However, further intervention may be indicated if significant obstruction remains. If the right ventricular pressure exceeds 75 % of the systemic pressure, there may be indication for intervention.

Low Cardiac Output Syndrome

Acute right ventricular dysfunction may occur in the immediate post-intervention period and can present with low cardiac output syndrome, increased central venous pressure, hepatomegaly, hypotension, arrhythmias, and progression to right ventricular and circulatory failure. Initial efforts to support cardiac output and systemic oxygen delivery in the face of RV dysfunction should be to optimize heart rate and rhythm and preload, maintain normothermia to decrease myocardial oxygen consumption, and monitor ventilator and arterial blood gas parameters to ensure the lowest possible pulmonary vascular resistance. Additionally, inhaled nitric oxide and ventilator strategies may also be used to decrease pulmonary vascular resistance. In general, diastolic dysfunction predominates and should be managed with the administration of phosphodiesterase inhibiters like milrinone or calcium channel blocker like levosimendan. If there is coexisting systolic dysfunction, modest inotropic support may be indicated. Epinephrine is often used in this situation because, at lower doses (<0.05 mcg/kg/min), epinephrine is a pulmonary vasodilator and may decrease right ventricular afterload. Some patients with RVOTO may have cardiomyopathy and require a longer duration of support in the postoperative period. This may be associated with biventricular hypertrophy and dysfunction and may be associated with genetic syndromes like Noonan syndrome. Severe right ventricle dysfunction with critical impairment of systemic oxygen delivery may necessitate mechanical circulatory support in the form of extracorporeal membrane oxygenation (ECMO). Some patients may require, as an intermediate step, the creation of an atrial "pop-off" (surgical or by cardiac catheterization) in order to relieve the strain on the right-sided heart and optimize systemic stroke volume, although at the expenses of lower saturations.

Pulmonary Valve Insufficiency

Pulmonary insufficiency is rarely present in children in the absence of stenosis or following an intervention for pulmonary stenosis. These patients may include patients that have had percutaneous balloon valvotomy. Pulmonary valve insufficiency was noted in 80–90 % patients, but most of these patients do not develop significant right ventricular volume overload [22]. One report documented the development of clinically significant pulmonary insufficiency in 6 (6 %) of 107 patients at late follow-up. Some of these patients required pulmonary valve replacement [23]. The incidence of pulmonary insufficiency following surgical valvotomy has been reported as high as 60–90 % [24]. However, improved techniques in surgical valvotomy likely result in significantly better results that the historical results above. The degree of insufficiency may be limited by the decreased compliance and resultant higher end-diastolic pressure of the hypertrophied right ventricle. However, as the right ventricular compliance improves after relief of obstruction, the degree of insufficiency may increase and become more clinically evident. Long-term effects of pulmonary valve regurgitation result in right ventricular dilation and dysfunction and decreased exercise capacity and development of important atrial and ventricular arrhythmia [10, 25].

Outcomes and Long-Term Follow-Ups

Right Ventricular Outflow Tract

Outcomes for patients who undergo surgical intervention on the right ventricular outflow tract below the pulmonary valve are excellent. After relief of the pulmonary stenosis, long-term medical management is rarely necessary. However, depending on the clinical situation and presence of associated defects, the patient should continue to be followed by a congenital cardiologist. Occasionally, Holter monitoring can be useful to detect silent arrhythmias. Recurrence of pulmonary stenosis is not uncommon and may require re-intervention.

Pulmonary Valve and Main and Branch Pulmonary Arteries

Outcomes for repair of supravalvar stenosis and main/branch pulmonary arteries depend on the initial severity of the disease and the etiology. The most important factors to determine outcome are the effectiveness of the intervention and the presence and severity of any residual pulmonary valve insufficiency or stenosis across the valve or into the branch pulmonary arteries. Patients who have isolated pulmonary valve stenosis without dysplastic, thickened leaflets generally have excellent long-term outcomes after intervention, whether surgical or catheter-based, and typically the single intervention is all the patient will need. Thickened dysplastic pulmonary valve leaflets are more problematic, and these patients are at higher risk of the need for re-intervention or replacement of the valve due to recurrent stenosis and/or insufficiency. Interventions on the branch pulmonary arteries may include surgical arterioplasty or catheter-based therapy including balloon dilation with or without stent placement. Long-term outcomes are dependent on the ability to expand the stenotic area to as close to normal diameter as possible.

Medical management for patients who have had intervention on their pulmonary valve and/or pulmonary arteries is typically conservative, with few patients requiring long-term medication usage. After initial recovery from surgery or catheterization, patients should have yearly follow-up in outpatient clinic with echocardiogram. All patients who have had intervention on their pulmonary valve or branch pulmonary arteries should have follow-up with a cardiologist. Choosing the appropriate timing for re-intervention or replacement of the pulmonary valve is challenging but should be considered if the right ventricle becomes dilated or hypertrophied or if systolic function deteriorates. Other indications include significant tricuspid insufficiency or important, usually atrial, arrhythmia, or else the documentation of concerning signs in the ECG reflecting a high risk for sudden death in older patients. Re-intervention for branch pulmonary stenosis can either be combined with a needed pulmonary valve surgery, when patch augmentation can be performed, or can be performed in the cardiac catheterization laboratory when stenosis is felt to be severe enough to impact growth of the vessel or when stenosis in one branch causes a disproportionate flow to the opposing lung.

Conclusion

Right ventricular outflow tract obstruction (RVOT), with or without associated regurgitation, consists in a wide variety of anomalies. The vast majority of patients with RVOT pathologies may currently benefit from surgical or interventional procedures with reassuring results, although the incidence or residual abnormalities or recurrent lesions remain of concern. Patients with chromosomal anomalies or syndromes may be at a higher risk for re-intervention. Future directions will likely be focused on the development of interventional strategies and devices for selected patients. Surgery and probably hybrid approaches will, however, remain the sole alternative for other patients.

References

1. Armstrong EJ, Bischoff J (2004) Heart valve development: endothelial cell signaling and differentiation. Circ Res 95(5):459–470
2. Wilson PD, Correa-Villasenor A, Loffredo CA, Ferencz C (1993) Temporal trends in prevalence of cardiovascular malformations in Maryland and the district of Columbia, 1981–1988. The Baltimore-Washington infant study group. Epidemiology 4:259–265
3. Jorge AA, Malaquias AC, Arnhold IJ, Mendonca BB (2009) Noonan syndrome and related disorders: a review of clinical features and mutations in genes of the RAS/MAPK pathway. Horm Res 71(4):185–193
4. Libby P, Bonow RO, Mann DL, Zipes DP (2007) Braunwald's heart disease: a textbook of cardiovascular medicine, 8th edn. Saunders, Philadelphia
5. Nishimura RA, Gersony WM et al (1993) Second natural history study of congenital heart defects. Circulation 87:89–137
6. Hayes CJ, Gersony WM, Driscoll DJ, Keane JF, Kidd L, O'Fallon WM, Pieroni DR, Wolfe RR, Weidman WH (1993) Second natural history study of congenital heart defects. Results of treatment of patients with pulmonary valvar stenosis. Circulation 87:I28–I37
7. Yerbakan C, Klopsch C, Niefeldt S, Zeisig V, Vollmar B, Liebold A, Sandica E, Steinhoff G (2010) Acute and chronic response of the right ventricle to surgically induced pressure and volume overload – an analysis of pressure volume relations. Interact Cardiovasc Thorac Surg 10(4):519–525
8. Geva T, Sandweiss BM, Gauvreau K, Lock JE, Powell AJ (2004) Factors associated with impaired clinical status in long-term survivors of tetralogy of Fallot repair evaluated by magnetic resonance imaging. J Am Coll Cardiol 43:1068–1074
9. Kane C, Kogon B, Pernetz M, McConnell M, Kirshbom P, Rodby K, Book W (2011) Left ventricular function improves after pulmonary valve replacement in patients with previous right ventricular outflow tract reconstruction and biventricular dysfunction. Heart Inst J 38(3):234–237
10. Bouzas B, Kilner PJ, Gatzoulis MA (2005) Pulmonary regurgitation: not a benign lesion. Eur Heart J 26(5):433–439
11. Zoghbi WA et al (2003) Recommendations for evaluation of the severity of native valvular regurgitation with two-dimensional and Doppler echocardiography. J Am Soc Echocardiogr 16(7):777–802
12. Voet A, Rega F, de Bruaene AV, Troost E, Gewillig M, Van Damme S (2012) Long-term outcome after treatment of isolated pulmonary valve stenosis. Int J Cardiol 156(1):11–15
13. Tabatabaei H, Boutin C, Nykanen DG, Freedom RM, Benson LN (1996) Morphologic and hemodynamic consequences after percutaneous balloon valvotomy for neonatal pulmonary stenosis: medium-term follow-up. J Am Coll Cardiol 27:473–478
14. Ladusans EJ, Qureshi SA, Parsons JM, Arab S, Baker EJ, Tynan M (1990) Balloon dilatation of critical stenosis of the pulmonary valve in neonates. Br Heart J 63:362–367
15. Hanley FL, Sade RM, Freedom RM, Blackstone EH, Kirklin JW (1993) Outcomes in critically ill neonates with pulmonary stenosis and intact ventricular septum. J Am Coll Cardiol 22:183–192
16. O'Connor BK, Beekman RH, Lindauer A, Rocchini A (1992) Intermediate-term outcome after pulmonary balloon valvuloplasty: comparison with a matched surgical control group. J Am Coll Cardiol 20(1):169–173
17. Alva C, Ho SY, Lincoln CR, Rigby ML, Wright A, Anderson RH (1999) The nature of obstructive muscle bundles in double chambered right ventricle. J Thorac Cardiovasc Surg 117:1180–1187

18. Pongiglione G, Freedom RM, Cook D et al (1982) Mechanism of acquired right ventricular outflow tract obstruction in patients with ventricular septal defect: an angiocardiographic study. Am J Cardiol 50:776–780

19. Hachiro Y, Takagi N, Koyanagi T et al (2001) Repair of double chambered right ventricle: surgical results and long-term follow-up. Ann Thorac Surg 72:1520–1522

20. Said SM, Burkhart HM, Dearani JA, O'Leary PW, Ammash NM, Schaff HV (2012) Outcomes of surgical repair of double-chambered right ventricle. Ann Thorac Surg 93:197–200

21. Stulak JM, Dearani JA, Burkhart HM, Connolly HM, Warnes CA, Suri RM, Schaff HV (2010) The increasing use of mechanical pulmonary valve replacement over a 40-year period. Ann Thorac Surg 90: 2009–2015

22. Rao PS, Galal O, Patnana M (1998) Results of three to 10 year follow up of balloon dilatation of the pulmonary valve. Heart 80(6):591–595

23. Berman W, Fripp RR, Raisher BD, Yabek SM (1999) Significant pulmonary valve incompetence following oversize balloon pulmonary valvotomy in small infants: a long-term follow-up study. Catheter Cardiovasc Interv 48(1):61–65; discussion 66

24. McNamara DG, Latson LA (1982) Long-term follow-up of patients with malformations for which definitive surgical repair has been available for 25 years or more. Am J Cardiol 50(3):560–568

25. Harrild DM, Powell AJ, Tran TX, Geva T, Lock JE, Rhodes J, McElhinney DB (2010) Long-term pulmonary regurgitation following balloon valvuloplasty for pulmonary stenosis risk factors and relationship to exercise capacity and ventricular volume and function. J Am Coll Cardiol 55(10):1041–1047

Congenital Aortic Valve Stenosis and Regurgitation

90

Viktor Hraška, Joachim Photiadis, Peter Zartner, and Christoph Haun

Abstract

Congenital aortic valve stenosis, defined as an obstruction to outflow from the left ventricle by an abnormal aortic valve, represents a spectrum of anatomical and clinical variations from critical to noncritical aortic stenosis. Congenital aortic insufficiency due to absence or underdevelopment of the aortic cusps is extremely rare; however, post-procedural aortic insufficiency with residual aortic stenosis is often seen.

The diagnosis is generally easily established by echocardiography. The decision-making process and treatment management is challenging due to heterogeneous makeup of patients. All available treatment options provide palliation, rather than cure.

The most appropriate management of critical aortic stenosis remains controversial. Both balloon dilatation of aortic valve and open valvotomy are firmly established as effective initial treatments with encouraging survival benefits. Morphology of the valve usually determines the need for re-intervention. Conceivably, if three cusps could be constructed, open valvotomy may provide superior long-term outcomes in comparison with ballooning regarding preservation of the native aortic valve.

In older children, reconstruction of the aortic valve is an attractive option, which preserves growth potential of the native valve, stabilizes

Electronic Supplementary Material: The online version of this chapter (doi:10.1007/978-1-4471-4619-3_23) contains supplementary material, which is available to authorized users.

V. Hraška (✉) • J. Photiadis • P. Zartner
German Pediatric Heart Center, Asklepios Clinic Sankt Augustin, Sankt Augustin, Germany
e-mail: v.hraska@asklepios.com

C. Haun
Neonatal and Pediatric Cardiac Intensive Care, German Pediatric Heart Center, Sankt Augustin, Germany

geometry of the left ventricle, and does not rule out the future valve replacement options. In some children, the best alternative is to use a pulmonary autograft or prosthetic valve, despite the well-known drawbacks of these procedures. The Ross procedure has the capacity for growth, but durability limitations become apparent by the end of the first postoperative decade, in particular in younger patients. Prosthetic mechanical valves are durable; however, anticoagulation therapy is required, which is attended by the problems of thromboembolism and bleeding. Bioprosthetic valves and heterografts in children do not require anticoagulation, but there is no growth potential and particularly the durability is limited requiring early reoperations. Anatomy, pathophysiology, clinical signs and symptoms as well as indications, timing of intervention or surgical correction, and long-term outcomes are described in detail for each lesion.

Keywords

Aortic regurgitation • Aortic stenosis • Balloon dilatation of aortic valve • Critical aortic stenosis • Left ventricular outflow tract obstruction • Low cardiac output syndrome • Open valvotomy • Reconstruction of aortic valve • Replacement of aortic valve • Ross–Konno procedure • Ross procedure • Surgical repair

Introduction

Brief Historical Background

Congenital etiology of aortic stenosis was first recognized by Paget in 1844 [1].

In 1958, Spencer and colleagues performed the first open valvotomy in inflow occlusion, followed by aortic valvotomy utilizing cardiopulmonary bypass [2]. Later in 1983, Lababidi reported the first balloon dilatation of congenital aortic stenosis [3].

Definitions

Congenital Aortic Valve Stenosis

Congenital aortic valve stenosis, defined as an obstruction to outflow from the left ventricle by an abnormal aortic valve, constitutes about 5 % of all congenital cardiac malformation, with incidence in males up to five times higher than in females [4].

Congenital aortic valve stenosis represents a spectrum of anatomical and clinical variations from critical to noncritical aortic stenosis. Critical aortic stenosis in newborns is a challenging situation with severe obstruction at valvar level, with ductal-dependent systemic circulation and symptoms of heart failure.

Noncritical aortic valve stenosis occurs in the setting of either a malformed valve (unicuspid or bicuspid) or a tricuspid valve with commissural fusion [5, 6].

Aortic Insufficiency

Congenital aortic insufficiency due to absence or underdevelopment of the aortic cusps is extremely rare with an incidence of 0.3 % of congenital heart disease [7].

Aortic valve insufficiency may result from any procedure for aortic valve stenosis. Otherwise, aortic insufficiency is associated with certain congenital heart diseases (ventricular septal defect, common truncus arteriosus, tetralogy of Fallot, sub-aortic membrane, supra-valvar aortic stenosis, and others). Aortic valve insufficiency also occurs in the setting of malformed aortic valve, or may be the result of dilatation of the aortic root due to a connective tissue disorder (Marfan, Loeys–Dietz, Ehlers–Danlos, Turner syndromes) [8, 9].

Anatomy

Critical Aortic Stenosis

A reduced cross-section area in critical aortic stenosis is the result of deficiency in, or absence of, one or more commissures, leading to a unicuspid, bicuspid, or tricuspid valve with fused commissures. This is often accompanied by myxomatous changes and thickening of the valve cusps, with or without commissural fusion, and hypoplasia of the valvar annulus [10].

Noncritical Aortic Stenosis

Most frequently seen (in about 70 % of cases) is bicuspid valve with the two commissures arranged as anterior and posterior. There may be a third false commissure (raphe). There are usually variable degrees of peripheral fusion of one or both commissures creating a stenosis [11]. If the free edges of both thickened bicuspid cusps are taut with no extra length and equal in length to the diameter of the aortic root, they cannot open completely and thereby produce obstruction. Abnormal tricuspid aortic valves may not be obstructive during early infancy, but may become stenotic later in life due to cusps thickening and calcification.

Aortic Insufficiency

Prolapse is the most frequent cusp pathology in pure aortic insufficiency. This pathology may also coexist with root dilatation [12–14]. Predominant morphological factors contributing to aortic insufficiency after the balloon-dilated aortic valve include a combination of anterior commissural

avulsion, cusp dehiscence with retraction, cusp tear or cusp perforation, central incompetence due to calcified cusps and sinus of Valsalva dilation, deficient cusps, and free cusp edge adhesion to the aortic wall [10, 15, 16].

Physiology and Pathophysiology

Critical Aortic Stenosis

The postnatal course depends on the combination of the severity of outflow tract obstruction and the function and development of the left ventricle and shunts on the atrial and ductal level.

In the neonate with critical aortic stenosis, both systemic and coronary perfusions may be dependent on the patent ductus arteriosus. As the ductus arteriosus begins to close after birth, signs of circulatory collapse develop with hypotension, oliguria, and metabolic acidosis [10, 17].

In older children, valvar aortic stenosis causes increased ventricular afterload, resulting in increased ventricular wall stress and workload. This provides the stimulus for left ventricle concentric hypertrophy in order to normalize left ventricle wall stress, keeping an appropriate left ventricle ejection fraction. The pressure gradient across the stenotic valve causes a mismatch between coronary perfusion pressure and myocardial perfusion pressure, potentially leading to subendocardial myocardial ischemia, arrhythmias, and infarction. Endocardial fibroelastosis, a focal or diffuse cartilage-like fibroelastic thickening of the endocardium and papillary muscles, may develop as a consequence of chronic in utero or postnatal subendocardial ischemia. This process could severely impair the systolic and diastolic function of the left ventricle. If left ventricle hypertrophy is incapable of normalizing wall stress, afterload mismatch develops. During exercise, there may be development of subendocardial ischemia, causing angina-like symptoms, or ineffective increase of cardiac output leading to syncope [10].

Increased left ventricle end-diastolic pressure results in impaired cardiac output especially at exercise. The left ventricle compensates for this by dilation, which further increases wall stress. Eventually the dilation will result in decreased systolic function and further deterioration of cardiac output. At this point, it is unlikely that relief of the aortic stenosis will result in complete recovery of ventricular function.

Aortic Insufficiency

Chronic aortic regurgitation represents a condition of combined volume and pressure overload. The balance between afterload excess, preload reserve, and hypertrophy cannot be maintained indefinitely in many patients, and afterload mismatch and/or depressed contractility ultimately results in a reduction in ejection fraction, first into the low normal range and then below normal. With time, during which the ventricle develops progressive chamber enlargement and a more spherical geometry, depressed myocardial contractility predominates over excessive loading as the cause of progressive systolic dysfunction. At this point, relief of the insufficiency may not result in return of normal left ventricular morphology or function, and, consequently, long-term survival may be impaired [18].

Diagnosis

Clinical Sign and Symptoms

Critical Aortic Stenosis

Neonates and infants with critical aortic valve stenosis and ductus-dependent circulation present with varying degrees of cyanosis and reduced peripheral perfusion. Systolic ejection murmur may or may not be present, depending on left ventricular function and the amount of blood flow across the aortic valve. Occasionally, a neonate will present with circulatory collapse following spontaneous ductal closure.

Neonates and infants with severe, noncritical aortic stenosis, without ductal dependency, may present within the first weeks of life with a history of irritability, failure to thrive, and poor feeding.

Noncritical Aortic Stenosis

Older children are usually asymptomatic and have a systolic murmur or a systolic ejection click. With progression of stenosis, symptoms of breathlessness, syncope, and angina might develop. There is constant risk of bacterial endocarditis. Undetected, severe aortic valve stenosis is a known cause of sudden death and accounts for approximately 1 % of all causes of sudden death in young people [10].

Aortic Insufficiency

The majority of children with aortic insufficiency remain asymptomatic. With the progression of declining systolic function or elevated filling pressures of the left ventricle, breathlessness, syncope, and angina might develop. There is constant risk of bacterial endocarditis.

Electrocardiogram

The electrocardiogram (ECG) demonstrates the left ventricular hypertrophy, with left ventricular strain or ischemia (Fig. 90.1).

Chest X-Ray

Chest radiography may reveal cardiomegaly with pulmonary venous congestion, primarily in neonates who present with critical aortic stenosis; otherwise, the heart size is usually normal. Post-stenotic dilatation of the ascending aorta may be visible.

Echocardiography

Echocardiography usually provides complete diagnostic and hemodynamic information. In determining actual valve morphology, it is

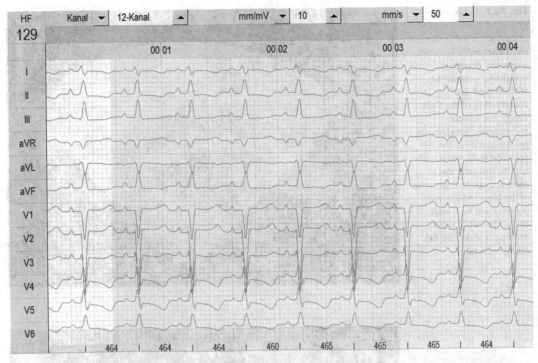

Fig. 90.1 ECG of a newborn with critical aortic valve stenosis short after birth. It shows significant dominance of the left ventricular leads (S in V1 and R in V6) with alteration of the repolarization (including positive T-waves in V1/V2 and negative T-wave in V4 to V6 with mildly descending ST segments)

important to determine cusps thickness, mobility, the annular diameter at hinge points, and the height difference between cusp margin and aortic insertion in the long-axis view. The Doppler gradient across the stenotic aortic valve can be greatly underestimated in a situation of low cardiac output with depressed left ventricle contractility and right-to-left shunt at ductal level. In patients with normal ventricular function, the severity of aortic stenosis is graded according to well-established peak Doppler gradient measurements, as mild (< 40 mmHg), moderate (< 60 mmHg), and severe (> 60 mmHg) [19].

Aortic regurgitation is best seen in apical and parasternal long-axis view. Regurgitation is graded according to a composite assessment scale as nontrivial, mild (no left ventricle dilation, no retrograde flow in the descending aorta, and proximal jet width <2.5 mm/m^2), moderate (left ventricular end-diastolic volume z-score >2 but <4, with or without retrograde flow in the descending aorta, and proximal jet width >2.5 but <3.5 mm/m^2), or severe (left ventricular end-diastolic volume z-score >4, retrograde flow in the descending aorta, and proximal jet width >3.5 mm/m^2), with emphasis placed on jet width if criteria are inconsistent (Figs. 90.2 –90.5).

Cardiac Catheterization

Cardiac catheterization is usually performed in anticipation of balloon aortic valve dilatation, in the presence of significant symptoms (syncope, fainting episode, ECG changes), or in the presence of additional defects and multilevel stenosis. Peak-to-peak systolic gradient measured in the catheterization laboratory with the patient under sedation or anesthesia may be significantly less than that estimated by Doppler echocardiography (Figs. 90.6–90.9).

Fig. 90.2 Echocardiography of a newborn with critical aortic valve stenosis short after birth. It shows a severely depressed left ventricular contractility with dilation and compression of the right ventricular cavum, endocardial fibroelastosis predominantly at the posterior wall, and a white papillary muscle due to chronic ischemia. Because of the high end-diastolic pressure and high wall stress, the mitral valve opening is short and the filling reduced

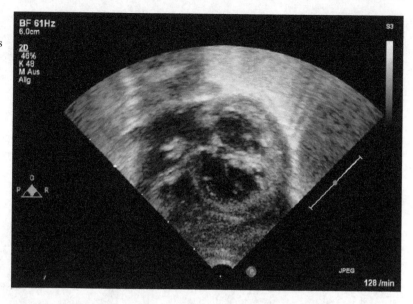

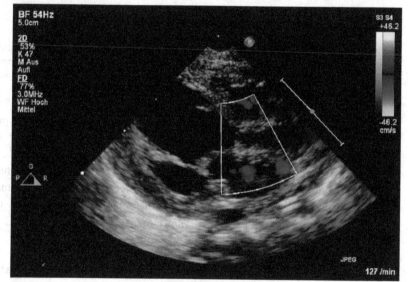

Fig. 90.3 Long-axis view of the same patient. The aortic valve is dysplastic mildly thickened with a small central loophole and a dorsal orientated asymmetric jet

Cardiac Magnetic Resonance

Cardiac magnetic resonance (cMRI) provides precise information on left ventricular function, ejection fraction, and regional wall dysfunction and can also provide reliable information on the functional evaluation of the valvar dysfunction; however, to date, echocardiography and three-dimensional echocardiography assess aortic valve morphology better than cMRI. Obtaining a cardiac magnetic resonance of infants and young children may require sedation which further limits the applicability.

Exercise Stress Testing

In those patients with mild to moderate stenosis, exercise stress testing could be helpful in eliciting symptoms or objective measures of ischemia that

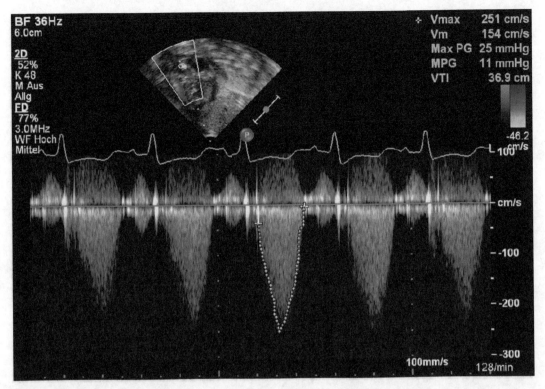

Fig. 90.4 Trans-aortic Doppler flow profile in the same patient. Because of the bad left ventricular function, the calculated transvalvular pressure gradient does not reflect to actual severity of the stenosis

may not be evident from routine history or evaluation. In most situations, exercise stress testing is most often helpful when positive in the asymptomatic patient.

Decision Making

Critical Aortic Stenosis

In the neonate with ductal-dependent systemic circulation, the key issue is to decide whether left-sided structures are adequate to sustain the systemic circulation and, if so, what kind of treatment is the most beneficial [20–23]. In very borderline situations, the hybrid approach might stabilize the circulation and help to select proper treatment plan later on [24]. Proposed formulas [23, 25–27] have limited clinical value, and at this point there is no agreement on what combination of left-sided structures would be adequate to perform biventricular correction [28].

The decision-making protocol for critical aortic stenosis [20] emphasizes the assessment of the fixed morphological parameters. Aortic stenosis is associated with abnormalities of the mitral valve apparatus including supra-mitral valve ring, mitral valve hypoplasia or stenosis, and abnormalities of the sub-mitral valve apparatus including single papillary muscle, parachute, or mitral valve arcade. Abnormalities of the left ventricle include left ventricular hypoplasia, non-compaction, and subendocardial fibroelastosis. Additional abnormalities of the left ventricular outflow tract include diffuse tunnel or fibrous sub-aortic ring and aortic arch hypoplasia and coarctation of the aorta. In the majority of cases, fixed morphological parameters of the mitral valve apparatus are surgically uncorrectable at least in the neonatal period. Reduced dimension of the mitral valve orifice is a well-recognized risk factor for death [23, 26]. Therefore, if the mitral valve annulus diameter is <7 mm in a neonate, or < −2 z-score, or if there

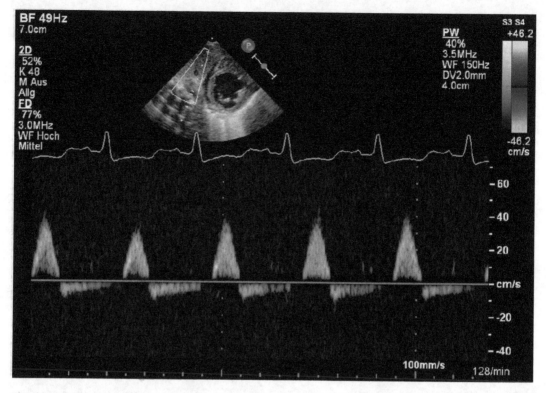

Fig. 90.5 Sys-diastolic flow pattern of the descending aorta in the same patient. The peak flow velocity is low, while the systolic antegrade flow only short. Because of the reduced stroke volume, there is a diastolic reversed flow as the blood redistributes to the upper limbs and through the open duct to the lungs

is severe inflow obstruction, some caregivers may considerer single ventricular palliation with possible attempts to promote the growth of inflow, if the remaining part of left ventricle is well developed or surgically repairable. The left ventricular outflow tract structures, such as hypoplasia of the aortic annulus (<5 mm), ratio of left and right ventricular lengths <0.8, a cardiac apex not formed by the left ventricle, and the presence of endocardial fibroelastosis, may be relative contraindications for simple aortic valvotomy [25, 26]. Aortic valvotomy is ineffective to address any of these morphologic issues. However, these morphological parameters are correctable, and biventricular repair is still feasible with a Ross or Ross–Konno operation [29, 30]. The Ross or Ross–Konno option is considered, if there is failure of the balloon valvuloplasty or the open valvotomy as well.

Predominantly retrograde flow in the ascending aorta is suggestive of severely hypoplastic left heart structures, and most often a single-ventricle palliation will be necessary.

However, the presence of total or predominant antegrade blood flow in the ascending aorta and transverse aortic arch correlates with survival after a biventricular type of repair [31].

Noncritical Aortic Stenosis

Intervention for aortic valve stenosis is indicated in symptomatic patients, when the peak Doppler gradient exceeds 40 mmHg, and LV hypertrophy and/or changes in repolarization in the resting ECG and pathological findings in the stress test are notable.

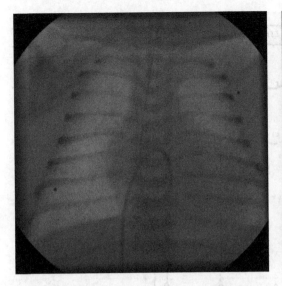

Fig. 90.6 Angiography in a hydropic preterm (32nd week of gestation) with critical aortic valve stenosis. The patient (bodyweight 1.9 kg) was brought to the cathlab at 1 h after birth while on high-frequency ventilation. Atrial contrast injection demonstrates massive atrial dilation and severely impaired left ventricular function. There is a short appearance of the left-sided pulmonary veins

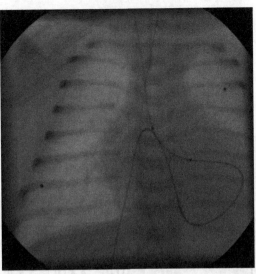

Fig. 90.8 Antegrade balloon dilation. A 4-mm coronary balloon, followed by a 5-mm balloon, is inflated within the aortic valve. Echocardiographic shortening fraction improved from 6 % to 22 % the following day. The patient underwent Ross operation at the age of 3.5 years and developed normal during follow-up

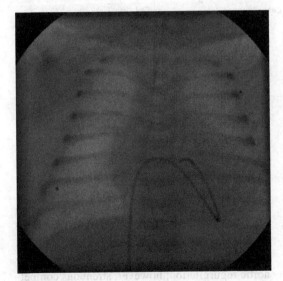

Fig. 90.7 Antegrade demonstration of the critical aortic valve stenosis. A 4-French Behrmann Wedge catheter is placed under the aortic valve. Contrast application reveals a thin jet through the valve to the aorta ascendens. This catheter is further used to place a coronary guide wire through the valve to advance a balloon catheter

In asymptomatic patients, a peak gradient of more than 60 mmHg is an indication for intervention. Although each patient should be evaluated individually, evidence suggests that early intervention before the left ventricle develops myocardial changes might be beneficial [10, 17].

Aortic Insufficiency

The timing for surgery in patients with chronic aortic regurgitation is controversial. Accepted indications are the presence of symptoms, increasing left ventricle dilation with or without dysfunction, or both, in the setting of moderate or even worse aortic regurgitation. In order to achieve complete recovery of the left ventricular function, surgery should be performed before the z-score of the preoperative left ventricular end-diastolic dimension is no greater than 4 [10].

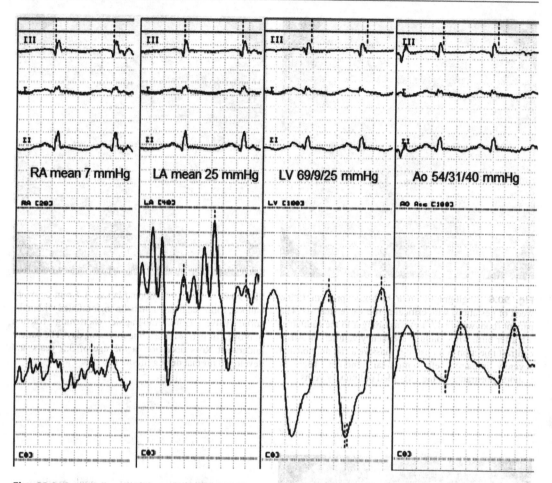

RA mean 7 mmHg | LA mean 25 mmHg | LV 69/9/25 mmHg | Ao 54/31/40 mmHg

Fig. 90.9 Intracardiac pressure curves before balloon dilation. The left atrial pressure is severely elevated, which is caused by the left ventricular low output and elevated diastolic and end-diastolic pressures. The trans- aortic peak gradient of 15 mmHg is misleading as the aortic opening is like a pinhole and causes the left ventricle to fail

Medical Management

Critical Aortic Stenosis

Critically ill neonates are stabilized by aggressive resuscitation (ventilatory and inotropic support, correction of acidosis and protection of multiorgan function), while patency of the ductus is maintained by prostaglandins. A trial discontinuation of prostaglandins should be undertaken. Intervention (balloon valvuloplasty or surgery) is indicated on a semi-elective basis if ductal closure is tolerated. Dependency on the ductal circulation is a clear indication for semi-urgent intervention.

Noncritical Aortic Stenosis and Aortic Insufficiency

Prophylaxis against the development of endocarditis is indicated for all patients undergoing procedures associated with bacteremia. Exercise and participation in sports are not restricted for those asymptomatic patients with stable gradient of less than 40 mmHg and/or no more than moderate aortic regurgitation; however, strenuous competitive level activities should be avoided. In any case, the annual evaluation should be done. In aortic regurgitation, afterload reduction might improve left ventricular volume and left ventricle mass, thus temporarily preserving left ventricle function. However, in patients with severe aortic regurgitation, afterload reduction may lead to impaired coronary perfusion by decreasing diastolic blood pressure and should be used with caution. β-Blockers are used in patients with the risk of dilatation of the aortic root, because of structural abnormalities of the aortic wall, or after Ross procedure.

Surgical and Interventional Management

Neonatal Critical Aortic Stenosis

At these authors' institution, the German Pediatric Cardiac Center, Sankt Augustin, an interdisciplinary consensus-based approach, as follows, is preferable:

1. If the left ventricle function is depressed, a ballooning with a balloon not larger than 70 % of diameter of the aortic annulus is performed to slightly increase the effective orifice area of the aortic valve, creating a minimal risk of regurgitation. This so-called "gentle" balloon dilatation of the aortic valve is used as an intermittent step to stabilize the patient before open valvotomy. If the left ventricle function is not severely depressed, open valvotomy is the method of choice, unless there is a clearly symmetric non-myxomatous valve, which could be considered for ballooning [20].

2. If the left ventricle function is severely depressed and the left ventricle is dilated, apart from "gentle ballooning," balloon atrial septostomy is recommended to partially decompress the left atrium and left ventricle. Patency of the ductus arteriosus is maintained by prostaglandins.

3. If decompression of the left ventricle is ineffective, an open valvotomy with bilateral pulmonary artery banding and atrial septectomy may be considered first, with the aim of decompressing the left ventricle, while maintaining the right ventricular contribution to systemic perfusion via the ductus arteriosus. However, caregivers ought to keep in mind that manipulation around the patent ductus arteriosus (dissection of the left pulmonary artery and the ascending aorta) can trigger ductal narrowing, necessitating a stent implantation afterwards.

4. If mechanical circulatory support of a failing left ventricle is necessary, recovery can be expected within 5–7 days. Afterwards, the situation should be reevaluated, and the strategy eventually changed, so as not to miss the proper timing for either a Ross–Konno or single-ventricle pathway.

The proposed protocol fits to the concept of a hybrid procedure, which serves as a bridge to a more definitive repair for patients with a borderline left ventricle and/or borderline left ventricular function [20, 24]. This concept may significantly reduce the risk of a definitive procedure by providing patients more time to grow, mature, and "declare themselves" as either one- or two-ventricle candidates [32].

Surgical Management: Open Valvotomy for Critical Aortic Stenosis

A detailed description of this technique is shown on Video 90.1 [33, 34].

Interventional Management for Critical Aortic Stenosis

In critical aortic stenosis balloon dilation can be performed using an antegrade or retrograde route. In order to minimize the risk of post-procedural aortic regurgitation, it is recommended to start with a small balloon, i.e., with a balloon/valve ratio of 0.6. If the valve thickness is less than 1/3 of the valve radius, recommended balloon/valve ratio is between 0.7 and 0.9. In asymmetric, but tricuspid valves, balloon/valve ratio between 0.6 and 0.8 is recommended (Figs. 90.10–90.14).

Noncritical Aortic Stenosis

Interventional Management for Noncritical Aortic Stenosis

The technique used is identical with ballooning in neonates. To minimize post-procedural valvar

Video 90.1

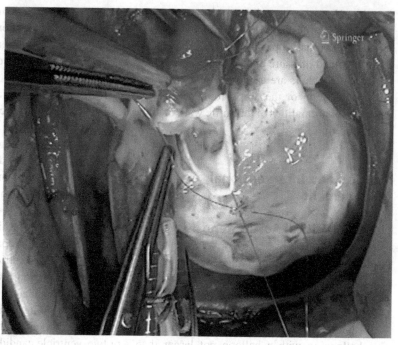

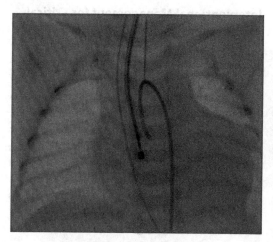

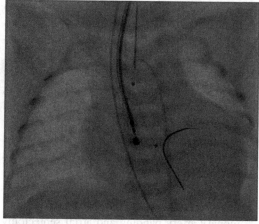

Fig. 90.10 Retrograde angiography of the ascending aorta in a full-term newborn with critical aortic stenosis. The valve is asymmetric with a dominant right leaflet and adhesions between the two other smaller leaflets. The antegrade flow is reduced and towards the descending aorta compensated through open duct. Coronary arteries show a reduced excursion reflecting the severely reduced left ventricular function

Fig. 90.11 Balloon valvuloplasty using a coronary balloon with 4 mm diameter. Using a 4-French arterial short sheath for an access, the stenotic valve was retrogradely passed with a coronary soft-tipped guide wire. The coronary balloon was then placed within the valve and a short inflation up to 12 atm performed

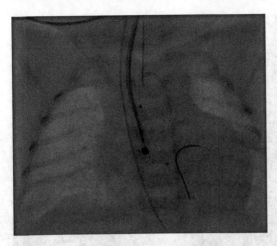

Fig. 90.12 Re-dilation with a 5-mm coronary balloon. A stepwise increase of the balloon diameters was chosen to reduce the risk of unnecessary regurgitation

Fig. 90.14 Ascendogram in comparison to the initial picture. The right-sided aortic leaflet shows improved mobility. The antegrade aortic perfusion is better and supported by the regained contractility of the left ventricle. There is only a minimal regurgitation at valve. Surgical reconstruction of the valve in this patient was performed 2 months later when the trans-aortic gradient started to rise again

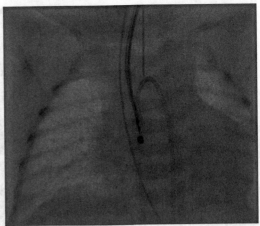

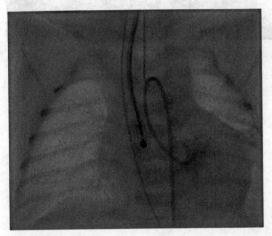

Fig. 90.13 Post-interventional left ventricular angiogram. Immediately after the balloon valvuloplasty, the left ventricle shows improved contractility. The aortic valve imposes thickened with stiff left-sided valves. Antegrade flow has improved markedly, and there is a partially inversion of the shunt flow across the open duct with contrastation of the pulmonary arteries

regurgitation, rapid ventricular pacing via a temporary wire placed in the right ventricle, as well as avoiding of oversized balloons, is recommended.

Reconstructive Surgery for Noncritical Aortic Stenosis and Aortic Regurgitation

The proper coaptation of the aortic valve depends on the aortic annulus, the sinotubular dimension, and the height and position of each commissure in relation to the other commissures. The effective height of cusps and the crescent-shaped portion of the leaflet's free edge form the area of coaptation. The cusp height, that is, the distance from insertion to free margin in its central portion in the children, ranges from 4 mm to 9 mm and in the adults from 7 mm to 12 mm [14].

The first step of the operation is to relieve the commissural fusion and extensive thinning and shaving of the valve cusps. Afterwards, the appropriate technique of repair is chosen based on the underlying pathology. There are several possibilities:

1. In bicuspid valves, in order to maximize effective orifice area, the commissurotomy can be extended in circumferential fashion beyond the commissures into the aortic wall, splitting the aortic wall into two layers [35]. Incision into a raphe should be avoided; however, debridement of the raphe usually improves mobility of the cusps with subsequent enlargement of the effective orifice area of the valve.

Video 90.2

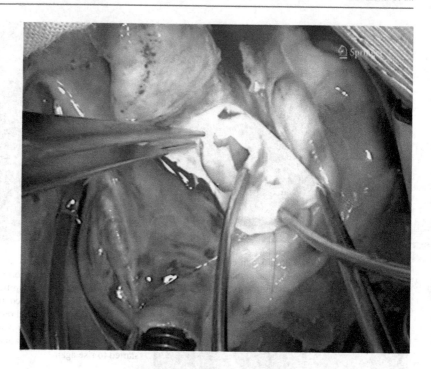

2. Perforations or tears in the aortic cusps are repaired either with a direct suture or with pericardial patches.

3. Redundant tissue is corrected by shortening the coaptation edge to match the adjacent cusps. Shortening is provided by either triangular resection or plication of redundant tissue.

   If correction of the cusp's length does not result in the correction of prolapsed, the free edge reinforcement is performed by an over and over running suture, suspending both ends of suture at the level of corresponding commissures, thus reinforcing and shortening the free edge.

4. More extensive cusp destruction, with deficient cusps, requires an extension procedure using a pericardial patch. First, cusps are shaved leaving their base and unaffected body intact, than pericardial extensions are fashioned to fit the specific architecture of each cusp, but slightly oversized in depth (10–15 %) and lengths (up to 25 %). Each neocusp's free edge is leveled with

the sinotubular bar at the commissural level [36, 37].

5. Dysplastic unicuspid or bicuspid aortic valve is suitable for "tricuspidalization" using most of the available native tissue for creation of two adjacent cusps while adding a third cusp from pericardium. A detailed description of this technique is shown on Video 90.2 [34].

Another alternative is the incision of the raphe creating two unsupported cusps. Subsequently, the pericardial triangle patch is folded and sutured along both edges of the divided raphe and vertically to the aortic wall to provide support in the diastole, preventing cusp prolapse [38].

Mild dilatation of the annulus can be managed with a sub-commissural annuloplasty [39].

The trans-esophageal echocardiography (TEE) is an essential tool for assessment of the LV function, residual gradients, and insufficiency of the aortic valve after weaning from pump. If a peak gradient >40 mmHg and aortic

Video 90.3

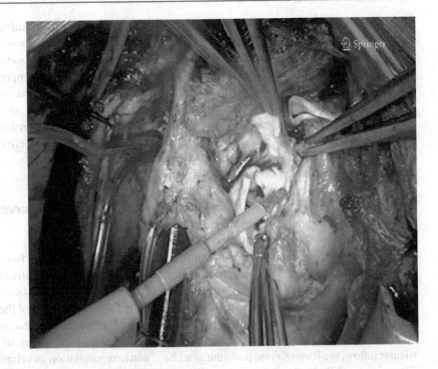

insufficiency is moderate or more, attempts to reduce these residuals should be considered. In general, residual stenosis is better tolerated than insufficiency [40–42].

Mechanical Aortic Valve Replacement
The standard technique of mechanical aortic valve replacement is used.

Ross Operation
In children, a standard technique of complete root replacement is used. A detailed description of this technique is shown on Video 90.3 [34, 43].

Aortic Root Replacement Using an Aortic Homograft
Homograft aortic root replacement is currently used for treatment of complicated bacterial endocarditis with aortic root abscesses and in the management of complex left ventricular outflow tract obstructions, when Ross–Konno is not an option and the root is too small for a mechanical valve [44].

Complications and Critical Care Management

Postsurgical Complications

Critical Aortic Stenosis
Early mortality for critical aortic stenosis is reported between 6 % and 19 % and is associated with adverse prognostic factors for critical aortic stenosis, such as mitral stenosis, a small-sized left ventricle, a small aortic annulus, depressed left ventricle fractional shortening, a low aortic gradient, endomyocardial fibroelastosis, and other coexisting defects [20, 33, 45–47]. Pre-procedural resuscitation by prostaglandin (PGE$_1$) and myocardial recovery render tendency to better survival postsurgically.

The risk of post-procedural aortic regurgitation is quite low; however, mild to moderate aortic valve gradient is typically seen, and associated de novo aortic insufficiency, although usually trivial, may impact risks and management.

Postoperatively, atrial rhythm is essential for fill-ing of the more or less restrictive left ventricle. Temporary pacemaker support may be required. Persistent pulmonary hypertension and low car-diac output, manifested by poor peripheral circu-lation, impaired tissue perfusion, and acidosis, are seen particularly in neonates with poor pre-operative left ventricle function and associated lesions. They are best managed with meticulous assessment and correction of low blood volume and filling pressures, inotropes, ventilation aiming for a slightly alkalotic pH, and inhaled nitric oxide as required. Failure of pulmonary hypertension to resolve and continued low car-diac output indicates morphological and or func-tional limitations of left-sided heart structures. Pure functional deterioration of the left ventricle might require mechanical circulatory support by extracorporeal membrane oxygenation or a left ventricular assist device. With adequate left ven-tricular inflow, the Ross–Konno procedure can be lifesaving for failed valvotomy with persistence of outflow tract obstruction, severe aortic insuffi-ciency, or extensive endocardial fibroelastosis. Overall borderline left ventricle, incapable to support systemic circulation, should be converted to single-ventricle physiology with Norwood-type repair, or the patient should be listed for a heart transplant.

Noncritical Aortic Stenosis and Aortic Regurgitation

Early mortality for valve reconstruction and aor-tic valve replacement is approaching zero percent even in complex reconstructions. Postopera-tively, preserved or even hyperactive left ventric-ular systolic function is observed frequently. This should not divert attention to a variable extent of diastolic dysfunction related to myocardial hypertrophy, subendocardial ischemic precondi-tions like endocardial fibroelastosis (EFE), or both. Despite a cursory glance at high systemic pressures and precordial activity, meticulous assessment and correction of low blood volume and filling pressure is required first. Only after confirmation of balanced circulatory volume and filling, medication for afterload reduction may be considered to avoid high-pressure gradients on

freshly reconstructed valve tissues, as well as β-blockade, usually hours after recovery from ischemic operative episode. Conduction abnor-malities including complete heart block and arrhythmias represent the most serious early post-operative complication, especially if the patient required complex reconstruction. Again, ensur-ing sinus rhythm and effective atrioventricular synchrony is important.

Catheter-Based Intervention Complications

Early mortality in the largest series of balloon valvuloplasty for neonatal critical aortic stenosis is reported as 9–14 % [48–51]. Mortality is asso-ciated with hypoplasia of the left heart structures and the presence of endocardial fibroelastosis in neonates [50]. Incidence of moderate or severe aortic regurgitation developing shortly after bal-looning is reported to be between 15 % and 33 % [25, 51, 52]. Importantly, the necessity of emer-gent aortic valve replacement with a Ross proce-dure or Ross–Konno procedure for severe aortic regurgitation after a balloon valvuloplasty has a very high mortality rate and has been reported as high as 80 % at 1 year post-intervention [53]. The procedure-related morbidity is not trivial with balloon aortic valvuloplasty. There is up to 15 % incidence of aortic wall injury, around 3 % incidence of procedural femoral artery damage, and up to 2 % incidence of injuries to the heart itself, such as rupture of valves or myocardial perforation [48, 54].

Outcomes and Long-Term Follow-Ups

Critical Aortic Stenosis

The most appropriate management of critical aortic stenosis remains controversial. Both bal-loon dilatation of aortic valve and open valvotomy are firmly established as effective ini-tial treatments with encouraging survival bene-fits. Improved early results depend more upon better understanding of the limits of biventricular repair than on the method of treatment. Valvotomy of any kind is a palliative procedure and re-intervention remains frequent. Patients undergoing open valvotomy are more likely to have residual stenosis, particularly in unicuspid or bicuspid valves [20, 23, 25, 45, 47–52, 55, 56]. On the other hand, those patients undergoing ballooning are more likely to develop aortic regurgitation and are at the risk of progressive aortic regurgitation and ventricular dysfunction with the need for earlier aortic valve replacement [55, 57, 58].

Balloon Dilatation of the Aortic Valve

Overall survival is between 75 % and 85 % at 1 year and usually remains unchanged at 5 years and 10 years of follow-up [49–51, 55]. The risks of sudden death and congestive heart failure are low [49]. Typically, procedural aortic regurgitation progresses in severity over time [58]. Freedom from moderate to severe aortic regurgitation is about 60 % at 10 years [51, 59].

Neonates with critical aortic stenosis have a significantly higher hazard of repeated interventions due to residual aortic stenosis than older patients with isolated aortic stenosis. Freedom from death or re-intervention at 10 years is 29–50 % [49].

Freedom from aortic valve surgery or aortic valve replacement is between 50 % and 79 % at 10 years and is longer in patients with lower post-dilation gradients and less severe post-dilation aortic regurgitation. There is an ongoing steady hazard of aortic valve replacement [49–51].

Open Surgical Valvotomy

Overall survival is between 70 % and 91 % at 1 year and usually remains unchanged at 10 years and 20 years of follow-up [20, 45–47, 56].

Overall, the 10-year event-free survival for critical neonates is between 50 % and 70 % [34, 47, 56]. These figures compared favorably with 29–50 % event-free survival at 10 years reported after ballooning [48, 49, 51].

Valve morphology determines the need for re-intervention. Unicuspid and bicuspid valves by definition have fundamental morphological and functional abnormalities; the number of re-interventions and patients needing an aortic valve replacement is therefore higher. If three cusps could be constructed without producing significant aortic regurgitation, the need for any re-intervention for recurrent stenosis is less than in patients with bicuspid valves [46]. The tricuspid valve morphology showed exceptional outcomes with event-free survivals of 90 % and 100 % freedom from aortic valve replacement at 20 years of follow-up. These figures suggest superior long-term outcomes of open valvotomy in comparison with ballooning regarding preservation of the native aortic valve [20].

Noncritical Aortic Stenosis and Aortic Insufficiency

Balloon Dilatation of Congenital Aortic Stenosis

Aortic stenosis, treated later in life, differs from critical aortic stenosis in many aspects. Overall survival is between 90 % and 95 % at 15 and 20 years, respectively. There is an ongoing steady hazard for aortic valve surgery with 50–30 % freedom from aortic valve replacement at 15–20 years. Post-interventional aortic regurgitation is progressive. Suboptimal post-interventional outcome, including both higher residual gradient (> 35 mmHg) and higher grade of aortic regurgitation (>mild), is independently associated with shorter freedom from aortic valve surgery. On the other hand, age and patients with isolated aortic stenosis treated between 1 year and 10 years of age have significantly better outcomes. The long-term aortic valve outcomes are primarily a function of the underlying aortic valve disease and post-procedural physiology. Secondary aortic valve surgery seems to be inevitable for a significant number of patients [49, 52, 59].

Surgical Management

Surgical options in children with aortic valve disease remain limited. There is no ideal valve substitute; therefore, valve repair, which preserves growth of native tissue with no need for anticoagulation, is preferred as long as aortic valve stenosis can be significantly reduced and valve competence preserved. Furthermore, aortic valve repair does not preclude any future replacement strategies [36, 60].

Open surgical valvotomy for noncritical stenosis can be performed with very low mortality (2–3 %). However, there remains a relatively high rate of reoperation (30–40 % at 15–20 years) [61].

If a more complex reconstruction is required, the best results are obtained when sufficient native aortic tissue, including the hinge point of the native leaflet, remains prior to cusp extension. Conversion of congenitally bicuspid aortic valves to tricuspid arrangement might confer better outcomes, probably due to reduction in cusps stress load and improved flow patterns, by providing optimal effective orifice area. Reconstruction is safe, with early mortality approaching zero and with five-year freedom from valve replacement up to75 % [16, 36, 37, 40–42, 60, 63].

In general, early valve function after reconstruction is excellent; however, long-term durability of repair is unknown.

Aortic Valve Replacement

Any aortic valve substitute in children has certain drawbacks. The Ross procedure is an attractive alternative to a mechanical prosthesis, but is not a cure for aortic valve disease. The great advantages of the Ross procedure are the superior hemodynamic performance, the growth potential, the low endocarditis risk, low thrombogenicity, and the lack of need for anticoagulant therapy [64].

The main concern is progressive neo-aortic root dilation [36, 62, 65]. Durability limitations become apparent by the end of the first postoperative decade, in particular in younger patients [66]. Only 82 % freedom from autograft reoperation at 15 years of follow-up was reported from a large single institution study [67]. Prominent mechanism for development of aortic regurgitation is dilatation of the Valsalva sinus and sinotubular junction. In general, the autograft valve cusps are thin but preserved [68]. Autograft dilation and valve dysfunction are more common in patients in whom the autograft was placed for predominant aortic valve insufficiency as

opposed to stenosis or in patients in whom there was a significant size mismatch between the native valve annulus and autograft. Modifications of the root replacement, which include annular and sinotubular junction reduction and stabilization, might reduce incidence of late autograft failure [69–71]. The presence of a native bicuspid aortic valve might be an additional risk factor for autograft dysfunction due to an inherent abnormality of the pulmonary annulus, or valves with mucocystic degeneration of the stroma [72–75]. The risk of autograft failure in these specific subsets of patients remains to be determined, and mechanical valve replacement should be considered as a reasonable option [16]. The histology of the pulmonary artery wall when placed at high pressure demonstrates fracture of elastin fibers and a general disorganization. This mechanical adaptation phenomenon in the wall of the autograft might be another potential risk factor for Ross failure. The reduction of autograft wall stress with aggressive postoperative control of blood pressure with β-blockers and afterload reduction drugs may decrease the risk of autograft dilation [76–79]. The rate of autograft deterioration is reported at 1.69 %/patient-year in a mixed pediatric population [66].

Freedom from pulmonary homograft replacements after the Ross procedure is 90 % at 12-year follow-up [80] with a right ventricular outflow tract deterioration rate of 1.66 %/patient-year [66].

Overall, the risk of reoperation is approximately 10 % at 10 years, on either the autograft or the right ventricular conduit [80, 81]. The rate of reoperation on the autograft is higher than for the right ventricle to pulmonary artery valve conduit, except in younger pediatric patients who are expected to outgrow their conduits [82, 83].

Mechanical valve replacement in children is complicated by the need for systemic anticoagulation, by the lack of annular growth, and by patient-prosthesis mismatch. Operative mortality is low, ranging between 0 % and 5 % [10, 84, 85], and is associated with poor preoperative status. Long-term survival rates range from 85 % to 64 % at 20-year follow-up, reflecting the complexity of the underlying congenital disease, being more favorable for isolated aortic stenosis [86, 87].

Freedom from reoperation in pediatric patients is between 85 % and 90 % at 10 years, which is comparable to the Ross procedure [81, 86].

Other alternatives for valve replacement are unappealing, including a tissue valve with rapid degeneration in children or an allograft with no growth potential and limited durability.

Future Developments

Better understanding of fetal–maternal interaction, together with improved technologies and definitions of indications for intrauterine intervention, including prenatal aortic valve dilatation, may improve outcomes in the future. It remains to be seen whether trans-catheter aortic valve implantation used in adults will be applicable for older children as a temporary solution before aortic valve replacement. The future of aortic valve surgery is the development of scaffolds or grafts, populated with autologous cells that are organized into normal structural aortic valve tissue. These tissue-engineered grafts may eventually be capable of growth, remodelling, healing, and adaptation [88].

References

1. Paget J (1844) On obstruction of the branches of the pulmonary artery. Med Chir Trans 27:162
2. Spencer FC, Neill CA, Sank L et al (1960) Anatomical variation in 46 patients with congenital aortic stenosis. Am Surg 26:204–216
3. Labadibi Z (1983) Aortic balloon valvuloplasty. Am Heart J 106:751–752
4. Samanek M, Slavik Z, Zborilova B et al (1989) Prevalence, treatment and outcome of heart disease in live-born children: a prospective analysis of 91, 823 live-born children. Pediatr Cardiol 10:205
5. Roberts WC, Ko JM (2005) Frequency by decades of unicuspid, bicuspid, and tricuspid aortic valves in adults having isolated aortic valve replacement for aortic stenosis, with or without associated aortic regurgitation. Circulation 11:920–925
6. Lewin MB, Otto CM (2005) The bicuspid aortic valve: adverse outcomes from infancy to old age. Circulation 111:832–834
7. Donofrio MT, Engle MA, O'Loughlin JE et al (1992) Congenital aortic regurgitation. J Am Coll Cardiol 20:366–372
8. Bonderman D, Gharehbaghi-Schnell E, Wollenek G et al (1999) Mechanisms underlying aortic dilatation in congenital aortic valve malformation. Circulation 99:2138–2143
9. Dervanian P, Mace L, Folliguet TA, Di Virgilio A (1998) Surgical treatment of aortic root aneurysm related to Marfan syndrome in early childhood. Pediatr Cardiol 19:369–373
10. Hraska V, Photiadis J (2009) Angeborene Anomalien des linksventrikulären Ausflusstrakts. In: Ziemer G, Haverich A (eds) Herzchirurgie, 3rd edn. Springer, Berlin\Heidelberg\New York, pp 421–459
11. Roberts WC (1973) Valvular, subvalvular and supravalvar aortic stenosis. Cardiovasc Clin 5:97–126
12. de Kerchove L, Glineur D, Poncelet A et al (2008) Repair of aortic leaflet prolapse: a ten-year experience. Eur J Cardiothorac Surg 34:785–791
13. Jeanmart H, de Kerchove L, Glineur D et al (2007) Aortic valve repair: the functional approach to leaflet prolapse and valve-sparing surgery. Ann Thorac Surg 83:S746–S751
14. Bierbach BO, Aicher D, Abu Issa O et al (2010) Aortic root and cusp configuration determine aortic valve function. Eur J Cardiothorac Surg 38:400–406
15. Solymar L, Sudow G, Berggren H et al (1992) Balloon dilation of stenotic aortic valve in children. An intraoperative study. J Thorac Cardiovasc Surg 104:1709–1713
16. Bacha EA, Satou GM, Moran AM et al (2001) Valve-sparing operation for balloon-induced aortic regurgitation in congenital aortic stenosis. J Thorac Cardiovasc Surg 122:162–168
17. Jonas RA (2004) Left ventricular outflow tract obstruction: aortic valve stenosis, subaortic stenosis, supravalvular aortic stenosis. In: Jonas RA (ed) Comprehensive surgical management of congenital heart disease. Arnold, London, pp 320–340
18. Bonow RO, Carabello B, de Leon Jr AC (1998) Guidelines for the management of patients with valvular heart disease: executive summary A report of the American College of Cardiology/American Heart Association Task Force on Practice Guidelines (Committee on Management of Patients with Valvular Heart Disease). Circulation 98:1949–1984
19. Hossack KF, Neutze JM, Lowe JB et al (1980) Congenital valvar aortic stenosis. Natural history and assessment for operation. Br Heart J 43:561–573
20. Hraska V, Sinzobahamvya N, Haun C et al (2012) The long-term outcome of open valvotomy for critical aortic stenosis in neonates. Ann Thorac Surg 94:1519–1526
21. Corno AF (2005) Borderline left ventricle. Eur J Cardiothorac Surg 27:67–73

22. Emani SM, Bacha EA, McElhinney DB et al (2009) Primary left ventricular rehabilitation is effective in maintaining two-ventricle physiology in the borderline left heart. J Thorac Cardiovasc Surg 138:1276–1282

23. Colan SD, McElhinney DB, Crawford EC et al (2006) Validation and re-evaluation of a discriminant model predicting anatomic suitability for biventricular repair in neonates with aortic stenosis. J Am Coll Cardiol 47:1858–1865

24. Brown C, Boshoff D, Eyskens B et al (2009) Hybrid approach as bridge to biventricular repair in a neonate with critical aortic stenosis and borderline left ventricle. Eur J Cardiothorac Surg 35:1080–1082

25. Lofland GK, McGrindle BW, Williams WG et al (2001) Critical aortic stenosis in the neonate: a multi-institutional study of management, outcomes, and risk factors. J Thorac Cardiovasc Surg 121:10–27

26. Hickey EJ, Caldarone CA, Blackstone EH et al (2007) Critical left ventricular outflow tract obstruction: the disproportionate impact of biventricular repair in borderline cases. J Thorac Cardiovasc Surg 134:1429–1437

27. Alsoufi B, Karamlou T, McCrindle BW et al (2007) Management options in neonates and infants with critical left ventricular outflow tract obstruction. Eur J Cardiothorac Surg 31:1013–1021

28. Eicken A, Georgiev S, Balling G et al (2010) Neonatal balloon aortic valvuloplasty-predictive value of current risk score algorithms for treatment strategies. Catheter Cardiovasc Interv 76:404–1

29. Aszyk P, Thiel C, Sinzobahamvya C et al (2012) Ross-Konno procedure in infants – mid-term results. Eur J Cardiothorac Surg 42:687–694

30. Hraska V, Lilje C, Kantorova A et al (2010) Ross-Konno procedure in children. World J Pediatr Congenit Heart Surg 1:28–33

31. Kovalchin JP, Brook MM, Rosenthal GL et al (1998) Echocardiographic hemodynamic and morphometric predictors of survival after two-ventricle repair in infants with critical aortic stenosis. J Am Coll Cardiol 32:237–244

32. Davis CK, Pastuszko P, Lamberti J et al (2011) The hybrid procedure for the borderline left ventricle. Cardiol Young 21:26–30

33. Hraska V, Photiadis J, Arenz C (2008) Open valvotomy for aortic valve stenosis in newborns and infants. Multimedia Manual of Cardiothoracic Surgery. Available at http://mmcts.oxfordjournals.org/content/2008/0915/mmcts.2008.003160.full.pdf+html

34. Hraska V, Murin P (2012) Surgical management of congenital heart disease I: complex transposition of great arteries right and left ventricular outflow tract obstruction. Ebstein's anomaly. A video manual. Springer, Berlin

35. Ilbawi MN, DeLeon SY, Wilson WR Jr et al (1991) Extended aortic valvuloplasty: a new approach

36. Polimenakos AC, Sathanandam S, Blair C et al (2010) Selective tricuspidization and aortic cusp extension valvuloplasty: outcome analysis in infants and children. Ann Thorac Surg 90:839–847

37. Caspi J, Ilbawi MN, Roberson DA et al (1994) Extended aortic valvuloplasty for recurrent valvular stenosis and regurgitation in children. J Thorac Cardiovasc Surg 107:1114–1120

38. Tolan MJ, Daubeney PE, Slavik Y et al (1997) Aortic valve repair of congenital stenosis with bovine pericardium. Ann Thorac Surg 63:465–469

39. Cosgrow DM, Rosenkranz ER, Hender WG et al (1991) Valvuloplasty for aortic insufficiency. J Thorac Cardiovasc Surg 102:571–576

40. Tweddell JS, Pelech AN, Frommelt PC et al (2005) Complex aortic valve repair as a durable and effective alternative to valve replacement in children with aortic valve disease. J Thorac Cardiovasc Surg 129:551–558

41. Tweddell JS, Pelech AN, Jaquiss RDB et al. (2005) Aortic valve repair. Semin Thorac Cardiovasc Surg Pediatr Card Surg Annu 8:112–121

42. Alsoufi B, Karamlou T, Bradley T et al (2006) Short and midterm results of aortic valve cusp extension in the treatment of children with congenital aortic valve disease. Ann Thorac Surg 82:1292–1300

43. Hraska V, Photiadis J, Poruban R et al. (2008) Ross-Konno operation in children. Multimedia Manual of Cardiothoracic Surgery. Available at http://mmcts.ctsnetjournals.org/cgi/content/full/2008/0915/mmcts.2008.003160

44. Clarke DR (1991) Extended aortic root replacement with cryopreserved allografts: do they hold up? Ann Thorac Surg 52:669–675

45. Agnoletti G, Raisky O, Boudjemline Y et al (2006) Neonatal surgical aortic commissurotomy: predictors of outcome and long-term results. Ann Thorac Surg 82:1585–1592

46. Bhabra MS, Dhillon R, Bhudia S et al (2003) Surgical aortic valvotomy in infancy: impact of leaflet morphology on long-term outcomes. Ann Thorac Surg 76:1412–1416

47. Miyamoto T, Sinzobahamvya N, Wetter J et al (2006) Twenty years experience of surgical aortic valvotomy for critical aortic stenosis in early infancy. Eur J Cardiothorac Surg 30:35–40

48. Ewert P, Bertram H, Breuer J et al (2011) Balloon valvuloplasty in the treatment of congenital aortic valve stenosis — A retrospective multicenter survey of more than 1000 patients. Int J Cardiol 149:182–185

49. Brown DW, Dipilato AE, Chong EC et al (2010) - Aortic valve reinterventions after balloon aortic valvuloplasty for congenital aortic stenosis: intermediate and late follow-Up. J Am Coll Cardiol 56:1740–1749

50. Han RK, Gurofsky RC, Lee KJ et al (2007) Outcome and growth potential of left heart structures after

neonatal intervention for aortic valve stenosis. J Am Coll Cordiol 50(25):2406–2414

51. McElhinney DB, Lock JE, Keane JF et al (2005) Left heart growth, function, and reintervention after balloon aortic valvuloplasty for neonatal aortic stenosis. Circulation 111:451–458

52. Reich O, Tax P, Marek J et al (2004) Long term results of percutaneous balloon valvoplasty of congenital aortic stenosis: independent predictors of outcome. Heart 90:70–76

53. Hickey EJ, Yeh T, Jacobs JP et al (2010) Ross and Yasui operations for complex biventricular repair in infants with critical left ventricular outflow tract obstruction. Eur J Cardiothorac Surg 37:279–288

54. Brown DW, Chong EC, Gauvreau K (2008) Aortic wall injury as a complication of neonatal aortic valvuloplasty: incidence and risk factors. Circ Cardiovasc Interv 1:53–59

55. McCrindle BW, Blackstone EH, Williams WG et al (2001) Are outcomes of surgical versus transcatheter balloon valvotomy equivalent in neonatal critical aortic stenosis? Circulation 104(12 suppl I):I152–I158

56. Alexiou C, Langley SM, Dalrymple-Hay MJR et al (2001) Open commissurotomy for critical isolated aortic stenosis in neonate. Ann Thorac Surg 71:489–493

57. Karamlou T, Shen I, Alsoufia B et al (2005) The influence of valve physiology on outcome following aortic valvotomy for congenital bicuspid valve in children: 30-year results from a single institution. Eur J Cardiothorac Surg 27:81–85

58. Balmer C, Beghetti M, Fasnacht M (2004) Balloon aortic valvuloplasty in paediatric patients: progressive aortic regurgitation is common. Heart 90:77–81

59. Fratz S, Gildein HP, Balling G et al (2008) Aortic valvuloplasty in pediatric patients substantially postpones the need for aortic valve surgery: a single-center experience of 188 patients after up to 17.5 years of follow-up. Circulation 117:1201–1206

60. McMullan DM, Oppido G, Davies B et al (2007) Surgical strategy for the bicuspid aortic valve: tricuspidization with cusp extension versus pulmonary autograft. J Thorac Cardiovasc Surg 134:90–98

61. Brown JW, Ruzmetov M, Vijay P et al (2003) Surgery for aortic stenosis in children: a 40-year experience. Ann Thorac Surg 76:1398–1411

62. Odim J, Laks H, Allada V et al (2005) Results of aortic valve sparing and restoration with autologous pericardial leaflet extension in congenital heart disease. Ann Thorac Surg 80:647–654

63. Mavroudis C, Backer CL, Kaushal S (2009) Aortic stenosis and aortic insufficiency in children: impact of valvuloplasty and modified Ross-Konno procedure. Semin Thorac Cardiovasc Surg Pediatr Card Surg Annu 12:76–86

64. Al-Halees Z, Pieters F, Qadoura F et al (2002) The Ross procedure is the procedure of choice for congenital aortic valve disease. J Thorac Cardiovasc Surg 123:437–442

65. Elkins RC, Lane MM, McCue C (1996) Pulmonary autograft reoperation: incidence and management. Ann Thorac Surg 62:450–455

66. Takkenberg JJ, Klieverik LM, Schoof PH et al (2009) The Ross procedure: a systematic review and meta-analysis. Circulation 119:222–228

67. Alsoufi B, Fadel B, Bulbul Z (2012) Cardiac reoperations following the Ross procedure in children: spectrum of surgery and reoperation results. Eur J Cardiothorac Surg 42:25–3

68. Hörer J, Hanke T, Stierle U (2009) Neoaortic root diameters and aortic regurgitation in children after the Ross operation. Ann Thorac Surg 88:594–600

69. Brown JW, Ruzmetov M, Shahriari AP (2010) Modification of the Ross aortic valve replacement to prevent late autograft dilatation. Eur J Cardiothorac Surg 37:1002–1007

70. Al Rashidi F, Bhat M, Höglund P et al (2010) The modified Ross operation using a Dacron prosthetic vascular jacket does prevent pulmonary autograft dilatation at 4.5-year follow-up. Eur J Cardiothorac Surg 37:928–933

71. Slater M, Shen I, Welke K et al (2005) Modification to the Ross procedure to prevent autograft dilatation. Semin Thorac Cardiovasc Surg Pediatr Card Surg Annu 8(1):181–184

72. Garg V, Muth AN, Ransom JF et al (2005) Mutations in NOTCH1 cause aortic valve disease. Nature 437:270–274

73. Alsoufi B, Manlhiot C, Fadel B (2010) The Ross procedure in children: preoperative haemodynamic manifestation has significant effect on late autograft re-operation. Eur J Cardiothorac Surg 38:547–555

74. Laudito A, Brook MM, Suleman S et al (2001) The Ross procedure in children and young adults: a word of caution. J Thorac Cardiovasc Surg 122:147–153

75. David TE, Omran A, Webb G et al (1996) Geometric mismatch of the aortic and pulmonary roots causes aortic insufficiency after the Ross procedure. J Thorac Cardiovasc Surg 112:1231–1239

76. Hraska V, Krajci M, Haun C et al (2004) Ross and Ross-Konno procedure in children and adolescents: mid-term results. Eur J Cardiothorac Surg 25:742–747

77. Carr-White GS, Afoke A, Birks EJ et al (2000) Aortic root characteristic of human pulmonary autografts. Circulation 102(Suppl III):III-15–III-21

78. De Sa M, Moshkovitz Y, Butany J et al (1999) Histologic abnormalities of the ascending aorta and pulmonary trunk in patients with bicuspid aortic valve disease: clinical relevance to the Ross procedure. J Thorac Cardiovasc Surg 118:588–596

79. Ishizaka T, Devaney EJ, Ramsburgh SR et al (2003) Valve sparing aortic root replacement for dilation of the pulmonary autograft and aortic regurgitation after the Ross procedure. Ann Thorac Surg 75:1518–1522

80. Elkins RC, Lane NM, McCue C (2001) Ross operation in children: late results. J Heart Valve Dis 10:736–741

81. Gaynor JW, Alexiou C, McDonald A et al (2000) Aortic valve replacement in children: are mechanical prostheses a good option? Eur J Cardiothorac Surg 17:125–133

82. Hazekamp MG, Grotenhuis HB, Schoof PH et al (2005) Results of the Ross operation in a pediatric population. Eur J Cardiothorac Surg 27:975–979

83. Pasquali SK, Cohen MS, Shera D et al (2007) The relationship between neo-aortic root dilation, insufficiency and reintervention following the Ross Procedure in children and young adults. J Am Coll Cardiol 49:1806–1812

84. Ibrahim M, Cleland J, O'Kane H et al (1994) St Jude medical prosthesis in children. J Thorac Cardiovasc Surg 108:52–56

85. Mazzitelli D, Guenther T, Schreiber C (1998) Aortic valve replacement in children: are we on the right track? Eur J Cardiothorac Surg 13:565–571

86. Alexiou C, McDonald A, Langley SM et al (2000) Aortic valve replacement in children are mechanical prostheses a good option? Eur J Cardiothorac Surg 17:125–133

87. Champsaur G, Robin J, Tronc F (1997) Mechanical valve in aortic position is a valid option in children and adolescents. Eur J Cardiothorac Surg 11:117–122

88. Hopkins R (2007) Cardiac surgeon's primer: tissue-engineered cardiac valves. Semin Thorac Cardiovasc Surg Pediatr Card Surg Annu 10(1):125–135

Sub-aortic Stenosis

Johann Brink and Christian Brizard

Abstract

The left ventricular outflow tract is a complex of integrated anatomical structures that constitute subvalvar, valvar, and supravalvar components. Congenital left ventricular outflow tract obstruction can occur at a single level in isolation or at multiple levels. This condition affects 3–10 % of individuals with congenital heart disease and accounts for 0.25 for every 100 live births. Congenital subaortic stenosis represents a heterogeneous spectrum of lesions that cause obstruction in the left ventricular outflow tract beneath the aortic valve and is present in 8–30 % of patients with left ventricular outflow tract obstruction. The spectrum of obstruction ranges from a discrete localized fibrous or fibromuscular subaortic membrane with varying degrees of extension to a complete long diffuse fibrous tunnel subaortic stenosis. Another form of left ventricular outflow tract obstruction is a pure muscular form of hypertrophic obstructive cardiomyopathy. Infrequently, subaortic stenosis may also be the consequence of anomalous septal insertion of the mitral valve, accessory mitral valve tissue, abnormal papillary muscle insertion or muscle bands, and posterior displacement of the infundibular septum in the absence of a ventricular septal defect (with or without a subaortic membrane). Albeit the necessity for surgical intervention is well delineated, surgical timing and technique remain controversial. This chapter will focus on the three forms of subaortic stenosis (discrete form, the subaortic tunnel, and the hypertrophic obstructive cardiomyopathy) with an emphasis on surgical management.

J. Brink • C. Brizard (✉)
Cardiac Surgery, The Royal Children's Hospital,
Melbourne, VIC, Australia
e-mail: johann.brink@rch.org.au;
Christian.Brizard@rch.org.au

E.M. da Cruz et al. (eds.), *Pediatric and Congenital Cardiology, Cardiac Surgery and Intensive Care*,
DOI 10.1007/978-1-4471-4619-3_24, © Springer-Verlag London 2014

Keywords

Aortic valve • DSS • HOCM • Hypertrophic obstructive cardiomyopathy • Konno procedure • Left ventricle • Membrane resection • Mitral valve • Modified Konno procedure • Myectomy • Outflow tract • Ross-Konno procedure • Ross procedure • Subaortic stenosis • Tunnel subaortic stenosis • Ventriculoseptoplasty

Introduction

The left ventricular (LV) outflow tract is a complex of integrated anatomical structures that constitute subvalvar, valvar, and supravalvar components. Congenital LV outflow tract obstruction can occur at a single level in isolation or at multiple levels. This condition affects 3–10 % of individuals with congenital heart disease and accounts for 0.25 for every 100 live births [1–3]. Congenital subaortic stenosis represents a heterogeneous spectrum of lesions that cause obstruction in the LV outflow tract beneath the aortic valve and is present in 8–30 % of patients with LV outflow tract obstruction [4]. The spectrum of obstruction ranges from a *discrete localized* fibrous or fibromuscular *subaortic membrane* with varying degrees of extension to a complete long *diffuse fibrous tunnel subaortic stenosis*. Discrete subaortic stenosis was initially described by Chevers in 1842 [5]. The diffuse tunnel subaortic stenosis was coined by Spencer and later reintroduced by Reis, Morrow and colleagues in 1971 [6]. Another form of LV outflow tract obstruction is a pure muscular form of *hypertrophic obstructive cardiomyopathy*. This dynamic obstruction results from a bulging interventricular septum and the systolic anterior excursion of the anterior mitral valve leaflet. Infrequently, subaortic stenosis may also be the consequence of anomalous septal insertion of the mitral valve, accessory mitral valve tissue, abnormal papillary muscle insertion or muscle bands, and posterior displacement of the infundibular septum in the absence of a ventricular septal defect (with or without a subaortic membrane) [7]. Left ventricular outflow tract obstruction is a continuum of disease.

Surgical management and timing of intervention remain a therapeutic challenge. Subaortic obstruction is found most often in isolation with normal left ventricular and aortic arch structures. This group of patients then requires surgical relief of the obstruction allowing for biventricular repair. However, severe obstruction at multiple levels (Shone's complex) [8] can occur, including varying degrees of hypoplasia of the left heart structures as well as the aortic valve and aortic arch that coalesce into the spectrum of hypoplastic left heart syndrome, leading to a single ventricle pathway. Albeit the necessity for surgical intervention is well delineated, surgical timing and technique remain controversial. This chapter will focus on the three forms of subaortic stenosis (discrete form, the subaortic tunnel, and the HOCM) with an emphasis on surgical management.

Anatomy

The *cause* of subaortic stenosis has not been completely elucidated. However, plausible explanations for this lesion are well justified in the literature. Normal cardiac morphological growth and development is a continuous and dynamic process subjected to normal fluid dynamic forces and shear stress. The development of discrete subvalvar lesions is based upon abnormal flow patterns in the left ventricular outflow tract. These flow patterns account for significant flow acceleration, turbulence, and vortex formation that lead to an imbalance of shear forces. The rheological damage on the endocardium may cause a transfer of shear stress from elastin to collagen, which triggers gene

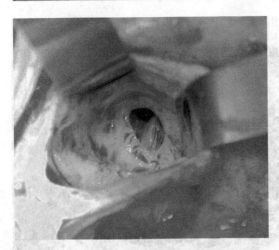

Fig. 91.1 Discrete subaortic membrane several years after a Ross procedure. This operative picture demonstrates the acquired character of this disease

expression of tissue growth factors. Cellular proliferation ensues and induces the discrete fibrous membrane [9, 10]. A small morphological aberration in the LV outflow tract can produce a significant increase in septal shear stress. In 1997, Cape and colleagues demonstrated that a smaller aortoseptal angle dramatically increased septal shear stress and was even more significant in the presence of a ventricular septal defect (VSD). Subaortic stenosis may also be the result of posterior projection of the conal septum into the LV outflow tract in a posterior malaligned VSD. Rosenquist et al. [11] demonstrated an increased distance between the mitral and aortic valves in patients with subaortic stenosis. This consistent finding led to postulate that an alteration in the direction of blood flow close to the crest of the interventricular septum may cause differentiation of embryonic cells into a fibrotic tissue variant [11]. Discrete subaortic stenosis is rarely diagnosed antenatally or during infancy but becomes evident in the first decade of life presenting with features of progressive LV outflow tract obstruction. A discrete subaortic membrane is therefore more of an acquired lesion rather than congenital (Fig. 91.1). Other rare morphological causes for subaortic stenosis include excessive endocardial tissue, valvular tags, chordae, or papillary muscle on the

ventricular surface of the anterior mitral valve leaflet attached to the septum [12], or septal bands low in the LV outflow tract [13].

A *localized discrete subaortic membrane* is a thin fibromuscular ridge or crescent beneath the aortic valve arising from the interventricular septum and is initially separated from the aortic valve. Being subjected to the vicious cycle of obstruction and turbulence, the ridge will evolve into a more prominent fibrous shelf of various thicknesses that extends toward the anterior mitral valve leaflet to become a circumferential ring. The resulting concentric left ventricular hypertrophy usually presents with a projection of the muscular septal bulge into the LV outflow tract (Fig. 91.2).

At the severe end of the spectrum, progressive fibromuscular proliferation causes this circumferential ring to extend apically for the distance of 10–30 mm [14] creating a *tunnel subaortic stenosis*. The anterior mitral valve leaflet often becomes incorporated in the tunnel by fibrous strands originating from the interventricular septum. A tunnel subaortic stenosis may also be the consequence of excessive fibrosis after previous resection of a subaortic membrane.

In most instances, the *aortic valve* is tricuspid and normal in appearance. Damage to the aortic valve may occur due to turbulence with subsequent cusp thickening. The fibrous ridge extends in height and becomes adherent to the undersurface of the aortic valve cusps, causing inadequate coaptation and retraction, with subsequent aortic valve regurgitation. Rarely, supravalvar and valvar aortic stenoses occur in conjunction with discrete subvalvar stenosis. In contrast, the tunnel subaortic obstruction is associated with small aortic annular dimensions and normal valvar appearance [14]. A bicuspid aortic valve is present in 23 % of patients with subaortic stenosis [15].

Concentric *left ventricular hypertrophy* is usually present in subaortic stenosis. The left ventricular cavity is small and subendocardial fibrosis is a frequent finding. Some patients with tunnel subaortic stenosis have excessive asymmetric hypertrophy of the septum (compared to

Fig. 91.2 Echocardiography showing a discrete subaortic membrane and demonstrating the distance between the membrane and the aortic valve at an early stage of the disease

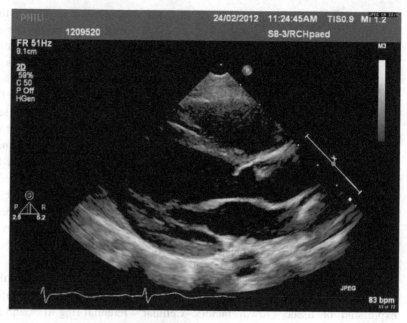

Fig. 91.3 Echocardiography showing a severe HOCM in tele-systole

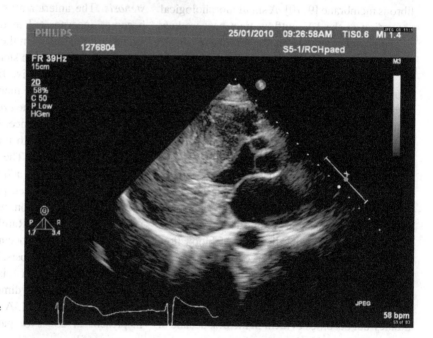

the posterior ventricular wall) and muscle fiber disarray [14]. These features are pathognomonic of hypertrophic obstructive cardiomyopathy (HOCM), a pure dynamic form of subaortic stenosis (Fig. 91.3) [16, 17]. HOCM is a monogenic autosomal dominant disease with considerable genetic heterogeneity. More than 1,000 distinct sarcomere protein gene mutations encoding for specific contractile proteins have been identified and the majority of these were found only in one or a few families. These sarcomeric proteins include β-myosin heavy chain, myosin-binding protein, troponin T, α-tropomyosin, myosin regulatory light chain, myosin essential light chain, and cardiac actin. More than 50 % of human mutations occur in β-myosin heavy chain and myosin-binding protein [18].

Congenital discrete subaortic stenosis may occur in isolation or be associated with *coexisting cardiac anomalies*. A concomitant VSD is present in 32 % of this population [19]. Other conditions include aortic coarctation, interrupted aortic arch, and atrioventricular septal defects.

Subvalvar obstruction may also be part of *multi-level obstructions of left heart* structures as in *Shone's complex*, which includes supramitral valve ring, parachute mitral valve, and coarctation of the aorta [20].

Pathophysiology

A wide spectrum of pathophysiological mechanisms is responsible for the heterogeneous anatomical composition in patients with subaortic stenosis. Physiologically, *localized discrete subaortic stenosis* behaves similarly to aortic valve stenosis. The obstruction is rarely evident in infancy, but becomes more severe over time, confirming the progressive nature of the disease. The localized discrete membrane impedes LV ejection causing an increased afterload and intraventricular pressure. The load on any region of the myocardium at any given point is expressed by the equation according to the Law of Laplace: (pressure × radius)/(2 × wall thickness). Thus, to maintain normal ejection fraction, any increase in pressure will need to be equalized by an increase in wall thickness at the cost of increased peak intraventricular pressure. This mechanical stress induces gene transcription and eventually an increase of the number of force-generating units (sarcomeres) in the myocyte. In the in vivo heart, an increase in the afterload causes an increase in myosin heavy chain synthesis by 35 % within only a few hours [20]. The biochemical consequences include re-expression of immature fetal cardiac genes that modify motor unit composition, energy metabolism, and genes that encode for hormonal pathways of, for example, atrial natriuretic peptide and angiotensin-converting enzyme [21]. The progressive increase in myocardial mass is accompanied by increased collagen deposition within the myocardium causing diminished ventricular compliance. The end result of concentric hypertrophy is an increased intraventricular peak systolic pressure relative to aortic systolic pressure with an elevated LV end-diastolic pressure. The above factors cause an imbalance between myocardial oxygen demand and delivery, resulting in decreased LV perfusion pressure and subendocardial ischemia, infarction, and fibrosis that lead to decreased systolic function.

Increased turbulence and blood flow velocity in the LV outflow tract may cause a progressive extension of a discrete localized subaortic membrane to the ventricular surface of the aortic valve cusps causing regurgitation. A jet lesion on the cusp in itself might cause thickening or damage making the valve vulnerable to infective endocarditis. The localized membrane may progress to tunnel subaortic stenosis. This form of obstruction, as in HOCM, may demonstrate disproportionate ventricular septal thickening and abnormal systolic anterior mitral valve leaflet motion (SAM). The mechanism of SAM was initially explained by the Venturi effect. Accelerated flow during LV systole over the anterior leaflet of the mitral valve caused a sucking force, pulling the tip of the leaflet into the LV outflow tract resulting in a dynamic form of obstruction. This mechanism has been challenged by the *drag theory*. Sherrid and colleagues proved that at the onset of SAM, LV outflow tract flow velocity was normal. Venturi forces were present, but at much less magnitude than previously postulated. The data demonstrated that SAM was the consequence of a hydrodynamic push force of flow, called *drag* [22]. Another explanation for the initiation of SAM is the combination of a redundant anterior mitral valve leaflet and anterior displacement of the papillary muscles producing chordal relaxation. Thus, the mitral valve is situated more anterior in the LV as appose to its normal central position, and flow sweeps up the leaflet and pushes it toward the septum [23]. Dynamic obstruction is mostly demonstrated in the pure muscular forms of hypertrophic obstructive cardiomyopathy by a large muscle mass, located deep in the LV cavity and causing a mid-cavity obstruction [24].

Diagnosis

Clinical

Mild obstruction is usually present early in life and symptomatic features are uncommon. Due to the progressive nature of this disease, obstruction becomes more severe with age—however, still presenting with only mild symptomatology. Approximately 25 % of patients requiring surgical intervention are asymptomatic. When the narrowing becomes very severe, presenting symptoms include fatigue, exercise intolerance, syncope, and angina. Congestive cardiac failure features much later in life, and very rarely, cardiac arrest with sudden death results without preexisting clinical symptoms. Tunnel subaortic stenosis displays a much more rapid progression than a discrete localized subaortic membrane and often presents during infancy.

The physical signs are similar to valvar stenosis. A carotid thrill and prominent left ventricular apex impulse may be present. A systolic ejection murmur without an ejection click is audible at the left sternal border over the aortic valve area. An early diastolic decrescendo murmur may be present at the left lower sternal edge in the presence of aortic valve regurgitation.

Electrocardiogram

The ECG may show varying degrees of left ventricular hypertrophy and in severe obstruction it may display evidence of left ventricular strain patterns.

Imaging

Chest x-ray is usually normal and non-diagnostic; however, left ventricular and left atrial enlargement may be evident in advanced disease.

Echocardiography is the gold standard diagnostic method for subaortic stenosis. Two-dimensional cross-sectional imaging in the parasternal long axis demonstrates the distinct ridge in the left ventricular outflow tract. Tunnel subaortic stenosis presents a long diffuse circular tunnel. Surgical timing, indication, and decision-making are dependent on a detailed assessment of the full extent of the lesion, including aortic and mitral valve involvement. Good quality images are therefore imperative and transoesophageal and three-dimensional echocardiograms are an invaluable diagnostic option to consider. Color Doppler-derived ultrasound assesses the level and severity of the LV outflow tract obstruction and quantifies the aortic valve regurgitation. Peak flow velocity is an accurate measurement to determine the degree of obstruction and cardiac catheterization is rarely indicated in the diagnostic evaluation of subaortic stenosis. Echocardiography may also reveal the presence of severe systolic septal bulging in the mid-cavity of the LV outflow tract, as well as SAM of the anterior mitral valve leaflet toward the septum. Evidence of these dynamic forms of obstruction is essential in surgical decision-making (Fig. 91.4).

Decision-Making

In the 1970s, discrete subvalvar aortic stenosis was considered to be a rapidly progressive disease and some centers have considered its presence alone or a gradient as little as 30 mmHg to justify surgical intervention [15]. The rationale for such an aggressive approach, especially during infancy and in young childhood, is the progressive nature of the disease as well as prevention of the aortic valve regurgitation. Subsequent data has demonstrated that the

Fig. 91.4 Echocardiography showing a severe HOCM in tele-diastole (Same patient as in Fig. 91.3)

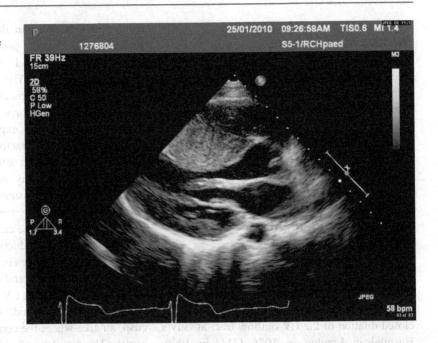

rate of progression is variable and that the aortic valve regurgitation was often worse after surgery and with less progressive lesions than thought [25]. The timing of surgery and surgical indications remain controversial; however, the keystone decision-making factors are *age at presentation*, a *significant or progressive gradient in the LV outflow tract*, *LV hypertrophy*, and the *status of the aortic valve*. These authors' approach to surgical intervention includes the following guidelines: due to the rapid rate of progression of the lesion at early age [26], a mean Doppler gradient greater than 30 mmHg during infancy or in a very young child requires surgery whatever the status of the aortic valve. If the mean gradient is less than 30 mmHg and the aortic valve is normal, then this population should be followed up serially for progressive increase in gradient and aortic valve involvement, provided that the LV hypertrophy remains stable. Due to the high recurrence rate after surgical intervention at an early age (5–10 years) [27], some groups have advocated for deferring surgery beyond the age of 10 years, or when the mean gradient is 40–50 mmHg [12]. However, Barkhordarian et al. have proved

that operating children between 1 and 10 years restores the geometry of the aortoseptal angle and remodels the LV outflow tract. This ability is lost when the patient is operated at an older age [28]. Surgery is recommended in progressive LV outflow tract gradients and LV hypertrophy. The presence of aortic valve regurgitation or a new onset of regurgitation justifies surgery. Progressive extension of a discrete membrane, with or without a significant gradient, might also justify surgery. Geva et al. have proved that independent risk factors for reoperation for recurrence are an initial peak gradient greater or equal to 60 mmHg and those patients who required peeling of the membrane from the mitral or aortic valve [29].

Tunnel subaortic stenosis is a more complex lesion that requires a much more aggressive surgical approach. It is therefore reasonable that a peak Doppler gradient of 50–60 mmHg, significant LV hypertrophy, and new aortic valve regurgitation warrant surgical intervention [30]. However, our surgical indications are similar to that of a discrete localized membrane and the anatomy in tunnel stenosis selects the surgical procedure.

Medical Management

The use of medical therapy in subaortic stenosis is limited to symptomatic treatment of congestive cardiac failure in advanced disease only. Interventional therapy has little, if any, role in the treatment of subaortic stenosis, and attempts with balloon dilation or stenting of the LV outflow tract have proved potentially hazardous.

Surgical Management

History

Almost 15 years after the first description of discrete subaortic stenosis, Brock attempted closed dilation of the LV outflow tract at Guy's Hospital in London in 1956 [31]. In 1960, Spencer reported surgical treatment of this lesion on cardiopulmonary bypass [32]. Fifteen years later, Rastan and Konno introduced the aortoventriculoplasty as treatment for diffuse subaortic stenosis that included valve replacement [33, 34]. The modified Konno operation made possible achieving complete relief of diffuse LV outflow tract obstruction while preserving the aortic valve in 1978 [4], Vouhé and colleagues described an aortoseptal approach in 1984 [35] and in 1986 Cooley reported ventricular septoplasty with aortic valve conservation [36]. Cooley also introduced the apico-aortic valved conduit as a surgical option for complicated forms of left ventricular outflow tract obstruction [37].

Discrete Subaortic Membrane

The surgical approach is through a median sternotomy. Cardiopulmonary bypass is established by cannulation of the aorta high just below the takeoff of the innominate artery. A single venous cannula is often used and the left heart is vented via the right superior pulmonary vein after limited dissection of the interatrial groove. The aorta is clamped and blood

cardioplegia is given in the aortic root. In the presence of significant aortic regurgitation, the aorta is opened and direct intracoronary cardioplegia is given. The aorta is opened with a "hockey stick" incision extended into the noncoronary sinus, and three traction sutures are applied to aid in the exposure of the valve. A malleable ribbon retractor is used to visualize the membrane. Careful attention focuses at all times not to cause any damage to the aortic cusps. Meticulous assessment is made when evaluating the extent of the membrane and its proximity to the aortic valve cusps, the mitral valve, and the area of the conduction system. Attention is also directed to the area below the membrane to identify septal bulging and a possible secondary membrane deeper in the LV cavity. The resection starts below the left side of the non-coronary cusp, an area where the conduction tissue is not at risk. The membrane is retracted with a micro tooth forceps and the cleave plane is dissected in an anti-clockwise direction using an 11 blade or an ophthalmic blade. Once the plane is developed, the membrane can easily be separated from the muscle. The membrane is then separated in an anti-clockwise direction toward the mitral valve. The area below the right and non-coronary commissure, at the inferior margin of the membranous septum, is where the conduction tissue lies, and meticulous attention should be taken not to resect muscle in this area. This is done with a combination of blunt and sharp dissection. If the membrane involves the aortic valve, it should be separated carefully from the undersurface of the cusp. The membrane is then separated from the mitral valve. Once the membrane is removed, attention is drawn to the distant LV cavity to exclude an additional second membrane [12] and to evaluate the presence of a muscular septal bulge.

Additional Septal Myectomy

A myectomy is performed in the septum below the aortic valve between the left half of the right coronary cusp and the right half of the left coronary cusp. Resection beyond this point toward the right could result in complete heart block and should be avoided. Two radial incisions are made with an 11 blade at these points. A quadrangular wedge is then resected down to the level of the papillary muscles with sharp-tip scissors. The depth of resection can be judged from the septal thickness measured on the echocardiogram before the surgery. Too liberal resection may result in an iatrogenic ventricular septal defect.

The need for septal myectomy is still controversial. Incomplete relief of the obstruction and residual LV outflow tract gradient has been believed to be a major risk factor for recurrence. Some groups advocate for additional myectomy as an essential technique for complete relief of the stenosis and prevention of recurrent obstruction [2, 38]. Reduced flow velocity and turbulence in the outflow tract results in less shear stress and reduces the incidence of recurrent fibrosis. Others have argued that an additional myectomy adds little value to the outcome and may even form a substrate for recurrent scaring [39]. At the Royal Children's Hospital, Melbourne, a myectomy after the membrane resection is systematically added.

The aortotomy and left atrium vent are closed and the heart is de-aired. The cross clamp is removed and the patient is weaned from cardiopulmonary bypass. Routine intraoperative transesophageal or epicardial echocardiogram is performed to evaluate for residual gradient in the LV outflow tract, aortic and mitral valve competence, and possibly an interventricular septal defect. Under anesthetic conditions and during the initial stages post bypass, hyperdynamic cardiac function may falsely overestimate the true residual LV outflow obstruction, and direct needle pressure measurement in the left ventricle and aorta may be a more accurate method of assessment for residual obstruction. The hyperdynamic state of the heart could be attenuated by sufficient volume preload, optimal hematocrit, minimal use of inotropic agent, and/or afterload reduction therapy. However, it is our practice not to hesitate to return on bypass and perform additional relief of the obstruction if a residual gradient is of any significance.

Tunnel Subaortic Stenosis and HOCM

The decision-making process and surgical strategy for tunnel subaortic stenosis and HOCM are much more complicated than in discrete subaortic stenosis. A detailed echocardiographic anatomical and physiological analysis is crucial in order to select the appropriate surgical procedure to adequately relieve the LV outflow tract obstruction, and the required surgical strategy is often invasive. The determining anatomical factors have been adopted from the multi-level approach described by Vouhé [40] and include the extent of the stenotic lesion (localized or diffuse), multi-level obstruction (supravalvar, valvar, and subvalvar obstruction), aortic valve function, aortic annular size, and mitral valve involvement.

Using a median sternotomy, the subaortic tunnel is approached with the technique described above. Diffuse subaortic stenosis is managed with the aortoseptal approach [40, 41]. A vertical aortotomy is performed and extended down to the intercoronary commissure. The aortic valve and subvalvar anatomy are inspected.

Normal Aortic Valve Cusps and Normal Size Annulus

Normal aortic annular orifice and valve cusps warrant preservation of the aortic root and a modified Konno operation/ventriculoseptoplasty should be the procedure of choice to yield adequate relief of the obstruction and prevent future reoperation [36, 42]. This operation provides complete relief of the LVOT gradient. It is very appropriate for the tunnel subaortic obstruction. In the authors' unit, however, its usage has been extended to the HOCM patients that require surgical intervention. The procedure begins with the resection of the subaortic membrane when it is present, with a myectomy as described above. Then, a right angle instrument is inserted at the cephalad extremity of the myectomy through the aortic valve and directed from below the anterior trigone into the

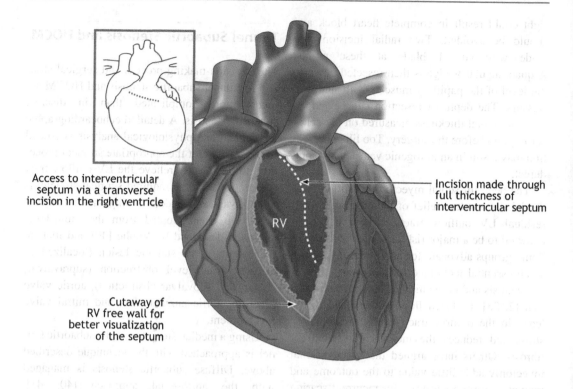

Access to interventricular
septum via a transverse
incision in the right ventricle

RV

Incision made through
full thickness of
interventricular septum

Cutaway of
RV free wall for
better visualization
of the septum

Fig. 91.5 Principle of the ventriculoseptoplasty, longitudinal view

interventricular septum to a point visualized through infundibular incision. Meticulous care should be taken to prevent injury to the aortic valve. A longitudinal septostomy is performed at this point below the pulmonary valve and extended obliquely *toward the apex of the left ventricle* to a level below the tip or even close to the base of the papillary muscles (Fig. 91.5). The left side margin *and only the left side* of the ventriculotomy is thinned out to prevent injury to the conduction tissue (Figs. 91.6 and 91.7). The incision is then extended proximally into the intercoronary sub-commissural triangle. The septal incision provides proper exposure to perform adequate resection of fibrotic and excessive muscular tissue in the LV outflow tract. Care should be taken not to perform any resection in the inferior/rightward edge in order to prevent injury to the conduction tissue. The mitral and aortic valve should be cleared from any fibrous tissue. Then, the septal incision is closed with a polytetrafluoroethylene (PTFE) augmentation

patch secured with interrupted pledgeted sutures (Figs. 91.8 and 91.9). Closure of the distal trabeculated portion of the septum should be performed with reinforced pledgeted-supported sutures to prevent a residual interventricular septal defect [43]. Circumferential augmentation of the LV outflow tract is achieved with the septal incision, resection of excess fibrotic tissue, muscle resection, thinning of the septum on the left side of the incision, and insertion of the patch (Figs. 91.10 and 91.11). The right ventriculotomy is closed directly or with a glutaraldehyde-treated autologous pericardial patch with a continuous running suture. The aorta is closed directly.

The ventriculoseptoplasty, despite its apparent complexity, yields excellent result with rare complications. The subaortic gradient is usually totally abolished. Complications can be complete heart block or trifascicular block, which would require the insertion of a pacemaker. The relative diastolic dysfunction associated with the hypertrophy requires a DDD pacing system.

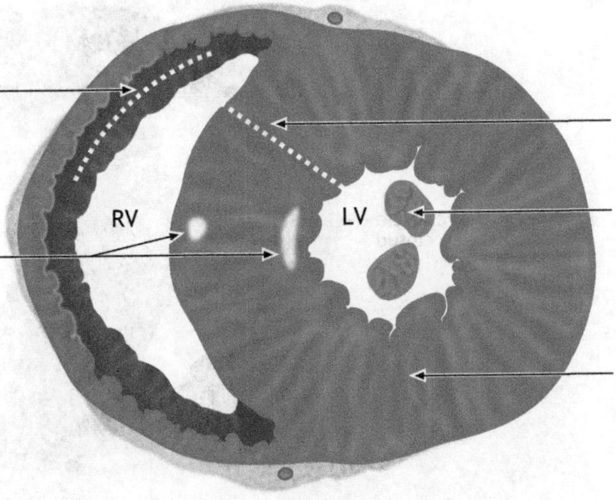

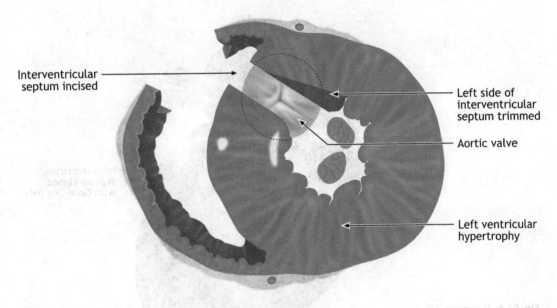

Fig. 91.6 Principle of the ventriculoseptoplasty, transverse cut

Fig. 91.7 Principle of the ventriculoseptoplasty, transverse cut

Aortic regurgitation can be created by direct injury to the valve or distortion of the right left commissure. Residual left side gradient can be seen if the resection or the extent of the septostomy is insufficient; this should trigger an immediate reoperation. Residual right-sided gradient can be seen if the right ventriculotomy has been closed directly [44]. At the Royal Children's Hospital, Melbourne, the indication for ventriculoseptoplasty is six times more common for HOCM than for subaortic tunnel, which is a very rare entity in the program. Metton et al. also report the utilization of the ventriculoseptoplasty in half of their patients, whereas other series with the modified Konno procedure use this technique exceptionally for the HOCM [44]. This is probably related to the age of the patients, as the Morrow-Bigelow myectomy is a more simple and well-accepted technique for the surgical management of the HOCM in adults

Fig. 91.8 Reconstruction
stages of the
ventriculoseptoplasty

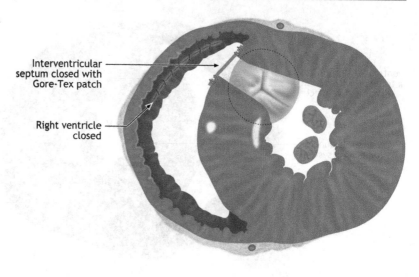

Interventricular
septum closed with
Gore-Tex patch

Right ventricle
closed

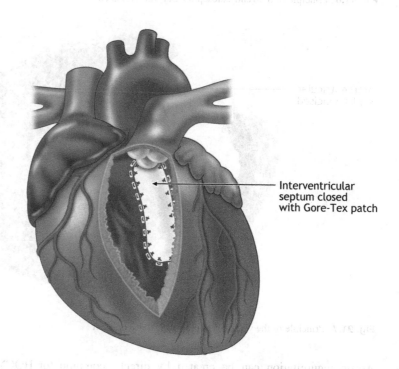

Interventricular
septum closed
with Gore-Tex patch

Fig. 91.9 Reconstruction
stages of the
ventriculoseptoplasty

in North America. It is, however, much more difficult to provide with a complete elimination of the gradient than with the modified Konno procedure.

The indications in a tunnel subaortic obstruction are simply dictated by the mean gradient, whereas the indication in HOCM must adhere to the guidelines provided by the experts [45],

namely, symptoms resistant to medical therapy or the presence of a mitral valve regurgitation created by the SAM.

In the presence of aortic valve regurgitation not accessible to repair and/or hypoplastic aortic annulus, the ventriculoseptoplasty is not suitable. The relief of the subaortic obstruction has to be associated with the replacement of the aortic

Fig. 91.10 Postoperative echocardiography (short axis) of the ventriculoseptoplasty in diastole. The patch is well visible at the superior aspect of the trench in the septum

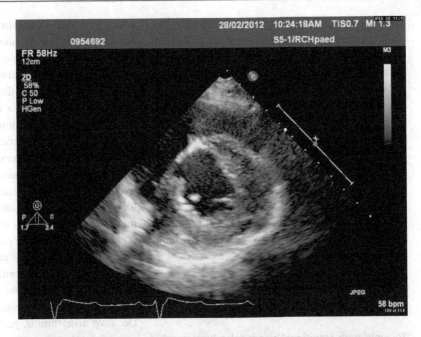

Fig. 91.11 Postoperative echocardiogram (short axis) of the ventriculoseptoplasty in systole. Most of the lumen existing in the cavity is within the trench in the septum

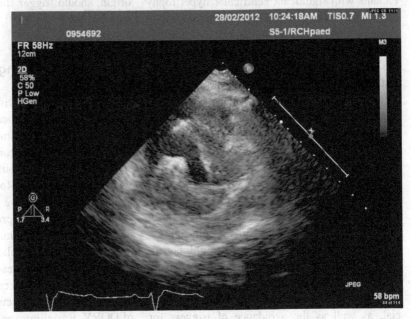

valve. In the pediatric age group, this is best done with the combination of the pulmonary autograft transposition or Ross procedure and the Konno procedure: the so-called Ross-Konno procedure. The combination of the two procedures is logical and the harvest of the pulmonary autograft makes the exposure to the infundibular septum very easy. Reddy et al. have proposed to use a flap of the infundibulum attached to the autograft to eventually cover the incision in the interventricular septum [46]. At the Royal Children's Hospital, Melbourne, this technique is rarely used in the context of critical aortic stenosis. On the other hand, at an older age, the Ross-Konno procedure is used every time the valve cannot be salvaged. These authors are very opposed to the utilization of right ventricular infundibulum free wall to cover the septal cut at any age. The non-vascularized patch of RV free wall is thin and will dilate, withdrawing support to the neo-pulmonary valve and thus allowing for the billowing of one or two sinuses of the autograft and adding a second mechanism secondary for the pulmonary autograft failure. At the Royal Children's Hospital, Melbourne, it is preferred to use a Gore-Tex® patch to provide a reliable support to the autograft. Generally, with the Ross procedure, the earlier the age it is performed, the less stable the pulmonary autograft [47, 48], and the same principle applies to the Ross-Konno procedure.

Postoperative Management

Patients with significant ventricular hypertrophy may benefit from a left atrial pressure monitoring in the postoperative course to allow for appropriate preload and volume management, although this may be institution dependent. Otherwise, a standard comprehensive monitoring of cardiac metrics and markers of tissue perfusion is of vital importance. After these complex interventions, patients who are hemodynamically stable and free of bleeding and arrhythmias may progress rapidly toward extubation. Monitoring of the left atrial pressure and tissue perfusion markers during the ventilator weaning process may be useful in assessing patient reserves and the impact of positive pressure in the patient's physiology; along these lines, some patients might benefit from extubation to non-invasive positive pressure in the form of CPAP, BiPAP, or analogous modalities. Adequate sedation and pain control is crucial, as well as the avoidance of triggers for tachycardia that may impact the diastolic filling of hypertrophic ventricles. As much as maintenance of an even or slightly negative fluid balance is important, particular attention ought to be paid to the fact that these patients require relatively elevated filling pressures to maintain proper hemodynamic conditions and tissue perfusion, needless to say that dehydration must be avoided. Cardiovascular support is usually provided with

a combination of milrinone (for its inotropic, lusitropic, and vasodilator effect) and low-dose dopamine or epinephrine as needed. Caregivers need to find a balance between the benefit of these drugs and the potential disadvantages in terms of induction of tachycardia and increased myocardial oxygen consumption. At the Royal Children's Hospital, Melbourne, we also use very low-dose vasoconstrictors to increase the coronary perfusion pressure of the excessively hypertrophied myocardium. Arrhythmias ought to be proactively prevented (i.e., rectification of metabolic disturbances) and aggressively treated if present. It is mandatory to warrant normal atrioventricular conduction and to consider interventricular re-synchronization strategies in patients with unstable hemodynamics and unresponsive to conventional medical therapy. De novo arrhythmias, particularly of ventricular origin, should trigger studies for potential coronary lesions.

Outcomes and Long-Term Follow-Up

The long-term results with discrete subaortic stenosis suggest a recurrence rate of 10–35 % without additional myectomy and less than 5 % with myectomy. Recurrence after resection should be treated with either a repeated resection with myectomy or a Ross-Konno procedure if a significant aortic valve involvement is present. If the aortic valve is preserved and the lesion has extended to a tunnel subaortic stenosis, then a ventriculoseptoplasty is indicated. Recurrence after repeated resection is possible and mostly encountered in complex reconstructions involving the left ventricular outflow tract (repair of DORV, Rastelli procedure).

The long-term results of the ventriculoseptoplasty are outstanding with virtually no recurrence of the gradient and no long-term mortality. In HOCM however, if the relief of the symptoms is usually achieved, the risk of sudden death seems not to be modified. The decision-making process for the implantation of defibrillators in these patients can be very challenging.

The long-term results of the Ross-Konno procedure are dominated by the autograft dilation and function. Implantation at a very young age is associated with poor function of the neo-aortic valve.

References

1. Hoffman JI, Christianson R (1978) Congenital heart disease in a cohort of 19,502 births with long-term follow-up. Am J Cardiol 42(4):641–647
2. Rayburn ST, Netherland DE, Heath BJ (1997) Discrete membranous subaortic stenosis: improved results after resection and myectomy. Ann Thorac Surg 64(1):105–109
3. Grech V (2001) Incidence and management of subaortic stenosis in Malta. Pediatr Cardiol 22(5):431
4. (null) (2003) Cardiac surgery. Kirklin JW, Barrat-Boyes BG (eds) Churchill Livingstone, New York
5. Chevers N (1842) Observations on the diseases of the orifices and valves of the aorta. Guy Hosp Rep 7:387–442
6. Reis RL, Peterson LM, Mason DT, Simon AL, Morrow AG (1971) Congenital fixed subvalvular aortic stenosis. An anatomical classification and correlations with operative results. Circulation 43(5 Suppl): I11–I18
7. Marasini M, Zannini L, Ussia GP, Pinto R, Moretti R, Lerzo F et al (2003) Discrete subaortic stenosis: incidence, morphology and surgical impact of associated subaortic anomalies. Ann Thorac Surg 75(6):1763–1768
8. Brauner RA, Laks H, Drinkwater DC Jr, Scholl F, McCaffery S (1997) Multiple left heart obstructions (Shone's anomaly) with mitral valve involvement: long-term surgical outcome. Ann Thorac Surg 64(3):721–729
9. Cape EG, Vanauker MD, Sigfússon G, Tacy TA, del Nido PJ (1997) Potential role of mechanical stress in the etiology of pediatric heart disease: septal shear stress in subaortic stenosis. J Am Coll Cardiol 30(1):247–254
10. Ferrans VJ, Muna WF, Jones M, Roberts WC (1978) Ultrastructure of the fibrous ring in patient with discrete subaortic stenosis. Lab Invest 39(1):30–40
11. Rosenquist GC, Clark EB, McAllister HA, Bharati S, Edwards JE (1979) Increased mitral-aortic separation in discrete subaortic stenosis. Circulation 60(1):70–74
12. Jonas RA (ed) (2004) Comprehensive management of surgical management of congenital heart disease. Hodder Arnold, London
13. Gewillig M, Daenen W, Dumoulin M, Van der Hauwaert L (1992) Rheologic genesis of discrete subvalvular aortic stenosis: a Doppler echocardiographic study. J Am Coll Cardiol 19(4):818–824
14. Maron BJ, Redwood DR, Roberts WC, Henry WL, Morrow AG, Epstein SE (1976) Tunnel subaortic stenosis: left ventricular outflow tract obstruction produced by fibromuscular tubular narrowing. Circulation 54(3):404–416
15. Brauner R, Laks H, Drinkwater DC, Shvarts O, Eghbali K, Galindo A (1997) Benefits of early surgical repair in fixed subaortic stenosis. J Am Coll Cardiol 30(7):1835–1842
16. (null) (2003) Cardiac surgery. Kirklin JW, Barrat-Boyes BG (eds) 3rd edn. Churchill Livingstone, New York, pp 1013–1034
17. Maron BJ, Ferrans VJ, Henry WL, Clark CE, Redwood DR, Roberts WC et al (1974) Differences in distribution of myocardial abnormalities in patients with obstructive and nonobstructive asymmetric septal hypertrophy (ASH). Light and electron microscopic findings. Circulation 50(3):436–446
18. Seidman CE, Seidman JG (2011) Identifying sarcomere gene mutations in hypertrophic cardiomyopathy: a personal history. Circ Res 108(6):743–750
19. Kitchiner D, Jackson M, Malaiya N, Walsh K, Peart I, Arnold R et al (1994) Morphology of left ventricular outflow tract structures in patients with subaortic stenosis and a ventricular septal defect. Br Heart J 72(3):251–260
20. Imamura T, McDermott PJ, Kent RL, Nagatsu M, Cooper G, Carabello BA (1994) Acute changes in myosin heavy chain synthesis rate in pressure versus volume overload. Circ Res 75(3):418–425
21. Lorell BH, Carabello BA (2000) Left ventricular hypertrophy: pathogenesis, detection, and prognosis. Circulation 102(4):470–479
22. Sherrid MV, Arabadjian M (2012) Echocardiography to individualize treatment for hypertrophic cardiomyopathy. Prog Cardiovasc Dis 54(6):461–476
23. Klues HG, Maron BJ, Dollar AL, Roberts WC (1992) Diversity of structural mitral valve alterations in hypertrophic cardiomyopathy. Circulation 85(5):1651–1660
24. Falicov RE, Resnekov L (1977) Mid ventricular obstruction in hypertrophic obstructive cardiomyopathy. New diagnostic and therapeutic challenge. Br Heart J 39(7):701–705
25. Leigter DA, Sullivan ID, Gersony WM (2001) Discrete subvalvar aortic stenosis: natural history and hemodynamics. J Am Coll Cardiol 14:1539–1544
26. Gersony WM (2001) Natural history of discrete subvalvar aortic stenosis: management implications. J Am Coll Cardiol 38(3):843–845
27. Wright GB, Keane JF, Nadas AS, Bernhard WF, Castaneda AR (1983) Fixed subaortic stenosis in the young: medical and surgical course in 83 patients. Am J Cardiol 52(7):830–835
28. Barkhordarian R, Wen-Hong D, Li W, Josen M, Henein M, Ho SY (2007) Geometry of the left ventricular outflow tract in fixed subaortic stenosis and intact ventricular septum: an echocardiographic study in children and adults. J Thorac Cardiovasc Surg 133(1):196–203

29. Geva A, McMahon CJ, Gauvreau K, Mohammed L, del Nido PJ, Geva T (2007) Risk factors for reoperation after repair of discrete subaortic stenosis in children. J Am Coll Cardiol 50(15):1498–1504

30. Jonas RA (2002) Modified Konno procedure for the tunnel subaortic obstruction. Oper Tech Thorac Cardiovasc Surg 7:176–180

31. Brock R, Fleming PR (1956) Aortic subvalvar stenosis; a report of 5 cases diagnosed during life. Guys Hosp Rep 105(4):391–408

32. Spencer FC, Neill CA, Sank L, Bahnson HT (1960) Anatomical variations in 46 patients with congenital aortic stenosis, Am Surg 26:204–216

33. Rastan H, Koncz J (1975) Plastic enlargement of the left ventricular outflow tract. A new operative method (author's transl). Thoraxchir Vask Chir 23(3):169–175

34. Konno S, Imai Y, Iida Y, Nakajima M, Tatsuno K (1975) A new method for prosthetic valve replacement in congenital aortic stenosis associated with hypoplasia of the aortic valve ring. J Thorac Cardiovasc Surg 70(5):909–917

35. Vouhe PR, Poulain H, Bloch G, Loisance DY, Gamain J, Lombaert M et al (1984) Aortoseptal approach for optimal resection of diffuse subvalvular aortic stenosis. J Thorac Cardiovasc Surg 87(6):887–893

36. Cooley DA, Garrett JR (1986) Septoplasty for left ventricular outflow obstruction without aortic valve replacement: a new technique. Ann Thorac Surg 42(4):445–448

37. Cooley DA, Norman JC, Reul GJ, Kidd JN, Nihill MR (1976) Surgical treatment of left ventricular outflow tract obstruction with apicoaortic valved conduit. Surgery 80(6):674–680

38. Altarabsheh SE, Dearani JA, Burkhart HM, Schaff HV, Deo SV, Eidem BW et al (2013) Outcome of septal myectomy for obstructive hypertrophic cardiomyopathy in children and young adults. ATS Elsevier 95(2):663–669

39. Ashraf H, Cotroneo J, Dhar N, Gingell R, Roland M, Pieroni D et al (1985) Long-term results after excision of fixed subaortic stenosis. J Thorac Cardiovasc Surg 90(6):864–871

40. Vouhé PR, Neveux J-Y (1991) Surgical management of diffuse subaortic stenosis: an integrated approach. ATS Soc Thorac Surg 52(3):654–661

41. Vouhe PR, Poulain H, Vouron J, Loisance DY, Bloch G, Cachera JP (1984) Surgical treatment of aortic subvalvular obstruction. Experimental study of a new approach. Arch Mal Coeur Vaiss 77(3):307–313

42. Vouhe PR, Ouaknine R, Poulain H, Vernant F, Mauriat P, Pouard P et al (1993) Diffuse subaortic stenosis: modified Konno procedures with aortic valve preservation. Eur J Cardiothorac Surg 7(3):132–136

43. Caldarone CA, Van Natta TL, Frazer JR, Behrendt DM (2003) The modified Konno procedure for complex left ventricular outflow tract obstruction. Ann Thorac Surg 75(1):147–151, –discussion151–2

44. Metton O, Ali WB, Raisky O, Vouhe PR (2008) Modified Konno operation for diffuse subaortic stenosis. Multimed Manual Cardio-Thorac Surg 2008 (0915):1–6

45. Maron BJ, Dearani JA, Ommen SR, Maron MS, Schaff HV, Gersh BJ et al (2004) The case for surgery in obstructive hypertrophic cardiomyopathy. J Am Coll Cardiol 44(10):2044–2053

46. Reddy VM, Rajasinghe HA, Teitel DF, Haas GS, Hanley FL (1996) Aortoventriculoplasty with the pulmonary autograft: the "Ross-Konno" procedure. J Thorac Cardiovasc Surg 111(1):158–165

47. Ruzmetov M, Geiss DM, Shah JJ, Buckley K, Fortuna RS (2013) The Ross-Konno is a high-risk procedure when compared with the Ross operation in children. ATS Elsevier 95(2):670–675

48. Pasquali SK, Cohen MS, Shera D, Wernovsky G, Spray TL, Marino BS (2007) The relationship between neo-aortic root dilation, insufficiency, and reintervention following the Ross procedure in infants, children, and young adults. J Am Coll Cardiol 49(17):1806–1812

Supravalvar Aortic Stenosis

Max B. Mitchell and Eduardo M. da Cruz

Abstract

Supravalvar aortic stenosis is the least common form of left ventricular outflow tract obstruction, caused by an elastin arteriopathy that occurs in Williams-Beuren syndrome, familial elastin arteriopathy, and "sporadic" elastin arteriopathy. All three populations have a microdeletion involving the elastin precursor gene on chromosome 7 (7q11.23). In patients with Williams-Beuren syndrome, the elastin gene is deleted or disrupted together with a number of neighboring genes that probably are important for the other features of the syndrome (elfin face, mild mental retardation, hypercalcemia), whereas in patients with familial, non-Williams supravalvar aortic stenosis, the elastin gene only is subjected to a loss-of-function translocation or point mutation. Patients with "sporadic" supravalvar aortic stenosis are members of a family either carrying an elastin gene mutation with a subclinical phenotype or carrying the elastin gene defect as a new mutation. Defective elastin production leads to obstructive lesions in the large elastin-containing arteries. Other sites of arterial obstruction that occur with elastin arteriopathy include the pulmonary arteries, aortic arch branches, the abdominal aorta, and the renal arteries. The patterns and severity of arterial disease are highly variable; consequently, supravalvar aortic stenosis occurs across a large clinical spectrum. This chapter will provide an overview of the anatomy, pathophysiology, management, and outcomes of this entity.

M.B. Mitchell (✉)
Department of Surgery, Heart Institute, The Children's
Hospital Colorado, University of Colorado at Denver,
School of Medicine, Aurora, CO, USA
e-mail: mitchell.max@childrenscolorado.org

E.M. da Cruz
The Heart Institute, Department of Pediatrics, Children's
Hospital Colorado, University of Colorado School of
Medicine, Aurora, CO, USA
e-mail: eduardo.dacruz@childrenscolorado.org;
orgdacruz.eduardo@tchden.org

E.M. da Cruz et al. (eds.), *Pediatric and Congenital Cardiology, Cardiac Surgery and Intensive Care*,
DOI 10.1007/978-1-4471-4619-3_25, © Springer-Verlag London 2014

Keywords

Brom's repair • Chromosome 7 deletion • Coronary ischemia • Doty patch aortoplasty • Elastin arteriopathy • Familial elastin arteriopathy • Hypertrophic cardiomyopathy • Sporadic elastin arteriopathy • Supravalvar aortic stenosis • McGoon's single-sinus patch aortoplasty • Williams-Beuren syndrome

Historical Background

Supravalvar aortic stenosis (SVAS) first came to significant attention when Williams described four patients with this unusual form of left ventricular outflow tract obstruction in association with mild mental retardation and distinctive elf-like facial appearance [1]. Shortly thereafter Beuren reported similar patients with obstructive pulmonary arterial lesions with and without SVAS [2]. Subsequently, this condition was termed Williams-Beuren syndrome [3]. The heritable nature of this syndrome suggested a genetic basis for this form of congenital cardiovascular disease that was subsequently linked to a deletion on chromosome 7 resulting in abnormal elastin production. Interestingly, SVAS and other obstructive cardiovascular lesions associated with Williams-Beuren syndrome also occur in nonsyndromic patients who are otherwise normal. Nonsyndromic patients share the underlying defect in the elastin precursor gene, but adjacent genes responsible for the other features common to Williams-Beuren syndrome are not affected. Surgical correction for SVAS was first accomplished in the late 1950s, shortly after the development of cardiopulmonary bypass. Since that time, numerous SVAS repairs have been reported. The first reported repair was McGoon's single-sinus patch aortoplasty [4]. In 1977, the Doty 2-sinus inverted bifurcated patch aortoplasty technique was described [5]. In 1988, Brom reported the first 3-sinus repair [6]. In 1993, Myers and Chard separately introduced similar all-autologous 3-sinus repairs [7, 8]. Over the past decade, there has been a resurgence of interest in surgery for SVAS as evidenced by numerous recent publications.

Introduction

SVAS is the least common form of left ventricular outflow tract obstruction (LVOTO). It is caused by an elastin arteriopathy and occurs in three defined populations: Williams-Beuren syndrome, familial elastin arteriopathy, and "sporadic" elastin arteriopathy [9]. All three populations have a microdeletion involving the elastin precursor gene on chromosome 7 (7q11.23) [10, 11]. In patients with Williams-Beuren syndrome, the elastin gene is deleted or disrupted together with a number of neighboring genes that probably are important for the other features of the syndrome (elfin face, mild mental retardation, hypercalcemia), whereas in patients with familial, non-Williams SVAS, the elastin gene only is subjected to a loss-of-function translocation or point mutation. Patients with "sporadic" SVAS are members of a family either carrying an elastin gene mutation with a subclinical phenotype or carrying the elastin gene defect as a new mutation. Defective elastin production leads to obstructive lesions in the large elastin-containing arteries. Other sites of arterial obstruction that occur with elastin arteriopathy include the pulmonary arteries, aortic arch branches, the abdominal aorta, and the renal arteries. The patterns and severity of arterial disease are highly variable; consequently, SVAS occurs across a large clinical spectrum.

Anatomy

Clinical reports divide SVAS into two categories based on the degree of involvement of the ascending aorta: "discrete" disease and "diffuse"

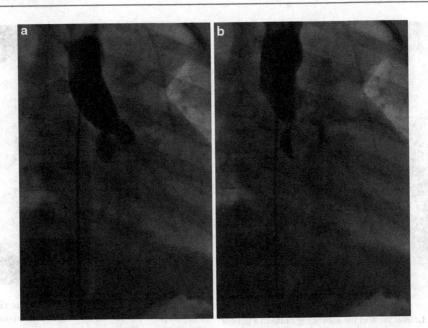

Fig. 92.1 Discrete supravalvar aortic stenosis visualized during diastole at angiography in a patient with severe stenosis (**a**). Same patient depicted during systole (**b**). The degree of stenosis is more apparent during systole. In this case, a tri-leaflet aortic valve with markedly thickened leaflets was noted at surgery. Excursion of the thickened leaflets was limited by the supravalvar ring, and both valvar and aortic wall components contributed to stenosis. This is apparent from the filling defect at the supravalvar level visualized during systole compared to the narrowing present during diastole

disease [12–19]. Discrete SVAS is characterized by a localized ringlike thickening at the sinotubular junction that results in an hourglass-shaped aortic root (Fig. 92.1a, b). Discrete disease occurs in approximately 75 % of patients in surgical series. Diffuse disease is characterized by tubular hypoplasia and thickening of the entire ascending aorta (Fig. 92.2). In more severe cases, aortic thickening and luminal hypoplasia extend through the aortic arch and can even extend past the iliac bifurcation. Diffuse disease complicates the management of SVAS, and this is the most common problematic feature encountered in patients with SVAS. However, even in the discrete form, SVAS is often deceptively complex. In addition to anatomic distortion at the sinotubular junction, concomitant primary and secondary lesions of the left ventricular outflow tract are common to both the discrete and diffuse forms of SVAS. These features include membranous subaortic and/or muscular subaortic obstruction, bicuspid aortic valve, and dysplastic thickening of tri-leaflet aortic valve [9, 14, 20].

Valvar aortic stenosis and/or insufficiency can occur with bicuspid valves and may also occur with tri-leaflet valves that have significant dysplastic changes. Other significant associated anatomic anomalies include concomitant coronary artery obstruction and/or severe right heart outflow tract obstruction. Thistlethwaite et al. classified coronary artery obstructions associated with SVAS into three morphologic types. *Type I obstruction* is characterized by medial thickening of the aorta and proximal coronary artery that results in circumferential ostial stenosis confined to the origin of the coronary artery. This is the most common form of coronary obstruction associated with SVAS. *Type II obstruction* occurs with partial fusion of the aortic valve cusp to the thickened ridge at the sinotubular junction above the level of the coronary artery ostium. Rarely, fusion of the valve cusp to the aortic wall can totally isolate the sinus and coronary ostium from the aortic lumen [21]. *Type III obstruction* is characterized by diffuse long-segment narrowing of the proximal coronary artery. All three types of

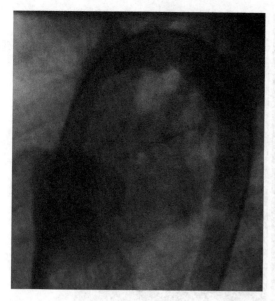

Fig. 92.2 Lateral view of the ascending aorta in a patient with diffuse supravalvar aortic stenosis involving the entire ascending aorta

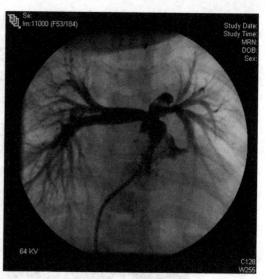

Fig. 92.3 Supravalvar pulmonary stenosis visualized at angiography in an infant with concomitant diffuse supravalvar aortic stenosis

coronary artery obstruction most frequently involve the left system [22]. In these patients, accelerated atherosclerotic lesions of the coronary arteries may also occur even during childhood.

Physiology and Pathophysiology

Myocardial perfusion is uniquely and adversely affected by SVAS compared to other forms of LVOTO. Unlike other forms of LVOTO, obstruction with SVAS occurs distal to the origin of the coronary ostia. Consequently, perfusion during systole occurs at significantly higher pressure which may in part explain the significant incidence of associated obstructive coronary lesions. In addition, obstruction at the sinotubular junction can limit myocardial perfusion during diastole. Severe left ventricular hypertrophy commonly accompanies SVAS in patients coming to surgical correction. Myocardial oxygen supply and demand is delicately balanced, and these patients are notoriously susceptible to severe hemodynamic instability and cardiovascular collapse that is difficult to recover. In patients

with coronary artery involvement, coronary obstruction also contributes to myocardial ischemic damage, and the balance of myocardial oxygen supply and demand is even more precarious. It is therefore of paramount importance to avoid sudden decreases in systemic vascular resistances, particularly when administering anesthetic drugs or any drug with vasodilator effects (see "Medical Management").

Concomitant right heart obstruction occurs in 10–30 % of cases [12, 13, 18, 23]. Right-sided obstruction may occur at the infundibulum, main pulmonary artery, branch pulmonary arteries, or any combination of these levels. Patients with severe biventricular pressure overload develop biventricular hypertrophy and are at significantly increased risk for myocardial ischemia and sudden cardiac arrest [13, 14, 19, 23, 24].

A rare and underappreciated group of patients with elastin arteriopathy present with supravalvar pulmonary stenosis (SVPS) characterized by a ringlike obstruction at the sinotubular junction of the pulmonary valve (Fig. 92.3). This entity closely mirrors the pathology seen with SVAS. Patients with SVPS have severe right heart pressure overload and marked right ventricular hypertrophy. In the author's experience, patients with

SVPS present primarily in infancy, and SVPS may present with or without SVAS. Patients with combined SVAS and SVPS almost always have the diffuse form of SVAS. Significant hypoplasia of the proximal branch pulmonary arteries is commonly present in this subgroup. Biventricular obstruction results in the development of severe biventricular hypertrophy. Myocardial oxygen supply and demand in these patients is balanced poorly, and these patients are among the most susceptible to cardiac arrest. Coronary artery obstruction may also occur in patients with combined SVPS and SVAS. Given the young age at presentation and complexity of pathology, patients with combined SVAS and SVPS are at very high risk for adverse events.

Diagnosis

Clinical Presentation

Patients with Williams-Beuren syndrome exhibit a characteristic elf-like facial appearance, a lack of social inhibition, and varying degrees of intellectual impairment. Although readily recognized during infancy, the distinctive facial appearance may be easily missed at birth. Other stigmata of this entity may be a prominent forehead, long philtrum, enamel hypoplasia, hyperacusia, and unusual affinity for music. Nonsyndromic patients have a normal appearance and intelligence. Patients with SVAS are usually asymptomatic. Dyspnea, syncope and angina, or signs of significant congestive heart failure may occur but are uncommon. Aside from the characteristic appearance seen with Williams-Beuren syndrome, typical physical findings include a laterally displaced apical heartbeat, suprasternal and carotid thrills, and systemic hypertension. Systolic hypertension is frequent and may be more pronounced in the right arm; the latter may be related to the Coanda effect or may result from stenosis of the origin of the contralateral subclavian artery. At auscultation a loud systolic ejection murmur with radiation into the neck is heard. In the presence of associated right-sided obstruction or peripheral

pulmonary stenosis, diffuse systolic murmurs of varied degrees may be identified.

Electrocardiogram

The electrocardiogram (ECG) demonstrates voltage criteria for left ventricular hypertrophy. In the case of biventricular obstruction, right ventricular hypertrophy is evident and right axis deviation is present. T-wave changes occur as a late finding.

Chest X-Ray

Chest x-ray typically demonstrates normal lung fields and mild to moderate cardiomegaly.

Echocardiography

Echocardiogram is the primary diagnostic modality used to evaluate SVAS, and it often suffices to provide the information required to plan surgery. It allows the documentation of the detailed anatomy of the left- and right-sided obstructions and their impact on the systolic and diastolic function of both ventricles. Echocardiography also evaluates coronary anatomy and rules out potential associated anomalies. Parasternal and apical long-axis views best display the supra-aortic narrowing, while the suprasternal view best shows the diffuse hypoplasia of the ascending aorta and the aortic arch. The morphology of the aortic valve and the gradient across the obstruction should be investigated. Similarly, the left and right ventricular pressures should be evaluated.

Echocardiography is the primary modality used for long-term assessment of patients with SVAS. In following these patients, it is important to understand the limitations of Doppler-derived gradient estimates. The Bernoulli equation is relatively accurate for focal narrowing but is less useful when following longer-segment narrowing of a vessel. In the latter case, Bernoulli-derived calculations significantly overestimate the degree of obstruction. This limitation is important in following patients with diffuse disease and infants in particular. Persistent gradients are more common in these patients, and it is necessary to follow changes over time as well as other indicators such as myocardial mass and estimates of pulmonary artery pressure.

Cardiac Catheterization

Preoperative cardiac catheterization to define arch branch vessel involvement, coronary artery obstruction, and branch pulmonary artery anatomy may be helpful in selected cases. Nevertheless, the benefit of this complementary study ought to be counterbalanced with the risks associated with invasiveness, toxicity of contrast products, and the need for anesthesia and its significant risks in this population. This author's bias is to utilize cardiac catheterization with ECMO standby. Angiography provides superior coronary artery imaging, particularly in small children, and the emergency institution of ECMO is more practical in the catheterization suite compared to the environments associated with other forms of imaging.

Cardiac MRI and CT Scan

MR and CT angiography provide good anatomic detail in elastin arteriopathy. However, patients with SVAS are at increased risk of sudden death with any drop in coronary perfusion pressure [9, 13, 16, 18, 23, 25, 26]. As for cardiac catheterization, risks related to anesthesia or sedation are not negligible. If so required, anesthesia should be performed by cardiovascular anesthesiologists and in a setting where rapid cardiovascular resuscitation can be effectively accomplished.

Decision-Making

The goal of surgery for SVAS is to relieve obstruction and prevent secondary degeneration of the aortic valve. These indications do not differ on the basis of age. Surgery is recommended for persistent peak LVOT gradients greater than 50 mmHg [16]. Aortic valve insufficiency, coronary artery involvement, and concomitant severe right heart obstructive disease may indicate surgery at lesser gradients [14, 15, 18, 23]. Ideally, intervention should be undertaken prior to the development of severe ventricular hypertrophy and secondary lesions of the aortic valve leaflets and coronary ostia. Surgical correction of pulmonary artery involvement may be more difficult to achieve than relief of left heart obstruction, particularly with regard to peripheral pulmonic stenosis, and residual right heart pressure overload is common. In the presence of concomitant pulmonary artery disease, obstructive lesions proximal to the lobar branch level should be addressed at the time of SVAS repair. In unusual circumstances, severe right heart obstruction occurs with only mild or moderate SVAS. In this circumstance, surgical intervention for the right heart obstruction is indicated, and addressing even mild or moderate SVAS is advisable in order to improve perioperative myocardial oxygen balance and reduce the likelihood of subsequent need to address SVAS.

Indications for surgical intervention of elastin arteriopathy-associated pulmonary artery obstruction are not well established. Spontaneous regression of mild to moderate pulmonary artery obstruction is likely [21]. However, spontaneous regression of severe pulmonary artery obstruction is not well documented, and these patients are more likely to require surgical intervention [23]. There is no evidence that supravalvar pulmonary stenosis improves spontaneously. Patients who come to surgery for SVAS should undergo repair of correctible central pulmonary artery stenosis at the time of SVAS repair. Balloon dilation of lobar-level pulmonary artery lesions is advisable for patients who require operation for SVAS [9]. Patients with supravalvar pulmonary stenosis and correctable central pulmonary artery lesions should undergo correction when significant right ventricular hypertrophy develops. The decision to intervene on patients with the most severe forms of pulmonary artery obstruction must be individualized. Patients with severely hypoplastic pulmonary arteries may exhibit diffuse narrowing extending into the lobar branches, and beyond this is not amenable to surgical correction.

Medical Management

Because SVAS is a fixed anatomic obstruction, medical management primarily consists of careful serial monitoring for progression of severity. Surgical correction is the only effective treatment, and there is no role for interventional catheterization in the management of SVAS. In some cases, discrete pulmonary artery stenosis of one or both branch pulmonary arteries may respond to balloon angioplasty. However, if SVAS repair is indicated, surgical patch angioplasty of the central pulmonary arteries is advised, and balloon angioplasty with or without stent placement is typically reserved for intraparenchymal lesions that are not readily approachable at operation. Because the myocardium in patients with SVAS is particularly at risk of ischemia, blood pressure control with afterload-reducing agents should be avoided.

Any intervention requiring anesthesia in patients with SVAS ought to be carefully evaluated. Patients with Williams-Beuren syndrome and nonsyndromic SVAS should be regarded as at high risk during anesthesia, especially if there is bilateral outflow tract obstruction or evidence of myocardial ischemia [27]. There is insufficient data in the literature to support a specific anesthetic technique for congenital SVAS. The goal of anesthetic management is meticulous attention to myocardial oxygen supply and demand, and it is also important to keep in perspective right ventricular oxygen balance in patients with associated pulmonary artery stenosis [28, 29]. The hemodynamic goals for SVAS during anesthesia are to:

1. Maintain normal heart rate: avoiding tachycardia to optimize filling time for the hypertrophic ventricles.
2. Maintain sinus rhythm: for the above reason, atrioventricular synchrony is capital.
3. Maintain adequate preload: excessive preload in the context of decreased ventricular compliance may lead to significant elevations in left ventricular end-diastolic pressure and left atrial pressure with consequent pulmonary edema, whereas inadequate preload may lead to a marked decrease in stroke volume and low cardiac output.
4. Maintain ventricular contractility: ventricular function can vary from hyperdynamic to severely depressed.
5. Maintain left ventricular afterload.

Diastolic hypotension in these patients may decrease coronary perfusion pressure. In contrast to valvar aortic stenosis, the presence of an obstructive lesion above the coronary ostia aggravates the adverse effect of hypotension. For patients with pulmonary artery stenosis, the hemodynamic goals are the same, except that a decrease in pulmonary vascular resistance is desirable in maintaining right ventricular output. Control of ventilation to avoid hypoxia, hypercarbia, and acidosis and to maintain adequate lung volume may be advantageous in the more fragile patient with pulmonary artery stenoses. Also, some patients may benefit from the use of selective pulmonary vasodilators like nitric oxide.

Surgical Management

Surgical procedures to treat SVAS have evolved from early simple operations to more recent complicated reconstructions of the aortic root (Video 1). The simplest repair of SVAS is *McGoon's single-sinus patch aortoplasty* (Fig. 92.4). A longitudinal incision oriented at the midpoint of the noncoronary sinus is extended proximally just above the aortic valve annulus and distally above the sinotubular junction. A diamond-shaped patch is then inserted to relieve the area of stenosis.

The most common repair is the two-sinus *Doty patch aortoplasty* (Fig. 92.5). A longitudinal incision is made in the ascending aorta directly above the right-left aortic valve commissure. This incision is then bifurcated proximally into the noncoronary and right coronary sinuses. The incision in the right coronary sinus is directed to the left of the right coronary ostium. The resulting defect is then reconstructed using a dumbbell-shaped patch.

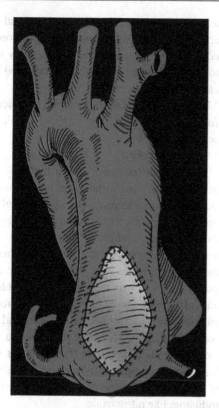

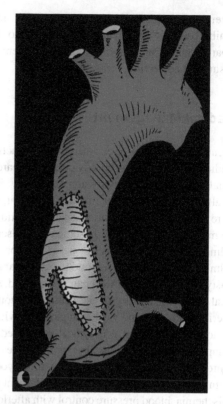

Fig. 92.4 McGoon's single-sinus patch aortoplasty for supravalvar aortic stenosis. Relief of supravalvar aortic stenosis is achieved with a diamond-shaped patch inserted into the noncoronary sinus

Fig. 92.5 Doty inverted bifurcated two-sinus patch aortoplasty. Relief of supravalvar aortic stenosis is achieved with dumbbell-shaped patch enlarging the right and noncoronary sinuses

Brom's repair is the most commonly employed three-sinus technique (Fig. 92.6). The ascending aorta is transected just above the point of maximal narrowing. Incisions are made into each of the three sinuses. The incision in the left sinus is directed to the right of the coronary ostium, and the incision in the right sinus is directed to the left of the coronary ostium. Separate shield-shaped patches are used to enlarge each sinus, thereby symmetrically enlarging the sinotubular junction. It is often necessary to enlarge the distal aorta which is most easily accomplished with a single anteriorly placed triangular patch. The aorta is then re-approximated. The Myers approach is an all-autologous three-sinus repair. The author refers to this procedure as the autologous slide aortoplasty (Fig. 92.7a, b) [18].

Acceptable results have been achieved with all of these techniques; however, three-sinus repairs have gained increasing acceptance due to more

recent appreciation of the functional anatomy of the aortic root [12–14, 17–20]. Single- and two-sinus repairs result in persistent geometric distortion of the aortic root, and secondary effects on the leaflets may theoretically compromise long-term aortic valve function. There are two putative advantages to reconstructing all three sinuses [12, 13, 17–19]. First, the right and left coronary sinuses are enlarged which should improve coronary perfusion to both coronary systems. Second, restoring normal aortic root anatomy should minimize secondary aortic leaflet injury and improve long-term durability of the aortic valve [20]. Whether or not three-sinus repairs actually achieve these objectives has not been established. Nevertheless, the recent literature is strongly biased toward three-sinus repairs, and the Brom technique in particular has gained considerable popularity.

Techniques employing inert patch augmentation carry potential disadvantages that may be of

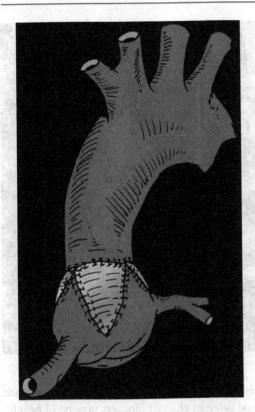

Fig. 92.6 Brom's repair of supravalvar aortic stenosis. The aorta transected and each sinus is enlarged with a shield-shaped patch followed by re-approximation of the aorta

particular concern in small children. Distortion with somatic growth could lead to recurrent stenosis or aortic insufficiency as a result of asymmetric valve geometry. Theoretically, all-autologous techniques may avoid these issues and provide important growth potential in smaller children. When the author's center recognized that a significant number of our patients with SVAS were presenting for repair early in childhood, the Myers slide aortoplasty technique was adopted [18]. This shift occurred in the late 1990s, and other centers appear to have had a similar interest in this procedure [13, 14, 18]. The results were satisfactory, but this technique is no longer favored. Slide aortoplasty is technically challenging in smaller children, and it has been necessary to add additional patch materials in 25–50 % of attempted cases obviating the potential advantage [9, 13, 14, 18]. In the authors' experience, additional patch augmentation was

necessary only in very young patients, while older patients, in whom avoidance of inert patch material was of less theoretic benefit, were well suited for slide aortoplasty. These authors' group and others concluded that all-autologous techniques are best suited for patients with discrete disease [7, 18, 30]. Because younger patients more frequently exhibit diffuse disease, the slide aortoplasty technique is not advisable in infants, and there is little advantage to this procedure in older patients in whom growth potential is of less concern. Thus, these authors currently favor the Brom technique at all ages [31, 32].

The Brom technique is particularly useful in infants and smaller patients. In addition to the theoretical benefits of thee-sinus reconstruction, transection of the aorta greatly improves exposure that is maintained throughout reconstruction of the proximal root. This exposure permits easier examination of the aortic valve leaflets compared to the Doty and McGoon techniques facilitating leaflet thinning and valvuloplasty techniques when required. The distance between the aortic valve commissures and coronary ostia is often minute in young infants, particularly on the left. Transecting the aorta aids in precise placement of the incisions in the right and left sinuses. In contrast, sliding the distal aorta into these incisions with the all-autologous techniques can be very challenging because exposure of the right coronary artery origin and nearby leaflet becomes progressively limited. When diffuse disease involves the transverse arch or beyond, the entire arch must be augmented. The Brom technique is readily adapted to these cases. For the most severe cases in which the descending aorta is also involved, the best that can be achieved is to decompress the ascending aorta into the arch branches by augmenting the arch to a level beyond the left subclavian artery.

Postoperative Management

The management of patients undergoing correction of SVAS is similar to other aortic root procedures. Following most aortic root operations, blood pressure is carefully limited to avoid

Fig. 92.7 (a, b) Myers slide aortoplasty repair of supravalvar aortic stenosis. The aorta is transected. Incisions are made into each sinus. Counter-incisions are made in the distal ascending aorta above each commissure. The aorta is then re-approximated with autologous flaps of the ascending aorta functioning to enlarge the area stenosis

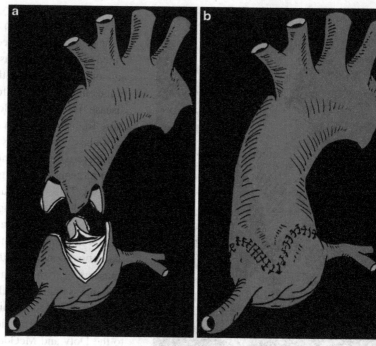

bleeding from fresh aortic suture lines. However, any degree of hypotension poses significant risk early following SVAS repair and should be avoided. Early after repair of SVAS, the myocardium in these patients remains vulnerable to ischemia, and significant ischemia can occur at perfusion pressures that would be considered optimal for most other postoperative patients. Several factors explain this observation. Undetected or untreatable obstructive lesions in the coronary arteries may be present. The coronary arteries in patients with diffuse SVAS are commonly quite small compared to patients of similar size with other lesions. Because severe ventricular hypertrophy is common, the foregoing factors are a setup for inadequate coronary perfusion during the early postoperative phase. Lastly, patients with Williams-Beuren syndrome are also prone to perturbations in calcium metabolism, and these patients may be more susceptible to coronary spasm. For these reasons, cardiac output and adequate perfusion pressures should be carefully maintained. Intravenous nitroglycerine is commonly, but cautiously, used to promote coronary perfusion. Sedative and afterload-reducing agents may be required but must be

used with appropriate caution. Beta blockade and calcium channel blockers may be of benefit, but there is no data to guide therapeutic recommendations for these agents. The ECG should be carefully monitored for signs of ischemia. Ventricular ectopy may be an early warning of ischemia, and its presence should prompt efforts to optimize myocardial blood supply.

The above premises design the frame for the postoperative course.

Standard monitoring is based on continuous ECG, invasive arterial and central venous pressure, and oxygen saturation. Some patients may return from the operating room with a left atrial catheter as well. Very importantly, markers of tissue perfusion require close follow-up; these include serial lactate levels, intermittent or continuous monitoring of mixed venous saturation, and near-infrared spectroscopy (NIRS). Patients are maintained free of pain and sedated with opioids titrated to minimal efficient dose associated with benzodiazepines. A word of caution is necessary though regarding the latter, as these agents may induce significant hypotension. In the authors' experience, dexmedetomidine offers an attractive alternative, if titrated to minimal necessary doses and avoiding the use of boluses. This drug is all the more interesting that it may help blunt the stress response in these patients. Some patients with Williams-Beuren syndrome may be challenging to sedate. Ketamine infusion combined with low-dose benzodiazepines proves useful in achieving adequate sedation while preserving systemic vascular resistance. Minimal intervention and establishment of a "normal" day-and-night biological cycle, including sleep induction as required, are capital principles.

Inotropic and lusitropic drugs are consistently used and usually combine milrinone and low-dose dopamine or epinephrine. Significant myocardial dysfunction may occur (see below). As much as the benefit of these drugs has been extensively studied, caregivers must be aware of the impact on myocardial oxygen consumption and must remain attentive to induction of tachycardia that may poorly impact the diastolic filling of severely hypertrophic ventricles. Some patients require the use of vasopressin, phenylephrine, or other α-agonists in order to maintain systemic vascular resistances high enough to adequately perfuse coronary arteries. Significant hypertension may also occur though, exposing the patients to the risks of bleeding. In such scenarios, infusion of selective systemic vasodilators like sodium nitroprusside or nicardipine may be useful.

Prevention of arrhythmias (i.e., compensation of electrolytic disturbances, administration of magnesium sulfate, and avoidance of triggering factors) and aggressive management of de novo rhythm anomalies are of paramount importance. The same applies to atrioventricular and interventricular synchrony that may be ensured by the use of external pacemakers. Most patients return from the operating room with atrial and ventricular pacing wires, which facilitates the task. Atrial pacing wires may also be useful in clarifying the etiology and type of arrhythmia, which proves very useful when designing a goal-oriented therapy.

De novo ventricular arrhythmias or evidence of ischemic changes in the ECG justify prompt investigation focused on the coronary anatomy, including an echocardiography and eventually cardiac catheterization and/or surgical exploration.

Mechanical ventilation ought to take into account cardiopulmonary interactions for both left- and right-sided heart. The usual trend is to extubate these patients as soon as deemed safe, usually during the first 24 h and once hemodynamic stability and bleeding are under control. Patients with significant right heart dysfunction may benefit from strategies that reduce right afterload, both ventilatory and pharmacological. Details about these principles may be found in a specific chapter dedicated to cardiopulmonary interactions elsewhere in this book.

Intravenous and oral diuretics are administered based on the overall hemodynamic conditions and fluid balance. Caregivers should be careful with aspects discussed above with regard to the need for adequate preload in the presence of significantly hypertrophic ventricles, with diastolic dysfunction and poor compliance.

Last but not least, proactive nutritional support and mobilization make a difference in the acute and midterm convalescence of these patients.

Complications

Patients with SVAS are more susceptible to postoperative bleeding than many other patients due to the need to maintain higher blood pressure. Significant myocardial dysfunction may occur due to several reasons. Inadequate decompression of LVOTO may occur, particularly in cases with the diffuse form of the disease. Coronary compromise may occur due to missed lesions or technical difficulties in relieving coronary lesions, particularly in infants. Advanced ventricular and/or biventricular hypertrophy may compromise adequate myocardial preservation. In addition, residual distal pulmonary artery obstruction may limit the efficacy of right heart decompression compromising postoperative right ventricular function. Because the aortic valve is commonly abnormal, relief of SVAS may be accompanied by new onset of aortic insufficiency. In addition, oversizing of corrective patches can lead to central insufficiency due to splaying of the aortic valve leaflets.

Patients who progress toward refractory low cardiac output or inadequate tissue perfusion are candidates for extracorporeal life support strategies.

Controversies

For many years it has been thought that SVAS tends to worsen with time, eventually requiring surgical intervention in most patients, while pulmonary lesions tend to improve over time and commonly will not require treatment. Recently, Hickey and colleagues have questioned this thinking [16]. In a large number of patients followed to a mean of 8 years from the time of SVAS diagnosis, these authors found that many patients with mild to moderate SVAS, particularly those with Williams syndrome, improved with time and never required surgical intervention. Conversely, there is more evidence for spontaneous regression of elastin arteriopathy-related pulmonary artery obstructions. It is important to recognize that the series that have reported the tendency for spontaneous regression of pulmonary artery obstruction are dominated by patients with mild to moderate disease. There is little if any evidence supporting spontaneous regression of severe pulmonary artery obstruction in patients with elastin arteriopathy. This is particularly true for patients with supravalvar pulmonary stenosis. Consequently, pursuing a nonoperative approach for patients with severe right heart pressure overload should be reserved only for patients with noncorrectible diffuse pulmonary artery hypoplasia.

The most controversial topic related to SVAS is the most appropriate surgical procedure. In the past decade, there is a clear surgical bias favoring 3-sinus techniques. However, this bias is based almost entirely on theoretical grounds. In fact, the largest surgical series in the literature reported excellent results with extended single-sinus repairs [15]. Another very recent series from the University of Michigan also reported excellent outcomes with the extended single-sinus repair [33]. Only a large multicenter outcome study is likely to provide a definitive answer as to the ideal surgical approach for the correction of SVAS.

Outcomes and Long-Term Follow-up

The results of repair of SVAS are generally quite good with excellent short-term and good long-term survivals. Although there is disagreement in the literature, there is reasonable short- and long-term data favoring multi-sinus repairs (i.e., two- and three-sinus repairs considered collectively) over the classic McGoon technique [13, 15, 17, 19]. However, there is no data that definitively demonstrates the superiority of three-sinus repairs over the Doty two-sinus repair.

Risk factors predicting the need for reintervention include diffuse disease, bicuspid aortic valve, and subaortic stenosis [13, 14, 18, 19]. Because diffuse disease and other complex coexisting lesions are more common in infants, the results in this subset of patients are significantly worse. Stamm and colleagues from the Children's Hospital Boston group published one of the largest series of surgical patients with congenital SVAS [13]. In this series, diffuse disease was a clear risk factor for surgical mortality. In addition, diffuse disease was the only variable that independently predicted decreased long-term survival. Diffuse disease was also associated with a higher risk of subsequent reoperation. This study did not correlate younger age at surgical presentation with a higher prevalence of diffuse disease, but the methods reported do not indicate that age was considered in their analysis. At Children's Hospital Colorado, patients with diffuse disease tend to present for SVAS repair at smaller size and younger age compared to patients with discrete disease [18]. In our report, six of eight patients operated at weight <10 kg had diffuse disease, while 16 of 17 patients ≥10 kg had localized disease. Only one patient with diffuse disease underwent SVAS at age greater than 2 years, and most patients were infants at the time of repair. Eronen et al. also reported that a significant majority of infants undergoing surgery for SVAS had diffuse disease (60 %) [34]. Given that nearly all reports demonstrate that patients with diffuse disease comprise between 20 % and 30 % of patients undergoing SVAS repair, this report and our findings suggest that patients who present at young age are more likely to have diffuse disease and are therefore more likely to have less optimal long-term outcomes.

There are few data reporting on the outcomes of patients with biventricular obstruction. Patients with severe right heart obstruction and moderate to severe SVAS are at significantly higher risk of early death compared to patients with SVAS alone [9, 21, 23]. In the Children's Hospital Boston report, there were seven early deaths in 75 patients undergoing repair of SVAS (9 %) [13]. These investigators subsequently reported that six of these early deaths occurred in the subgroup of 33 patients with SVAS who also had right heart obstruction (18 %) [23]. Although the earlier report from Boston did not identify right heart obstruction as a risk factor for early death following SVAS repair, the fact that six of the seven early deaths in their reports had biventricular obstruction strongly suggests that these patients are at higher risk. Not surprisingly, patients with more generalized obstructive pulmonary vascular disease were more likely to have the diffuse form of SVAS. Importantly, these authors noted that patients with severe right heart obstructive lesions were referred for surgery at significantly younger age compared to patients with SVAS alone and that the severity of right heart obstruction had a strong inverse correlation with age at primary assessment. Patients with significant biventricular obstruction have precarious myocardial perfusion. Consequently, these patients are at significantly increased risk of hemodynamic collapse during the induction of anesthesia. In two literature reviews of congenital SVAS and sudden death associated with anesthesia, biventricular obstruction was present in approximately 30 % of reported cases. Notably, 60 % were infants and 80 % were age 2 years or less [25, 26].

Significant obstructive coronary artery lesions occur in 5–10 % of patients with SVAS. Intuitively, associated coronary artery involvement increases the risk of surgery in patients with SVAS. However, no report has demonstrated that coronary artery disease increases operative risk. This is most likely due to the fact that single-center series have too few patients to definitively demonstrate the impact of coronary lesions in these patients. Individual case descriptions from recent surgical series do suggest that infants with coronary disease distal to the ostia are at higher risk of death [17]. The technical challenges of coronary artery reconstruction are made more difficult by the small coronary artery lumen and aortic root sizes in infants compared to older patients. Several case reports describe left main coronary artery arterioplasty performed at the time of SVAS repair, but these reports primarily involve cases in older children and teenagers [35, 36].

Repair of coronary obstructions is feasible even in young infants. Thistlethwaite et al. reported superb results in nine patients who underwent concomitant procedures for SVAS and coronary artery obstruction [22]. Importantly, five of nine patients in Thistlethwaite's series were 2 years of age or younger at the time of surgical presentation, and three of the five patients with type I lesions (ostial obstruction) were infants. Although rare, right coronary obstruction also occurs. Concomitant coronary disease logically increases the risk of surgery for SVAS, particularly in infants. Furthermore, coronary artery involvement is strongly correlated with increased risk of sudden death occurring with anesthesia, and a large proportion of reported cases involve infants and children under the age of 2 years [25, 26].

Future Developments

The management of SVAS is well established and overall outcomes are reasonably good. Patients with severe diffuse disease have the poorest outcomes both early following surgery and in long-term follow-up. Unfortunately, better strategies to improve outcome in these patients seem limited by the nature of the disease in these patients. Because elastin arteriopathy is linked to an autosomal dominant microdeletion on chromosome 7 (7q11.23), genetic counseling should be advised for all patients diagnosed with SVAS. Therapies directed at treating or correcting the underlying elastin deficiency are conceivable, but there are no such clinical applications currently available.

References

1. Williams JCP, Barratt-Boyes BG, Lowe JB (1961) Supravalvular aortic stenosis. Circulation 24:1311–1318
2. Beuren AJ, Apitz J, Harmjanz D (1962) Supravalvular aortic stenosis in association with mental retardation and a certain facial appearance. Circulation 26:1235–1240
3. Beuren AJ, Schulze C, Eberle P et al (1964) The syndrome of supravalvular aortic stenosis, peripheral pulmonary stenosis, mental retardation and similar facial appearance. Am J Cardiol 13:471–483
4. McGoon DC, Mankin HT, Vlad P et al (1961) The surgical treatment of supravalvular aortic stenosis. J Thorac Cardiovasc Surg 41:125–133
5. Doty DB, Polansky DB, Jenson CB (1977) Supravalvular aortic stenosis. Repair by extended aortoplasty. J Thorac Cardiovasc Surg 74:362–371
6. Brom GG (1988) Obstruction of the left ventricular outflow tract. In: Khonsari S (ed) Cardiac surgery: safeguards and pitfalls in operative technique. Lippincott Williams & Wilkins, Rockville
7. Chard RB, Cartmill TB (1993) Localized supravalvar aortic stenosis: a new technique for repair. Ann Thorac Surg 55:782–784
8. Myers JL, Waldhausen JA, Cyran SE et al (1993) Results of surgical repair of congenital supravalvular aortic stenosis. J Thorac Cardiovasc Surg 105:281–287, discussion 287–288
9. Stamm C, Friehs I, Ho SY et al (2001) Congenital supravalvar aortic stenosis: a simple lesion? Eur J Cardiothorac Surg 19:195–202
10. Li DY, Toland AE, Boak BB et al (1997) Elastin point mutations cause an obstructive vascular disease, supravalvular aortic stenosis. Hum Mol Genet 6:1021–1028
11. Meng X, Lu X, Li Z et al (1998) Complete physical map of the common deletion region in Williams syndrome and identification and characterization of three novel genes. Hum Genet 103:590–599
12. Hazekamp MG, Kappetein AP, Schoof PH et al (1999) Brom's three-patch technique for repair of supravalvular aortic stenosis. J Thorac Cardiovasc Surg 118:252–258
13. Stamm C, Kreutzer C, Zurakowski D et al (1999) Forty-one years of surgical experience with congenital supravalvular aortic stenosis. J Thorac Cardiovasc Surg 118:874–885
14. McElhinney DB, Petrossian E, Tworetzky W et al (2000) Issues and outcomes in the management of supravalvar aortic stenosis. Ann Thorac Surg 69:562–567
15. Brown JW, Ruzmetov M, Vijay P et al (2002) Surgical repair of congenital supravalvular aortic stenosis in children. Eur J Cardiothorac Surg 21:50–56
16. Hickey EJ, Jung G, Williams WG et al (2008) Congenital supravalvular aortic stenosis: defining surgical and nonsurgical outcomes. Ann Thorac Surg 86:1919–1927; discussion 1927
17. Metton O, Ben Ali W, Calvaruso D et al (2009) Surgical management of supravalvular aortic stenosis: does Brom three-patch technique provide superior results? Ann Thorac Surg 88:588–593
18. Scott DJ, Campbell DN, Clarke DR et al (2009) Twenty-year surgical experience with congenital supravalvar aortic stenosis. Ann Thorac Surg 87:1501–1507; discussion 1507–1508
19. Kaushal S, Backer CL, Patel S et al (2010) Midterm outcomes in supravalvular aortic stenosis demonstrate the superiority of multisinus aortoplasty. Ann Thorac Surg 89:1371–1377
20. Stamm C, Li J, Ho SY et al (1997) The aortic root in supravalvular aortic stenosis: the potential surgical relevance of morphologic findings. J Thorac Cardiovasc Surg 114:16–24
21. Wren C, Oslizlok P, Bull C (1990) Natural history of supravalvular aortic stenosis and pulmonary artery stenosis. J Am Coll Cardiol 15:1625–1630
22. Thistlethwaite PA, Madani MM, Kriett JM et al (2000) Surgical management of congenital obstruction of the left main coronary artery with supravalvular aortic stenosis. J Thorac Cardiovasc Surg 120:1040–1046
23. Stamm C, Friehs I, Moran AM et al (2000) Surgery for bilateral outflow tract obstruction in elastin arteriopathy. J Thorac Cardiovasc Surg 120:755–763
24. Vaideeswar P, Shankar V, Deshpande JR et al (2001) Pathology of the diffuse variant of supravalvar aortic stenosis. Cardiovasc Pathol 10:33–37
25. Bird LM, Billman GF, Lacro RV et al (1996) Sudden death in Williams syndrome: report of ten cases. J Pediatr 129:926–931
26. Burch TM, McGowan FX Jr, Kussman BD et al (2008) Congenital supravalvular aortic stenosis and sudden death associated with anesthesia: what's the mystery? Anesth Analg 107:1848–1854
27. Gupta P, Tobias JD, Goyal S, Miller MD, Melendez E, Noviski N, De Moor MM, Mehta V (2010) Sudden cardiac death under anesthesia in pediatric patient with Williams syndrome: a case report and review of literature. Ann Card Anaesth 13:44–48
28. Horowitz PE, Akhtar S, Wulff JA, Al Fadley F, Al Halees Z (2002) Coronary artery disease and anesthesia-related death in children with Williams syndrome. J Cardiothorac Vasc Anesth 16:739–741
29. Shanewise JS, Hug JCC (2000) Anesthesia for adult cardiac surgery. In: Miller RD (ed) Anesthesia,

5th edn. Churchill Livingstone, Philadelphia, pp 1753–1804

30. Seo D, Shin H, Park J et al (2007) Modified simple sliding aortoplasty for supravalvar aortic stenosis. Ann Thorac Surg 83:2248–2250

31. Mitchell MB, Goldberg SP (2011) Brom repair for supravalvar aortic stenosis. Oper Tech Thorac Cardiovasc Surg Comp Atlas 16:70–84

32. Mitchell MB, Goldberg SP (2011) Supravalvar aortic stenosis in infancy. Semin Thorac Cardiovasc Surg Pediatr Card Surg Annu 14:85–91

33. Kavarana MN, Riley M, Sood V et al (2012) Extended single-patch repair of supravalvar aortic stenosis: a simple and effective technique. Ann Thorac Surg 93:1274–1279

34. Eronen M, Peippo M, Hiippala A et al (2002) Cardiovascular manifestations in 75 patients with Williams syndrome. J Med Genet 39:554–558

35. Martin MM, Lemmer JH Jr, Shaffer E et al (1988) Obstruction to left coronary artery blood flow secondary to obliteration of the coronary ostium in supravalvular aortic stenosis. Ann Thorac Surg 45:16–20

36. Shin H, Katogi T, Yozu R et al (1999) Surgical angioplasty of left main coronary stenosis complicating supravalvular aortic stenosis. Ann Thorac Surg 67:1147–1148

Coarctation of the Aorta

93

Melissa Lee, Yves d'Udekem, and Christian Brizard

Abstract

The aortic arch is a beautiful structure distributing oxygenated blood to the brain, to the upper and lower limbs, and to all organs as well as being a significant component of the ventriculo-arterial couple. A narrowing of the aortic arch has profound physiological consequences. This chapter explores the condition of coarctation of the aorta, its history, clinical presentation and diagnosis, management, early and late outcomes, and important points to consider for long-term follow-up.

Keywords

Aorta • Aortic arch • Anastomosis • Balloon angiography • Coarctation of the aorta • Discrete coarctation of the aorta • End to end anastomosis • End-to-side anastomosis • Extra-anatomical bypass • Hypertension • Hypoplasia of the aortic arch • Native coarctation of the aorta • Re-obstruction • Tubular hypoplasia

Introduction

Coarctation of the aorta is often regarded as a benign condition. In the current era, improved pre- and postoperative care and refined surgical techniques have seen excellent short-term outcomes after early surgical repair of aortic coarctation. Because of these excellent early results, many consider this surgical repair as a "cure." However, it is clear that many of these patients will go on to develop hypertension early in life, the consequences of which can be devastating. Furthermore, there is still debate regarding the optimal surgical repair technique for aortic coarctation, of which there are many, thoracotomy or sternotomy approach, resection, end-to-side anastomosis or, less so, subclavian flap, and what to do when there is associated hypoplasia of the aortic arch. What is clear, however, is that coarctation of the aorta can no longer be regarded as a benign condition and that the quality of the decision-making and the surgical treatment is paramount for the future well-being of the patient.

M. Lee • Y. d'Udekem • C. Brizard (✉)
Cardiac Surgery, The Royal Children's Hospital,
Melbourne, VIC, Australia
e-mail: Christian.Brizard@rch.org.au

E.M. da Cruz et al. (eds.), *Pediatric and Congenital Cardiology, Cardiac Surgery and Intensive Care*,
DOI 10.1007/978-1-4471-4619-3_27, © Springer-Verlag London 2014

Definition

Coarctation of the aorta is a congenital narrowing of the aortic isthmus, between the left subclavian artery (proximally) and the ductus arteriosus (distally). The lumen of the aorta may be atretic in the most severe cases, but the walls of the aorta are still in continuity, as opposed to interrupted aortic arch where there is a lack of continuity between the proximal and distal segments of the aortic arch.

Historical Considerations

The first report of coarctation of the aorta is attributed to Morgagni who described the anomaly from an autopsy in 1760, and Paris was the first to describe the full pathological features almost 30 years later. However, it was not until 1944 that the first coarctation repair was performed by Crafoord and Nylin [1], and the introduction of prostaglandin E_1 (PGE_1) that followed in the mid-1970s dramatically changed the medical management and stabilization of these patients, allowing the repair of coarctation in neonates to become more successful [2].

Prevalence and Genetics

Aortic coarctation occurs in 3–4 per 10,000 live births [3], accounting for 7 % of anomalies in live-born children with congenital heart defects [4], and has a higher occurrence in males [5].

Coarctation of the aorta generally shows multifactorial inheritance, but its inheritance has also been reported as an autosomal dominant trait [6].

Morphology

Aortic coarctation constitutes a spectrum of lesions generally including variable degrees of aortic arch hypoplasia. On one end of the spectrum is a narrowing of the aortic arch so severe it is almost indistinguishable from interrupted aortic arch and arch hypoplasia (Fig. 93.1), and on

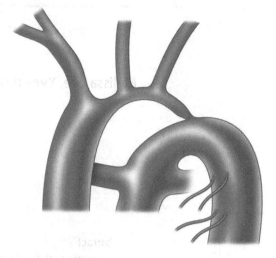

Fig. 93.1 Coarctation with severe aortic arch hypoplasia almost indistinguishable from interrupted aortic arch and arch hypoplasia

the other end of the spectrum there is *discrete coarctation* (Fig. 93.2) where there is a localized shelflike lesion within the aortic arch lumen often with a proximal tapering of the arch towards the obstruction. A uniform tubelike narrowing of part of the aortic arch can also be present (*tubular hypoplasia*).

In many infants with aortic coarctation, a smaller than normal transverse arch – in addition to the localized isthmic stenosis – can be present (Fig. 93.3) [7]. The incidence of this hypoplastic arch of varying severity in patients with coarctation is between 40 % and 80 % [8–11], depending on the definition used.

Furthermore, it is important to define the specific segment of aortic arch in question. The proximal transverse arch is between the brachiocephalic or innominate artery and the left common carotid artery, and the distal transverse arch between the left common carotid artery and the left subclavian artery.

There is no true consensus on the precise definition of aortic arch hypoplasia. Moulaert and associates described an arch as hypoplastic if the diameter of the proximal arch, distal arch, or isthmus was less than 60 %, 50 %, or 40 % of the diameter of the ascending aorta, respectively [12]. This was the most commonly used criterion for aortic arch hypoplasia by studies in the

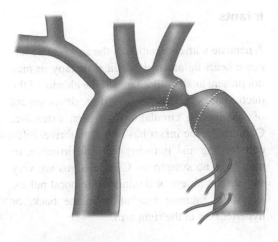

Fig. 93.2 Discrete coarctation

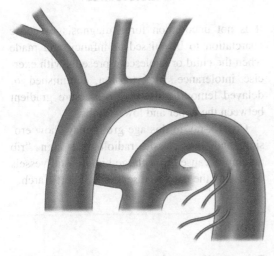

Fig. 93.3 Aortic arch hypoplasia associated with coarctation

literature. However, because the ascending aorta can often be small in addition to the arch itself, such as in aortic atresia and other anomalies, it is difficult to define a hypoplastic arch using solely the ratio of the ascending aorta [13].

A more practical definition by Karl et al. has been used widely and describes the aortic arch as hypoplastic if the cross-sectional diameter of the transverse arch plus 1 mm is less than the patient's weight in kilograms [14]. Although the ease of this definition makes it attractive for everyday use, it does not provide much scientific meaning. Today, most centers examine the proximal and distal arch in terms of z-scores to

diagnose arch hypoplasia [13, 15, 16]. These values represent the number of standard deviations from the expected dimensions obtained from normal populations. Aortic arch z-scores of −2 or lower indicate hypoplasia of the arch, independent of the size of other aortic parts.

Despite existing debate regarding the criteria of hypoplasia, most have acknowledged that aortic coarctation patients with hypoplastic arch represent a challenging group compared to patients with isolated aortic coarctation.

Associated Anomalies

Coarctation of the aorta may coexist with a number of cardiac anomalies. It is most commonly associated with bicuspid aortic valve, occurring in up to 60 % of patients [17]. Up to 20 % of coarctation patients may require aortic valve repair for stenosis [17]. A patent ductus arteriosus may be present in more than one third of neonates with aortic coarctation and is rarely associated with a coarctation beyond the neonatal period [18]. Ventricular septal defect is commonly found with coarctation including in 48 % of the 326 coarctation patients reviewed by the Congenital Heart Surgeons' Society [19]. Not uncommonly, arch hypoplasia is associated with a bovine trunk where a single trunk comprising the innominate artery and left common carotid artery arises from the ascending aorta, and the distal arch is long and hypoplastic. An anomalous right subclavian artery is present in 1 % of aortic coarctation patients, and it was recently identified as a risk factor for late aortic arch re-obstruction [17, 20]. Rarely, coarctation can be found in neonates with tetralogy of Fallot [18].

Less commonly, coarctation with varying degrees of arch hypoplasia can be associated with complex cardiac conditions including Taussig-Bing anomaly, transposition of the great arteries, hypoplastic left heart syndrome, and single ventricle with systemic outflow obstruction such as tricuspid atresia with transposed great arteries. Coarctation of the aorta is present in more than 80 % of patients with hypoplastic left heart syndrome [21].

Clinical Presentation and Diagnosis

The modes of presentation depend heavily on the severity of the aortic coarctation and the prevalence and severity of associated cardiac anomalies.

Neonates

A critical neonatal coarctation occurs when a severe constriction of the aorta results in profound circulatory collapse, and a significant number of these patients present within the first week of life. In utero, flow to the arch vessels is provided by the left ventricle while the right ventricle maintains circulation to the descending aorta and the rest of the body via the ductus arteriosus, and its patency is dependent on high pulmonary resistance and circulating prostaglandin. Following birth, as the neonate begins self-ventilation and the level of prostaglandin plummets, the pulmonary resistance falls and the ductus arteriosus closes. If a severe coarctation is present, the closure of the ductus will impede blood flow to the lower body segment, resulting in diminished or absent femoral pulses and compromised tissue perfusion in the territories perfused by the descending aorta. There may also be a pressure gradient between the upper and lower limbs on blood pressure measurement or Doppler investigation. The neonate is said to have a ductal-dependent systemic circulation. The neonate becomes acutely unwell, with signs and symptoms of heart failure and circulatory collapse including tachypnea, paleness, lethargy, and liver enlargement.

Chest x-ray demonstrates an enlarged heart and congested lung fields.

Analysis of arterial blood gas exposes a worsening and progressive metabolic (lactic) acidosis. Uncorrected metabolic acidosis results in the neonate developing signs of organ failure including shock, renal failure, necrotizing enterocolitis, and seizures and will ultimately lead to death.

Infants

A neonate with coarctation of the aorta may overcome heart failure with medical therapy or may not present at all until infancy if the closure of the ductus has occurred slowly or if the development of a collateral circulation has been extensive. Commonly, the infant has failure to thrive, difficult feeding and is tachypneic and irritable, or may have no symptoms. Clinical signs are very suggestive: absent or diminished femoral pulses, a systolic murmur irradiating in the back, or hypertension in the right arm.

Childhood and Adolescence

It is not uncommon for a diagnosis of aortic coarctation to be missed at infancy and made when the child or adolescent presents with exercise intolerance, hypertension, diminished or delayed femoral pulses, or a pressure gradient between the upper and lower limbs.

Chest x-ray in this age group may show erosion and the classic radiological sign "rib notching" caused by enlarged intercostal vessels bypassing the narrowed segment of aortic arch.

Imaging

Echocardiography

Two-dimensional echocardiography is the diagnostic method of choice in neonates and infants. The aortic arch is best visualized from the suprasternal notch in the superior paracoronal view, a consequence of a thymus that is usually large and envelops the aortic arch. As the thymus involutes after infancy, the transverse arch becomes more enveloped by the lung than thymus, and thus the assessment of severity of coarctation becomes increasingly difficult using this method of imaging.

Doppler ultrasound is useful for the assessment of maximal velocity and thus pressure across the aortic arch and descending aorta and can be used to diagnose first-time or *native* coarctation or re-obstruction. The diastolic runoff distal to the aortic coarctation is a good correlation of the severity of the stenosis. It may be the only visible sign of the coarctation and should trigger further morphologic imaging.

Cardiac Catheterization and Angiography

Although cardiac catheterization provides a very accurate assessment of the coarctation, in the vast majority of cases, a diagnosis of coarctation and management plan can be made from history, examination, and noninvasive investigations. It is of limited value in the delineation of the anatomy and generates no or little additional information. It is also associated with significant morbidity. Hence, it may be more appropriate to proceed to a cardiac catheterization in cases of re-coarctation, when the diagnosis is confirmed at the time of the catheterization aiming proceed to elective interventional therapy.

Computerized Tomography and Magnetic Resonance Imaging

Although transthoracic echocardiography is the diagnostic method of choice in neonates and infants, there may be instances when segments of the aorta cannot be visualized very clearly and the extent of associated anomalies is uncertain. Computerized tomography (CT) or magnetic resonance imaging (MRI) may be required for clarification of the diagnosis, assessment of the severity of disease, detection of associated anomalies, and for clear visualization of three-dimensional anatomy before surgery. MRI provides much better images than echocardiography in the older child and adolescent. It is also an excellent tool for the assessment of collateral development and for assessment of postoperative repair. The calculation of gradient across the aortic coarctation area is very accurate.

Although the assessment of the aortic arch and descending aorta is excellent by MRI, its use is limited in smaller children because of the need for

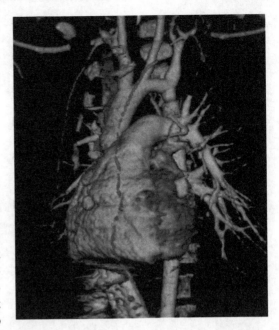

Fig. 93.4 A cardiac CT scan demonstrating coarctation of the aorta

sedation or anesthesia. In addition, MRI cannot be used as a follow-up investigation in those patients with metallic prosthesis such as a pacemaker.

CT is an excellent tool for the assessment of aortic coarctation as there is rarely a need for anesthesia and it offers the highest resolution among noninvasive imaging modalities (Fig. 93.4) [22]. In particular, cardiac CT angiography is excellent at detecting associated anomalies and with the lowest acquisition time among noninvasive imaging modalities [23], but is a contraindication in those patients with allergy to contrast media and also may cause contrast-induced nephropathy.

Medical Therapy

The introduction of PGE_1 has seen the preoperative status of neonates presenting with acute severe arch obstruction dramatically improve. Intravenous administration of PGE_1 maintains patency of the ductus arteriosus, allowing for resuscitation and restoration of organ perfusion in these compromised infants. If the coarctation is diagnosed in utero, then preventive administration of PGE$_1$ at low dose will avoid closure of the duct. Apnea needs to be closely monitored in these children. When neonates present acutely, high doses of PGE$_1$ may be required to reopen the ductus and relax the ductal tissue in the isthmus. Ventilation is required for the resuscitation and administration of inotropic agents such as dopamine or milrinone (once the efficiently ductus is reopened by the prostaglandins) to optimize cardiac output may also be needed. Medical therapy should be continued until the child is stabilized with restoration of urine output; normal acid–base, electrolytes, and creatinine; and full recovery of the multiorgan compromise.

Interventional Therapy

There is an ongoing controversy regarding the suitability of balloon angioplasty for native coarctation despite increasing evidence that balloon angioplasty is inferior to surgical intervention in native coarctation [24]. Some authors may argue that it is a safer intervention than surgery, but there remains the concern that this is an inadequate treatment of arch hypoplasia and that the abnormal ductal tissue is not removed. Furthermore, balloon angioplasty still carries a risk of paraplegia [25] or primary or secondary aortic rupture with hemothorax that may be lethal. The complication of aneurysm formation after balloon angioplasty is well documented with rates reported as high as 43 % [26]. This intervention has to be associated with stenting most of the time and is therefore a technical conundrum in neonates, infants, and small children. Extensive discussion of interventional strategies in the aorta can be found in a specific chapter elsewhere in this textbook.

Timing for Surgery

Neonates with ductal-dependent circulation will need relief of their aortic coarctation within one or two days of presentation once they are stabilized medically. Today, even neonates born with coarctation and very low birth weight of less than 2 kg can undergo surgical repair with a low mortality and acceptable rates of re-obstruction [27].

For asymptomatic patients with aortic coarctation, it is advised that surgical repair be ideally carried out before 1 year of life or as soon as possible to reduce the risk of developing late hypertension [28]. In the largest follow-up study to date of 646 patients with aortic coarctation by Cohen et al., it was found that hypertension occurred in 7 % of patients operated on as infants, as opposed to 33 % of patients who had repair performed after the age of 14 [29]. The study also found age at the time of initial repair to be the most important predictor of hypertension. At the Royal Children's Hospital, Melbourne, these authors advocate that aortic coarctation patients who present acutely should be operated as soon as stabilization is achieved, but no sooner. The clinically stable patient with well-tolerated gradients or obstruction should be operated no later than 1–2 months after diagnosis and certainly before 6 months of life. Diagnosis later in life commands an intervention within 6 months.

Techniques for Surgical Repair

The first successful case of coarctation repair by surgical treatment was achieved in 1944 by Crafoord and Nylin using resection and end-to-end anastomosis [1]. Since then, several repair techniques have evolved to treat this congenital anomaly. Furthermore, the surgical management of coarctation today is made even more complex by the choice of surgical approaches. Arch repair can be achieved either from a left thoracotomy or a median sternotomy. The left thoracotomy approach is traditionally used for repair of isolated coarctation, with or without mild distal arch hypoplasia. In comparison, sternotomy repair is typically reserved for coarctation patients requiring a one-stage repair of associated cardiac lesions [9, 14]. However, because sternotomy allows a more proximal anastomosis and therefore a more extensive arch repair, there is an increasing trend to operate from the front in patients with associated proximal

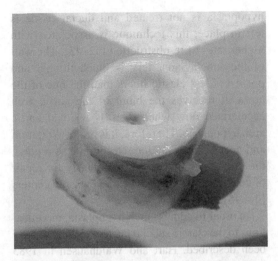

Fig. 93.5 Pathology specimen demonstrating a segment of the aortic arch resected for coarctation of the aorta

arch hypoplasia, even in the absence of associated anomalies [30]. Sternotomy is now also suggested for coarctation patients with other concerning associated arch morphologies such as anomalous right subclavian artery [20] or common brachiocephalic trunk [20].

The aortic arch can be surgically repaired by a number of different techniques and approaches, as discussed below.

Resection and End-to-End Anastomosis

The approach is from a left thoracotomy in the third or fourth intercostal space. The ductus arteriosus is ligated and divided. The proximal part of the arch vessels and the descending aorta are then dissected and mobilized. Adequate mobilization of the descending aorta and proximal vessels is required to create an anastomosis without tension following resection of the coarctation. The ligamentum arteriosum is ligated and the aorta clamped before the coarctation is completely and largely resected to include all ductal tissue (which is not macroscopically visible within the aorta) (Fig. 93.5). The aorta is re-approximated with the distal arch and the descending aorta anastomosed in an end-to-end fashion (Fig. 93.6).

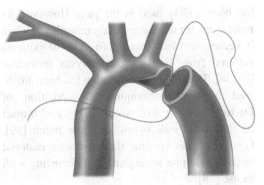

Fig. 93.6 End-to-end anastomosis

Over the past two decades, a modified version of this technique, the extended end-to-end anastomosis, has gradually replaced end-to-end anastomosis, but the latter is still being advocated by some [15, 31]. It has been suggested that adequate growth of the aortic arch occurs with simple resection and end-to-end anastomosis, even when associated with a hypoplastic aortic arch [15]. However, it has been previously demonstrated that adequate growth of the arch does not occur after end-to-end repair [32].

Patch Graft Aortoplasty

In the ensuing years following simple resection and end-to-end anastomosis, the high incidence of re-coarctation post-end-to-end anastomosis repair [33] drove Vossschulte to pioneer patch aortoplasty in 1957 [34].

The approach is as for end-to-end anastomosis, but patch aortoplasty can also be achieved from sternotomy. After clamping of the aorta above and below the area of coarctation, a longitudinal incision is made in the left anterior face of the narrowed aortic region. A patch of synthetic material made of Dacron® (polyethylene terephthalate) or Gore-Tex® (polytetrafluoroethylene) is then used to enlarge the opened area.

This technique requires minimal dissection and a short clamp time while effectively enlarging the narrowed aortic segment and has a low re-coarctation rate [36]. It is for these reasons that it has been widely used in the past. However, its indications for use were greatly diminished when it became evident that up to 7 % of patients suffered from late aortic aneurysm formation [37, 38]. The aneurysm formation has been attributed to the noncompliant composition of Dacron® creating excessive tension and impact on the aortic wall opposite to the patch [39]. Gore-Tex® has become the prosthetic material of choice despite aneurysms still occurring with its use [38].

Patch aortoplasty is still used in older patients where a tension-free end-to-end anastomosis may not be easily achieved [31]. Patch repair may remain an appropriate technique in some patients with long tubular hypoplasia.

Subclavian Flap Aortoplasty

Subclavian flap aortoplasty was introduced by Waldhausen and Nahrwold in 1966 as an alternative technique of repair to patch aortoplasty [40]. These two techniques were popularized in the 1970s.

Approach to subclavian flap aortoplasty is as for end-to-end anastomosis. The left subclavian artery is ligated distally, followed by an incision made along the lateral border of the artery into its base and along the aorta to well below the coarctation. This subclavian flap is then turned down and positioned within the margins of the aortic incision without removing the abnormal ductal tissue.

This repair technique avoids the extensive mobilization of the descending aorta and the circumferential suture line that is required by other techniques. Subclavian flap repair causes interruption to the arterial supply of the left upper limb and is generally avoided beyond infancy due to the inadequate development of collateral vessels necessary for compensation of this interruption. It has been found, however, that there is growth retardation of the arm even with repair in infancy, with these patients reporting discomfort and even claudication in the left arm [41]. Furthermore, because

hypoplasia is not treated and ductal tissue is left in place, this technique is associated with higher rates of re-obstruction [42, 43]. The wall of the subclavian artery is much thinner and possesses less elastic fibers than the one of the aorta. It receives the blunt of the aortic arch accelerated flow when there is residual aortic arch hypoplasia. Therefore, it is prone to dilation and aneurysm formation. Despite these reports, the use of subclavian flap aortoplasty for repair of coarctation is still advocated by some centers [44, 45].

In order to address arch hypoplasia, modifications to the classic subclavian flap technique have been described. Hart and Waldhausen in 1983 proposed a modified reverse subclavian flap technique [46]. However, this technique still requires the left subclavian artery supply to the left arm to be severed. Another modification was designed in the mid-1980s in which the base of the left subclavian artery was still used as a flap to augment the repair but the artery itself was reimplanted onto the arch [47]. At the Royal Children's Hospital, Melbourne, these authors strongly believe that this technique should be abandoned.

Extended End-to-End Anastomosis

There was great concern about the capacity of the techniques of previous eras to adequately address associated aortic arch hypoplasia. This speculation led Amato et al. to describe extended end-to-end anastomosis repair in 1977 to aid repair of arch hypoplasia [48].

The classic approach is as for end-to-end anastomosis, but extended end-to-end repair can also be achieved from sternotomy. After the coarctation segment is excised and the ductal tissue resected, an incision is made along the inner curvature of distal aortic arch. A wide oblique anastomosis is then created between the distal arch and the descending aorta (Fig. 93.7).

Extended end-to-end anastomosis is reported to be an effective repair technique for relieving the obstruction caused by distal transverse arch hypoplasia [7, 9, 10]. Furthermore, this

Fig. 93.7 Extended end-to-end anastomosis

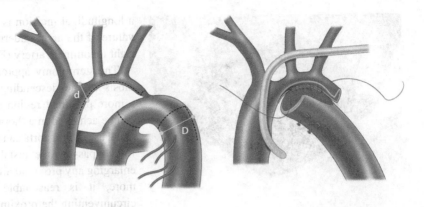

Fig. 93.8 End-to-side anastomosis

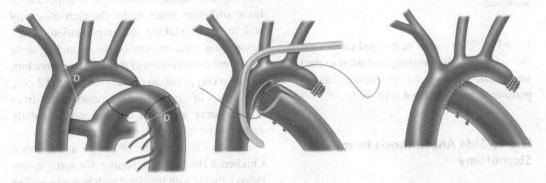

technique preserves the subclavian artery and uses autologous tissue to allow growth of the arch, hence avoiding the use of prosthetic material [36]. For these reasons, extended end-to-end repair has become the technique of choice for neonates and infants with aortic coarctation, with or without mild arch hypoplasia, in many centers worldwide [30]. However, many centers advocate that extended arch repair be reserved for patients with severe arch hypoplasia [38, 49].

Despite its popularity, there is concern over the capacity of extended end-to-end repair to address proximal arch hypoplasia [10, 16, 32]. At the Royal Children's Hospital, Melbourne, it has been recognized that the limiting diameter is one of the initial arches (D in Fig. 93.6). Because a much larger anastomosis than this diameter is not hemodynamically useful and is time consuming during cross clamp, it is preferred to tying the isthmus and performing a circular anastomosis in

the proximal inner curvature of the arch. From the side, it is reasonable to expect to be able to implant the descending aorta below the takeoff of the left carotid artery (Fig. 93.8). This procedure is called end-to-side anastomosis).

End-to-Side Anastomosis from Thoracotomy

Approach is as for resection and end-to-end anastomosis. An incision just longer than the circumference of the descending aorta is made into the underside of the arch. An anastomosis is then created directly between the descending aorta and the incision, and the distal arch is ligated to form an end artery joining into the left subclavian artery [10, 50].

Several centers worldwide have advocated for this technique [10, 14, 16]. When the diameter

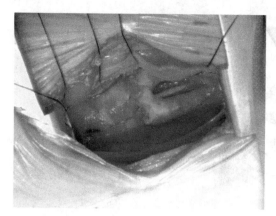

Fig. 93.9 End-to-side anastomosis being performed via sternotomy

(as in Fig. 93.8) cannot be bridged safely from the side without compromising perfusion to the right innominate artery, the procedure has to be performed from the front (Fig. 93.9).

End-to-Side Anastomosis from Sternotomy

In the present day, however, several centers argue that end-to-side anastomosis repair from sternotomy is the most effective technique for surgical repair of coarctation and aortic arch hypoplasia [10, 16]. End-to-side anastomosis was first described by Trusler in 1975 [51] for interrupted aortic arch repair and was adopted for aortic coarctation due to the low rate of re-coarctation observed through the use of this technique [10].

A routine median sternotomy incision is performed and the patient put on cardiopulmonary bypass. Extensive dissection of the arch and supra-aortic vessels is done. After ligation and division of the duct, the descending aorta is aggressively mobilized with division of the three first pairs of intercostal arteries. The anastomosis is performed with aortic cross clamp and selective perfusion of the right innominate artery. A clamp is applied to the descending aorta allowing pulling it up towards the proximal part of the inner curvature of the arch. All head vessels are snared. The distal aortic arch is ligated and

a longitudinal incision is made in the inner curvature of the arch, underneath the takeoff of the right innominate artery (Fig. 93.10).

The sternotomy approach allows the anastomosis of the descending aorta to be made to a more proximal region of the aortic arch than can be achieved in a thoracotomy approach. The distal ascending aorta can even be reached, therefore bypassing the distal arch and extensively enlarging any proximal arch hypoplasia. Furthermore, it is reasonable to assume that by circumventing the proximal arch hypoplasia, the likelihood of residual or recurrent obstruction will be minimized. However, it is important to leave sufficient space under the arch concavity and to avoid making the implantation of the descending aorta too low on the ascending aorta to prevent compression of the left main bronchus, a known complication of this technique [52, 53]. The use of end-to-side anastomosis from a sternotomy approach unfortunately regularly damages the left recurrent laryngeal nerve.

This is the technique of choice at the Royal Children's Hospital, Melbourne, for aortic coarctation patients with proximal arch hypoplasia. The use of end-to-side repair from sternotomy in the absence of associated cardiac anomalies has only been promoted in several centers, but the results reported have been promising thus far [10, 16].

Extra-Anatomical Bypass Grafts

In the adult-sized patient, the use of an extra-anatomical graft via sternotomy to bypass the whole aortic arch and isthmus has been demonstrated to be more effective at relieving arch obstruction than the conventional techniques described above [54]. In patients with previous arch surgery or with very complex anatomy, this approach can be preferred to a direct aortic arch surgery. However, when the anatomy is simple, a direct anastomosis from the front or a patch augmentation with continuous perfusion of the right innominate artery during cross clamp is a simple and very effective surgery. When the extra-anatomical bypass is selected, it is important to closely monitor chest drain losses

Fig. 93.10

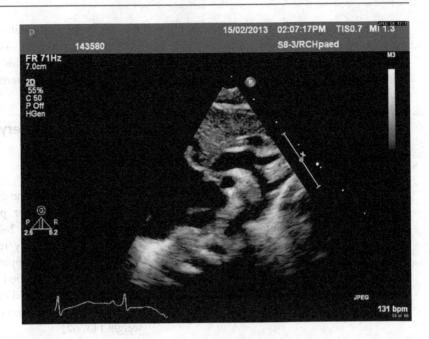

postoperatively as there is potential for prolonged postoperative drainage of mediastinal and pleural effusions. This prolonged effusion drainage is thought to be related to the transudation of plasma through the Dacron grafts. A preliminary report with a newer third-generation Dacron graft has yielded promising results [55].

Postoperative Complications and Critical Care Management

Hemorrhage

The most common cause of significant hemorrhage is related to excessive tension on individual sutures resulting in tearing. The preferential use of a running suture technique particularly posteriorly can minimize this risk.

Chylothorax

Postoperatively the nature of the chest tube drainage should be analyzed when profuse serous or milky drainage is produced. High level of triglycerides and chylomicrons is found in chylous effusions. The chest tube should be left in place until the cessation of the chyle.

Left Recurrent Laryngeal Nerve Palsy

It is important to visualize the left recurrent laryngeal nerve during mobilization of the ligamentum arteriosum and to take particular care when dissecting out this area in the case of reoperation. Additionally, to avoid injury to the vagus nerve, great care should be taken when mobilizing the medial pleural flap.

Paraplegia

Paraplegia is by far the most feared and devastating complication reported with surgery for aortic coarctation. Paraplegia can only occur when insufficient or no collateral circulation is present. It does not occur when the coarctation is atretic. In neonates and infants, the risk is high when the right subclavian artery is abnormal and coming from the descending aorta. In that situation, the proximal clamp will interrupt flow to both vertebral arteries and therefore the supply to the superior part of the spinal cord in addition to the interruption of the of flow to the Adamkiewicz artery [56].

At the Royal Children's Hospital, Melbourne, any surgical cure of coarctation when the risk of paraplegia is high is done under partial bypass between the main pulmonary artery and the descending aorta. To evaluate the need for partial bypass, the descending aorta distal to the coarctation is clamped temporarily and the residual pressure is needled. Pressure less than 30–40 mmHg would command partial bypass. The patients at greater risk are those with re-coarctation after balloon dilation when the collateral circulation has subsided or coarctation with moderate gradient. Neonates are not at risk unless the anatomy is as mentioned above.

Paradoxical Hypertension

Paradoxical hypertension is extremely common after coarctation repair and tends to occur in two phases. The initial phase over the first 24–48 h is likely a consequence of reduced stretch of the baroreceptors in the aortic arch and carotid arties resulting in a noradrenergic storm [57].

The second phase of elevated blood pressure is likely secondary to increased renin levels [58], though intense arterial vasospasm and endothelial ischemia resulting from sudden exposure of the distal vascular bed to higher pressures after surgery has also been implicated [57]. Treatment is medical which includes relaxation of smooth musculature, inhibition of angiotensin-converting enzyme, and the use of β-blockers. In the postoperative period, the choice of esmolol may be safer than other akin medications all the more that it allows titration. Once patients are stabilized, esmolol can be easily replaced by oral propranolol. Most commonly used drugs to modulate systemic hypertension in the immediate postoperative period are sodium nitroprusside and intravenous calcium inhibitors, like nicardipine. It has been shown that the commencement of a β-blocker prior to surgery reduces both postoperative blood pressure and activity of rennin [59]. As yet, there is no clear relationship between this transient paradoxical hypertension and long-term hypertension [60].

Outcomes of Surgery

Early Survival

Hospital mortality in the current era is low with operative mortality for patients with discrete coarctation as small as 2–4 % [10, 20, 36]. The causes of death usually result from continuing heart failure, poor preoperative status, or management errors. Identified risk factors for early death include associated cardiac anomalies [10, 11, 14], early era surgery [61], and low birth weight [43, 62].

Late Survival

Overall late survival based on adult and pediatric repair of aortic coarctation can range from 60 to 100 % depending on the length of follow-up [8, 10, 11, 16, 29, 61]. The few reports on repair of discrete coarctation in the first year of life have found 10-year survival of 92–99 % [28, 63].

Late survival is lower in reports on adult patients. In a large series of 229 patients at 40 years of follow-up after coarctation repair, only 69 % of patients were alive 40 years after surgery [61]. The landmark study by Cohen et al. examining late outcomes in 646 patients operated on as early as 1948 found 30-year survival to be only 72 % [29]. In adult patients, the main causes of death are cardiovascular diseases such as ischemic heart disease and cerebrovascular disease, which are likely accelerated by hypertension.

Aortic Arch Re-obstruction

Studies on the outcomes after neonatal repair of aortic coarctation in patients have revealed a wide range of results regarding the incidence of re-obstruction, ranging between 2 % and 33 % [11, 14, 16]. Elgamal et al. showed very promising results after end-to-side repair via a median sternotomy, as only 2 % of patients had arch re-obstruction 5 years after repair [16]. It was recently demonstrated that a third of all patients with arch hypoplasia suffered from arch re-obstruction [64]. It is suspected that the size of the transverse aortic arch in these much older patients was overestimated at the time of surgical repair planning and some would have benefited from a more extensive arch repair from a sternotomy.

There is no standard definition for arch re-obstruction making comparisons between studies difficult. However, there is a general agreement that re-obstruction be defined as a blood pressure difference of more than 20 mmHg between upper and lower limbs. On echocardiogram, a peak gradient of more than 25 mmHg is typically accepted. Interestingly, Smith Maia et al. examined the occurrence of re-obstruction in infants and children using three noninvasive methods, clinical examination of right arm-leg gradient, Doppler echocardiography, and magnetic resonance imaging, and showed that none of these methods used alone was able to diagnose re-obstruction in every case, suggesting that these methods should be used in combination [65].

Despite the lack of consensus on the definition of arch re-obstruction, today it is well accepted that there is a higher incidence of re-obstruction after classical repair techniques such as end-to-end anastomosis [66], patch repair [67], and subclavian flap repair [68]. Consequently, the use of more extensive techniques has now been advocated to repair aortic coarctation. There have been encouraging results reported after end-to-side repair via sternotomy, with freedom from obstruction at 10 years at 91.6 %, compared with only 61.2 % for extended end-to-end repair [64]. Interestingly, the incidence of re-obstruction after extended end-to-end repair was found to be so significant that this technique is reported to be a significant predictive factor for late obstruction, along with end-to-end anastomosis repair and patch repair.

Aortic Arch Growth

For many decades, it has been believed that a hypoplastic aortic arch will grow after conventional repair of coarctation [7, 15, 49, 69]. However, the evidence for this notion has been drawn from studies that have reported relatively short-term outcomes, with poor distinction between whether proximal or distal arch hypoplasia was examined, and an obvious lack of definition defining optimal growth. The proximal and distal arch should be analyzed separately, as the growth of these two segments may not be uniform. It was recently been demonstrated that while the distal transverse arch grows reliably after coarctation repair, the proximal transverse arch remained small in one third of patients [32].

Today, there is growing suspicion that arch hypoplasia requires enlargement during coarctation surgery to promote postoperative growth.

Hypertension

Systemic hypertension is the most concerning late outcome after successful repair of coarctation, and its development is a grave concern in this patient population because it is directly linked to mortality at a young age [29, 61]. Literature across pediatric and adult repair of coarctation has shown that late hypertension occurs in 17–75 % of patients [15, 28, 29, 43, 65, 70–73]. The studies focused on the prevalence of resting hypertension after neonatal repair has found hypertension to occur in 17–30 % of patients [28, 70, 71, 73]. Unfortunately, the proportion of patients with hypertension only increases as the patient ages [29].

The definition of hypertension used in many studies is very liberal, with only blood pressures more than 160/90 mmHg considered hypertensive. This very lenient definition of hypertension, combined with the fact that many of these studies only examined resting blood pressure and not ambulatory blood pressure, is why the prevalence of hypertension after coarctation is probably underestimated.

The few reports on 24-h ambulatory blood pressure after coarctation repair have demonstrated hypertension to be prevalent in 28–60 % of patients depending on the length of follow-up time [70, 71, 73]. These studies also found that arch re-obstruction only accounted for a minority of hypertensive cases and an inability of resting blood pressure measurements to detect hypertension in every case.

Risk factors identified for the development of hypertension after coarctation repair include older age at time of surgery [28, 29, 72], the use of surgical repair techniques from an early era [38, 72], having a resulting "non-Roman aortic arch shape" after repair [74], arch re-obstruction [72], and intrinsic vascular abnormalities including increased intima-media thickness of the pre-stenotic arteries, reduced vasoreactivity, and increased stiffness [75, 76].

It is still unclear what the best management for this late hypertension is, and large randomized control studies investigating this are needed.

Long-Term Follow-Up

Patients who have undergone aortic coarctation repair are no longer considered "cured" and must be followed up for their entire life. In particular, annual 24-h ambulatory blood pressure monitoring after approximately 10 years of age when the child can tolerate the investigation for a 24-h period, echocardiogram imaging including measurements of the proximal and distal arch and conversion to z-score, and Doppler measurement of the peak gradient across the descending aorta should be mandatory for these patients, as these tests are more sensitive than resting blood pressure measurements and clinical limb gradient assessment, respectively.

References

1. Crafoord C, Nylin G (1945) Congenital coarctation of the aorta and its surgical treatment. J Thorac Surg 14:347–361

2. Elliott RB, Starling MB, Neutze JM (1975) Medical manipulation of the ductus arteriosus. Lancet 1:140–142

3. Hoffman JI, Kaplan S (2002) The incidence of congenital heart disease. J Am Coll Cardiol 39:1890–1900

4. Samanek M, Voriskova M (1999) Congenital heart disease among 815,569 children born between 1980 and 1990 and their 15-year survival: a prospective Bohemia survival study. Pediatr Cardiol 20:411–417

5. Campbell M, Polani PE (1961) The aetiology of coarctation of the aorta. Lancet 1:463–468

6. Beekman RH, Robinow M (1985) Coarctation of the aorta inherited as an autosomal dominant trait. Am J Cardiol 56:818–819

7. Myers JL, McConnell BA, Waldhausen JA (1992) Coarctation of the aorta in infants: does the aortic arch grow after repair? Ann Thorac Surg 54:869–874; discussion 74–75

8. Hager A, Schreiber C, Nutzl S et al (2009) Mortality and restenosis rate of surgical coarctation repair in infancy: a study of 191 patients. Cardiology 112:36–41

9. Conte S, Lacour-Gayet F, Serraf A et al (1995) Surgical management of neonatal coarctation. J Thorac Cardiovasc Surg 109:663–674; discussion 74–75

10. Thomson JD, Mulpur A, Guerrero R et al (2006) Outcome after extended arch repair for aortic coarctation. Heart 92:90–94

11. Lacour-Gayet F, Bruniaux J, Serraf A et al (1990) Hypoplastic transverse arch and coarctation in neonates. Surgical reconstruction of the aortic arch: a study of sixty-six patients. J Thorac Cardiovasc Surg 100:808–816

12. Moulaert AJ, Bruins CC, Oppenheimer-Dekker A (1976) Anomalies of the aortic arch and ventricular septal defects. Circulation 53:1011–1015

13. Pigula FA (2007) Surgery for aortic arch disease in the neonate. Pediatr Cardiol 28:134–143

14. Karl TR, Sano S, Brawn W et al (1992) Repair of hypoplastic or interrupted aortic arch via sternotomy. J Thorac Cardiovasc Surg 104:688–695

15. Brouwer RM, Erasmus ME, Ebels T et al (1994) Influence of age on survival, late hypertension, and recoarctation in elective aortic coarctation repair. Including long-term results after elective aortic coarctation repair with a follow-up from 25 to 44 years. J Thorac Cardiovasc Surg 108:525–531

16. Elgamal MA, McKenzie ED, Fraser CD Jr (2002) Aortic arch advancement: the optimal one-stage approach for surgical management of neonatal coarctation with arch hypoplasia. Ann Thorac Surg 73:1267–1272; discussion 72–73

17. Roos-Hesselink JW, Scholzel BE, Heijdra RJ et al (2003) Aortic valve and aortic arch pathology after coarctation repair. Heart 89:1074–1077

18. Gutgesell HP, Barton DM, Elgin KM (2001) Coarctation of the aorta in the neonate: associated conditions, management, and early outcome. Am J Cardiol 88:457–459

19. Quaegebeur JM, Jonas RA, Weinberg AD et al (1994) Outcomes in seriously ill neonates with coarctation of the aorta. A multiinstitutional study. J Thorac Cardiovasc Surg 108:841–851; discussion 52–54

20. Kaushal S, Backer CL, Patel JN et al (2009) Coarctation of the aorta: midterm outcomes of resection with extended end-to-end anastomosis. Ann Thorac Surg 88:1932–1938

21. Elzenga NJ, Gittenberger-de Groot AC (1985) Coarctation and related aortic arch anomalies in hypoplastic left heart syndrome. Int J Cardiol 8:379–393

22. Gopal A, Loewinger L, Budoff MJ (2010) Aortic coarctation by cardiovascular CT angiography. Catheter Cardiovasc Interv 76:551–552

23. Wyers MC, Fillinger MF, Schermerhorn ML et al (2003) Endovascular repair of abdominal aortic aneurysm without preoperative arteriography. J Vasc Surg 38:730–738

24. Cowley CG, Orsmond GS, Feola P et al (2005) Long-term, randomized comparison of balloon angioplasty and surgery for native coarctation of the aorta in childhood. Circulation 111:3453–3456

25. Ussia GP, Marasini M, Pongiglione G (2001) Paraplegia following percutaneous balloon angioplasty of aortic coarctation: a case report. Catheter Cardiovasc Interv 54:510–513

26. Forbes TJ, Kim DW, Du W et al (2011) Comparison of surgical, stent, and balloon angioplasty treatment of native coarctation of the aorta: an observational study by the CCISC (Congenital Cardiovascular Interventional Study Consortium). J Am Coll Cardiol 58:2664–2674

27. Sudarshan CD, Cochrane AD, Jun ZH et al (2006) Repair of coarctation of the aorta in infants weighing less than 2 kilograms. Ann Thorac Surg 82:158–163

28. Seirafi PA, Warner KG, Geggel RL et al (1998) Repair of coarctation of the aorta during infancy minimizes the risk of late hypertension. Ann Thorac Surg 66:1378–1382

29. Cohen M, Fuster V, Steele PM et al (1989) Coarctation of the aorta. Long-term follow-up and prediction of outcome after surgical correction. Circulation 80:840–845

30. Wright GE, Nowak CA, Goldberg CS et al (2005) Extended resection and end-to-end anastomosis for aortic coarctation in infants: results of a tailored surgical approach. Ann Thorac Surg 80:1453–1459

31. Stark J, de Leval M, Tsang V (2006) Surgery for congenital heart defects. Wiley, London

32. Liu JY, Kowalski R, Jones B et al (2010) Moderately hypoplastic arches: do they reliably grow into adulthood after conventional coarctation repair? Interact Cardiovasc Thorac Surg 10:582–586

33. Schuster SR, Gross RE (1962) Surgery for coarctation of the aorta. A review of 500 cases. J Thorac Cardiovasc Surg 43:54–70

34. Vossschulte K (1961) Surgical correction of coarctation of the aorta by an "isthmusplastic" operation. Thorax 16:338–345

35. Abbruzzese PA, Aidala E (2007) Aortic coarctation: an overview. J Cardiovasc Med (Hagerstown) 8:123–128

36. Backer CL, Mavroudis C, Zias EA et al (1998) Repair of coarctation with resection and extended end-to-end anastomosis. Ann Thorac Surg 66:1365–1370; discussion 70–71

37. Bromberg BI, Beekman RH, Rocchini AP et al (1989) Aortic aneurysm after patch aortoplasty repair of coarctation: a prospective analysis of prevalence, screening tests and risks. J Am Coll Cardiol 14:734–741

38. Walhout RJ, Lekkerkerker JC, Oron GH et al (2003) Comparison of polytetrafluoroethylene patch aortoplasty and end-to-end anastomosis for coarctation of the aorta. J Thorac Cardiovasc Surg 126:521–528

39. Rheuban KS, Gutgesell HP, Carpenter MA et al (1986) Aortic aneurysm after patch angioplasty for aortic isthmic coarctation in childhood. Am J Cardiol 58:178–180

40. Waldhausen JA, Nahrwold DL (1966) Repair of coarctation of the aorta with a subclavian flap. J Thorac Cardiovasc Surg 51:532–533

41. van Son JA, van Asten WN, van Lier HJ et al (1990) Detrimental sequelae on the hemodynamics of the upper left limb after subclavian flap angioplasty in infancy. Circulation 81:996–1004

42. Dodge-Khatami A, Backer CL, Mavroudis C (2000) Risk factors for recoarctation and results of reoperation: a 40-year review. J Card Surg 15:369–377

43. Toro-Salazar OH, Steinberger J, Thomas W et al (2002) Long-term follow-up of patients after coarctation of the aorta repair. Am J Cardiol 89:541–547

44. Barreiro CJ, Ellison TA, Williams JA et al (2007) Subclavian flap aortoplasty: still a safe, reproducible, and effective treatment for infant coarctation. Eur J Cardiothorac Surg 31:649–653

45. Pandey R, Jackson M, Ajab S et al (2006) Subclavian flap repair: review of 399 patients at median follow-up of fourteen years. Ann Thorac Surg 81:1420–1428

46. Hart JC, Waldhausen JA (1983) Reversed subclavian flap angioplasty for arch coarctation of the aorta. Ann Thorac Surg 36:715–717

47. de Mendonca JT, Carvalho MR, Costa RK et al (1985) Coarctation of the aorta: a new surgical technique. J Thorac Cardiovasc Surg 90:445–447

48. Amato JJ, Rheinlander HF, Cleveland RJ (1977) A method of enlarging the distal transverse arch in infants with hypoplasia and coarctation of the aorta. Ann Thorac Surg 23:261–263

49. Siewers RD, Ettedgui J, Pahl E et al (1991) Coarctation and hypoplasia of the aortic arch: will the arch grow? Ann Thorac Surg 52:608–613; discussion 13–14

50. Rajasinghe HA, Reddy VM, van Son JA et al (1996) Coarctation repair using end-to-side anastomosis of descending aorta to proximal aortic arch. Ann Thorac Surg 61:840–844

51. Trusler GA, Izukawa T (1975) Interrupted aortic arch and ventricular septal defect. Direct repair through a median sternotomy incision in a 13-day-old infant. J Thorac Cardiovasc Surg 69:126–131

52. Serraf A, Lacour-Gayet F, Robotin M et al (1996) Repair of interrupted aortic arch: a ten-year experience. J Thorac Cardiovasc Surg 112:1150–1160

53. Tlaskal T, Hucin B, Kostelka M et al (1998) Successful reoperation for severe left bronchus compression after repair of persistent truncus arteriosus with interrupted aortic arch. Eur J Cardiothorac Surg 13:306–309

54. Brink J, Lee MG, Konstantinov IE et al (2013) Complications of extra-anatomic aortic bypass for complex coarctation and aortic arch hypoplasia. Ann Thorac Surg 95:676–681

55. De Paulis R, Scaffa R, Maselli D et al (2008) A third generation of ascending aorta Dacron graft: preliminary experience. Ann Thorac Surg 85:305–309

56. Setty SP, Brizard CP, d'Udekem Y (2007) Partial cardiopulmonary bypass in infants with coarctation and anomalous right subclavian arteries. Ann Thorac Surg 84:715; author reply 15–16

57. Sealy WC (1990) Paradoxical hypertension after repair of coarctation of the aorta: a review of its causes. Ann Thorac Surg 50:323–329

58. Parker FB Jr, Streeten DH, Farrell B et al (1982) Preoperative and postoperative renin levels in coarctation of the aorta. Circulation 66:513–514

59. Gidding SS, Rocchini AP, Beekman R et al (1985) Therapeutic effect of propranolol on paradoxical hypertension after repair of coarctation of the aorta. N Engl J Med 312:1224–1228

60. Fox S, Pierce WS, Waldhausen JA (1980) Pathogenesis of paradoxical hypertension after coarctation repair. Ann Thorac Surg 29:135–141

61. Hoimyr H, Christensen TD, Emmertsen K et al (2006) Surgical repair of coarctation of the aorta: up to 40 years of follow-up. Eur J Cardiothorac Surg 30:910–916

62. Karamlou T, Bernasconi A, Jaeggi E et al (2009) Factors associated with arch reintervention and growth of the aortic arch after coarctation repair in neonates weighing less than 2.5 kg. J Thorac Cardiovasc Surg 137:1163–1167

63. Wood AE, Javadpour H, Duff D et al (2004) Is extended arch aortoplasty the operation of choice for infant aortic coarctation? Results of 15 years' experience in 181 patients. Ann Thorac Surg 77:1353–1357; discussion 57–58

64. Rakhra SS, Lee M, Iyengar AJ et al (2013) Poor outcomes after surgery for coarctation repair with hypoplastic arch warrants more extensive initial surgery and close long-term follow-up. Interact Cardiovasc Thorac Surg 16:31–36

65. Smith Maia MM, Cortes TM, Parga JR et al (2004) Evolutional aspects of children and adolescents with surgically corrected aortic coarctation: clinical, echocardiographic, and magnetic resonance image analysis of 113 patients. J Thorac Cardiovasc Surg 127:712–720

66. Kappetein AP, Zwinderman AH, Bogers AJ et al (1994) More than thirty-five years of coarctation repair. An unexpected high relapse rate. J Thorac Cardiovasc Surg 107:87–95

67. Backer CL, Paape K, Zales VR et al (1995) Coarctation of the aorta. Repair with polytetrafluoroethylene patch aortoplasty. Circulation 92:II132–II136

68. Brouwer MH, Kuntze CE, Ebels T et al (1991) Repair of aortic coarctation in infants. J Thorac Cardiovasc Surg 101:1093–1098

69. Jahangiri M, Shinebourne EA, Zurakowski D et al (2000) Subclavian flap angioplasty: does the arch look after itself? J Thorac Cardiovasc Surg 120:224–229

70. O'Sullivan JJ, Derrick G, Darnell R (2002) Prevalence of hypertension in children after early repair of coarctation of the aorta: a cohort study using casual and 24 hour blood pressure measurement. Heart 88:163–166

71. de Divitiis M, Pilla C, Kattenhorn M et al (2003) Ambulatory blood pressure, left ventricular mass, and conduit artery function late after successful repair of coarctation of the aorta. J Am Coll Cardiol 41:2259–2265

72. Hager A, Kanz S, Kaemmerer H et al (2007) Coarctation Long-term Assessment (COALA): significance of arterial hypertension in a cohort of 404 patients up to 27 years after surgical repair of isolated coarctation of the aorta, even in the absence of restenosis and prosthetic material. J Thorac Cardiovasc Surg 134:738–745

73. Lee MG, Kowalski R, Galati JC et al (2012) Twenty-four-hour ambulatory blood pressure monitoring detects a high prevalence of hypertension late after coarctation repair in patients with hypoplastic arches. J Thorac Cardiovasc Surg 144:1110–1116

74. Ou P, Bonnet D, Auriacombe L et al (2004) Late systemic hypertension and aortic arch geometry after successful repair of coarctation of the aorta. Eur Heart J 25:1853–1859

75. de Divitiis M, Rubba P, Calabro R (2005) Arterial hypertension and cardiovascular prognosis after successful repair of aortic coarctation: a clinical model for the study of vascular function. Nutr Metab Cardiovasc Dis 15:382–394

76. Ou P, Celermajer DS, Mousseaux E et al (2007) Vascular remodeling after "successful" repair of coarctation: impact of aortic arch geometry. J Am Coll Cardiol 49:883–890

Interrupted Aortic Arch

94

Melissa Lee, Yves d'Udekem, and Christian Brizard

Abstract

Interrupted aortic arch is often regarded as the most severe form of coarctation and this is certainly a good way of viewing it. This chapter will explore the history of interrupted aortic arch, the different types and associated anomalies, the surgical and medical management, the outcomes after surgery, and recommendations for long-term follow-up of patients with interrupted aortic arch.

Keywords

24-h ambulatory blood pressure monitoring • Aberrant right subclavian artery • Anastomosis • Aortic arch • Balloon angioplasty • Bronchocompression • Cardiac surgery • Congenital heart disease • DiGeorge syndrome • End-to-side anastomosis • Hypertension • Interrupted aortic arch • Left carotid artery turndown • Left ventricular outflow tract obstruction • Patch • Prostaglandin E_1 • Re-intervention • Re-obstruction • Subaortic stenosis • Type A • Type B • Type C

Definition

IAA is a complete anatomic and luminal lack of continuity between the proximal and distal segments of the aortic arch.

Introduction

Although interrupted aortic arch (IAA) is a rare condition, it represents an extreme and life-threatening form of congenital heart disease that can be treated using several different management strategies. In the current era, improved pre- and perioperative care and the use of prostaglandin E_1 (PGE_1) have seen the outcomes of patients with IAA shift from the early and mid-term to the long-term life span. Refined surgical technique has demonstrated excellent outcomes in the management of this anomaly, but there continues to be room for improvement.

M. Lee (✉) • Y. d'Udekem • C. Brizard
Cardiac Surgery, The Royal Children's Hospital,
Melbourne, VIC, Australia
e-mail: Christian.Brizard@rch.org.au

E.M. da Cruz et al. (eds.), *Pediatric and Congenital Cardiology, Cardiac Surgery and Intensive Care*,
DOI 10.1007/978-1-4471-4619-3_28, © Springer-Verlag London 2014

Historical Considerations

The first description of IAA is credited to Steidele who described the anomaly consisting of an absent aortic isthmus in 1778 [1]. The absence of more proximal sections of the arch was described much later. In 1818, the absence of the segment between the left subclavian and left common carotid arteries was described by Seidel [2], and in 1948 the absence of the segment between the left common carotid and innominate arteries was reported by Weisman and Kesten [3]. By 1959, Celoria and Patton introduced the classification of interrupted aortic arch according to the site of obstruction into types A, B, and C (described in detail in the subsection dedicated to morphology) [4].

The first successful surgical repair for IAA was done by Samson and described by Merrill in 1955, with the patients' two ventricular septal defects (VSD) closed 4 years later [5]. It was not until 1970 that the first simultaneous repair of interrupted aortic arch and VSD closure was performed successfully by Barratt-Boyes using deep hypothermic circulatory arrest, to connect a 12-mm polyester conduit via both a thoracotomy and sternotomy approach [6]. Five years later, in 1975, Trusler reported the first simultaneous IAA and VSD repair via a median sternotomy without the use of a prosthetic graft [7]. However, it was not until the introduction of PGE$_1$ in 1976 by Elliot and colleagues that the treatment of IAA was revolutionized [8].

Prevalence and Genetics

IAA occurs in 0.03/10,000 live births [9], accounting for just over 1 % of anomalies in live-born children with congenital heart defects [10].

There is a known association between IAA and the deletion of chromosome 22q11-, or DiGeorge syndrome. Roughly two thirds of those patients with DiGeorge syndrome have type B IAA, but only one third of those with type B IAA have DiGeorge syndrome.

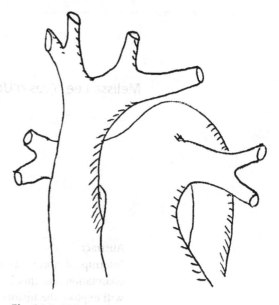

Fig. 94.1 IAA type A

Morphology

Type A interruption is described when the interruption is distal to the left subclavian artery (Fig. 94.1).

Type B interruption occurs between the left common carotid and left subclavian arteries. It is by far the most common type of IAA, occurring in 60–70 % of cases (Fig. 94.2).

Type C interruption is described when the interruption occurs between the innominate and left common carotid arteries. This type is the rarest of the three, occurring in less than 5 % of cases of IAA [11] (Fig. 94.3).

All IAA types have ductal-dependent perfusion to the lower body.

Associated Anomalies

IAA may coexist with a number of cardiac anomalies. The most commonly associated anomaly is a large ventricular septal defect (VSD), found in almost all cases. This large VSD may cause protrusion of muscle and posterior deviation of the infundibular septum into the subaortic region, resulting in left ventricular outflow tract

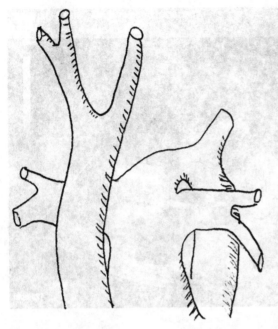

Fig. 94.2 IAA type B

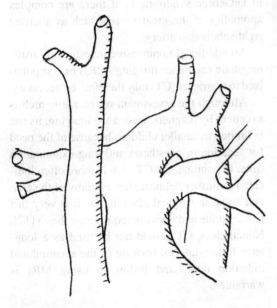

Fig. 94.3 IAA type C

relevant as the ascending aorta and aortic valve only have to carry the flow to both carotid arteries before any correction. Their size is reduced in accordance to this flow during fetal life and may not be sufficient for the whole cardiac output after correction. The deviation of the infundibular septum creates a spectrum of left ventricular outflow tract (LVOT) obstruction in the IAA type B. IAA is commonly associated with bicuspid aortic valve, occurring in approximately 30–50 % of patients with IAA. Subaortic stenosis may be present or develop after repair as a consequence of the anatomy described above.

Less commonly, IAA can be associated with lesions such as truncus arteriosus, transposition of the great arteries, and aortopulmonary window.

Clinical Presentation and Diagnosis

Unless diagnosed antenatally and unlike coarctation of the aorta, IAA almost always presents in the neonatal period as the ductus arteriosus closes. The neonate becomes acutely unwell with poor perfusion of the body and profound metabolic (lactic) acidosis. If left untreated, the metabolic acidosis results in the neonate developing shock, liver failure, renal failure, necrotizing enterocolitis, and seizures and ultimately dying.

On clinical examination, there may be diminished or absent femoral pulses depending on the type of IAA. Post-ductal saturations are low.

Chest x-ray demonstrates an enlarged heart and pulmonary congestion.

Analysis of arterial blood gas exposes a worsening and progressive lactic acidosis.

Imaging

Two-dimensional echocardiography is the diagnostic method of choice, as the exact location of the aortic arch interrupted can be well determined (Figs. 94.6 and 94.7); echocardiography also documents the presence of an associated VSD or other cardiac anomalies.

narrowing (Fig. 94.4). An aberrant right subclavian artery, which originates as a fourth brachiocephalic branch from the descending thoracic aorta, commonly occurs in type B (Fig. 94.5). This association is particularly

Fig. 94.4 A 2D echocardiographic image demonstrating a large VSD

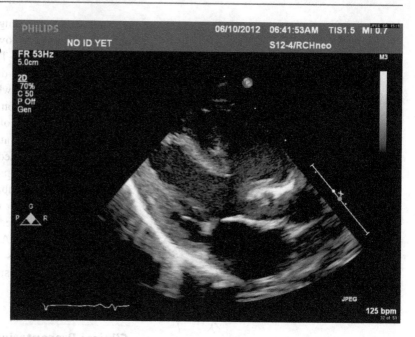

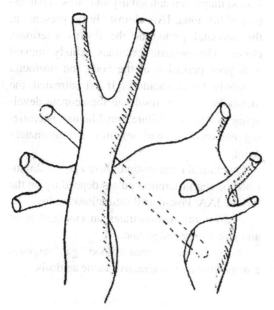

Fig. 94.5 Aberrant right subclavian artery and IAA type B

Similarly to coarctation of the aorta, cardiac catheterization is not required in the vast majority of cases. However, echocardiography may be unconvincing in some circumstances, if there is no acoustic window because of a lack of thymus in DiGeorge syndrome or if there are complex anomalies of the great vessels such as aberrant right subclavian artery.

An additional noninvasive investigation using magnetic resonance imaging (MRI) or computerized tomography (CT) may therefore be necessary.

Although the assessment of the aortic arch is excellent by magnetic resonance imaging, its use is limited in smaller children because of the need for sedation or anesthesia and long examination time. In contrast, the CT scan is more often indicated to further delineate the anatomy of the arch and assist in surgical planning, as it is very fast and accurate and does not require anesthesia [12]. Nonetheless, CT should not be used as a long-term follow-up tool because of the accumulated radiation dose, and follow-up using MRI is warranted.

Medical Therapy

The introduction of PGE$_1$ radically improved the preoperative management of neonates presenting with IAA [8]. Intravenous administration of PGE$_1$ maintains patency of the ductus arteriosus,

Fig. 94.6 A 2D echocardiographic image demonstrating IAA

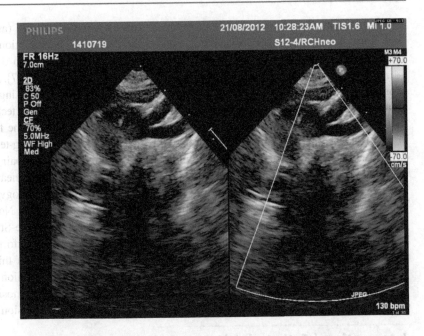

Fig. 94.7 Colour Doppler ultrasound demonstrating IAA

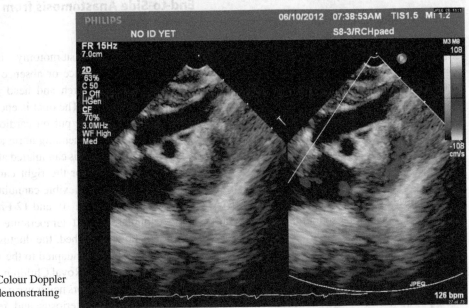

allowing for resuscitation and restoration of organ perfusion in these compromised infants. It is important to maximize pulmonary resistance by minimizing the administration of oxygen, as this will increase systemic blood flow, which will in turn improve end-organ perfusion and limit the development of associated generalized acidosis.

It is generally advised to intubate the child as a precaution to the potential apneic episodes triggered by PGE$_1$, although there is no evidence to suggest that this is the best practice. The child may also require mechanical ventilation and administration of inotropic agents such as dopamine to optimize cardiac output. Medical therapy should be continued until the child is stabilized with normal acid–base, electrolytes and creatinine, and recovery of the multiorgan function.

As part of these patients' preoperative workup, a chromosomal analysis for 22q11- deletion using fluorescent in situ hybridization (FISH test) should be performed. Given the high prevalence of DiGeorge syndrome in children with IAA, it is reasonable to presume that the patient has DiGeorge syndrome and thus abnormalities with T cells. It is therefore important to use irradiated blood in all instances of transfusion, including cardiopulmonary bypass, to avoid the possibility of graft-versus-host disease caused by transfused lymphocytes. After surgery, rotational antibiotics or other immune therapy may be required to overcome susceptibility to infection.

Interventional Catheterization

Interventional catheterization has no place in the initial management of IAA. It may be used after surgical repair to provide relief across a direct anastomosis if stenotic. In that situation, the recurrence is usually due to some residual ductal tissue at the anastomotic site and recurrence of stenosis after balloon angioplasty may occur.

Surgical Management

All neonates will require surgical repair for IAA within 1 or 2 days of presentation, once they are stabilized medically.

Since the first successful case of IAA repair by surgical treatment was achieved in 1955 using end-to-end anastomosis (as described in ▶ Chap. 93, "Coarctation of the Aorta"), several repair techniques have been tried to treat this anomaly. These interventions include from a repair using a carotid flap with banding of the pulmonary trunk [13] to a single-stage complete repair using a graft (as described in 1972) [6] or without the use of synthetic material [7]. Currently, almost all centers perform the repair of IAA and noncomplex associated anomalies in a single-stage approach with direct end-to-side

anastomosis [14–16] (as also illustrated in ▶ Chap. 93, "Coarctation of the Aorta"). The benefits of the addition of a patch to the repair remain controversial [17]. At the Royal Children's Hospital, Melbourne, a single-stage repair using an end-to-side anastomosis technique without an additional patch has been the favored approach since 1985 with excellent long-term results [18].

If a biventricular repair is not possible such as with hypoplastic left heart syndrome or other single ventricle physiology with IAA, reconstruction of the arch with a Norwood-like procedure including Damus-Kaye-Stansel associated with a shunt should be performed (both techniques described elsewhere in this book). In the latter case, a patch augmentation of the arch rather than the end-to-side anastomosis is required to avoid left bronchial compression.

End-to-Side Anastomosis from Sternotomy

A routine median sternotomy incision is performed. The presence or absence of thymus is noted. The aortic arch and head vessels are extensively dissected. The duct is encircled with a snare. The patient is put on cardiopulmonary bypass between the ascending aorta and the two venae cavae. The aorta is cannulated at the foot of the right innominate or the right carotid artery with a 6- or 8-French flexible cannula. The vena cava is cannulated with 10- and 12-French right-angle cannulas. Target temperature is 24 °C. When half flow is reached, the ductus arteriosus is ligated and the flow adapted to the right radial artery pressure. At the Royal Children's Hospital, Melbourne, these authors never use a second cannula in the ductus arteriosus and rely on the collateral circulation for the perfusion of the lower body. The duct is divided and a clamp is applied onto the descending aorta. The descending aorta is extensively mobilized with dissection and division of three pairs of intercostal arteries. Checking from the inside and on the aspect of the aortic wall section, all ductal tissue is resected. The transition between the thick, fragile, and gelatinous ductal tissue and the thin souple and resistant aortic wall is obvious once that transition has been crossed. It is absolutely paramount that this resection is done without any compromise. Absolutely all ductal tissue has to be removed and this often reduces the length of what operators would like to rely on to perform a tension-free anastomosis by a significant amount (approximately 1 cm). The remainder of the aortic arch surgery is performed as for the end-to-side anastomosis as described in ▶ Chap. 93, "Coarctation of the Aorta". The anastomosis has to be made as posterior and superior as possible and may need to extend into the posterior aspect of the left carotid artery. It is important to leave sufficient space under the arch concavity and to avoid making the implantation of the descending aorta too low on the ascending aorta to prevent compression of the left main bronchus, a known complication of this technique [16, 19]. The use of end-to-side anastomosis from a sternotomy approach regularly damages the left recurrent laryngeal nerve, but this is most of the time reversible within months.

Left Carotid Artery Turndown Procedure (LCATD)

Alternative approaches to the repair of IAA that are advocated by some authors include a staged approach with the left carotid artery turndown procedure (LCATD) [20, 21]. The approach is from a left thoracotomy in the fourth intercostal space. The left carotid artery is divided and anastomosed to the descending aorta. Pulmonary artery banding is also performed in cases with associated VSD.

Although early outcomes with this technique may be acceptable, long-term outcomes including greater survival and freedom from arch re-intervention are more favorable after end-to-side repair than after LCATD [18]. This technique is not suitable for patients with complex lesions, including d-transposition of the great arteries, truncus arteriosus, and hypoplastic left heart syndrome [21]. This technique has not been used at the Royal Children's Hospital, Melbourne, for more than 18 years.

Postoperative Complications and Critical Care Management

The complications of IAA and coarctation are all interchangeable (please consult the chapter on aortic coarctation by these authors). In IAA in particular, it is important to examine the residual gradient across the repair to ensure that the newly anastomosed arch does not have a residual narrowing before leaving the operating room. This is best done with an epicardial echocardiography study after the removal of the aortic cannula or less easily with the transesophageal echography.

Chylothorax

Intraoperatively, care should be given to lymphostasis with fine suture of any lymphatic leaking area during the dissection and before chest closure. Postoperatively, the nature of the chest tube drainage should be monitored for profuse serous or milky drainage, most likely to be chyle. The chest tube should be left in place until the cessation of the chylothorax.

Left Recurrent Laryngeal Nerve Palsy

It is important to protect the left recurrent laryngeal nerve during mobilization of the descending thoracic aorta; specifically, operators should avoid forceps making contact with the nerve during diathermy of the deep structures. Despite extra caution, the use of end-to-side repair, as previously mentioned, frequently injures the left recurrent laryngeal nerve. This lesion is often transitory and will recover after a few months.

Left Bronchial Compression

The compression of the left bronchus is a well-known complication of the end-to-side anastomosis in IAA. It is due to stretching of the descending aorta crossing over the left bronchus when it is brought anteriorly for the anastomosis. The elasticity of the aorta applies a downward force on the superior and posterior aspect of the left main bronchus. Narrowing or occlusion of the left main bronchus can occur acutely after surgery or progressive reduction of the lumen is also seen. This complication is prevented by the extensive mobilization and the performance of the anastomosis as posteriorly as possible. The adherence to these principles has almost eliminated this complication at the Royal Children's Hospital, Melbourne. When it does occur, the treatment can be graded. If the compression is mild, it is acceptable to watch the evolution over the first 3–5 years of life and it may disappear completely. An acute occlusion in the postoperative period may be relieved with a more extensive mobilization of the descending aorta and aortopexy through a left thoracotomy. If this is not sufficient, then a Gore-Tex graft interposition in the descending aorta will provide a definitive solution in all cases. At the Royal Children's Hospital, Melbourne, this complication has been encountered in the past and successfully treated using this graded strategy. The replacement of the graft to an adult-sized diameter in the second decade of life is usually a fairly straightforward procedure [22].

Left Ventricular Outflow Tract Obstruction

The potential for left ventricular outflow tract (LVOT) obstruction exists in IAA types B and C as described above. Historically, this has led to many authors describing various modifications of the VSD closure technique to prevent or modify the posterior deviation of the infundibular septum [11, 23–26]. Even more, the Damus-Kaye-Stansel operation was initially described to bypass a potentially obstructive aortic valve in precisely this group of patients (Yasui procedure) [23], but it has been shown to be a procedural risk factor for mortality [14]. In practice, all modifications of the VSD closure technique seem to have very little impact, and the potential

obstruction with aortic valve less than 6 mm in diameter invariably translates postoperatively to normal LVOT velocities. Postoperatively, the patients who do have gradients are very rare. The strategy that seems to generate the less mortality and morbidity is to treat the potential LVOT obstruction by neglect and then monitor the valvar and subaortic velocities postoperatively. A small proportion of patients, less than 5 %, may develop a gradient within the first few months of life. They should be treated secondarily with a Ross-Konno procedure when the gradient warrants this surgery.

A review of 112 patients with repaired IAA from as early as 1985 found that there was a higher risk of arch obstruction and subsequent re-intervention in patients who required reoperation for LVOT obstruction [18]. This is likely related to the physiology described previously, where the restriction of blood flow through the LVOT obstruction causes underdevelopment of left-sided structures, including the aorta, and correlates with more significant disease.

Other Postoperative Issues

Patients with 22q11- deletion ought to be carefully managed with regard to metabolic disturbances and especially concerning the risks for persistent hypocalcemia; more often than not, these patients need a continuous infusion of calcium chloride in the postoperative phase and replacement therapy afterwards.

Outcomes of Surgery

Early Survival

Hospital mortality for neonatal IAA repair in the current era is approximately 7–10 % [18, 20, 27]. Reported risk factors for early mortality include preoperative complications [28], earlier year of surgery with better survival for those undergoing primary repair rather than palliation [28], and lack of VSD closure [18].

Late Survival

Overall late survival of IAA can range from 47 % to 94 % [14, 17, 18, 20, 21, 27, 29]. One hundred and twelve patients with IAA from the Royal Children's Hospital, Melbourne, were reviewed recently [18]. Eighty-five percent of patients had undergone end-to-side repair. Hospital survivors achieved an 18-year survival of 92 %. It was also found that the 18-year survival after end-to-side repair was 97 %, while it was 74 % after other procedures. These figures are far more favorable than the 16-year overall survival of 59 % found in the Congenital Heart Surgeons Society study of 472 neonates with IAA [17]. Although many have shown improvement of overall mortality with time [17, 27], they are yet to reach the outcomes obtained by the Royal Children's Hospital, which should serve as a benchmark for other institutions.

Reported risk factors for mortality include low birth weight, outlet and trabecular VSD, subaortic narrowing, Damus-Kaye-Stansel procedure, and subaortic myotomy or myectomy for subaortic stenosis [14].

Arch Re-Obstruction and Re-Intervention

Arch re-obstruction and arch re-intervention are common following IAA repair with the largest series reporting that after 16 years, 28 % of patients required an arch re-intervention [17], while the Royal Children's Hospital, Melbourne, series showed an 18-year freedom from re-obstruction and re-invention rate of 78 % and 69 %, respectively [18]. The Royal Children's Hospital also demonstrated that patients with an aberrant right subclavian artery, those operated on with a procedure other than end-to-side anastomosis, and those needing further relief of LVOT obstruction had higher chances of recurrent arch obstruction. Specifically, the 18-year freedom from arch re-intervention after end-to-side repair was 78 %, while the LCATD study reported a 15-year freedom from arch re-intervention of only 57 % [21].

There is still debate regarding the best method of treating the arch re-obstruction. The Royal Children's Hospital study reported that 19 patients required an arch re-intervention. Eleven patients underwent balloon dilatation of the arch and one underwent balloon dilatation and stenting, only to have three of these procedures fail and the patients requiring surgery. Seven patients were sent directly to surgery.

Hypertension

Although there are increasing concerns regarding late occurrence of systemic hypertension in patients who have undergone coarctation repair, there is very little information known regarding the incidence of hypertension among patients undergoing repair of interrupted aortic arch [30, 31]. In the series of 112 patients with IAA, 92 were followed, and only five patients were found to have resting hypertension at last follow-up [18]. The 18-year freedom from resting hypertension was 88 %.

The prevalence of hypertension may be underestimated as resting blood pressure measurements have a lower sensitivity than 24-h ambulatory blood pressure monitoring [32, 33]. Studies investigating the prevalence of hypertension using 24-h ambulatory blood pressure monitoring after IAA repair and its effects are warranted.

Long-Term Follow-Up

Patients who have undergone IAA repair must be followed up for the entirety of life. In particular, annual 24-h ambulatory blood pressure monitoring after approximately 10 years of age when the child can tolerate the investigation for a 24-h period and echocardiogram imaging including measurements of the aortic arch and conversion to z-score, and Doppler measurement of the peak gradient across the repaired section of the arch, should be mandatory for these patients, as these tests are more sensitive than resting blood pressure measurements and clinical limb gradient assessment, respectively.

References

1. Steidele R (1778) Samml chir med beob, Vol. 2. Vienna, p 114
2. Seidel J (1818) Index musei anatomici kiliensis. CF Mohr, Kiel, p 61
3. Weisman D, Kesten HD (1948) Absence of transverse aortic arch with defects of cardiac septums; report of a case simulating acute abdominal disease in a newborn infant. Am J Dis Child 76:326–330
4. Celoria GC, Patton RB (1959) Congenital absence of the aortic arch. Am Heart J 58:407–413
5. Merrill DL, Webster CA, Samson PC (1957) Congenital absence of the aortic isthmus; report of a case with successful surgical repair. J Thorac Surg 33:311–320
6. Barratt-Boyes BG, Nicholls TT, Brandt PW et al (1972) Aortic arch interruption associated with patent ductus arteriosus, ventricular septal defect, and total anomalous pulmonary venous connection. Total correction in an 8-day-old infant by means of profound hypothermia and limited cardiopulmonary bypass. J Thorac Cardiovasc Surg 63:367–373
7. Trusler GA, Izukawa T (1975) Interrupted aortic arch and ventricular septal defect. Direct repair through a median sternotomy incision in a 13-day-old infant. J Thorac Cardiovasc Surg 69:126–131
8. Elliott RB, Starling MB, Neutze JM (1975) Medical manipulation of the ductus arteriosus. Lancet 1:140–142
9. Collins-Nakai RL, Dick M, Parisi-Buckley L et al (1976) Interrupted aortic arch in infancy. J Pediatr 88:959–962
10. Fyler D, Buckley D, Hellendrand W et al (1980) Report of the New England Regional Infant Cardiac Program. Pediatrics 65:375–461
11. Van Praagh R, Bernhard WF, Rosenthal A et al (1971) Interrupted aortic arch: surgical treatment. Am J Cardiol 27:200–211
12. Goo HW, Park IS, Ko JK et al (2005) Computed tomography for the diagnosis of congenital heart disease in pediatric and adult patients. Int J Cardiovasc Imaging 21:347–365; discussion 67
13. Sirak HD, Ressallat M, Hosier DM et al (1968) A new operation for repairing aortic arch atresia in infancy. Report of three cases. Circulation 37:II43–II50
14. Jonas RA, Quaegebeur JM, Kirklin JW et al (1994) Outcomes in patients with interrupted aortic arch and ventricular septal defect. A multiinstitutional study. Congenital Heart Surgeons Society. J Thorac Cardiovasc Surg 107:1099–1109
15. Tlaskal T, Chaloupecky V, Marek J et al (1997) Primary repair of interrupted aortic arch and associated heart lesions in newborns. J Cardiovasc Surg 38:113–118
16. Serraf A, Lacour-Gayet F, Robotin M et al (1996) Repair of interrupted aortic arch: a ten-year experience. J Thorac Cardiovasc Surg 112:1150–1160
17. McCrindle BW, Tchervenkov CI, Konstantinov IE et al (2005) Risk factors associated with mortality and interventions in 472 neonates with interrupted aortic arch: a Congenital Heart Surgeons Society study. J Thorac Cardiovasc Surg 129:343–350
18. Hussein A, Iyengar AJ, Jones B et al (2010) Twenty-three years of single-stage end-to-side anastomosis repair of interrupted aortic arches. J Thorac Cardiovasc Surg 139:942–947, 49; discussion 48
19. Tlaskal T, Hucin B, Kostelka M et al (1998) Successful reoperation for severe left bronchus compression after repair of persistent truncus arteriosus with interrupted aortic arch. Eur J Cardiothorac Surg 13:306–309
20. Brown JW, Ruzmetov M, Okada Y et al (2006) Outcomes in patients with interrupted aortic arch and associated anomalies: a 20-year experience. Eur J Cardiothorac Surg 29:666–673; discussion 73–4
21. Todman SH, Eltayeb O, Ruzmetov M et al (2013) Outcomes of interrupted aortic arch repair using the carotid artery turndown procedure. J Thorac Cardiovasc Surg 145:176–182
22. Bohuta L, Hussein A, Fricke TA et al (2011) Surgical repair of Truncus Arteriosus associated with interrupted aortic arch: long-term outcomes. Ann Thorac Surg 91:1473–1477
23. Yasui H, Kado H, Nakano E et al (1987) Primary repair of interrupted aortic arch and severe aortic stenosis in neonates. J Thorac Cardiovasc Surg 93:539–545
24. Luciani GB, Ackerman RJ, Chang AC et al (1996) One-stage repair of interrupted aortic arch, ventricular septal defect, and subaortic obstruction in the neonate: a novel approach. J Thorac Cardiovasc Surg 111:348–358
25. Jacobs ML, Chin AJ, Rychik J et al (1995) Interrupted aortic arch. Impact of subaortic stenosis on management and outcome. Circulation 92:II128–II131
26. Watanabe T, Tajima K, Sakai Y et al (1998) Everting closure for interrupted aortic arch, ventricular septal defect, and severe subaortic stenosis. Thorac Cardiovasc Surg 46:33–36
27. Morales DL, Scully PT, Braud BE et al (2006) Interrupted aortic arch repair: aortic arch advancement without a patch minimizes arch reinterventions. Ann Thorac Surg 82:1577–1583; discussion 83–4
28. Tlaskal T, Hucin B, Hruda J et al (1998) Results of primary and two-stage repair of interrupted aortic arch. Eur J Cardiothorac Surg 14:235–242
29. Sell JE, Jonas RA, Mayer JE et al (1988) The results of a surgical program for interrupted aortic arch. J Thorac Cardiovasc Surg 96:864–877
30. Hager A, Kanz S, Kaemmerer H et al (2007) Coarctation Long-term Assessment (COALA): significance of arterial hypertension in a cohort of 404 patients up to 27 years after surgical repair of isolated coarctation of the aorta, even in the absence of restenosis and prosthetic material. J Thorac Cardiovasc Surg 134:738–745

31. Ou P, Celermajer DS, Mousseaux E et al (2007) Vascular remodeling after "successful" repair of coarctation: impact of aortic arch geometry. J Am Coll Cardiol 49:883–890

32. Lee MG, Kowalski R, Galati JC et al (2012) Twenty-four-hour ambulatory blood pressure monitoring detects a high prevalence of hypertension late after coarctation repair in patients with hypoplastic arches. J Thorac Cardiovasc Surg 144:1110–1116

33. O'Sullivan JJ, Derrick G, Darnell R (2002) Prevalence of hypertension in children after early repair of coarctation of the aorta: a cohort study using casual and 24 h blood pressure measurement. Heart 88:163–166

Supramitral Stenosis

95

David Kalfa and Emile Bacha

Abstract

This chapter discusses the three main etiologies of supramitral stenosis: *cor triatriatum*, *supravalvar mitral ring*, and *coronary sinus obstruction*. These are characterized by similar hemodynamic and clinical patterns, related to pulmonary hypertension, venous obstruction, and limited left heart output. These entities are rare and most commonly associated with other congenital heart diseases, especially obstructive left-sided lesions. Their embryologic and anatomic features differ from each other and underlie their characteristics in terms of imaging and treatment. The surgical repair of these anomalies can be considered curative, and long-term prognostic is excellent.

Keywords

Accessory chamber • Atrial approach • Circumflex coronary artery • Cor triatriatum • Coronary sinus obstruction • Embryology • Endocardial cushion tissue • Left atrial appendage • Left atrium • Mitral valve • Normothermic cardiopulmonary bypass • Persistent left superior vena cava • Pulmonary hypertension • Pulmonary veins • Pulmonary venous obstruction • Supramitral ridge • Supramitral stenosis • Supravalvar mitral ring • Unroofed coronary sinus

Introduction

This chapter discusses the left atrial-level obstructive congenital malformations leading to supramitral stenosis. These lesions include *cor triatriatum*, *supravalvar mitral ring*, and *coronary sinus obstruction*.

In *cor triatriatum*, the pulmonary veins enter an accessory chamber that joins the left atrium through a narrow opening (Fig. 95.1). The prevalence of this rare disease is around 0.1–0.5 % of congenital heart patients [1] and is diagnosed more frequently in infancy than in adulthood [2–5].

The *supravalvar ring* is a fibrous ring situated just on the left atrial side of the mitral annulus and is often in continuity with the mitral valve

D. Kalfa (✉) • E. Bacha
Congenital and Pediatric Cardiac Surgery, Columbia University, Morgan Stanley Children's Hospital of New York-Presbyterian, New York, NY, USA
e-mail: eb2709@columbia.edu

Fig. 95.1 Echocardiography of supravalvar mitral ring. Note flow disturbance above mitral annulus

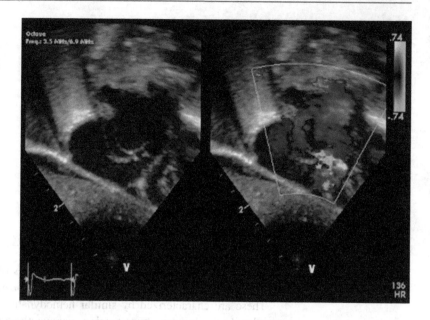

leaflets [6] (Fig. 95.2). The left atrial appendage enters the left atrium proximal to the ring, in contrast to the situation in cor triatriatum. Such an isolated congenital mitral valve disease is rare too, occurring in 0.4–0.6 % of congenital heart patients [7, 8], fewer than 100 cases having been reported in literature according to a recent review [9]. Supravalvar rings are a congenital heart abnormality, but postoperative "acquired" and recurrent progressive forms have been described [10, 11].

Finally, supramitral stenosis can also be a hemodynamic consequence of a *dilated coronary sinus*, related to a *persistent left superior vena cava*, creating a funnel-like obstruction onto the posterior atrial wall [12] (Fig. 95.3). Most left superior vena cava does not have such hemodynamic consequences, making this entity rare as well.

Myxoma of the left atrium that can cause supramitral stenosis will be discussed in another chapter.

Brief Historical Background

Church described the first cor triatriatum in 1868 [13]. Borst applied the name "cor triatriatum" for the first time in 1905 [14]. Vineberg and Gialloreto performed the first surgical correction 50 years later [15].

The first supramitral ring was described in 1902 by Fischer et al. [16]. Surgery of congenital mitral valve diseases started in the late 1950s [17].

Anatomy

Cor Triatriatum

Cor triatriatum and its variants seem to result from an incomplete absorption of the embryological common pulmonary vein into the left atrium. The classic cor triatriatum (cor triatriatum sinister) is characterized by a fibromembranous septum between an accessory atrial chamber ("proximal chamber," thick walled, receiving the pulmonary veins) and the left atrium ("distal chamber," thin walled, containing the mitral valve and left atrial appendage) [18]. The shape of this membrane, the size of the opening between the 2 chambers, the severity of hemodynamic stenosis, and the location and size of the foramen ovale are highly variable [2]. Figure 95.4 summarizes the anatomic classification of cor triatriatum by Van Praagh et al. [19].

Isolated forms of cor triatriatum are probably less common than cor triatriatum associated with other congenital heart malformations, such as atrial septal defect, partial or total anomalous pulmonary venous return [20, 21], persistent left

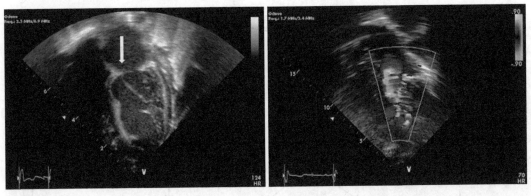

Fig. 95.2 Echocardiography of complex mitral valve disease. Note small mitral valve annulus and large left superior vena cava

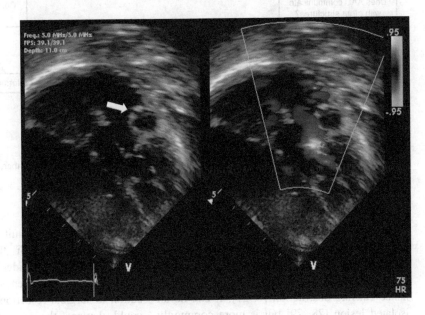

Fig. 95.3 Echocardiography of cor triatriatum

superior vena cava, ventricular septal defect, coarctation of the aorta, atrioventricular canal, transposition of great arteries [22], tetralogy of Fallot [1, 5, 18], or non-compaction of the left ventricle [23]. Microscopically, the membrane of cor triatriatum is a bilaminar muscular structure.

Supravalvar Mitral Ring

The embryologic origin of this rare disease is different from that one of cor triatriatum, since it could result from incomplete division of endocardial cushion tissue [24]. Its microscopical structure (a dense layer of sclerotic structure comparable to valve substrate) is thus different from the membrane of cor triatriatum [25]. This fibromembranous disc situated just proximal to the mitral annulus or valve leaflets is caused by accumulations of connective tissue that arise from the atrial surface of the mitral leaflets. The left atrial appendage enters the left atrium

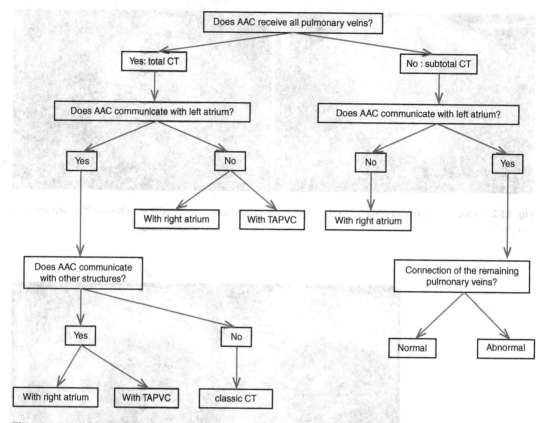

Fig. 95.4 Anatomic classification of cor triatriatum (CT). *AAC* accessory atrial chamber, *TAPVC* total anomalous pulmonary venous connection

proximal to the ring, in contrast to the situation in cor triatriatum. The ring is said supravalvar but often partially involves the mitral valve leaflets [26], preventing adequate opening of the leaflets, hence causing obstruction [6, 27]. It can be an isolated lesion [28, 29] but is more commonly associated with other obstructive left heart anomalies, such as parachute mitral valve, subvalvar or valvar aortic stenosis, or coarctation of the aorta [29–33], and less commonly with right-sided lesions (pulmonary stenosis and tetralogy of Fallot) [34–36]. Supravalvar mitral ring was classically described as one of the features of Shone's syndrome [33].

The supravalvar ring should be differentiated from another extremely rare supramitral structure: the *supramitral ridge*. This ridge consists of an isolated invagination of left atrial free wall immediately proximal to the mitral valve

and can mimic a supramitral ring. Nevertheless, and in contrast with the three previously described lesions, this ridge does not cause hemodynamic supramitral stenosis and is a contraindication to surgical resection; as such, a resection could damage the coronary vessel contained within the invaginated atrioventricular sulcus tissue.

Coronary Sinus Obstruction

This entity is directly related to the persistence of the left superior vena cava with coronary sinus dilation and posterior atrial wall deformation producing a funnel-like obstruction. The mitral valve and subvalvar apparatus are usually completely normal. Nevertheless, persistent left superior vena cava can be associated with left ventricular outflow tract obstruction and secondary subaortic stenosis [37].

Physiology and Pathophysiology

Obstruction of pulmonary venous return to the left atrium is the key hemodynamic feature of supramitral stenosis, whatever its anatomic substrate. Left atrial, pulmonary venous, and capillary pressures rise. Increased pulmonary venous pressure leads to pulmonary hypertension and attendant right heart failure and adversely affects mechanical and gas-exchanging properties of the lung. The severity of obstruction depends on multiple factors: the size of the fenestration in the membrane of cor triatriatum; location and width of the supramitral ring; presence, location, and size of an atrial septal defect; and associated cardiac lesions. Left atrial dilation, stretch, and progressive fibrosis are arrhythmogenic. Irreversible histological consequences of pulmonary hypertension, common in patients with left-to-right shunts, usually do not occur in children with supramitral stenosis [38]. Pulmonary hypertension related to congenital heart defects in children tends to resolve postoperatively less rapidly than in acquired diseases [39, 40].

Diagnosis

Clinical

The clinical presentation of patients with supramitral obstruction depends on the degree of stenosis and the growth rate of the patients [32, 41, 42]. In severe supramitral obstruction, symptoms and signs of low cardiac output predominate [43]: tachypnea, dyspnea, growth failure, and diminished peripheral perfusion and pulses [44]. Symptoms and signs of pulmonary venous obstruction and pulmonary overflow are usually associated (especially in the case of cor triatriatum with associated large ASD or total anomalous pulmonary venous connections): exhaustion at feeding, diaphoresis, pulmonary infections, loud second heart sound, right ventricular heave, and pulmonary systolic ejection click. Classic symptoms of postcapillary pulmonary hypertension can occur in children and young adults. Most patients with classic cor triatriatum

have onset of symptoms within the first few years of life. Nonetheless, some patients are asymptomatic until the second or third decade of life. Classic murmurs (systolic murmur of pulmonary overflow or mid-diastolic murmur at the mitral area) can be absent. Cor triatriatum can be misdiagnosed as chronic lung disease. Supravalvar ring can be completely asymptomatic and incidentally discovered by echocardiography or during surgery for other lesions.

Electrocardiography

ECG is nonspecific, displaying right ventricular and right atrial hypertrophy more frequently than left atrial hypertrophy.

Imaging

The chest X-ray is nonspecific for these entities. Cardiomegaly, pulmonary edema, pleural effusions, and pulmonary artery enlargement may be seen. A dilated accessory atrial chamber cannot be differentiated from an enlarged left atrium in other mitral stenosis.

Progress in echocardiography has improved the noninvasive diagnosis and evaluation of supramitral stenosis, making invasive imaging rarely necessary, unless major associated cardiac anomalies are suspected. Echocardiographic characteristics of the different types of supramitral stenosis are summarized in Table 95.1.

In all cases, mitral valve and subvalvar apparatus are normal, and venous obstruction can lead to dilation of right cavities and the pulmonary artery. Pulsed and color-flow Doppler can estimate the pressure gradient. A supravalvar ring should be suspected when the Doppler signal suggests turbulence beginning above the valve annulus. Transesophageal, 3D echocardiography [45], and contrast echocardiography can also be used to precise anatomy of supramitral stenosis, especially cor triatriatum in adults [46]. Supravalvar ring may be difficult to diagnose by transthoracic echocardiography; transesophageal echocardiography is particularly useful in the diagnosis.

Table 95.1 Echocardiographic characteristics of the different types of supramitral stenosis

Cor triatriatum	Supravalvar ring	Coronary sinus obstruction
Presence of a membrane = linear echo structure in the left atrium, above the mitral valve		No membrane
Curvilinear membrane, "wind sock"	At the base of MV leaflets	Dilation of the coronary sinus
Mobile: moves towards the mitral valve in diastole	Immobile or moves away from the valve in diastole	Immobile
Left atrial appendage: distal to the membrane	Left atrial appendage: proximal to the membrane	

Cardiac catheterization is not routinely necessary, unless the diagnosis is uncertain or major associated cardiac defects are suspected. It can demonstrate elevated pulmonary artery and pulmonary wedge pressures and a pressure gradient proximally and distally to the membrane/ring.

Other imaging modalities such as magnetic resonance imaging and computed tomography are less sensitive than echocardiography.

Decision Making

Cor Triatriatum

In cor triatriatum, an urgent operation is indicated in the following cases:

- Classic cor triatriatum with a restrictive connection between the two chambers associated with significant pulmonary hypertension in neonates or infants, as soon as the diagnosis is established, to avoid mortality in infancy. Without surgical treatment, 75 % of patients born with cor triatriatum die in infancy [47].
- Classic cor triatriatum with chronic symptoms in older patients.
- Atypical cor triatriatum with severe symptoms related to a restrictive patent foramen ovale in the neonatal period or infancy.

Supravalvar Ring and Coronary Sinus Obstruction

A semi-urgent operation is indicated in patients with symptoms or signs of pulmonary venous obstruction or hemodynamic documented pulmonary hypertension.

Medical Management

The treatment of such lesions is surgical by definition. In the patient with pulmonary edema or right heart failure, the usual medical management should be instituted, focused on the relief of symptoms and optimization of tissue perfusion and respiratory status. Particular attention ought to be paid to the prevention and management of arrhythmias. Any vasodilator or excessive afterload reduction should be avoided. Patients with these entities may tolerate respiratory infections rather poorly and may therefore need intensive care management in this context.

Surgical Management

Cor Triatriatum

Surgical excision of the cor triatriatum membrane under cardiopulmonary bypass is usually curative. This simple procedure has to be adapted to the intraoperative findings regarding the location of the membrane, the location and size of the atrial septal defect, and potential associated anomalous pulmonary venous connections and left superior vena cava. A right atrial approach is preferred in infants and small children, especially when the accessory atrial chamber is not enlarged. The enlargement of the right atrium related to a left-to-right shunt can make this surgical approach even easier. In larger patients with an enlarged accessory chamber, an incision of the right side of this chamber can allow the surgeon to perform the procedure. Before opening the heart, the drainage of all pulmonary and systemic veins and the presence or not of a left superior vena cava should always be checked. Moderate hypothermic or normothermic cardiopulmonary bypass using two venous cannulae is usually used; brief periods of low flow perfusion in hypothermic cardiopulmonary bypass can be used to optimize exposure in the smallest patients. When the right atrial approach is preferred, the first step is to enlarge the atrial septal defect in order to provide access to the left atrium. Then, the surgeon must check whether the accessory or main left atrial chamber has been entered, knowing that the accessory chamber contains the pulmonary venous orifices and the main left chamber, the mitral valve, and left atrial appendage. The second step is to resect the membrane, after having localized the hole within it and enlarged it for exposure of the adjacent structures than can be damaged during the resection of the membrane (orifice of the left inferior pulmonary vein and mitral valve). All pulmonary veins should be identified. The resection of the membrane should always be as large as possible. The opening in the atrial septum is then closed with a patch, taking care of a potential unroofed coronary sinus in case of a persistent left superior vena cava. When the left atrial approach is preferred, the accessory atrial chamber is opened through a vertical incision anterior to the right pulmonary veins, as for other mitral valve surgery, As through the right atrial approach, the positions of the hole within the membrane, the pulmonary veins, the mitral valve, and the atrial septum are identified, and the membrane is resected carefully. The right atrium should always be opened to ascertain the anatomy of the lesions. The remainder of the operation is completed in the usual fashion. This general surgical approach can be associated to treatment of associated potential lesions, such as repair of partial or total anomalous pulmonary venous connections or repair of unroofed coronary sinus syndrome.

Percutaneous balloon dilation using a double balloon technique [48] has been proposed, but is not the treatment of choice that remains surgical resection of the membrane as described above.

Supravalvar Ring

Cardiopulmonary bypass is conducted with moderate hypothermia or normothermia, using two venous cannulae. The left atrial approach is usually used: the left atrium is opened through a vertical incision anterior to the right pulmonary veins after limited dissection of the atrioventricular groove. Exposure of the mitral valve is enhanced with mattress sutures placed above each commissure and by insertion of an appropriately sized retractor or similar instrument. The surgical treatment consists in resecting the supravalvar membrane very carefully. In case of a large supravalvar mitral ring, the restrictive orifice has first to be identified, and stay sutures can be inserted in the membrane to apply traction and reveal the dissection plan between the ring and the mitral leaflet tissue. Such stay sutures are to be avoided in case of very thin and fragile ring in infants and small children. The initial incision is made perpendicularly to the mitral annulus and then extended to the level of the mitral annulus without damaging it. This initial incision is classically made above the anterior leaflet of the mitral valve for exposure reasons and to avoid damage to the circumflex coronary artery [49]. The whole membrane is then excised using blunt dissection in order to avoid damage to the underlying mitral valve tissue and the circumflex coronary artery. If the membrane is completely adherent to the mitral tissue, the procedure should be performed in two steps rather than damaging the mitral tissue. A systematic preoperative analysis of the mitral valve should always be performed, and significant associated congenital or iatrogenic mitral valve lesions should be treated. The finding of an eccentric anterolateral nonfibrous thickening directly proximal to the mitral valve can correspond to the differential diagnosis of supramitral ridge, which is a contraindication to surgery.

Coronary Sinus Obstruction

The surgical correction of an obstructive coronary sinus consists in resecting the roof of the dilated coronary sinus. This procedure requires adequate exposure either through a left atriotomy or a right atriotomy with enlargement of the atrial septal defect. A longitudinal incision is made in the enlarged sinus, and a segment of the wall can be excised. A probe can be passed from the coronary sinus ostium in right atrium to prevent stenosis of the coronary sinus during re-suture of the wall. The procedure of ligation of the left superior vena cava has been described but can be considered acceptable only in the case of small left superior vena cava and satisfactory innominate vein [12].

Postoperative Management

General principles of postoperative management should be followed and include particular attention to lung inflation, atrial arrhythmias, and the presence and early treatment of pulmonary hypertension. Patients usually progress towards extubation on a fast-track fashion and ought to be kept comfortable and free of pain with opioids and benzodiazepines as required, associated with non-opioid analgesia. Selected patients may benefit from an infusion of dexmedetomidine titrated to minimal efficient doses. Inotropic support, if needed, usually associates milrinone and low-dose dopamine. Hemodynamic instability or de novo arrhythmias should raise suspicion for the potential of coronary artery anomalies acquired during the intervention. Transesophageal echocardiography is helpful to determine adequacy of repair, status of ventricular function, and degree and presence of pulmonary hypertension. It is prudent to have nitric oxide available in the operating room. A left atrial pressure catheter could be placed at the time of operation in most severe patients.

Furthermore, atrial pacing wires are helpful in the diagnosis and treatment of atrial arrhythmias.

Early mobilization and nutritional support are crucial for a prompt convalescence.

Complications

Cor Triatriatum

Complications that can occur after surgical correction of cor triatriatum are related to:

- Residual lesions: nonoptimal resection of the membrane, residual atrial septal defect
- Iatrogenic lesions of the adjacent structures: mitral valve damage, rupture of the free atrial wall, hemorrhagic syndrome

- Atrial surgery: air embolism, supraventricular arrhythmias
- Pathophysiology: crises of pulmonary hypertension

Hospital deaths are uncommon after repair of classic cor triatriatum and are usually related to associated cardiac conditions in atypical cor triatriatum.

Supravalvular Mitral Ring and Coronary Sinus Obstruction

Surgical repair of these diseases can be complicated with residual intra-atrial gradient, perforation of the mitral valve leaflets, lesions of the circumflex coronary artery, air embolism, supraventricular arrhythmias, and crises of pulmonary hypertension.

Outcomes and Long-Term Follow-Up

Cor Triatriatum

Small series from the early 1990s reported a mortality rate between 8 % and 20 % [50–53]. Most reported deaths occurred in the youngest and most symptomatic patients and in atypical forms associated with other cardiac anomalies. In the current area, hospital deaths are uncommon after repair of isolated cor triatriatum, even in critically ill infants [54]. An early correction of classic cor triatriatum results in a life expectancy that approaches that of general population [52]. The severe pulmonary arterial changes that result in pulmonary hypertension have been reversible in the patients studied postoperatively. Long-term postoperative occurrence of pulmonary vein stenosis has been described and emphasizes the similar embryologic origin of both diseases [55]. Another long-term adverse event is the restenosis of the orifice between the two chambers, directly related to a nonoptimal original surgical procedure [56].

Supravalvular Mitral Ring

Hospital deaths are uncommon after resection of a supramitral valvar ring and are most commonly related to complex associated left heart lesions or comorbidities [26]. Complete relief of the diastolic gradient can be obtained after surgical repair of supravalvar ring, in contrast with other forms of mitral stenosis [40, 57, 58]. Recurrent or progressive forms of supravalvar ring have been described [10, 11], especially when a potential underlying anatomic anomaly (such as a preeminent coronary sinus) is left untreated. The "intramitral ring" is associated with a worse outcome compared to "supramitral ring" [11].

Conclusion

Supramitral stenosis, in its three main forms, is currently successfully managed surgically, with low morbidity and mortality. These anomalies may remain undiagnosed for years which may increase the perioperative risks in patients with progressive and unrevealed pulmonary hypertension. After repair, patients require a long-term follow-up for the possibility of recurrent obstruction, evolving pulmonary vein stenosis, and to document progression of associated cardiac anomalies.

References

1. Krasemann Z, Scheld IIII, Tjan TD et al (2007) Cor triatriatum: short review of the literature upon ten new cases. Herz 32:506–510
2. Niwayama G (1960) Cor triatriatum. Am Heart J 59:291–317
3. Udovicic M, Biocic S, Vincelj J et al (2012) Tetralogy of fallot with cor triatriatum dexter in an adult patient: a case report. Congenit Heart Dis. doi:10.1111/j
4. Vallakati A, Nerella N, Chandra P et al (2012) Incidental diagnosis of cor triatriatum in 2 elderly patients. J Am Coll Cardiol 59(22):e43
5. Van Praagh R, Corsini I (1969) Cor triatriatum: pathologic anatomy and a consideration of morphogenesis based on 13 postmortem cases and a study of normal development of the pulmonary vein and atrial septum in 83 human embryos. Am Heart J 78(3):379–405
6. Anabtawi IN, Ellison RG (1965) Congenital stenosing ring of the left atrioventricular canal (supravalvular mitral stenosis). J Thorac Cardiovasc Surg 49:994–1005
7. Hoffman JI, Kaplan S (2002) The incidence of congenital heart disease. J Am Coll Cardiol 39(12):1890–1900
8. Magovern JH, Moore GW, Hutchins GM (1986) Development of the atrioventricular valve region in the human embryo. Anat Rec 215(2):167–181
9. Mychaskiw G 2nd, Sachdev V, Braden DA et al (2002) Supramitral ring: an unusual cause of

10. Martin RP, Qureshi SA, Radley-Smith R (1987) Acquired supravalvar membranous stenosis of the left atrioventricular valve. Br Heart J 58(2):176–178
11. Toscano A, Pasquini L, Iacobelli R et al (2009) Congenital supravalvar mitral ring: an underestimated anomaly. J Thorac Cardiovasc Surg 137(3):538–542
12. Cochrane AD, Marath A, Mee RB (1994) Can a dilated coronary sinus produce left ventricular inflow obstruction? An unrecognized entity. Ann Thorac Surg 58(4):1114–1116
13. Church W (1967/1968) Congenital malformation of the heart: abnormal septum in left auricle. Trans Pathol Soc Lond 19:188
14. Borst H (1905) Ein cor tratriatum. Zentralbl Allg Pathol 16:812
15. Vineberg A, Gialloreto O (1956) Report of a successful operation for stenosis of common pulmonary vein (cor triatriatum). Can Med Assoc J 74(9):719–723
16. Fischer T (1902) Two cases of congenital disease of the left side of the heart. Br Med J 1:639
17. Starkey GW (1959) Surgical experiences in the treatment of congenital mitral stenosis and mitral insufficiency. J Thorac Cardiovasc Surg 38:336–352
18. Marin-Garcia J, Tandon R, Lucas RV Jr et al (1975) Cor triatriatum: study of 20 cases. Am J Cardiol 35(1):59–66
19. Geva T, van Praagh S (2008) Anomalies of the pulmonary veins. In: Moss A, Allen H (eds) Moss and Adams' heart disease in infants, children, and adolescents. Lippincott Williams & Wilkins, Philadelphia
20. Edwin F, Gyan B, Tettey M et al (2012) Divided left atrium (cor triatriatum) in the setting of common atrium. Ann Thorac Surg 94(2):e49–e50
21. Gonzalez-Ramirez N, Castillo-Castellon F, Kimura-Hayama E (2012) Cor triatriatum sinister versus bowed septum primum in an infant with total anomalous pulmonary venous connection: a difficult imaging distinction. Pediatr Radiol 42(10):1254–1258
22. Gupta SK, Saxena A (2012) Cor triatriatum sinister with an atrial septal defect: an unusual cause of lutembacher physiology. Pediatr Cardiol. 2012 Oct 25. [Epub ahead of print]
23. Singh N, Aga P, Singh R et al (2013) Non-compaction of the left ventricular myocardium with Cor-triatriatum and associated anomalies. BMJ Case Rep. [Epub ahead of print]
24. Srinivasan V, Lewin AN, Pieroni D et al (1980) Supravalvular stenosing ring of the left atrium: case report and review of the literature. Cardiovasc Dis 7(2):149–158
25. Oglietti J, Reul GJ Jr, Leachman RD et al (1976) Supravalvular stenosing ring of the left atrium. Ann Thorac Surg 21(5):421–424
26. Collison SP, Kaushal SK, Dagar KS et al (2006) Supramitral ring: good prognosis in a subset

of patients with congenital mitral stenosis. Ann Thorac Surg 81(3):997–1001

27. Davichi FMJ, Edwards JE (1971) Diseases of the mitral valve in infancy. Circulation 43:565

28. Chung KJ, Manning JA, Lipchik EO et al (1974) Isolated supravalvular stenosing ring of left atrium: diagnosis before operation and successful surgical treatment. Chest 65(1):25–28

29. Sullivan ID, Robinson PJ, de Leval M et al (1986) Membranous supravalvular mitral stenosis: a treatable form of congenital heart disease. J Am Coll Cardiol 8(1):159–164

30. Moller H (1974) Congenital causes of left ventricular inflow obstruction. In: Edwards JE (ed) The heart. Williams & Wilkins, Baltimore

31. Otsuji Y, Handschumacher MD, Liel-Cohen N et al (2001) Mechanism of ischemic mitral regurgitation with segmental left ventricular dysfunction: three-dimensional echocardiographic studies in models of acute and chronic progressive regurgitation. J Am Coll Cardiol 37(2):641–648

32. Ruckman RN, Van Praagh R (1978) Anatomic types of congenital mitral stenosis: report of 49 autopsy cases with consideration of diagnosis and surgical implications. Am J Cardiol 42(4):592–601

33. Shone JD, Sellers RD, Anderson RC et al (1963) The developmental complex of "parachute mitral valve," supravalvular ring of left atrium, subaortic stenosis, and coarctation of aorta. Am J Cardiol 11:714–725

34. Benry J, Leachman RD, Cooley DA et al (1976) Supravalvular mitral stenosis associated with tetralogy of Fallot. Am J Cardiol 37(1):111–114

35. Gupta SK, Ramakrishnan S, Doshi S (2012) Cor-triatriatum: an unusual cause of elevated pulmonary capillary wedge pressure in a child with tetralogy of fallot. Catheter Cardiovasc Interv. 2012 Nov 21. [Epub ahead of print]

36. Horn ARJK, Tamer DM (1968) Supravalvular mitral stenosis in a patient with tetralogy of Fallot. Am J Cardiol 22:733–737

37. Kalfa D, Ghez O, Kreitmann B et al (2007) Secondary subaortic stenosis in heart defects without any initial subaortic obstruction: a multifactorial postoperative event. Eur J Cardiothorac Surg 32(4):582–587

38. Endo M, Yamaki S, Ohmi M et al (2000) Pulmonary vascular changes induced by congenital obstruction of pulmonary venous return. Ann Thorac Surg 69(1):193–197

39. Benmimoun EG, Friedli B, Rutishauser W et al (1982) Mitral valve replacement in children. Comparative study of pre- and postoperative haemodynamics and left ventricular function. Br Heart J 48(2):117–124

40. Collins-Nakai RL, Rosenthal A, Castaneda AR et al (1977) Congenital mitral stenosis. A review of 20 years' experience. Circulation 56(6):1039–1047

41. Baylen BG, Joyce JJ (2005) Congestive heart failure in infants and children. In: Osborne LM, DeWitt DT,

First LR et al (eds) Pediatrics. Elsevier, Mosby, Philadelphia

42. Daoud G, Kaplan S, Perrin EV et al (1963) Congenital mitral stenosis. Circulation 27:185–196

43. Mendez AB, Colchero T, Garcia-Picart J et al (2013) Unusual case of new-onset heart failure due to cor triatriatum sinister. Eur J Heart Fail 15(2):237–239

44. Weinik AC, Gittenberger-de Goot AC, Brom AG (1986) Developmental considerations of mitral valve anomalies. Int J Cardiol 11:85

45. Seguela PE, Leobon B, Acar P (2013) Three-dimensional transthoracic echocardiographic assessment of supramitral ring in a young child. Cardiol Young 9:1–4

46. Einav E, Perk G, Kronzon I (2008) Three-dimensional transthoracic echocardiographic evaluation of cor triatriatum. Eur J Echocardiogr 9(1):110–112

47. Kouchoukos N, Blackstone E, Hanley F et al (2012) Cor triatriatum. In: Kirklin JW, Barratt-Boyes BG (eds) Cardiac surgery. Churchill Livingstone, New York

48. Kerkar P, Vora A, Kulkarni H et al (1996) Percutaneous balloon dilatation of cor triatriatum sinister. Am Heart J 132(4):888–891

49. Konstantinovi YT, Calderone C, Coles JG (2004) Supramitral obstruction of left ventricular inflow tract by supramitral ring. Oper Tech Thorac Cardiovasc Surg 9:47–251

50. Muhiudeen-Russell IA, Silverman NH (1997) Images in cardiovascular medicine. Cor triatriatum in an infant. Circulation 95:2700

51. Rodefeld MD, Brown JW, Heimansohn DA et al (1990) Cor triatriatum: clinical presentation and surgical results in 12 patients. Ann Thorac Surg 50(4):562–568

52. Salomone G, Tiraboschi R, Bianchi T et al (1991) Cor triatriatum. Clinical presentation and operative results. J Thorac Cardiovasc Surg 101(6):1088–1092

53. van Son JA, Danielson GK, Schaff HV et al (1993) Cor triatriatum: diagnosis, operative approach, and late results. Mayo Clin Proc 68(9):854–859

54. Johnson W, Kirklin J (2012) Left ventricular inflow obstruction: pulmonary vein stenosis, cor triatriatum, supravalvar mitral ring, mitral valve stenosis. In: Moller J, Hoffman J (eds) Pediatric cardiovascular medicine. Blackwell, London

55. Richardson JV, Doty DB, Siewers RD et al (1981) Cor triatriatum (subdivided left atrium). J Thorac Cardiovasc Surg 81(2):232–238

56. Jorgensen CRFR, Varco RL, Lillehei CW et al (1967) Cor triatriatum: review of the surgical aspects with a follow-up report on the first patient successfully treated with surgery. Circulation 36:101

57. Macartney FJ, Scott O, Ionescu MI et al (1974) Diagnosis and management of parachute mitral valve and supravalvar mitral ring. Br Heart J 36(7):641–652

58. Neirotti R, Kreutzer G, Galindez E et al (1977) Supravalvular mitral stenosis associated with ventricular septal defect. Am J Dis Child 131(8):862–865

Acquired Mitral Valve Stenosis and Regurgitation

96

Cécile Tissot, Sanjay Cherian, Shannon Buckvold, and Afksendyos Kalangos

Abstract

Mitral valve disease is not uncommon in children, with a prevalence of 1.8–2.4 % (Thomson et al. Heart 83:185–187, 2000; Brand et al. Am Heart J 123:177–180, 1992). The most common causes of acquired mitral disease among children are *rheumatic fever* and *Marfan syndrome*. The mitral valve is most commonly involved in children with rheumatic fever (Bahadur et al. Indian Heart J 55:615–618, 2003). *Bacterial endocarditis* can also cause mitral valve disease, mostly regurgitation. Children with metabolic diseases and those receiving anticancer therapy with cardiotoxic drugs (anthracycline, doxorubicin) can present with mitral regurgitation secondary to a cardiomyopathy.

Electronic Supplementary Material: The online version of this chapter (doi:10.1007/978-1-4471-4619-3_32) contains supplementary material, which is available to authorized users.

C. Tissot (✉)
Pediatric Cardiology Unit, Department of Pediatrics, University Children's Hospital of Geneva, Geneva, Switzerland
e-mail: cecile.tissot@hcuge.ch

S. Cherian
Cardiovascular Surgery Service, The University Hospital of Geneva, Geneva, Switzerland

Frontier Lifeline & Dr. K. M. Cherian Heart Foundation, Chennai, India
e-mail: sanjaycherian@hotmail.com

S. Buckvold
The Heart Institute, Department of Pediatrics, Children's Hospital Colorado, School of Medicine, University of Colorado, Denver, CO, USA
e-mail: shannon.buckvold@childrenscolorado.org

A. Kalangos
Cardiovascular Surgery Service, The University Hospital of Geneva, Geneva, Switzerland
e-mail: Afksendyos.Kalangos@hcuge.ch

This chapter will focus on the etiology, clinical presentation, and management of acquired mitral regurgitation and stenosis while outlining the two major related conditions responsible for mitral valve disease: rheumatic fever and Marfan syndrome.

Keywords

Marfan syndrome • Mitral valve • Mitral regurgitation • Mitral stenosis • Rheumatic heart disease • Rheumatic fever • Valvuloplasty

Abbreviations

GABHS	Group A beta-hemolytic streptococcus
LA	Left atrium
LV	Left ventricle
MFS	Marfan syndrome
MR	Mitral regurgitation
MS	Mitral stenosis
MVP	Mitral valve prolapse
MVR	Mitral valve replacement
RA	Right atrium
RF	Rheumatic fever
RV	Right ventricle

Introduction

The mitral valve is the most complex of cardiac valves and is the one most commonly associated with acquired disease. There are three main conditions that affect the valve, isolated or combined: obstruction (stenosis), leakage (regurgitation), and bulging backward during valve closure (prolapse). Prolapse is the most common, occurring in up to 5 % of the entire population, whereas stenosis is the least common.

Mitral Valve Anatomy and Physiology

The normal mitral valve apparatus consists of four components:

– The *annulus*
– The *leaflets*
– The *tendinous cords*
– The *papillary muscles*

The mitral valve is derived from the endocardial cushions with some contribution of myocardial cells. It consists of two leaflets, the anterior and the posterior leaflets, suspended from the fibrous mitral valve annulus at the level of the atrioventricular junction. The anterior leaflet guards approximately two-thirds of the left atrioventricular orifice but occupies only one-third of its circumference. The posterior leaflet guards approximately one-third of the left atrioventricular orifice but occupies two-thirds of its circumference. The posterior leaflet is subdivided into three sections or scallops (P1, P2, P3). The two leaflets coapt at the anterolateral and posteromedial commissures. Each scalloped section of the posterior leaflet (P1, P2, P3) coapts with the anterior leaflet in areas designated A1, A2, and A3 (Fig. 96.1 and Picture 96.1) [4]. For proper mitral valve function, the mitral valve leaflets require proper functioning of all eight areas of coaptation (two commissures and six leaflet sections). The valve leaflets are normally prevented from prolapsing into the left atrium by the tendinous cords attached to the underside of the valve that insert into the papillary muscles. The papillary muscles are normally symmetric, occupying the

MV Anatomy

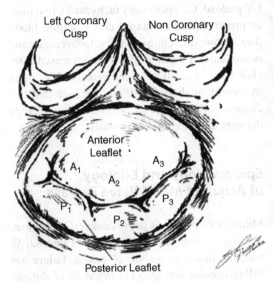

Fig. 96.1 Normal mitral valve anatomy with the anterior (A) and posterior (P) leaflets

anterolateral and posteromedial aspects of the LV below commissures, and they each typically have tendinous insertions that support both valve leaflets [4]. A dysfunction of any of these portions of the mitral valve apparatus can cause regurgitation or stenosis.

Mitral Regurgitation (MR)

In children, acquired mitral valve disease consists mostly of MR. In MR, blood is ejected into both the aorta and the low pressure LA [5, 6]. Dilatation of the LA from MR leads to elevated LA pressure and reduced pulmonary venous return to the LA, with consequent increased pulmonary venous pressure and reflex pulmonary arteriolar vasoconstriction. RV hypertension and dysfunction may result. Annular dilation occurs as a consequence of LA and LV dilatation, which further exacerbates MR. Severe LA dilation increases the risk of atrial arrhythmias and of respiratory compromise from left main stem bronchial compression, reduced lung capacity, and pulmonary edema from elevated pulmonary capillary hydrostatic pressure.

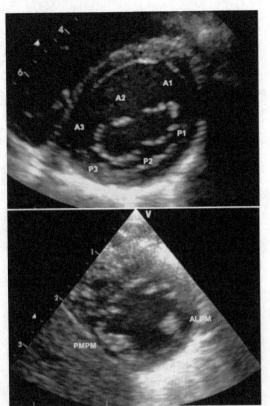

Picture 96.1 2D echocardiography short-axis view of the mitral valve, with the commissures and the scallops of the anterior (A) and posterior (P) leaflets identified: *A1-A2-A3* and *P1-P2-P3*. *Bottom* picture shows the anterolateral (ALPM) and posteromedial (PMPM) papillary muscles

Acute Mitral Regurgitation

Acute MR causes a sudden volume overload of the LA. Volume overload of the LV stretches the myocardial fibers and causes increased LV stroke volume. As MR progresses, the LV volume increases and the contractile function diminishes (Frank-Starling mechanism) leading to a decreased ejection fraction with reduced forward stroke volume and cardiac output [5, 6]. The regurgitant volume causes volume and pressure overload of the LA with increased pulmonary congestion and secondary pulmonary hypertension.

Chronic Compensated Mitral Regurgitation

In this phase, new sarcomeres are added to existing myocytes, thereby increasing individual myocardial fiber length and adjusting the length-tension relationship to allow the LV to bear the volume load, increase performance, and maintain forward cardiac output [5, 6]. Increased stroke volume of the LV induces eccentric hypertrophy. Children in this phase may be asymptomatic with normal exercise tolerance and may stay in this phase for years.

Chronic Decompensated Mitral Regurgitation

This phase is characterized by decreased LV contractility and stroke volume responsible for decreased forward cardiac output, increased end-systolic volume, increased LV filling pressure, and increased pulmonary venous congestion with symptoms of congestive heart failure. A normal ejection fraction can be a sign that heralds LV dysfunction. Indeed, intervention for MR should be considered prior to the onset of LV dysfunction, as it may not be reversible even with mitral valve surgery [5, 6]. Moreover, dilatation of the LV increases the mitral valve annulus and may worsen the degree of MR. Children in this phase present symptoms of heart failure and exercise intolerance.

Mitral Stenosis (MS)

In MS, the LV inflow is obstructed and causes LA dilation and hypertension in direct proportion to the severity of mitral obstruction. Progressive elevation in LA pressure leads to pulmonary venous hypertension and reflex pulmonary arteriolar vasoconstriction with RV hypertension and dysfunction. The pulmonary hypertension in MS is considered more readily reversible when compared with pulmonary hypertension associated with left-to-right shunt lesions. Severe LA dilation increases the risk of atrial arrhythmias (atrial flutter and fibrillation) and of respiratory compromise from left main stem bronchial compression, reduced lung capacity, and pulmonary edema from elevated pulmonary capillary hydrostatic pressure. In infants, congested bronchial veins may obstruct small bronchioles and cause further respiratory embarrassment through increased airway resistance. Outlet obstruction from the LA

leads to decreased cardiac output from decreased LV preload. Compensatory tachycardia functions to preserve cardiac output and systemic blood flow. However, compensatory tachycardia and neurohumoral mechanisms (e.g., increased catecholamine state) further compromise LV filling by shortening diastolic filling time such that cardiogenic shock follows, with reduced oxygen delivery and progressive acidosis.

Epidemiology and Etiology of Acquired Mitral Valve Disease

Mitral valve disease is not uncommon in children. A study in Turkish children showed that 8.6 % without clinical symptoms of cardiac failure had MR on echocardiography [7]. In a study of children aged 3–18 years old in Great Britain, the prevalence of MR was 1.8 % [1]. A prevalence of 2.4 % was found in another study in US children aged 0–14 years old [2]. The most common causes of acquired mitral valve disease among children are *rheumatic fever* and collagen vascular diseases including *Marfan syndrome, Ehlers-Danlos syndrome*, or *Loeys-Dietz syndrome*. MR is the most common cardiac anomaly found in children with rheumatic fever [3]. *Bacterial endocarditis* can also cause mitral valve disease, mostly regurgitation. In children, *metabolic* causes including mucopolysaccharidosis (Hurler syndrome or MPS type 1) should be thought. Children with *cancer* receiving cardiotoxic drugs (anthracycline, doxorubicin) can present with MR secondary to a cardiomyopathy. In this setting, asymptomatic MR is often the first sign of myocardial involvement [8].

Mitral Valve Prolapse (MVP)

The mitral valve annulus is nonplanar with a morphology that resembles a saddle. In a normal mitral valve, the leaflet edges are thrust together during ventricular systole, which involves papillary muscle contraction and tensing of the chordae along a small coaptation zone at the leaflet tips. MVP results when a leaflet edge slips past this coaptation zone.

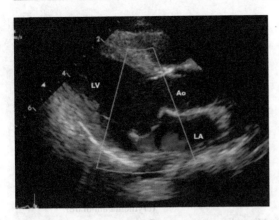

Picture 96.2 2D echocardiography long-axis view in Marfan syndrome with dilatation of ascending aorta, prolapsus of the anterior mitral leaflet with mild mitral regurgitation (*blue flow*). *Abbreviations: Ao aorta, LA left atrium, LV left ventricle*

The etiology of MVP is not clear and is probably multifactorial. Classic MVP is defined as leaflet displacement in systole exceeding the mitral valve annular plane by ≥2 mm, with leaflet thickening. Non-classic prolapse refers to leaflet displacement without valve thickening. It can result from excessive leaflet tissue (redundancy), myxomatous proliferation of the spongiosa, and elongation of the chordal apparatus and is seen in individuals with a wide range of congenital heart malformations as well as in acquired heart disease including collagen vascular disease (Marfan syndrome, Loeys-Dietz syndrome), ischemic heart disease, hypertrophic cardiomyopathy, and pectus excavatum, as well as in thin patients (Picture 96.2). MVP is a common finding in more than 50 % of patients with MFS [9]. MVP is usually diagnosed on the clinical basis of a mid-systolic click and a late systolic murmur of mitral regurgitation.

Rheumatic Fever (RF)

Rheumatic fever (RF) is a delayed nonsuppurative sequela of group A beta-hemolytic streptococcal (GABHS) pharyngitis in children. The disease has a delayed onset after the initial infection and presents with various manifestations including arthritis, carditis, chorea, subcutaneous nodules, or erythema marginatum.

The incidence of rheumatic heart disease has decreased dramatically in industrialized countries during the past several years related to the introduction of penicillin and a change in the virulence of the Streptococci. A dramatic decline in both the severity and mortality from acute RF has occurred in the past 30 years in these countries. The prevalence of rheumatic heart disease in the USA is now less than 0.05 per 1,000, with rare regional outbreaks [10, 11]. In contrast, RF and rheumatic heart disease have not decreased in developing countries. An estimated 5–30 million children and young adults are thought to have chronic rheumatic heart disease worldwide [12, 13]. Race and sex do not influence the disease incidence. Rheumatic disease in females is usually worse with a higher incidence of chorea and a worse prognosis of carditis. RF is principally a disease of childhood, occurring between 5 and 15 years, with a median age of 10 years at diagnosis. Rheumatic heart disease is still the major cause of acquired valve disease in the world [14].

However, the exact pathogenesis remains unclear; RF is believed to result from an autoimmune response. It develops following GABHS pharyngitis and almost only infections of the pharynx initiate or reactivate RF [15]. GABHS organisms are Gram-positive cocci which colonize the skin and oropharynx and are responsible for suppurative diseases (pharyngitis, impetigo, cellulitis, myositis, pneumonia, puerperal sepsis) and nonsuppurative diseases (RF, acute poststreptococcal glomerulonephritis).

The initial infection consists of sore throat, fever, malaise, and headache leading in a small percent of patients several weeks after to RF. Transmission of the organism is via direct contact with the secretions. Penicillin treatment shortens the clinical course of streptococcal pharyngitis and more importantly prevents the major sequelae [16].

Molecular mimicry between streptococcal and human proteins is thought to be the mechanism of the disease, together with a genetic susceptibility [17]. The observation that only a few M serotypes were implicated in outbreaks in the USA suggests a particular rheumatogenic potential of certain strains [10, 15, 18]. Anti-M antibodies against the streptococci may cross-react with heart tissue, causing infiltration of the heart by T lymphocytes [19]. Increased production of inflammatory cytokines is the final mechanism of the autoimmune reaction that causes damage to cardiac tissue.

Cardiovascular Involvement in RF

Acute rheumatic heart disease produces a pancarditis involving the pericardium, epicardium, myocardium, and endocardium. The most commonly affected valve is the mitral valve (65–70 % of patients), followed by the aortic (25 %) and the tricuspid (10 %) valves. The pulmonary valve is rarely affected. When pericarditis is present, it is usually self-limiting and rarely results in constrictive pericarditis. Recurrent episodes of RF may cause progressive damage to the valves. Severe scarring of the valves develops months to years after the initial episode of RF and is responsible for most cases of MS in adults.

Patients with previous RF are at a high risk of recurrence. The risk of recurrence increases within 5 years of the initial episode and with younger age at the time of the initial episode. The risk of carditis and severity of valve damage increases with each attack.

Clinical Presentation and Diagnostic Criteria

Acute RF is a systemic disease presenting with a large variety of symptoms. Antecedent of a sore throat 2–5 weeks prior to onset of symptoms is present in 70 % of patients. Systemic complaints are frequent including fever, fatigue, weight loss, headache, malaise, and pallor.

The major clinical manifestations are:
- Fever
- Arthritis: Polyarthritis is the most common symptom and frequently is the earliest manifestation (70–75 %). The arthritis involves usually the large joints, beginning in the lower extremities (knees, ankles) and migrating to other large joints in the upper extremities (elbows, wrists). The arthritis persists for about 1 week, is migratory, and responds dramatically to aspirin [20].

Table 96.1 Jones criteria for the diagnosis of acute rheumatic fever

Jones criteria	
Preceding streptococcal infection	Positive throat culture
	Rapid streptococcal antigen test
	Elevated or rising streptococcal antibody titer
Major diagnostic criteria	Carditis
	Polyarthritis
	Chorea
	Subcutaneous nodules
	Erythema marginatum (erythema annulare)
Minor diagnostic criteria	Fever
	Arthralgia
	Prolonged PR interval
	Elevated acute-phase reactants (ESR, CRP)

- Carditis: Pancarditis is the second most common complication (50 %). The classical clinical presentation is a new or changing murmur and tachycardia that is out of proportion to the fever. The murmurs of acute RF are from valve regurgitation (most commonly mitral or aortic) and the murmurs of chronic RF from stenosis, most commonly mitral. Dyspnea, edema, cough, and orthopnea are signs of congestive heart failure. Chest pain and a pericardial friction rub are signs of pericarditis. All degree of heart block can be seen, including:
  - Atrioventricular dissociation [21]
  - Sydenham chorea [22]
  - Pediatric autoimmune neuropsychiatric disorder (PANDAS) [23]
  - Erythema marginatum [24]
  - Subcutaneous nodules [25]
  - Arthralgias: cannot be considered a minor criteria if arthritis is present

The *modified Jones criteria* [26–28] provide guidelines for the diagnosis of RF and require evidence of a *previous GBHAS pharyngitis* as well as the presence of *two major or one major and two minor criteria* (Table 96.1). These criteria are not absolute, and the diagnosis can be made in patients with only confirmed streptococcal pharyngitis and chorea. The American Heart Association (AHA) guideline 2002 update [28] concluded that the role

Table 96.2 Antibodies tested in acute rheumatic fever

| Antistreptolysin O (ASO) |
| Anti-DNase B |
| Antihyaluronidase |
| Antistreptokinase |
| Antistreptococcal esterase |
| Anti-nicotinamide adenine dinucleotide (anti-NAD) |
| Antistreptococcal polysaccharide |
| Anti-teichoic acid |
| Anti-M protein |

of echocardiography in the diagnosis of RF was controversial in patients without cardiac findings on clinical exam. It was concluded that echocardiographic Doppler evidence of mitral or aortic regurgitation alone should not be either a major or a minor criterion in the diagnosis of RF.

Laboratory in RF

- **Throat culture for GABHS:** is usually negative in about 75 % of patients by the time RF appears [29].
- **Rapid antigen detection test:** has a specificity >95 % but a sensitivity of only 60–90 %. Thus, a throat culture should be obtained [30].
- **Antistreptococcal antibodies:** are at their peak at initial presentation and are useful for confirming previous GABHS infection [31, 32]. Table 96.2 summarizes the most common antibodies tested.
- **Acute-phase reactants:** C-reactive protein (CRP) and erythrocyte sedimentation rate (ESR) are elevated and have high sensitivity but low specificity [33].
- **Mild normochromic normocytic anemia**
- **Heart reactive antibodies:** rapid detection test for B-cell marker D8/17 by immunofluorescence is positive in 90 % of patients with RF [34].

Imaging Studies in RF

- Electrocardiogram
  Sinus tachycardia is a common finding. Alternatively, some children present sinus

bradycardia from increased vagal tone. First-degree atrioventricular block, probably related to localized myocardial inflammation of the atrioventricular node, is a common finding and is one of the Jones criteria. Second- and third-degree atrioventricular have been described.

- Echocardiography
  In individuals with acute rheumatic heart disease, echocardiography identifies and quantitates valve insufficiency and ventricular dysfunction. In patients with mild carditis, Doppler evidence of MR may be present during the acute phase of disease and usually resolves in weeks to months. In contrast, patients with moderate-to-severe carditis may have persistent mitral or aortic regurgitation [35]. According to the 1992 revised Jones criteria, evidence of new MR from Doppler echocardiography, in the absence of accompanying auscultatory findings, is not sufficient for making the diagnosis of carditis [36, 37].

Three mechanisms of MR have been described with RF [38, 39]:
- Prolapse of the aortic leaflet
- Rupture of the tendinous chords
- Non-coapting retracted immobile mural leaflet (Picture 96.3)

Echocardiographic features of MR from acute rheumatic valvulitis are annular dilatation, elongation of the chordae to the anterior leaflet, and a posterolaterally directed mitral regurgitation jet. A distinctive feature of acute rheumatic valvular disease is focal nodular thickening of the tips and bodies of the leaflets [40]. LV dilation is frequently seen and contributes to MR.

In individuals with chronic rheumatic heart disease, echocardiography assesses the progression of valve stenosis. The leaflets of affected valves become thickened diffusely, with fusion of the commissures and chordae tendineae. Increased echodensity of the mitral valve is often seen.

Marfan Syndrome (MFS)

Marfan syndrome (MFS) is a heritable connective tissue disorder which may affect the eyes, cardiovascular system, skeletal system, lungs, spinal

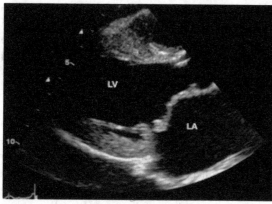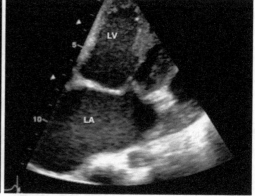

Picture 96.3 Color Doppler echocardiography long-axis and four-chamber views demonstrating a rheumatic mitral valve with thickened leaflet, absence of central coaptation, and marked left atrial dilation secondary to severe regurgitation. *Abbreviations: LA left atrium, LV left ventricle*

cord, skin, kidney, and other systems [41]. It results from fibrillin-1 (FBN1) gene mutations or deficiency, with consequences to the structural and regulatory function of FBN1, the glycoprotein constituent of extracellular microfibrils [42].

The diagnosis of MFS is clinical based on the identification of *major and minor diagnostic criteria* (Table 96.3). Cardiovascular complications in MFS have accounted for greater than 90 % of premature deaths related to aortic aneurysm since the era prior to open-heart surgery [43]. While nearly all patients with MFS continue to exhibit cardiovascular involvement, current anticipatory guidance and effective management have allowed those patients to achieve near-normal life expectancies [44].

The estimated incidence of MFS is 2–3 per 10,000 individuals [45], and the estimated prevalence is 1 in 5,000 individuals [42]. MFS exhibits autosomal dominant inheritance with complete penetrance but variable expression in 75 % of patients, while sporadic occurrence accounts for the remaining 25 % [44].

Cardiovascular Involvement in MFS

The most common cardiovascular abnormalities in pediatric MFS are dilation of the ascending aorta and MVP [46]. Fibrillin density is reduced and accompanied by partial fragmentation of the

longer fibrillin-coated elastic fibers, with abnormal globular change in the fibrillin coating of remaining portions of elastic fibers [47]. Both the anterior and posterior leaflets tend to become elongated and redundant, with some degree of thickening. Chordal elongation and rupture can occur. Progressive annular dilation and calcification can be demonstrated in 30 % of MFS patients [48].

All phases of MR have been described in neonates and children with MFS. As the anterior and posterior leaflets of the mitral valve become elongated, redundant, and somewhat thickened [48], prolapse of the anterior and/or posterior leaflet results [49]. MVP can be demonstrated in 17 % of children at age 5 years old, in 75 % of adolescents at age 15 years, and in 80 % of young adults at 30 years of age [46, 48]. It has been suggested that 100 % of children with evolving phenotypic expression of MFS will develop mitral valve dysfunction by 18 years of age and one-half of children with mitral valve dysfunction will develop MR before 25 years of age [46]. In fact, in the pediatric MFS population, mitral valve dysfunction and regurgitation contribute most to morbidity and mortality and have been suggested to be of prognostic significance [46, 48]. Severe MR in very young children is a feature of the infantile and neonatal expressions of MFS [50].

Endocarditis should be considered in any patient with MFS who presents with acutely

Table 96.3 Ghent diagnostic criteria. An index case must meet two major criteria in two organ systems and a minor criterion in a third system (Adapted from Stuart and Williams [41]). *Abbreviation: MFS = Marfan syndrome*

System	Major criteria	Minor criteria
Family history	MFS in parent, child, or sibling	
Genetics	Mutation of FBN1 gene	
Cardiovascular	Aortic root dilation	Mitral valve prolapse
	Dissection of ascending aorta	Calcification of the mitral valve (<40 years)
		Dilatation of the pulmonary artery
		Dilatation/dissection of descending aorta
Ocular	Ectopia lentis	Flat cornea elongated
		Globe myopia
Skeletal	Pectus excavatum needing surgery	Moderate pectus excavatum
	Pectus carinatum	High arched palate
	Pes planus	Typical facial features
	Positive wrist or thumb sign	Joint hypermobility
	Scoliosis >20° or spondylolisthesis	
	Armspan-height ratio >1.05	
	Protrusio acetabulae	
	Diminished extension elbows <170°	
Pulmonary		Spontaneous pneumothorax
		Apical bulla
Skin		Striae
		Recurrent or incisional herniae
Central nervous system	Lumbosacral dural ectasia	

progressive valvular disease, recurrent fever, or persistent constitutional symptoms of anorexia, weight loss, malaise, or personality changes. Perivalvular abscess can be associated with conduction abnormalities including complete heart block [51].

Clinical Presentation of MFS

MFS is most often suspected on the basis of skeletal and ophthalmic features that suggest the diagnosis. Because of its variability and tendency towards an evolving phenotype, the diagnosis of MFS is primarily clinical, made by applying the *Ghent criteria* (Table 96.3), but when the clinical diagnosis is less clear, a full range of diagnostic studies can be performed, and the objective findings can be assembled to make the diagnosis [41]. MFS exhibits a significant degree of clinical variability both within and among families. Albeit cardiovascular manifestations tend to develop in

adolescence, absence of manifestations until later in life has also been described. Severe phenotypes exist with significant valve dysfunction and/or rapidly progressive aortic root dilatation so-called neonatal MFS [52]. Mortality in infants with neonatal MFS can be as high as 95 % in the first year of life from relentlessly progressive, severe mitral, tricuspid, and/or aortic regurgitation that is often complicated by scoliosis, congenital pulmonary emphysema, and pulmonary hypertension [53]. In addition to the cardiac and pulmonary manifestations, neonatal MFS exhibits a distinctive neonatal phenotype [50, 52, 53].

Studies in MFS

- Electrocardiogram
  The resting ECG in MFS may include findings of atrial fibrillation, premature atrial or ventricular beats, long QT interval, and prolonged atrioventricular conduction

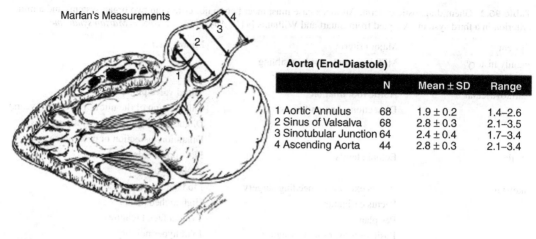

Marfan's Measurements

Aorta (End-Diastole)

	N	Mean ± SD	Range
1 Aortic Annulus	68	1.9 ± 0.2	1.4–2.6
2 Sinus of Valsalva	68	2.8 ± 0.3	2.1–3.5
3 Sinotubular Junction	64	2.4 ± 0.4	1.7–3.4
4 Ascending Aorta	44	2.8 ± 0.3	2.1–3.4

Fig. 96.2 Schematic representation of the normal aortic root by 2D echocardiogram long-axis view demonstrating the normal diameters of the (1) aortic annulus, (2) sinus of Valsalva, (3) sinotubular junction, and (4) ascending aorta

time [57]. Ventricular arrhythmias are associated with increased LV size, MVP, and abnormalities of repolarization and are an important cause of sudden death [54]. Complete heart block may be a presenting sign and symptom of endocarditis complicated by perivalvular abscess [51].

- Echocardiography
The clinical presentation of an aortic aneurysm in children with MFS is typically asymptomatic and is detected by serial echocardiographic evaluation with measurement of aortic root, sinus of Valsalva, sinotubular junction, and ascending aorta (Fig. 96.2) [55]. Echocardiography assessment of the mitral valve will be discussed in "Imaging Studies in RF".

Physical Evaluation

Mitral Regurgitation (MR)

The physical exam of a patient with MR is characterized by a pansystolic murmur loudest at the apex and radiating to the left axilla and to the back. The first heart sound is usually diminished and the second heart sound is split.

Other clinical features on physical examination often include:

- A displaced LV apical impulse
- An apical thrill, though significantly impaired LV function may attenuate this finding
- A loud second sound, in the setting of severe pulmonary hypertension
- An third heart sound, from the rapid, large volume flow into the LV
- A fourth sound, from flow into a noncompliant LV during atrial contraction

Mitral Stenosis (MS)

The physical exam of a patient with MS is characterized by a mid-diastolic rumbling murmur heard best at the apex. A loud first heart sound is often evident from abrupt closure of the mitral valve. In the case of RF, an opening snap is often present. When pulmonary hypertension is present, a loud second sound and a RV heave are present. In severe MS, decreased pulse amplitude may be appreciated due to the reduced stroke volume from significantly reduced LV filling.

Mitral Valve Prolapse (MVP)

The physical exam is characterized by a systolic click that varies with postural change.

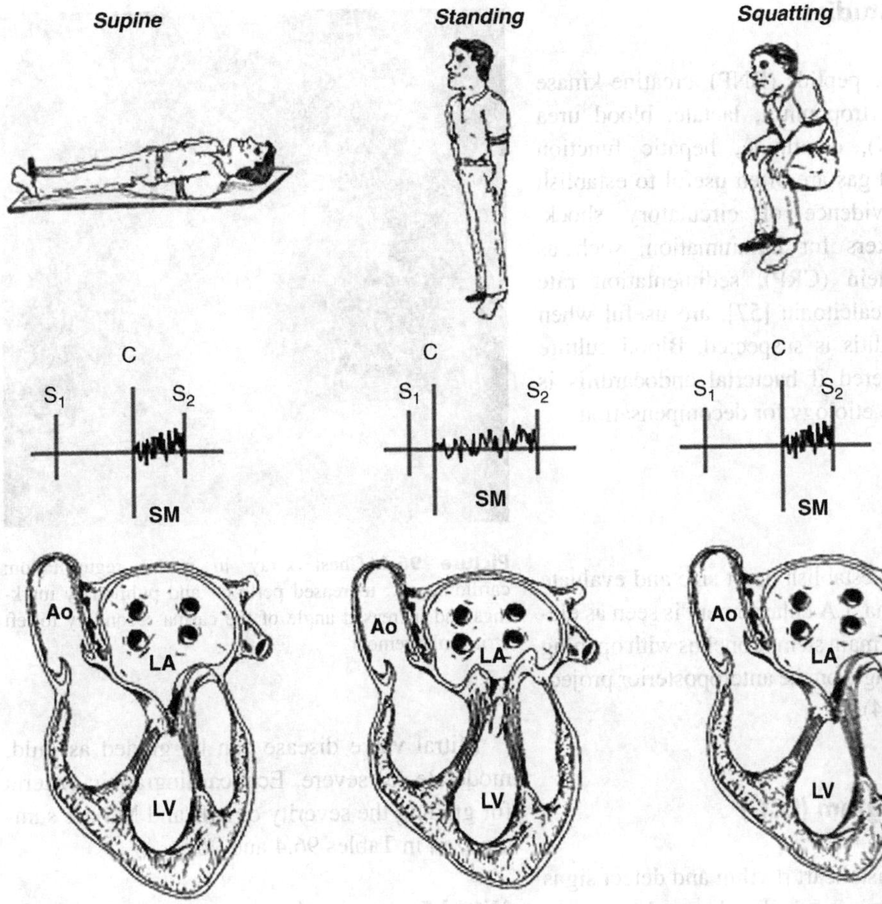

Fig. 96.3 Postural changes and auscultatory phenomena in patients with mitral valve prolapse, with alteration of systolic click and systolic murmur. As the left ventricular volume decreases (*upright* position), the systolic click moves towards the first heart sound and the murmur becomes more holosystolic. *Abbreviation: S1 = first heart sound, S2 = second heart sound, C = click, SM = systolic murmur, Ao = aorta, LA = left atrium, LV = left ventricle*

The systolic click moves towards the first heart sound with upright position and new click may appear. A MR murmur may be present only with the patient in the upright position. Rarely, a systolic precordial "honk" may be heard. Prompt squatting results in a movement of the systolic click away from the first heart sound and the systolic murmur of MR moves back to late systole. These postural changes are related primarily to change in LV volume, myocardial contractility, and heart rate (Fig. 96.3). LV volume is decreased in the upright position compared to the supine position, and reflex tachycardia occurs in the supine position [56].

Preoperative Management

Several diagnostic studies are likely to be valuable in guiding clinical management in patients who present with decompensated cardiac failure secondary to mitral valve disease, regardless of whether the etiology of mitral valve disease in MFS, RF, or congenital malformation.

Laboratory Studies

Brain natriuretic peptide (BNP), creatine kinase MB (CK-MB), troponin I, lactate, blood urea nitrogen (BUN), creatinine, hepatic function tests, and blood gas are often useful to establish biochemical evidence of circulatory shock. Serologic markers for inflammation, such as C-reactive protein (CRP), sedimentation rate (ESR), and procalcitonin [57], are useful when RF or endocarditis is suspected. Blood culture may be considered if bacterial endocarditis is suspected as the etiology for decompensation.

Chest X-Ray

Chest x-ray will establish heart size and evaluate pulmonary edema. LA enlargement is seen as elevation of the left main stem bronchus with opening of the carina's angle on the anteroposterior projection (Picture 96.4).

Electrocardiogram (ECG)

ECG will establish heart rhythm and detect signs of ischemia, strain, and chamber enlargement. Common ECG findings are:

- Signs of LA enlargement: P mitrale = bifid P wave (Picture 96.5)
- Signs of LV hypertrophy, strain, and/or enlargement (Picture 96.6)
- Signs of RV hypertrophy and strain suggestive of pulmonary hypertension

Transthoracic Echocardiography

Echocardiography will assess the valvar and subvalvar apparatus, measure the annulus size and mitral orifice area (Picture 96.7), and quantify the severity of MR or MS (Picture 96.8). It will give informations about LV and LA size and function, including wall motion abnormalities. It will allow estimation of mean mitral gradient (Picture 96.9) and RV and pulmonary artery pressures (Picture 96.10).

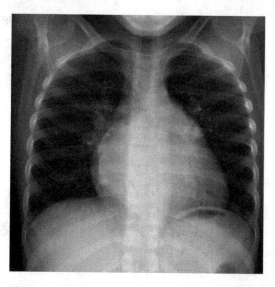

Picture 96.4 Chest x-ray in mitral regurgitation: cardiomegaly, increased perihilar and pulmonary markings and increased angle of the carina secondary to left atrial enlargement

Mitral valve disease can be graded as mild, moderate, or severe. Echocardiographic criteria for grading the severity of MR and MS are summarized in Tables 96.4 and 96.5.

Mitral Regurgitation

Echocardiography assesses the severity of mitral disease and the adaptive changes in cardiac chambers in response to MR [58, 59]. A chronic significant MR is usually accompanied by an increase in size of the left cardiac chambers, whereas significant regurgitation of acute onset may not result in this remodeling. While cardiac remodeling is not specific for the degree of regurgitation, its absence in the face of chronic regurgitation should imply a milder degree of MR.

Different techniques of Doppler echocardiography allow the evaluation of MR severity [58, 59]:

- *Color flow imaging* is the most common way to assess MR, even though this technique is not very reliable. It assumes that as the severity of MR increases, the size and extent of the jet into the LA increases. Theoretically, larger color jets that extend deep into the LA

Picture 96.5 Lead II ECG in mitral valve disease with enlarged and bifid P wave: P mitrale

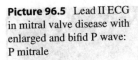
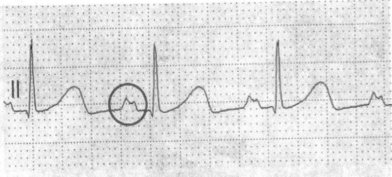

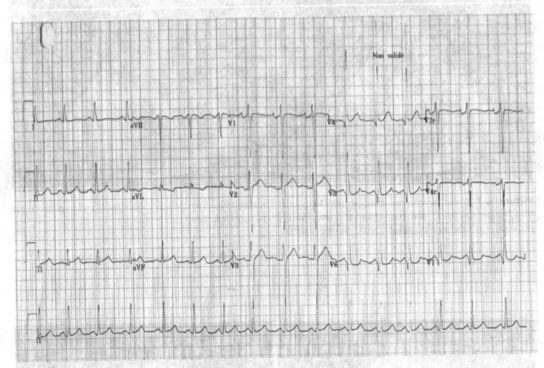

Picture 96.6 ECG in mitral valve disease with enlarged and bifid P wave and left ventricular enlargement and hypertrophy

represent more severe MR than small thin jets. Nevertheless, this method is not as accurate because for a similar severity of MR, patients with increased LA pressure, eccentric jets, or increased LA size may exhibit smaller jet area.

- The *vena contracta* is the area of MR jet as it leaves the regurgitant orifice. A vena contracta width <3 mm indicates mild MR and ≥7 mm defines severe MR.

- The *flow convergence method* is the most recommended method for evaluation of MR

severity and needs visualization of the proximal isovelocity surface area (PISA). The radius of the PISA is measured at mid-systole. Regurgitant volume and regurgitant opening surface (also called effective regurgitant orifice area = EROA) measurements allow for classification of the severity of MR.

- In the absence of MS, the increased *transmitral inflow* that occurs with increasing MR severity can be detected as higher Doppler flow velocities during early diastolic filling.

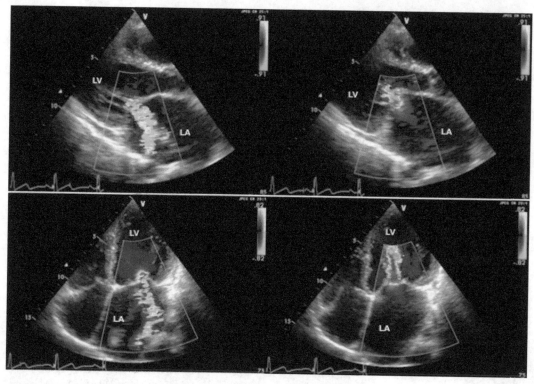

Picture 96.7 Color Doppler echocardiography long-axis view (*upper pictures*) and four-chamber view (*lower pictures*) in rheumatic fever with severe mitral regurgitation (*left pictures, blue flow*) and stenosis (*right pictures, red flow*)

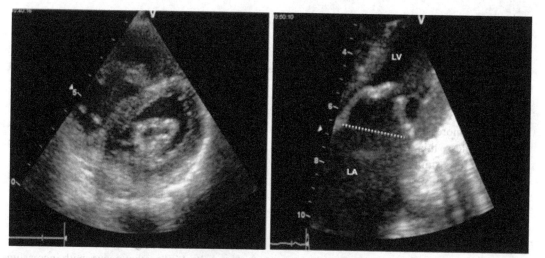

Picture 96.8 2D echocardiography short-axis and four-chamber views in rheumatic fever with thickened mitral leaflets thickening responsible for diminished opening and stenosis. Right picture shows decreased mitral valve area and left picture shows measurement of the mitral annulus (*doted yellow line*)

Picture 96.9 Doppler echocardiography in a patient with severe mitral regurgitation and stenosis (mean pressure gradient of 10 mmHg). Mitral E (early diastolic) and A (late diastolic) waves are not clearly discernable and DT (deceleration time) is increased. *Abbreviations: A = late diastolic (atrial contraction) wave, AVC = aortic valve closure, IVRT = isovolumic relaxation time, DT = deceleration time, E = early diastolic wave, MR = mitral regurgitation, MS = mitral stenosis*

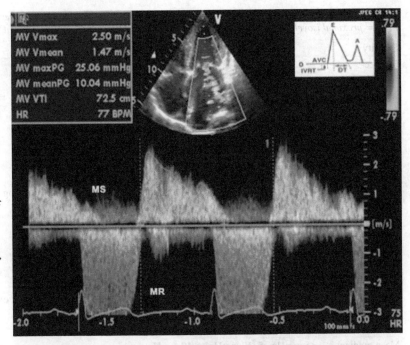

Picture 96.10 Doppler echocardiography in a patient with mitral rheumatic disease and tricuspid regurgitation (*TR*). Systolic pulmonary artery pressure (*SPAP*) can be estimated from the TR jet using the modified Bernoulli equation ($P = 4V^2$) and is estimated at 85 mmHg + RAP. *Abbreviations: P = pressure, RAP = right atrial pressure, SPAP = systolic pulmonary artery pressure, TRVmax = tricuspid regurgitation maximal velocity, V = velocity*

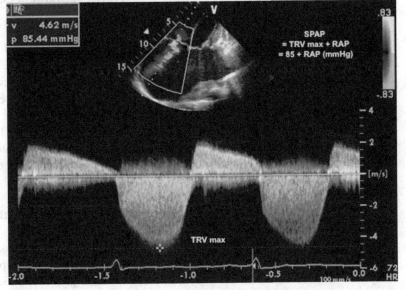

A peak E wave velocity of mitral inflow >1.5 m/s suggests severe MR. The pulsed Doppler mitral-to-aortic time velocity integral (TVI) ratio is also used as an easily measured index for the quantification of MR with a TVI ratio >1.4 suggestive of severe MR, whereas a TVI ratio <1 is in favor of mild MR.

– The *pulmonary venous flow* can also be used to grade MR in patients with normal diastolic function. With increasing severity of MR, there is a decrease of the S wave velocity with frank reversal in severe MR.

The *Carpentier's functional classification* of MR is often used, in particular in

Table 96.4 Estimation of mitral regurgitation severity by echocardiography. *Abbreviations: LA = left atrium, PISA = proximal isovelocity surface area of vena contracta, TVI = time velocity integral*

Severity	Mild	Moderate	Severe
LA size	≤4,0 cm	>4 cm	>4 cm
Jet surface	<4 cm²	4 à 8 cm²	>8 cm²
Jet length/width	<0,2	0,2–0,4	>0,4
Jet length/LA length	<1/3	1/3–2/3	>2/3
PISA: Proximal jet width	<0,3 cm	0,3 à 0,7 cm	≥0,7 cm
PISA: Regurgitant volume (R Vol)	<30 ml	30–60 ml	≥60 ml
Regurgitation opening surface	<0,2 cm²	0,2 à 0,4 cm²	≥0,4 cm²
Doppler mitral-to-aortic TVI ratio	<1	1–1.4	>1.4
Doppler mitral inflow	Systolic dominance	Systolic blunting	Systolic reversal
Doppler pulmonary vein flow	A wave dominance	variable	E wave dominance

Table 96.5 Severity of mitral stenosis assessed by echocardiography

Severity	Mild	Moderate	Severe
Mean gradient	<5 mmHg	5–10 mmHg	>10 mmHg
Mitral valve area	>1.5 cm²	1.0–1.5 cm²	<1.0 cm²

rheumatic disease when mitral valve repair is considered [60]:

– Type I: leaflet perforation (endocarditis) or annular dilatation
– Type II: excessive leaflet mobility accompanied by displacement of the free edge of one or both leaflets beyond the mitral annular plane (mitral valve prolapse)
– Type IIIa: restricted leaflet motion during both diastole and systole due to shortening of the chordae and/or leaflet thickening (rheumatic disease)
– Type IIIb: restricted leaflet motion only during systole

Mitral Stenosis

Echocardiography in MS shows thick and calcified mitral valve with narrow and "fish mouth"-shaped orifice and LA enlargement. Doppler echocardiography shows decreased opening of the mitral valve leaflets and increased blood flow velocity during diastole. The transmitral gradient as measured by Doppler echocardiography is the gold standard in the evaluation of the severity of MS.

Transesophageal Echocardiography (TEE)

TEE is a valuable tool for preoperative assessment of mitral valve disease, particularly in patients with poor windows. It is particularly useful when the patient is presenting atrial arrhythmia, to exclude the presence of LA or appendage's thrombi. Three-dimensional echocardiography is an emerging tool that should provide useful imaging of abnormal valves.

Cardiac Catheterization

Indications include assessment of pulmonary vascular reactivity in pulmonary hypertension or investigation of MS. Simultaneous left and right heart catheterization allows measurement of the mean pulmonary capillary wedge pressure (PCWP), which is a reflection of the LA pressure, and of the LV end-diastolic pressure, allowing for calculation of the pressure gradient between the LA and LV. The LA pressure can also be measured invasively and is elevated in either MS or MR. The primary hemodynamic consequence of MS is a pressure gradient

Fig. 96.4 Left heart catheterization in mitral stenosis with increased left atrial pressure and pressure gradient between the left atrium and left ventricle

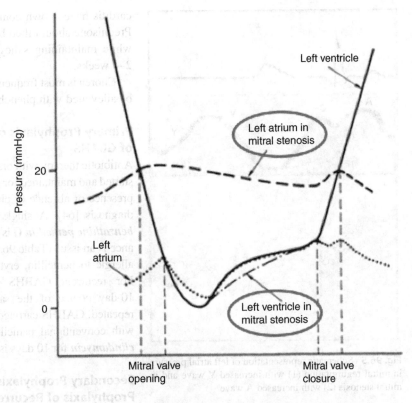

between the "A" wave of the LA and LV in diastole (Fig. 96.4).

The typical LA pressure tracing is composed of:

- The A wave (atrial contraction) follows the P wave of the electrocardiogram and is produced from the increased atrial pressure during the atrial contraction.
- The C wave (mitral valve closure) follows the QRS wave and result of the LV contraction and subsequent bulging of the mitral valve into the LA.
- The x descent (atrial diastole) occurs between the QRS and T waves and corresponds to atrial relaxation and rapid atrial filling.
- The V wave (ventricular contraction) occurs with the T wave and reflects passive venous filling of the left atrium when the mitral valve is closed. MR produces a prominent, tall V wave due to blood that is regurgitated into the LA during ventricular systole (Fig. 96.5). In chronic MR, the C wave may not be apparent: this has been termed a "C-V" wave.

- The diastolic y descent (atrial emptying) represents opening of the mitral valve and rapid filling of the ventricle. MS produces a markedly increased A wave and a gradual y descent (Fig. 96.5).

Cardiac Magnetic Resonance Imaging (MRI)

MRI can be used to generate cardiac volumetric data, to delineate ventricular function, and to demonstrate a panoramic view of the thoracic aorta in patients with MFS.

Medical Management

Medical Management of Rheumatic Fever (RF)

The goal of treatment consists of:
- Symptomatic relief of acute inflammation

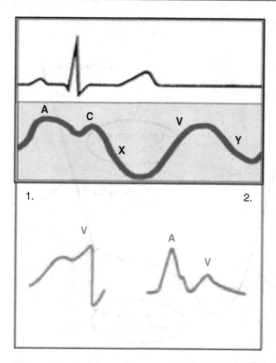

Fig. 96.5 Schematic representation of left atrial pressure in mitral regurgitation (1) with increased V wave and in mitral stenosis (2) with increased A wave

- Eradication of GABHS
- Prophylaxis against future infection to prevent recurrent cardiac disease
- Supportive treatment of heart failure

Anti-inflammatory Treatment of RF

Treatment of the inflammatory manifestations of acute RF uses salicylates and steroids. *Aspirin* in anti-inflammatory doses (80–100 mg/kg/day in children and 4–8 g/day in adults) effectively reduces all manifestations of the disease except chorea, and the response typically is dramatic [61]. Aspirin should be maintained at anti-inflammatory doses until the signs and symptoms of acute RF are resolved or residing (6–8 weeks) and the acute-phase reactants (CRP, ESR) have returned normal. When discontinuing therapy, aspirin should be withdrawn gradually over weeks while monitoring the CRP and ESR for rebound.

In patients with moderate-to-severe carditis, *oral prednisone* (2 mg/kg/day) is usually used for 2–4 weeks, but studies on the effect of corticosteroids in the treatment of rheumatic

carditis have shown conflicting results [62, 63]. Prednisone should then be tapered over 2 weeks while maintaining salicylates for an additional 2–4 weeks.

Chorea is most frequently self-limited but may be alleviated with phenobarbital or diazepam.

Primary Prophylaxis of RF: Eradication of GBAHS

Antibiotic therapy with oral *penicillin V* should be started and maintained for 10 days regardless of the presence or absence of pharyngitis at the time of diagnosis [64]. A single dose of intramuscular *benzathine penicillin G* is an alternative if compliance is an issue (Table 96.6). For patients who are allergic to penicillin, erythromycin can be used. For recurrent GABHS pharyngitis, a second 10-day course of the same antibiotic may be repeated. GABHS carriage is difficult to eradicate with conventional penicillin therapy. Thus, oral *clindamycin* for 10 days is recommended.

Secondary Prophylaxis of RF: Prophylaxis of Recurrence

Prophylactic therapy is indicated after RF to prevent recurrent streptococcal infection and further damage to the valves [18, 65]. Antibiotic prophylaxis should be started immediately after resolution of the acute episode [66]. Oral *penicillin V* or *benzathine penicillin G* intramuscularly every 3–4 weeks is the recommended regimen for most patients (Table 96.7) [67].

The duration of antibiotic prophylaxis is controversial. The American Heart Association currently recommends [66, 68] that patients with RF without carditis receive prophylactic antibiotics for 5 years or until aged 21 years, whichever is longer, that patients with carditis but no valve disease receive prophylactic antibiotics for 10 years or well into adulthood and that patients with carditis and valve disease receive antibiotics at least 10 years or until aged 40 years (Table 96.8).

Medical Management of Marfan Syndrome (MFS)

Many patients with MFS are on chronic beta-blockade therapy to decrease inotropy,

Table 96.6 Primary prophylaxis for rheumatic fever

Agent	Dose	Mode	Duration
Benzathine penicillin	≤27 kg: 600,000 U	Intramuscular	Once
	>27 kg: 1,200,000 U	Intramuscular	Once
Penicillin V	Children: 250 mg 2–3 times daily	Oral	10 days
	Adolescents/ adults: 500 mg 2–3 times daily	Oral	10 days
Allergy to penicillin:			
Erythromycin	20–40 mg/kg/ day 2–4 times daily (max 1 g/ day)	Oral	10 days

Table 96.7 Secondary prophylaxis of rheumatic fever

Agent	Dose	Mode
Benzathine penicillin	1,200,000 U every 4 week (every 3 week for high-risk patients)	Intramuscular
Penicillin V	Children: 250 mg twice daily	Oral
	Adults: 500 mg twice daily	
Allergy to penicillin:		
Erythromycin	250 mg twice daily	Oral

Table 96.8 Duration of secondary prophylaxis for rheumatic fever (RF)

Category	Duration
RF with carditis and residual heart disease	10 years or greater since last episode and at least until age 40, sometimes lifelong prophylaxis
RF with carditis but no residual heart disease	10 years or well into adulthood, whichever is longer
RF without carditis	5 years or until age 21, whichever is longer

chronotropy, ectopy, and aortic wall stress [69]. Chronic beta-blockade therapy may complicate the treatment of acute decompensated heart failure by rendering the myocardium less responsive to catecholamine infusion. For this reason, phosphodiesterase inhibitors, such as milrinone, and calcium sensitizers, such as levosimendan, may be preferable, as they increase contractility through increasing cAMP and improving the calcium-troponin C interaction, respectively, without specifically requiring adrenergic receptor stimulation.

Medical Management of Congestive Heart Failure

Treatment of congestive heart failure includes inotropic support, diuretics, afterload reduction, supplemental oxygen, bed rest, and sodium and fluid restriction. Patients with congestive heart failure from acute valve insufficiency will likely require continuous intravenous inotropic support. The beneficial role of *digoxin* in cardiac failure is controversial [70–72]. Digoxin should be started only after checking serum electrolytes due to the increased toxicity of digoxin with hypokalemia.

Diuretics frequently are used in conjunction with inotropic agents. *Furosemide* is usually the first choice. *Spironolactone* is often added in conjunction with furosemide as potassium-sparing diuretic.

Afterload reduction with angiotensin-converting enzyme inhibitors (ACEI) may be effective in improving cardiac output, particularly in the presence of mitral and aortic insufficiency [73]. *Captopril* is used in infants <6 months, while *enalapril* is usually preferred in older children due to more convenience related to its longer half-life. ACEI should be started carefully with a small, initial test dose as some patients have an abnormally large response to these agents with hypotension. ACEI should be administered only after correcting hypovolemia. When heart failure persists or worsens during the acute phase after aggressive medical therapy, surgery is indicated to decrease valve insufficiency.

Antibiotic Prophylaxis of Bacterial Endocarditis

Patients with rheumatic heart disease and valve damage require a single dose of antibiotics 1 hour before surgical and dental procedures to help prevent bacterial endocarditis [68, 73]. Patients who had RF without valve damage do not need endocarditis prophylaxis. Penicillin, ampicillin, or amoxicillin should not be used for endocarditis prophylaxis in patients already receiving penicillin for secondary prophylaxis due to an increased relative resistance of oral streptococci to penicillin and aminopenicillins. Alternate drugs recommended by the American Heart Association for these patients include oral *clindamycin*, *azithromycin*, or *clarithromycin*.

Interventional Management

Percutaneous Balloon Mitral Valvuloplasty

Approximately 40 % of patients with acute RF subsequently develop MS later in life. For patients with MS who require relief of obstruction, percutaneous balloon mitral valvuloplasty is the preferred treatment and gives results comparable to surgical commissurotomy [74]. 2D echocardiographic assessment of mitral valve morphology is the most important predictor of outcome. An echocardiographic score can be determined according to the valvar and subvalvar mitral anatomy, with a score <8 predicting good immediate and long-term results [75, 76].

The procedure involves a transseptal technique with a catheter placed into the LA and LV from a right atrial approach. Two techniques are available, the double balloon and the Inoue balloon, with the same results and comparable complications [77]. The procedure is guided by transesophageal echocardiogram. The drop in pulmonary vascular resistance is usually immediate after the valvuloplasty and patients feel immediately better. Percutaneous transmitral valvuloplasty has been shown to provide excellent intermediate-term palliation in children with rheumatic MS [78, 79]. Both percutaneous valvuloplasty and surgical commissurotomy yield comparable results and similar restenosis rates. The long-term result of the procedure still needs to be determined in small children, restenosis and moderate MR rate appearing to be higher in small children [78, 80].

Percutaneous Mitral Valve Repair

Percutaneous MR repair is an emerging area of interventional cardiology, but no data are available in children. Direct percutaneous repair of the mitral valve is undergoing trials using the Evalve mitral clip and Edwards mitral suture devices [81–83]. Further data are needed to evaluate the long-term outcome of these techniques.

Surgical Management

Optimal surgical management remains controversial. In MFS, the underlying connective tissue disorder is a risk factor for compromise of repair durability. Despite the important elastic fiber alterations in leaflet tissue and the multisystem involvement, mitral valve repair in MFS gives satisfactory long-term results in terms of freedom from reoperation in children and even in adults presenting with advanced valve pathology. In RF, early mitral valve surgery after the sudden onset of hemodynamically significant MR increases the likelihood of adequate repair and may be lifesaving in patients with heart failure resistant to medical treatment, whereas progression of the infectious and inflammatory reactions may affect valve tissue, thereby precluding optimum repair. In children, mitral valvuloplasty is preferred [84]. Valve replacement appears to be the preferred surgical option for patients with high rates of recurrent symptoms after annuloplasty or other repair procedures. Indications for mitral valve surgery in patients with mitral valve disease are summarized in Table 96.9.

Mitral Valve Repair

Many techniques have been described. Mitral valve repair without the use of prosthetic materials is feasible for the majority of patients and carries an appropriate growth pattern of the mitral valve annulus after surgery [85]. Rheumatic mitral valve repair has a greater rate of reoperation when compared to mitral valve replacement using a mechanical prosthesis, but

Table 96.9 Indications for surgery for chronic mitral regurgitation (Adapted from Bonow et al. [6]). *Abbreviations: LVEF = left ventricular ejection fraction, LVESD = left ventricular end-systolic dimension, NYHA = New York Heart Association dyspnea scale*

Symptoms	LVEF	LVESD
NYHA II–IV	>60 %	<45 mm
Asymptomatic or symptomatic	50–60 %	≥45 mm
Asymptomatic or symptomatic	<50 % or ≥45 mm	
Pulmonary artery systolic pressure ≥50 mmHg		

it provides better actuarial survival with fewer thromboembolic complications in children who are usually noncompliant to anticoagulation [86].

Several echocardiographic parameters can help to identify patients at risk of mitral valve repair failure: the presence of a large central regurgitant jet, severe annular dilatation (>50 mm), involvement of ≥3 scallops especially if the anterior leaflet is involved and extensive valve calcification.

This section will now focus more on the description of different mitral valve repair techniques that have to be performed according to the different mechanisms of mitral valve dysfunction based on Carpentier's classification.

– *Type I: Annular Dilatation*

MR due to pure type I dysfunction occurs usually during inflammatory pancarditis. Annular dilatation and deformity are corrected using either a traditional ring (like Carpentier-Edwards ring, metallic) or a biodegradable ring which becomes inevitable (Figs. 96.6 and 96.7), especially in pediatric sizes less than 26 mm, since smaller sizes are nonexistent in traditional rings and can be potentially stenotic at a later date in a growing child. The Kalangos-Bioring® consists of a partial ring made of 1,4-polydioxanone that is implanted directly into the valve annulus and is available in sizes down to 16 mm [87–89]. This ring is degraded and elicits a subendocardial fibrous reaction allowing for durable remodeling of the annulus. Kalangos et al. have published their pediatric mitral valve repair cohort using this biodegradable mitral annuloplasty

ring which has now reached 90 patients, with a mean follow-up of 27.3 ± 17.2 (1.8–60.5) months. Eighty-three patients (92 %) showed favorable outcome without significant failure, while seven patients have required reoperation within 1–20 months for mitral valve re-repair (n = 1) or replacement (n = 6) because of rheumatic (n = 4), congenital (n = 2), and degenerative (n = 1) mitral valve lesions [90].

Enlargement of the posterior leaflet or in exceptional cases of the anterior leaflet with a pericardial patch may permit the insertion of a larger traditional ring. In all cases of chronic rheumatic MR, concomitant mitral annuloplasty is mandatory due to the associated dilatation and deformity of the mitral annulus. Selection of the appropriate ring size is based on the surface area of the anterior leaflet or on the inter-trigonal distance.

– *Type IIa: Anterior Leaflet Prolapse*

Anterior leaflet prolapse is caused by rupture or elongation of anterior primary chordae tendineae and elongation of papillary muscle's heads. Rupture usually occurs during the active inflammatory phase of RF and frequently affects the paramedian anterior primary chordae tendineae. Anterior leaflet prolapse can be corrected using chordal shortening, chordal transfer techniques, or the use of artificial cords (Movie 96.1). Chordal shortening techniques include the split and tuck-in technique, chordal shortening at the free edge of the prolapsing anterior leaflet segment, and sliding shortening plasty of the elongated papillary muscle head. If the anterior leaflet prolapse is mainly due to elongation of the papillary muscle head on which thick, stiff, and short chordae tendineae are inserted, dislocation of the elongated head onto an adjacent site by suture fixation or sliding plasty of the papillary muscle head is effective in correcting prolapse.

– *Type IIa/IIIp: Anterior Leaflet Pseudo-prolapse and Restricted Posterior Leaflet Motion*

Contrary to true anterior leaflet prolapse in which the free edge of the anterior leaflet overrides the mitral annulus plane during systole

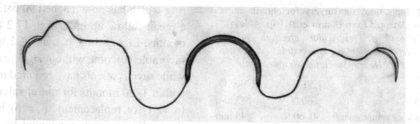

Fig. 96.6 *Characteristics of the biodegradable ring.* The biodegradable mitral annuloplasty ring (Kalangos-Bioring®) consists of a "C"-shaped segment of polymer, attached on either end to monofilament polyvinyl suture extensions, with a swaged stainless steel needle on each end. The suture is in continuity under the entire central portion of the polymer

on echocardiography, the free edge of the anterior leaflet does not override the mitral annulus plane with anterior leaflet pseudo-prolapse [39]. MR in type IIa/IIIp results mainly from the significant restricted motion of the posterior leaflet, allowing for the anterior leaflet to move up to the annular plane without overriding it. Repair techniques in the correction of the type IIa/IIIp mechanism are focused on increasing mobility or width of the restricted posterior leaflet, lowering of the coaptation point of the free edge of the anterior leaflet segment to the level of the corresponding coaptation point of the retracted posterior leaflet, and bringing the free edge of the retracted posterior leaflet segment up to the coaptation point of the opposite anterior leaflet segment. Resection of the posterior secondary and sometimes of primary chordae tendineae, shaving the thickened posterior leaflet, papillary muscle splitting at several sites, and commissurotomy can be effective in increasing mobility of the posterior leaflet. If the retraction of the posterior leaflet creates a "V" deformity between the P2 and P3 segments – as in the majority of cases – detachment of these retracted posterior segments from the native annulus and plication of the detached annulus and leaflet segments longitudinally can increase the width of the retracted posterior segments and their coaptation surface with the opposite anterior ones (Movie 96.2). Chordal shortening techniques and the use of artificial cords are effective in lowering the coaptation point of the anterior leaflet segments to that of the opposite posterior ones. Acceptable coaptation cannot always be obtained using standard repair techniques. A novel technique using suspension of the free edge of the retracted posterior leaflet segment to the opposite anterior annulus brings up this free edge to the level of the opposite anterior one, hence establishes a satisfactory coaptation surface between the corresponding opposite segments. This technique has been shown to allow for improved coaptation and resulted in avoidance or delay of valve replacement with an acceptable transvalvular gradient in most patients that did not significantly increase with growth [91].

– *Type III: Restricted Leaflet Motion*
  In the majority of cases, the restricted motion affects the leaflets' closure and generates MR. In some cases, it can affect leaflet opening during diastole due to commissural fusion and retraction of the subvalvular apparatus with fusion of the papillary muscles to the ventricular surface of the leaflet tissue resulting in mitral valve stenosis. Anterior and posterior commissurotomy associated with papillary muscle splitting, resection of the anterior and posterior secondary chordae and sometimes of the primary posterior chordae, shaving of the thickened tissue, and pericardial patch enlargement of the posterior and exceptionally of the anterior leaflet can potentially increase the mobility of both leaflets and offer a reasonable time period to the

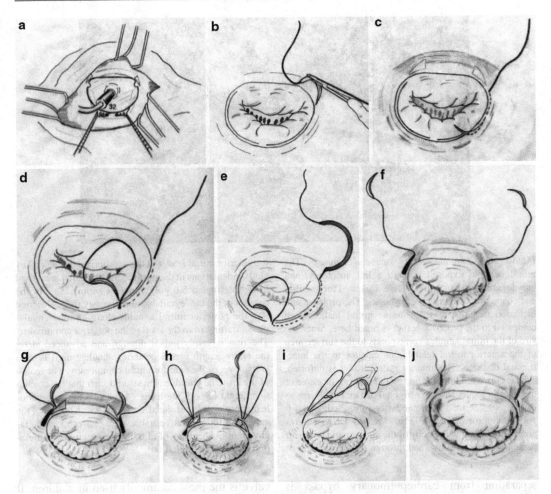

Fig. 96.7 *Biodegradable ring implantation.* (**a**) Sizing of annuloplasty ring – the anterior mitral leaflet is unfurled, and the corresponding size that matches the surface area of the anterior leaflet is chosen for annuloplasty ring implantation. (**b**) The biodegradable ring annuloplasty commences with the subendocardial insertion of the needle into the mitral annulus, at the level of the posterior commissure, 2 mm away from the hinge point, at a depth of 2–3 mm, and away from the mitral leaflet tissue. Care is taken not to orient the sutures deep towards the left atrioventricular groove, in order to prevent injury to the circumflex coronary artery. (**c**) The needle is advanced in an intra-annular plane, along the posterior segment of the mitral annulus, and exited 3–4 cm away from the point of entry. (**d**) The entry point of the next stitch is the same as the exit point of the previous stitch, thus moving the ring forward along the posterior mitral annulus. (**e**) Approximately three of such stitches advance the ring along the entire length of the posterior mitral annulus. (**f**) The last stitch exits at the level of the anterior commissure. (**g**) Annuloplasty ring fixation – the corresponding needles are passed into the anterior and posterior trigones. (**h**) The sutures are passed twice through the respective trigones, in order to double fix the ring firmly in place within the posterior mitral annulus. (**i**) The sutures are tied on themselves at the respective trigones. (**j**) Once the biodegradable ring implantation is complete, the posterior mitral annulus is well plicated, improving the coaptation between the anterior and posterior mitral leaflets. The entire annuloplasty ring lies embedded within the posterior annular tissue, with only the suture knots being visible at the anterior and posterior trigones

patients until progressive retraction over time renders mitral valve replacement inevitable.

Intraoperative assessment of the mitral valve competency is made by "floating" the mitral valve or by injecting and filling the left ventricle with iced saline solution to lift the valve leaflets and expose the valve function. A Hegar dilator is used to measure the mitral valve diameter to ensure normal orifice size for body weight. Transesophageal echocardiography following

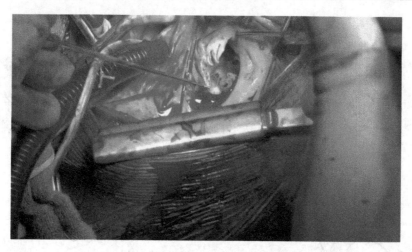

Movie 96.1 *Implantation of artificial chordae.* The mitral valve is exposed through a left atriotomy, and anterior and posterior mitral leaflets are tested for mobility and coaptation using two nerve hooks. The prolapse and increased mobility of the anterior mitral leaflet when compared to the posterior leaflet is noted here. Since the size of the mitral annulus corresponds to the surface area of the anterior mitral leaflet, this equates to the inter-trigonal distance. The anterior mitral leaflet is unfurled, and the corresponding size that matches the surface area of the anterior leaflet and inter-trigonal distance is chosen as the correct size for the annuloplasty ring. Pledgeted 4-0 polytetrafluoroethylene (PTFE; Goretex, USA) sutures are inserted through the body of the anterior and posterior papillary muscles below, and through the free margin of the anterior mitral leaflet at the appropriate distance. Any clefts/indentations in the posterior mitral leaflet are closed using interrupted 5-0 polypropylene sutures. One of the needles of the biodegradable annuloplasty ring is inserted into the posterior mitral annulus along an intra-annular plane, starting from the level of the posterior commissure. The ring is gently pulled through and advanced along the entire length of the posterior annulus, until it exits at the level of the anterior mitral commissure. The length of the artificial chordae is measured such that the coaptation height of both the leaflets is equal, and the anterior leaflet prolapse is corrected. Saline injection testing of the valve and intraoperative transesophageal echocardiography confirm adequacy of mitral valve repair and obliteration of mitral regurgitation

separation from cardiopulmonary bypass is imperative for the assessment of mitral valve function. Results for operative interventions in mitral regurgitation are generally more favorable than those for mitral stenosis.

Mitral Valve Replacement

Bioprosthetic and mechanical valves are indicated when reconstructive procedures have failed in young children. Tissue valves are available but are disadvantageous, as they calcify and degenerate at an accelerated rate in small children [92]. The respective sizes of the patient and the prosthetic valve are the greatest considerations in selecting an artificial mitral valve.

Limited mechanical prosthetic valves are available for use is children, particularly in small children [93]. The bileaflet mechanical valve is the most commonly used in children. It can be sutured in the supra-annular position. A special design with a supra-annular sewing cuff is available for small children, which allows an effective valvar orifice situated at the annular level. Anticoagulation is compulsory and Coumadin is used most commonly, with a target INR between 2.5 and 3.5. Unfortunately, complications are not uncommon. Indeed, mitral valve replacement in young children is associated with substantially increased risk of morbidity and mortality [94].

Minimally Invasive Surgery

Minimally invasive approaches have been increasingly described in adults and involve various modifications of the surgical approach, as in a small parasternal incision from the

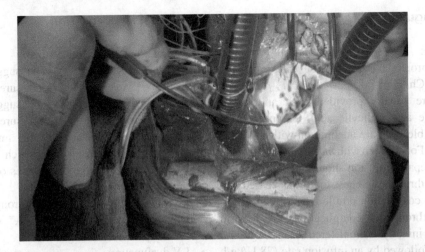

Movie 96.2 *Fundoplasty*. Inspection of the mitral valve using two nerve hooks demonstrates a typical stenotic "fish mouth" rheumatic valve, characterized by thickened, fibrotic leaflets with markedly limitation in mobility, and commissural fusion. Anterior and posterior commissurotomies are performed using a No. 11 blade, leaving a 2 mm margin between the incision and the annulus. Fused subvalvular tissue is also divided and released. Reinspection of the valves demonstrates retraction of the P2–P3 scallops of the posterior mitral leaflet. A 3–4 cm incision is made on the posterior mitral annulus, extending from P3 to P2, leaving a 2 cm rim away from the free margin of the posterior leaflet. Full thickness polypropylene sutures are taken through the 3 o'clock and 9 o'clock positions of the incision. Similarly, multiple interrupted sutures are taken through the 10 o'clock and 2 o'clock, 8 o'clock and 4 o'clock positions, etc. When these sutures are tied down, the orientation of this incision changes from a horizontal incision into a vertical incision, thereby improving the coaptation height of the P2 and P3 segments. The mitral annulus is then supported by conventional ring annuloplasty. Saline injection testing and intraoperative transesophageal echocardiography confirm adequacy of repair, with good leaflet coaptation and no mitral regurgitation

inferior border of the right second costal margin or a mini-thoracotomy. Cardiopulmonary bypass is provided via the femoral vessels, and the aorta is internally cross-clamped with a balloon occlusion cannula. Advantages are diminished pain and discomfort and earlier hospital discharge.

Postoperative Management

Postoperative Monitoring

The postoperative monitoring of patients following mitral valve surgery is an extension of the monitoring and vigilance required in the preoperative period, including anticipation of common postoperative complications following mitral valve surgery. As with preoperative monitoring, postoperative monitoring should include:

- Continuous cardiorespiratory, central venous, and arterial monitoring

- Continuous or intermittent mixed venous saturation to monitor adequacy of global tissue oxygen delivery
- NIRS (near-infrared spectroscopy) may be a useful tool to monitor changes in regional oxyhemoglobin saturation
- Continuous urine output monitoring via indwelling catheter
- Serial echocardiographic assessment, especially in the setting of severely compromised LV function

Additionally, postoperative monitoring following mitral valve surgery may also include:
- LA pressure monitoring to appreciate differences and alterations in the "A" and "V" pressure waveforms (Fig. 96.5)
- Epicardial atrial and ventricular pacing wires, which allow epicardial electrocardiogram and pacing
- Pulmonary artery pressure monitoring, particularly in patients at risk for pulmonary vascular reactivity as in those with MS

Anticoagulation

There is no evidence describing optimal thromboprophylaxis in children with prosthetic valves. Children with *biological prosthetic valves* are usually provided with antiplatelet agent like acetylsalicylic acid. Thromboembolism and bleeding are uncommon with this therapy [95]. For children with *mechanical prosthetic valves*, heparin infusion should be started when bleeding through the chest tubes has ceased and when the coagulation profile has normalized, to prevent thrombotic complications. A heparin bolus is initially administered (75 U/kg over 10 min) followed by an infusion rate (28 U/kg/h for <1 year old and 20 U/kg/h for >1 year old), targeting an aPTT of 60–85 s (assuming this reflect an anti-Xa level of 0.35–0.7) [95]. When the intracardiac lines, the chest tubes, and the pacing wires have been removed, transition to anti-vitamin K antagonists (AVKs) like oral Coumadin can be initiated with a loading dose of 0.2 mg/kg then adjusting the subsequent dose according to the INR [95]. The targeted INR should be between 2.5 and 3.5. For patients with contraindication to oral anticoagulation, low-molecular-weight heparin (LMWH) is a good alternative.

Postoperative Issues and Complications

Mitral valve surgery requires excellent technical surgical results if significant postoperative complications are to be averted. Transesophageal echocardiography should be performed in the operating room following separation from cardiopulmonary bypass so that the surgical result can be assessed and immediately addressed in case of residual lesion, particularly with associated LA hypertension. Consideration of the intravascular volume at the time of echocardiographic study is important, as hypovolemia leads to underestimation of the severity and hemodynamic consequence of residual lesions.

Left Atrial Hypertension

Causes of elevated LA pressure are:
- Residual MR, which may be suggested by giant "V" waves on the LA pressure tracing
- Residual MS, which may be suggested by large "A" waves on the LA pressure tracing
- Prosthetic mitral valve leaflet immobility, dysfunction, or thrombosis, which may also be suggested by large "A" waves on the LA pressure tracing
- Loss of atrioventricular synchrony, which may be suggested by canon "A" waves on the LA pressure tracing
- LV dysfunction
- Pericardial effusion with cardiac tamponade

Pulmonary Hypertension (PH)

In patients with long-standing MS or MR, the pulmonary vascular changes of medial thickening and intimal fibrosis associated with progressive pulmonary vascular disease may complicate the postoperative course. Standard therapy for PH should be considered as PH crises are common. In small children with valve replacement in supra-annular position, the relatively large prosthesis can impede pulmonary venous inflow or LV inflow, thereby promoting PH crises. In patients with PH and postoperative LV dysfunction or residual mitral valve dysfunction, cautious use of nitric oxide therapy is indicated, as the increased pulmonary venous return may worsen PH or LV dysfunction.

Low Cardiac Output Syndrome (LCOS)

LCOS can complicate any bypass surgery. Post MS repair, decreased LV compliance can lead to LCOS in the initial postoperative period. Post MR repair, adaptation of the LV volume overload can lead to LCOS. Additionally, LV function may be compromised by increased afterload secondary to

Picture 96.11 Serial chest x-rays on a patient with a #16 ATS prosthesis turned upside down in the mitral position. A malfunctioning posterior leaflet (*arrows*) is fixed in position and contributing to the patient's failure to progress from continuous positive airway pressure

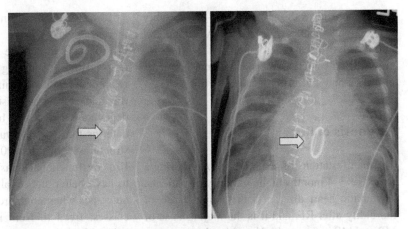

the newly competent mitral valve. Therapy consists of maintenance of optimal heart rate either with atrial pacing or isoproterenol as the cardiac output is highly rate dependent. Adequate preload should be maintained, but volume should be replaced slowly as excessive fluid infusion can lead to rapid LA pressure elevation and subsequent PH crisis.

Adequate LV filling pressure should be maintained to accommodate for diastolic dysfunction. Afterload reduction with milrinone infusion is beneficial to increase cardiac output, especially in patients with LV dysfunction. Afterload reduction may also be useful for reducing the hemodynamic consequences of residual MR.

Arrhythmia

Atrial flutter, atrial fibrillation, and multifocal atrial tachycardia secondary to atrial dilation can complicate the postoperative period. Atrial arrhythmias are not well tolerated especially when LV compliance is impaired. Management of such arrhythmia is essential in the early postoperative period in order to restore atrioventricular synchrony and optimize cardiac output.

Prosthetic Valve Malfunction

Proper function of the prosthetic valve should be carefully monitored, especially in small children with the prosthesis in a supraannular position. Leaflet malfunction may be suspected on the basis of serial chest x-rays in which leaflet position is fixed (Picture 96.11). When thrombosis is suspected, as in acute prosthetic valve dysfunction, streptokinase or tissue plasminogen activator therapy may be attempted. Chronic valve malfunction may be secondary to tissue entrapment of the valve leaflets. The surgical appearance is that of a pannus of tissue which encroaches upon the valve leaflets. The usual presentation is intermittent LA hypertension and absence of a valve click.

Long-Term Outcome

Prognosis of MFS

Long-term outcome in MFS patients is determined by the severity of cardiovascular manifestations. Neonates with phenotypic expression of MFS and cardiovascular involvement are most severely affected and often do not survive past 2 years of age without multiple valve replacements or heart transplantation. Children with MFS and mitral valve involvement can also have significantly limited life spans, particularly if valve dysfunction is rapidly progressive and accompanied by compromised ventricular function. Peri-surgical complications related to mitral valve replacement have the greatest risk of mortality in young patients with MFS. Alternatively, mitral valve disease can often be slowly progressive, with increased risk to female patients in the second and third decades of life.

Prognosis of RF

The manifestations of acute RF resolve during a period of 3–4 months in the majority of patients. Rheumatic heart disease is the major cause of morbidity after RF, and it is the major cause of MR and MS in the world. Variables that correlate with severity of valve disease are the number of previous attacks, the length of time between the onset of disease and beginning of treatment, and the sex, the prognosis being worse for females. Without recurrent attacks, valve insufficiency resolves in 70–80 % of patients. In patients with carditis and valve insufficiency, numerous factors (severity of initial carditis, presence of recurrences, time elapsed since rheumatic fever) affect the likelihood that valve abnormalities and the murmur will disappear. Following the development of antibiotics, the mortality rate in developed countries has decreased to nearly 0 % but has remained 1–10 % in developing countries. Prior to penicillin, 60–70 % of patients developed valve disease after acute rheumatic fever as opposed to 9–39 % nowadays.

Prognosis After Mitral Valve Repair

Prognosis after mitral valve repair is good with an event-free rate at 15 years of about 73 % [96]. The current risk of mitral valve reoperation in the pediatric age group is low, and the long-term results are satisfactory, irrespective of severe deformation of the mitral valve apparatus and associated complex cardiac anomalies [97]. Patients with significant associated congenital cardiac abnormalities are at a higher risk of early death after mitral reconstructive surgery. Mitral repair with a technique that allows annular growth is possible in most children with good long-term functional results [84].

Despite advances in repair techniques and increasing experience of surgeons over the last decade that have decreased the risk of reoperation following valve repair, the reoperation rate continues to remain higher in rheumatic valve disease compared to that of degenerative disease because of progressive deterioration of the valvular and subvalvular structures with time [90]. Type II and type IIa/IIIp dysfunctional classes have been shown to have better statistically significant long-term outcomes when compared to type I and type III classes: freedom from reoperation at 15 years being 92 % for type II and 89 % for type IIa/IIIp versus 64 % for type I and 62 % for type III. The incidence of thromboembolic complications is also low (0.2 %/pt/year) despite a high incidence of atrial fibrillation (2 %/pt/year) over the same follow-up period.

Prognosis After Mitral Valve Replacement (MVR)

MVR is an accepted alternative when the valve cannot be repaired, with a reported freedom from reoperation of 66–86 % [96, 98]. A multi-institutional study reported a 1-year survival of 79 %, a 5-year survival of 75 %, and a 10-year survival of 74 % for children <5 years of age [98]. The majority of deaths occur early after initial replacement, with little late attrition despite repeat MVR and chronic anticoagulation. Adverse outcome is common, particularly in the young child undergoing palliative surgery or requiring additional surgical procedures [99]. Complications include heart block requiring pacemaker, endocarditis, thrombosis, and stroke [98]. Complete atrioventricular canal, Shone's syndrome, and increased ratio of prosthetic valve size to patient weight increase the risk of adverse outcome. Reasons for second MVR are prosthetic valve stenosis in the majority of cases, thrombosis, or endocarditis [100]. Younger patients (<2 years), low weight, smaller prostheses (<20 mm), and greater ratio of prosthesis size to body size were risk factors for second MVR [100].

References

1. Thomson JD, Allen J, Gibbs JL (2000) Left sided valvar regurgitation in normal children and adolescents. Heart 83:185–187
2. Brand A, Dollberg S, Keren A (1992) The prevalence of valvular regurgitation in children with structurally normal hearts: a color Doppler echocardiographic study. Am Heart J 123:177–180
3. Bahadur KC, Sharma D, Shrestha MP et al (2003) Prevalence of rheumatic and congenital heart disease in schoolchildren of Kathmandu valley in Nepal. Indian Heart J 55:615–618
4. Asante-Korang A, O'Leary PW, Anderson RH (2006) Anatomy and echocardiography of the normal and abnormal mitral valve. Cardiol Young 16(Suppl 3):27–34
5. Bonow RO, Nikas D, Elefteriades JA (1995) Valve replacement for regurgitant lesions of the aortic or mitral valve in advanced left ventricular dysfunction. Cardiol Clin 13:73–83, 85
6. Bonow RO, Carabello B, De Leon AC Jr et al (1998) Guidelines for the management of patients with valvular heart disease: executive summary. A report of the American college of cardiology/American heart association task force on practice guidelines (committee on management of patients with valvular heart disease). Circulation 98:1949–1984
7. Ayabakan C, Ozkutlu S, Kilic A (2003) The Doppler echocardiographic assessment of valvular regurgitation in normal children. Turk J Pediatr 45:102–107
8. Allen J, Thomson JD, Lewis IJ, Gibbs JL (2001) Mitral regurgitation after anthracycline treatment for childhood malignancy. Heart 85:430–432
9. De Backer J, Loeys B, Devos D, Dietz H, De Sutter J, De Paepe A (2006) A critical analysis of minor cardiovascular criteria in the diagnostic evaluation of patients with Marfan syndrome. Genet Med 8:401–408
10. Stollerman GH (1997) Rheumatic fever. Lancet 349:935–942
11. Veasy LG, Wiedmeier SE, Orsmond GS et al (1987) Resurgence of acute rheumatic fever in the intermountain area of the United States. N Engl J Med 316:421–427
12. Carapetis JR (2007) Rheumatic heart disease in developing countries. N Engl J Med 357:439–441
13. Carapetis JR, McDonald M, Wilson NJ (2005) Acute rheumatic fever. Lancet 366:155–168
14. Marcus RH, Sareli P, Pocock WA, Barlow JB (1994) The spectrum of severe rheumatic mitral valve disease in a developing country. Correlations among clinical presentation, surgical pathologic findings, and hemodynamic sequelae. Ann Intern Med 120:177–183

15. Bessen DE, Sotir CM, Readdy TL, Hollingshead SK (1996) Genetic correlates of throat and skin isolates of group a streptococci. J Infect Dis 173:896–900
16. Denny FW, Wannamaker LW, Brink WR, Rammelkamp CH Jr, Custer EA (1950) Prevention of rheumatic fever; treatment of the preceding streptococcic infection. J Am Med Assoc 143:151–153
17. Patarroyo ME, Winchester RJ, Vejerano A et al (1979) Association of a B-cell alloantigen with susceptibility to rheumatic fever. Nature 278:173–174
18. Markowitz M, Gerber MA (1987) Rheumatic fever: recent outbreaks of an old disease. Conn Med 51:229–233
19. Cunningham MW, McCormack JM, Talaber LR et al (1988) Human monoclonal antibodies reactive with antigens of the group a streptococcus and human heart. J Immunol 141:2760–2766
20. Feinstein AR, Spagnuolo M (1993) The clinical patterns of acute rheumatic fever: a reappraisal. 1962. Medicine (Baltimore) 72:272–283, 262–3
21. Zalzstein E, Maor R, Zucker N, Katz A (2003) Advanced atrioventricular conduction block in acute rheumatic fever. Cardiol Young 13:506–508
22. Eshel G, Lahat E, Azizi E, Gross B, Aladjem M (1993) Chorea as a manifestation of rheumatic fever – a 30-year survey (1960–1990). Eur J Pediatr 152:645–646
23. Asbahr FR, Garvey MA, Snider LA, Zanetta DM, Elkis H, Swedo SE (2005) Obsessive-compulsive symptoms among patients with Sydenham chorea. Biol Psychiatry 57:1073–1076
24. Burke JB (1955) Erythema marginatum. Arch Dis Child 30:359–365
25. Baldwin JS, Kerr JM, Kuttner AG, Doyle EF (1960) Observations on rheumatic nodules over a 30-year period. J Pediatr 56:465–470
26. Jones criteria (revised) for guidance in the diagnosis of rheumatic fever (1965) Circulation 32:664–668
27. Guidelines for the diagnosis of rheumatic fever. Jones Criteria (1992 update). Special writing group of the committee on rheumatic fever, endocarditis, and Kawasaki disease of the council on cardiovascular disease in the young of the American Heart Association. JAMA 268:2069–2073
28. Ferrieri P (2002) Proceedings of the Jones criteria workshop. Circulation 106:2521–2523
29. McDonald M, Currie BJ, Carapetis JR (2004) Acute rheumatic fever: a chink in the chain that links the heart to the throat? Lancet Infect Dis 4:240–245
30. Mirza A, Wludyka P, Chiu TT, Rathore MH (2007) Throat culture is necessary after negative rapid antigen detection tests. Clin Pediatr (Phila) 46:241–246
31. Stollerman GH, Lewis AJ, Schultz I, Taranta A (1956) Relationship of immune response to group a streptococci to the course of acute, chronic and recurrent rheumatic fever. Am J Med 20:163–169
32. Rantz LA, Di Caprio JM, Randall E (1952) Antistreptolysin O and antihyaluronidase titers in

health and in various diseases. Am J Med Sci 224:194–200

33. Gupta RC, Badhwar AK, Bisno AL, Berrios X (1986) Detection of C-reactive protein, streptolysin O, and anti-streptolysin O antibodies in immune complexes isolated from the sera of patients with acute rheumatic fever. J Immunol 137:2173–2179

34. Khanna AK, Buskirk DR, Williams RC Jr et al (1989) Presence of a non-HLA B cell antigen in rheumatic fever patients and their families as defined by a monoclonal antibody. J Clin Invest 83:1710–1716

35. Kamblock J, N'Guyen L, Pagis B et al (2005) Acute severe mitral regurgitation during first attacks of rheumatic fever: clinical spectrum, mechanisms and prognostic factors. J Heart Valve Dis 14:440–446

36. Vijayalakshmi IB, Mithravinda J, Deva AN (2005) The role of echocardiography in diagnosing carditis in the setting of acute rheumatic fever. Cardiol Young 15:583–588

37. Marijon E, Ou P, Celermajer DS et al (2007) Prevalence of rheumatic heart disease detected by echocardiographic screening. N Engl J Med 357:470–476

38. Camara EJ, Neubauer C, Camara GF, Lopes AA (2004) Mechanisms of mitral valvar insufficiency in children and adolescents with severe rheumatic heart disease: an echocardiographic study with clinical and epidemiological correlations. Cardiol Young 14:527–532

39. Kalangos A, Beghetti M, Vala D et al (2000) Anterior mitral leaflet prolapse as a primary cause of pure rheumatic mitral insufficiency. Ann Thorac Surg 69:755–761

40. Vasan RS, Shrivastava S, Vijayakumar M, Narang R, Lister BC, Narula J (1996) Echocardiographic evaluation of patients with acute rheumatic fever and rheumatic carditis. Circulation 94:73–82

41. Pyeritz RE, Wappel MA (1983) Mitral valve dysfunction in the Marfan syndrome. Clinical and echocardiographic study of prevalence and natural history. Am J Med 74:797–807

42. von Kodolitsch Y, Robinson PN (2007) Marfan syndrome: an update of genetics, medical and surgical management. Heart 93:755–760

43. Murdoch JL, Walker BA, Halpern BL, Kuzma JW, McKusick VA (1972) Life expectancy and causes of death in the Marfan syndrome. N Engl J Med 286:804–808

44. Pyeritz RE (2000) The Marfan syndrome. Annu Rev Med 51:481–510

45. Judge DP, Dietz HC (2005) Marfan's syndrome. Lancet 366:1965–1976

46. van Karnebeek CD, Naeff MS, Mulder BJ, Hennekam RC, Offringa M (2001) Natural history of cardiovascular manifestations in Marfan syndrome. Arch Dis Child 84:129–137

47. Fleischer KJ, Nousari HC, Anhalt GJ, Stone CD, Laschinger JC (1997) Immunohistochemical abnormalities of fibrillin in cardiovascular tissues in Marfan's syndrome. Ann Thorac Surg 63:1012–1017

48. Bhudia SK, Troughton R, Lam BK et al (2006) Mitral valve surgery in the adult Marfan syndrome patient. Ann Thorac Surg 81:843–848

49. Fuzellier JF, Chauvaud SM, Fornes P et al (1998) Surgical management of mitral regurgitation associated with Marfan's syndrome. Ann Thorac Surg 66:68–72

50. Hennekam RC (2005) Severe infantile Marfan syndrome versus neonatal Marfan syndrome. Am J Med Genet A 139:1

51. Porter TR, Airey K, Quader M (2006) Mitral valve endocarditis presenting as complete heart block. Tex Heart Inst J 33:100–101

52. Morse RP, Rockenmacher S, Pyeritz RE et al (1990) Diagnosis and management of infantile Marfan syndrome. Pediatrics 86:888–895

53. Stuart AG, Williams A (2007) Marfan's syndrome and the heart. Arch Dis Child 92:351–356

54. Yetman AT, Bornemeier RA, McCrindle BW (2003) Long-term outcome in patients with Marfan syndrome: is aortic dissection the only cause of sudden death? J Am Coll Cardiol 41:329–332

55. Roman MJ, Rosen SE, Kramer-Fox R, Devereux RB (1993) Prognostic significance of the pattern of aortic root dilation in the Marfan syndrome. J Am Coll Cardiol 22:1470–1476

56. Boudoulas H, Kolibash AJ Jr, Baker P, King BD, Wooley CF (1989) Mitral valve prolapse and the mitral valve prolapse syndrome: a diagnostic classification and pathogenesis of symptoms. Am Heart J 118:796–818

57. Mueller C, Huber P, Laifer G, Mueller B, Perruchoud AP (2004) Procalcitonin and the early diagnosis of infective endocarditis. Circulation 109:1707–1710

58. Lancellotti P, Moura L, Pierard LA et al (2010) European association of echocardiography recommendations for the assessment of valvular regurgitation part 2: mitral and tricuspid regurgitation (native valve disease). Eur J Echocardiogr 11:307–332

59. Zoghbi WA, Enriquez-Sarano M, Foster E et al (2003) Recommendations for evaluation of the severity of native valvular regurgitation with two-dimensional and Doppler echocardiography. J Am Soc Echocardiogr 16:777–802

60. Villani M, Bianchi T, Locatelli G et al (1977) Congenital mitral valve malformations. Anatomical lesions and surgical treatment in paediatric age (author's transl). G Ital Cardiol 7:968–977

61. TREATMENT of acute rheumatic fever in children a co-operative clinical trial of A.C.T.H., cortisone, and aspirin (1955). A joint report by the rheumatic fever working party of the Medical Research Council of Great Britain and the subcommittee of principal investigators of the American Council on rheumatic fever and congenital heart disease, American Heart Association. Br Med J 1:555–574

62. Albert DA, Harel L, Karrison T (1995) The treatment of rheumatic carditis: a review and meta-analysis. Medicine (Baltimore) 74:1–12

63. Haffejee IE, Moosa A (1990) A double-blind pla-
cebo-controlled trial of prednisone in active rheumatic carditis. Ann Trop Paediatr 10:395–400
64. Dajani A, Taubert K, Ferrieri P, Peter G, Shulman S
(1995) Treatment of acute streptococcal pharyngitis
and prevention of rheumatic fever: a statement for
health professionals. Committee on rheumatic fever,
endocarditis, and Kawasaki disease of the council on
cardiovascular disease in the young, the American
heart association. Pediatrics 96:758–764
65. Shulman ST, Gerber MA, Tanz RR, Markowitz
M (1994) Streptococcal pharyngitis: the case for
penicillin therapy. Pediatr Infect Dis J 13:1–7
66. Dajani AS, Bisno AL, Chung KJ et al (1989) Prevention of rheumatic fever: a statement for health professionals by the committee on rheumatic fever,
endocarditis and Kawasaki disease of the council on
cardiovascular disease in the young, the
American heart association. Pediatr Infect Dis J
8:263–266
67. Lue HC, Wu MH, Wang JK, Wu FF, Wu YN
(1996) Three- versus four-week administration of
benzathine penicillin G: effects on incidence of streptococcal infections and recurrences of rheumatic
fever. Pediatrics 97:984–988
68. Dajani AS, Taubert KA, Wilson W et al (1997) Prevention of bacterial endocarditis. Recommendations
by the American heart association. Circulation
96:358–366
69. Yetman AT (2007) Cardiovascular pharmacotherapy
in patients with Marfan syndrome. Am J Cardiovasc
Drugs 7:117–126
70. Smith TW (1993) Digoxin in heart failure. N Engl
J Med 329:51–53
71. Tauke J, Goldstein S, Gheorghiade M (1994)
Digoxin for chronic heart failure: a review of the
randomized controlled trials with special attention
to the PROVED (prospective randomized study of
ventricular failure and the efficacy of digoxin) and
RADIANCE (randomized assessment of digoxin on
inhibitors of the angiotensin converting enzyme) trials. Prog Cardiovasc Dis 37:49–58
72. The effect of digoxin on mortality and morbidity in
patients with heart failure (1997) The Digitalis Investigation Group. N Engl J Med 336:525–533
73. Wilson W, Taubert KA, Gewitz M et al (2007) Prevention of infective endocarditis: guidelines from the
American heart association: a guideline from the
American heart association rheumatic fever, endocarditis, and Kawasaki disease committee, council on
cardiovascular disease in the young, and the council
on clinical cardiology, council on cardiovascular
surgery and anesthesia, and the quality of care and
outcomes research interdisciplinary working group.
Circulation 116:1736–1754
74. Berger M (2004) Natural history of mitral stenosis
and echocardiographic criteria and pitfalls in
selecting patients for balloon valvuloplasty. Adv
Cardiol 41:87–94
75. Wilkins GT, Weyman AE, Abascal VM, Block PC,
Palacios IF (1988) Percutaneous balloon dilatation of
the mitral valve: an analysis of echocardiographic
variables related to outcome and the mechanism of
dilatation. Br Heart J 60:299–308
76. Abascal VM, Wilkins GT, Choong CY et al (1988)
Echocardiographic evaluation of mitral valve structure and function in patients followed for at least
6 months after percutaneous balloon mitral
valvuloplasty. J Am Coll Cardiol 12:606–615
77. Gerardin B, Losay J, Leriche H, Piot D, Petit J,
Houyel L (1992) Percutaneous mitral valvulotomy:
comparison of 2 techniques in 100 matched-pair
patients. Arch Mal Coeur Vaiss 85:1799–1803
78. Kothari SS, Ramakrishnan S, Kumar CK, Juneja R,
Yadav R (2005) Intermediate-term results of percutaneous transvenous mitral commissurotomy in children less than 12 years of age. Catheter Cardiovasc
Interv 64:487–490
79. Arora R, Mukhopadhyay S, Yusuf J, Trehan V (2007)
Technique, results, and follow-up of interventional
treatment of rheumatic mitral stenosis in children.
Cardiol Young 17:3–11
80. Krishnamoorthy KM, Tharakan JA (2003) Balloon
mitral valvulotomy in children aged < or =12 years.
J Heart Valve Dis 12:461–468
81. Block PC (2006) Percutaneous transcatheter repair
for mitral regurgitation. J Interv Cardiol 19:547–551
82. Mack MJ (2006) New techniques for percutaneous
repair of the mitral valve. Heart Fail Rev 11:259–268
83. Silvestry FE, Rodriguez LL, Herrmann HC et al
(2007) Echocardiographic guidance and assessment
of percutaneous repair for mitral regurgitation with
the evalve MitraClip: lessons learned from
EVEREST I. J Am Soc Echocardiogr 20:1131–1140
84. Hillman ND, Tani LY, Veasy LG et al (2004) Current
status of surgery for rheumatic carditis in children.
Ann Thorac Surg 78:1403–1408
85. Honjo O, Ishino K, Kawada M, Akagi T,
Sano S (2006) Midterm outcome of mitral valve
repair for congenital mitral regurgitation in infants
and children. Interact Cardiovasc Thorac Surg
5:589–593
86. Chauvaud S, Fuzellier JF, Berrebi A, Deloche A,
Fabiani JN, Carpentier A (2001) Long-term (29
years) results of reconstructive surgery in rheumatic
mitral valve insufficiency. Circulation 104:I12–I15
87. Kalangos A, Sierra J, Vala D et al (2006)
Annuloplasty for valve repair with a new biodegradable ring: an experimental study. J Heart Valve Dis
15:783–790
88. Cikirikcioglu M, Pektok E, Myers PO, Christenson
JT, Kalangos A (2008) Pediatric mitral valve repair
with the novel annuloplasty ring: Kalangos-Bioring.
Asian Cardiovasc Thorac Ann 16:515–516
89. Cikirikcioglu M, Cherian S, Stimec B et al
(2011) Morphologic and angiographic analysis to
assess the safety of a biodegradable mitral
annuloplasty ring. J Heart Valve Dis 20:199–204

90. Kalangos A, Christenson JT, Beghetti M, Cikirikcioglu M, Kamentsidis D, Aggoun Y (2008) Mitral valve repair for rheumatic valve disease in children: midterm results and impact of the use of a biodegradable mitral ring. Ann Thorac Surg 86:161–168; discussion 168–9

91. Myers PO, Christenson JT, Cikirikcioglu M, Tissot C, Aggoun Y, Kalangos A (2010) Leaflet suspension to the contralateral annulus to address restriction or tethering-induced mitral and tricuspid regurgitation in children: results of a case–control study. J Thorac Cardiovasc Surg 140:1110–1116

92. Human DG, Joffe HS, Fraser CB, Barnard CN (1982) Mitral valve replacement in children. J Thorac Cardiovasc Surg 83:873–877

93. Spevak PJ, Freed MD, Castaneda AR, Norwood WI, Pollack P (1986) Valve replacement in children less than 5 years of age. J Am Coll Cardiol 8:901–908

94. Husain SA, Brown JW (2007) When reconstruction fails or is not feasible: valve replacement options in the pediatric population, Semin Thorac Cardiovasc Surg Pediatr Card Surg Annu 117–124

95. Monagle P, Chalmers E, Chan A et al (2008) Antithrombotic therapy in neonates and children: American college of chest physicians evidence-based clinical practice guidelines (8th edition). Chest 133:887S–968S

96. Wood AE, Healy DG, Nolke L, Duff D, Oslizlok P, Walsh K (2005) Mitral valve reconstruction in a pediatric population: late clinical results and predictors of long-term outcome. J Thorac Cardiovasc Surg 130:66–73

97. Yoshimura N, Yamaguchi M, Oshima Y et al (1999) Surgery for mitral valve disease in the pediatric age group. J Thorac Cardiovasc Surg 118:99–106

98. Caldarone CA, Raghuveer G, Hills CB et al (2001) Long-term survival after mitral valve replacement in children aged <5 years: a multi-institutional study. Circulation 104:I143–I147

99. Eble BK, Fiser WP, Simpson P, Dugan J, Drummond-Webb JJ, Yetman AT (2003) Mitral valve replacement in children: predictors of long-term outcome. Ann Thorac Surg 76:853–859; discussion 859–60

100. Raghuveer G, Caldarone CA, Hills CB, Atkins DL, Belmont JM, Moller JH (2003) Predictors of prosthesis survival, growth, and functional status following mechanical mitral valve replacement in children aged <5 years, a multi-institutional study. Circulation 108(Suppl 1):II174–II179

Acquired Tricuspid Stenosis and Regurgitation

97

Sanjay Cherian, Anuradha Sridhar, Raghavan Subramanyan, and Afksendyos Kalangos

Abstract

Acquired tricuspid valve diseases can occur due to structural or functional abnormality of the valve. Functional abnormality is the most common cause of tricuspid regurgitation in children and is secondary to annular dilatation caused by volume or pressure overload of the right heart. Two major conditions causing structural tricuspid valve diseases in children are rheumatic heart disease and infective endocarditis. When there is rheumatic involvement of the tricuspid valve, the mitral valve will invariably be involved and the condition is more common among children more than 15 years old. Bacterial endocarditis can cause tricuspid valve disease, mostly regurgitation, in any pediatric age group. This chapter includes etiology, pathophysiology, clinical presentation, and management of acquired tricuspid valve diseases.

Electronic Supplementary Material: The online version of this chapter (doi:10.1007/978-1-4471-4619-3_33) contains supplementary material, which is available to authorized users.

S. Cherian (✉)
Cardiovascular Surgery Service, The University Hospital of Geneva, Geneva, Switzerland

Frontier Lifeline & Dr. K. M. Cherian Heart Foundation, Chennai, India
e-mail: sanjaycherian@hotmail.com

A. Sridhar • R. Subramanyan
Frontier Lifeline & Dr. K. M. Cherian Heart Foundation, Chennai, India
e-mail: anuradhasridhar9@gmail.com;
cardio@frontierlifeline.com

A. Kalangos
Cardiovascular Surgery Service, The University Hospital of Geneva, Geneva, Switzerland
e-mail: Afksendyos.Kalangos@hcuge.ch

Keywords

Acquired heart disease • Biodegradable annuloplasty ring implantation •
Carcinoid • Cardiac surgery • Cardiopulmonary bypass • De Vega
annuloplasty • Fabry's disease • Infective endocarditis • Interventional
catheterization • Kay annuloplasty • Methysergide • Rheumatic heart
disease • Rigid ring annuloplasty • Tricuspid regurgitation • Tricuspid
stenosis • Tricuspid valve • Whipple's disease

Introduction

The tricuspid valve has a more complex morphology compared to the mitral valve due to the elaborate arrangement of its subvalvular apparatus. Tricuspid valve dysfunction can be divided into stenosis or regurgitation. Most stenotic valves will have clinical, echocardiographic, or angiographic evidence of regurgitation, whereas the dominantly regurgitant lesions are seldom associated with stenosis.

Anatomy and Function of the Tricuspid Valve

Anatomy

The tricuspid valve (TV) guards the right atrioventricular (AV) orifice which is surrounded by a fibrous ring. The tricuspid valve ring is part of the fibrous skeleton of the heart which surrounds both AV orifice and also the pulmonary and aortic orifices (Fig. 97.1). The fibrous ring of the right AV opening gives attachment to the cusps of the right AV valve and atrial and ventricular muscle [1].

The tricuspid valve is triangular or trapezoidal in shape and has three cusps connected by their bases to the fibrous ring surrounding the orifice and by their sides with one another, so as to form a continuous annular membrane round the margin of the opening. The cusps of the tricuspid valve are named after their position. The cusp which separates the right atrioventricular orifice from the infundibulum is the largest and most mobile and is called the anterior or infundibular or anterosuperior leaflet. The cusp lying on the

inferior wall of right ventricle is called the posterior or inferior or marginal leaflet. The septal or medial leaflet lies on the interventricular septum (Fig. 97.1).

The leaflets are formed by the endocardium, strengthened by a layer of fibrous tissue, which contains muscle fibers. The central part of each segment is thick and strong, whereas the lateral margins are thin and transparent. The free margins and the ventricular surface of all three leaflets have attachment to a number of delicate tendinous cords, the chordae tendineae.

The chordae are attached to the rounded muscular columns (Musculi papillares) [2] which project from nearly the whole of the inner surface of the ventricle, excepting near the opening of the pulmonary artery where the wall is smooth. The right ventricular papillary muscles originate in the ventricular wall and attach to the anterior, posterior, and septal leaflets of the tricuspid valve via the chordae tendineae.

The single most distinguishing feature of the tricuspid valve, however, is the attachment of the tendinous cords from the septal leaflet directly to the ventricular septum. This unique feature of septal attachment of the tricuspid valve helps to identify the valve in complex congenital heart diseases associated with atrioventricular discordance.

The chordae tendineae are attached to the valve leaflets in the following manner: (1) three or four reach the attached margin of each segment, where they are continuous with the AV tendinous ring; (2) four to six in number attached to the central thickened part of each segment; and (3) the most numerous and finest are connected with the marginal portion of each leaflet. The chordae are attached to the margins

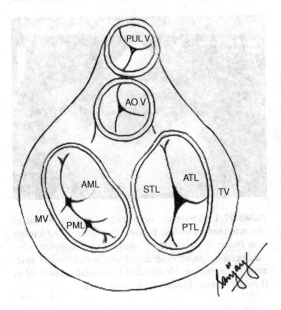

Fig. 97.1 The fibrous ring surrounding the right atrio-ventricular (AV) orifice is part of the fibrous skeleton of the heart which surrounds both AV orifices and also the pulmonary and aortic orifice. Note the relative position of the three leaflets of the Tricuspid valve. The anterior leaflet faces the infundibulum, the septal leaflet lies against the interventricular septum and the posterior leaflet is attached to the posterior margin of the AV fibrous ring. *AO V* aortic valve, *PUL V* pulmonary valve, *TV* tricuspid valve, *MV* mitral valve, *AML* anterior mitral leaflets, *PML* posterior mitral leaflet, *STL* septal tricuspid leaflet, *ATL* anterior tricuspid leaflet, *PTL* posterior tricuspid leaflet

and the ventricular surfaces of the cusps, whereas the atrial surfaces over which the blood flows are smooth.

Function

The TV allows blood to pass freely from the right atrium into the right ventricle in diastole and prevents regurgitation back to the right atrium during ventricular systole. The papillary muscle and chordae tendineae anchor the segments of the valve and prevent them from being forced through into the atrium. Structural alterations of the TV (congenital or acquired) can result in stenosis or regurgitation, whereas abnormal function of a structurally normal valve usually results in pure regurgitation [3, 4].

Classification of Tricuspid Valve Abnormalities

To aid in establishing the etiology, it is useful to divide the tricuspid valve anomalies into either stenotic or regurgitant types.

Tricuspid Stenosis

Stenotic tricuspid valves are always anatomically abnormal (fibrous thickening), and the causes are limited to a few conditions which include rheumatic heart disease, congenital abnormalities, metabolic or enzymatic abnormalities (carcinoid, Fabry's disease, Whipple's disease, methysergide therapy), and active infective endocarditis.

Rheumatic heart disease is the most common cause (>90 % cases) for tricuspid stenosis and is invariably accompanied by mitral valve involvement [5]. Congenital tricuspid stenosis is almost always associated with other anomalies like right ventricular outflow obstruction with secondary hypoplasia of the right ventricle and tricuspid valve [6]. Conditions mimicking tricuspid stenosis include right atrial myxomas, metastatic lung or renal cell carcinoma, and large thrombi causing supravalvar tricuspid stenosis, and primary or secondary tumors affecting the body of the right ventricles which are large enough to cause subvalvar obstruction [7].

Tricuspid Regurgitation

Isolated tricuspid regurgitation (TR) occurs either due to structural abnormality of the valve (congenital or acquired) or secondary to annular dilatation (functional tricuspid regurgitation) [4]. Functional tricuspid regurgitation can occur either due to pressure or volume overload of the right heart. Abnormalities of the tricuspid valve leading to TR can occur with rheumatic valvulitis, infective endocarditis, carcinoid syndrome, rheumatoid arthritis, radiation therapy, trauma, repeated endomyocardial biopsies, Marfan syndrome, tricuspid valve prolapse, tricuspid annular dilatation, or congenital disorders such as

Table 97.1 Causes of tricuspid valve (TV) dysfunction

Tricuspid regurgitation
　　Structural abnormality of the TV
　　　　Congenital
　　　　　　Ebstein's anomaly
　　　　　　TV dysplasia
　　　　　　TV hypoplasia
　　　　　　TV cleft
　　　　　　Double orifice TV
　　　　　　Unguarded TV orifice
　　　　Acquired
　　　　　　Endocarditis
　　　　　　Trauma
　　　　　　Carcinoid heart disease
　　　　　　Rheumatic heart disease
　　　　　　TV prolapse
　　　　　　Iatrogenic (radiation, drugs, biopsy, device lead)
　　Functional (morphologically normal leaflets with annular dilatation)
　　　　Idiopathic tricuspid annular dilatation
　　　　RV dysplasia
　　　　Endomyocardial fibrosis
　　　　Primary pulmonary hypertension (PHT)
　　　　Secondary PHT
　　　　Atrial septal defect
　　　　Anomalous pulmonary venous drainage

Tricuspid stenosis

Rheumatic heart disease

Congenital heart disease

Active infective endocarditis

Metabolic or enzymatic abnormalities (carcinoid, Fabry's disease, Whipple's disease, methysergide therapy)

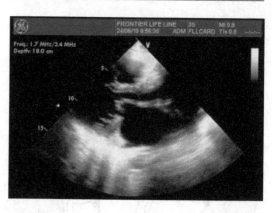

Video 97.1 Rheumatic heart disease of tricuspid valve: characterized by diffuse fibrous thickening of the leaflets with fusion of two or three commissures. Doppler echocardiography shows evidence of severe stenosis and moderate regurgitation. Mitral valve is invariably involved in rheumatic heart disease of tricuspid valve

Ebstein's anomaly or a cleft tricuspid valve as part of atrioventricular canal malformations. Anorectic drugs may also cause TR. The conditions causing tricuspid regurgitation are summarized in Table 97.1.

Pathophysiology of Acquired Tricuspid Valve Disease

Rheumatic Tricuspid Stenosis

Rheumatic involvement of the tricuspid valve is characterized by diffuse fibrous thickening of the leaflets with fusion of two or three commissures. The anteroseptal commissure is most commonly involved. Fusion of all three commissures leads to a diaphragm-like obstruction to flow by the valve (Video 97.1). The chordae tendineae of the tricuspid valve may thicken and shorten, but chordal fusion and chordal changes in general are not as severe as in rheumatic mitral valve stenosis. Also, in contrast to many stenotic mitral valves, the leaflet thickening in tricuspid stenosis is virtually always the result of fibrous tissue proliferation with no calcific deposits (Fig. 97.2). The absence of calcific deposits even in severely stenotic tricuspid valves should make them amenable to commissurotomy or repair procedure (surgical or transluminal balloon valvuloplasty) rather than replacement procedures. Unfortunately, the stenotic tricuspid valves are also moderately severe or severely regurgitant, therefore precluding successful commissurotomy procedures. Histologically, the leaflet tissue is comprised of dense collagen and elastic fibers, producing major distortion of the normal leaflet layers [8].

Infective Endocarditis of the Tricuspid Valve

Right-sided infective endocarditis is relatively uncommon, even among drug addicts. Large, infected vegetations obstructing the orifice of the tricuspid valve may occur following heart surgery in children with congenital heart disease [9] (Fig. 97.3) (Video 97.2).

Fig. 97.2 (a) Pathology specimen of Rheumatic tricuspid valve tissue showing leaflet thickening (*Arrow*) but no commissural fusion. (**b**) Rheumatic tricuspid valve tissue excised from a patient showing fibrous tissue proliferation and scarring but with no calcific deposits. *RA* Right atrium, *RV* Right ventricle

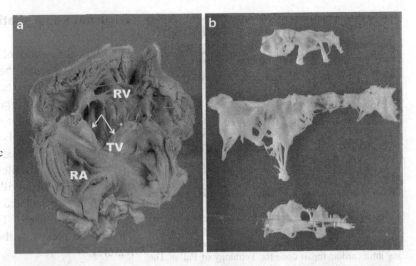

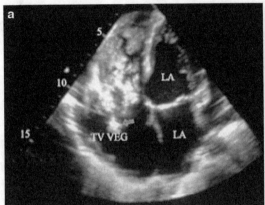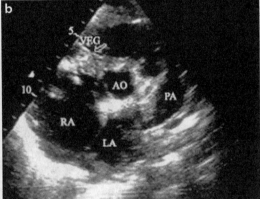

Fig. 97.3 (**a**) Apical 4 chamber view showing large vegetation arising from the tricuspid valve and extending into the right ventricle. (**b**) Parasternal short axis view showing a perimembranous VSD with vegetation of the tricuspid valve involving the defect margins (*green arrow*)

Carcinoid Disease of the Tricuspid Valve

Carcinoid lesions are fibrous white plaques located in the valvular and mural endocardium. The valve leaflets are thickened, rigid, and reduced in area (Video 97.3). Histologic examination discloses proliferation of fibrous tissue on atrial and ventricular surfaces of valve leaflets. The lesion is believed to reflect a direct effect on valvular and mural endocardium by vasoactive amines produced by the carcinoid tumor. About 50 % of patients with widespread lesions of carcinoid tumor develop various

combinations of right-sided valvular lesions (Fig. 97.4): tricuspid stenosis and/or regurgitation, and/or pulmonic stenosis and/or regurgitation [10]. These anomalies are extremely rare in childhood.

Clinical Manifestations

Tricuspid Stenosis

The clinical features of tricuspid stenosis include a giant *a* wave and diminished rate of *y* descent in the jugular venous pulse, a tricuspid opening

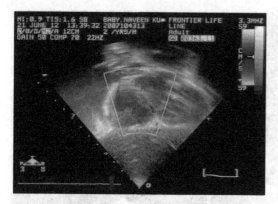

Video 97.2 Infective endocarditis: 2D and color Doppler echocardiography of a 4 year old child who had severe subacute infective endocarditis of tricuspid valve following intra cardiac repair done for Tetralogy of Fallot. The vegetation on the tricuspid valve is seen extending in to the right ventricular (RV) cavity, encroaching the ventricular septal patch and extending in to the RV outflow. There is moderate tricuspid regurgitation and stenosis

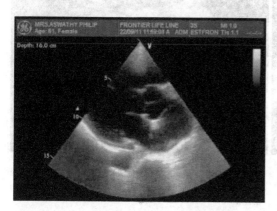

Video 97.3 Carcinoid involvement of tricuspid valve (TV). Apical 4-chamber view showing dilated right ventricle with tricuspid valve leaflets failing to coapt, resulting in constant semi open position. Fixed, retracted, and thickened tricuspid valve leaflets and associated chordae are seen. Color Doppler demonstrates severe tricuspid regurgitation into a dilated right atrium. Continuous-wave Doppler showing dagger-shaped profile of tricuspid regurgitation. (TR)

snap, and a murmur that is presystolic as well as mid-diastolic. The diastolic murmur characteristically increases on inspiration. In chronic rheumatic valve disease, the most common cause of tricuspid stenosis, there are almost always associated clinical findings of aortic and/or mitral valve disease.

Tricuspid Regurgitation

The clinical features of TR include abnormal systolic c-v waves in the jugular venous pulse, a lower left parasternal holosystolic murmur that may increase on inspiration (Carvallo's sign), a mid-diastolic murmur in severe regurgitation, and systolic hepatic pulsation. In rare instances, severe TR may produce systolic propulsion of the eyeballs, pulsatile varicose veins, or a venous systolic thrill and murmur in the neck. Other associated clinical features are related to the cause of TR. Moderate or severe TR may be present without the classic clinical features.

Investigations for Tricuspid Valve Dysfunction

Chest X-Ray

Chest X-ray is usually normal but, in advanced cases with RV hypertrophy or RV dysfunction-induced cardiac failure, it may show an enlarged superior vena cava, an enlarged right atrial or RV silhouette (behind the upper sternum in the lateral projection), or pleural effusion.

Electrocardiography

ECG is usually normal but, in advanced cases, may show tall peaked P waves caused by right atrial enlargement, a tall R or QR wave in V_1 characteristic of RV hypertrophy.

Echocardiography

Echocardiography is valuable in assessing tricuspid valve structure and motion, measuring annular size, and identifying other cardiac abnormalities that might influence tricuspid valve function. Doppler echocardiography permits estimation of the severity of TR, RV systolic pressure, and the tricuspid valve diastolic gradient. Although echocardiography is a valuable

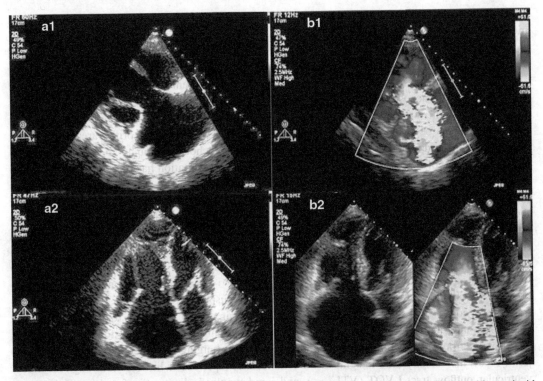

Fig. 97.4 (**a1** & **a2**) Two dimensional echocardiographic image in a patient with carcinoid heart disease – RV inflow view demonstrating thickened, retracted tricuspid valve leaflets. Color Doppler demonstrating severe tricuspid regurgitation. (**b1** & **b2**) Two dimensional echocardiographic image in a patient with carcinoid heart disease – Apical 4 chamber view demonstrating the marked leaflet retraction and lack of coaptation and dilated right atrium. Color Doppler demonstrating severe tricuspid regurgitation

diagnostic tool, it should be pointed out that clinically insignificant TR is detected by color Doppler imaging in many normal persons. This is not an indication for either routine follow-up or prophylaxis against bacterial endocarditis. Clinical correlation and judgment must accompany the echocardiographic results. Systolic pulmonary artery pressure greater than 55 mmHg is likely to cause TR with anatomically normal tricuspid valves, whereas significant TR occurring with systolic pulmonary artery pressures less than 40 mmHg is likely to reflect a structural abnormality of the valve apparatus. Systolic pulmonary artery pressure estimation combined with information about annular circumference will improve the accuracy of clinical assessment further.

The best view for recording TV Doppler velocities is parasternal long-axis angled posteriorly view or an apical four-chamber view. The forward flow velocities peak during rapid ventricular filling (peak E velocity) and atrial contraction (Peak A velocity). Generally, tricuspid valve peak E velocity is higher than the tricuspid valve peak A velocity and lower than the mitral peak E velocity. In normal fetus and neonates, however, the tricuspid peak A velocity is larger than the tricuspid valve peak E velocity, indicating greater reliance on the atrial contribution to right ventricular filling, probably as a result of diminished right ventricular compliance.

Assessment of Severity of Tricuspid Stenosis

Tricuspid stenosis refers to normal annulus size with obstruction to right ventricular inflow due to structural abnormalities in the valvular or subvalvular apparatus. In contrast a hypoplastic tricuspid valve is associated with small annulus.

Congenital tricuspid stenosis could be caused by either shortened and abnormal chordae, thickened and rolled TV leaflets with restricted lateral mobility, or supravalvar stenosing ring. A supravalvar stenosing ring or membrane is a rare anomaly and the membrane can be attached either close to the annulus or to the midportion of the leaflets.

The severity of tricuspid stenosis can be assessed by (1) measurement of peak and mean pressure gradients and pressure half-time across the tricuspid valve and (2) measurement of tricuspid valve area, either from continuity equation or from the proximal iso-velocity surface area method. The continuity equation method is independent of the transvalvar flow, whereas pressure gradients are dependent on the transvalvar flow.

The stenotic tricuspid valve area (CSA_{TV}) can be calculated from velocity time integral of the TS jet (VTI_{TV}), the velocity time integral of the left ventricular outflow tract LVOT (VTI_{LVOT}), and the cross-sectional area of the LVOT (CSA_{LVOT}), if the stroke volume is the same at both sites significant tricuspid regurgitation or aortic regurgitation [11]:

$$CSA_{TV} = [CSA_{LVOT} \times VTI_{LVOT}] / VTI_{TV}$$

Assessment of Severity of Tricuspid Regurgitation

Many of the techniques and approaches discussed in the section on quantitation of the severity of mitral regurgitation can also be applied to quantitation of the severity of tricuspid regurgitation. These methods include:

1. Measurement of right atrial volume and right ventricular end-diastolic and end-systolic volumes from two-dimensional echocardiography
2. Measurement of the spatial distribution of the tricuspid regurgitation jet on the color Doppler examination
3. Measurement of regurgitant volume, regurgitant fraction, and effective regurgitant

orifice area from the two-dimensional and Doppler echocardiography
4. Measurement of regurgitant volume and effective regurgitant orifice from the color Doppler examination

As with pulmonary regurgitation, the calculation of regurgitant volume, regurgitant fraction, and effective regurgitant orifice area from 2D and Doppler echocardiography in patients with tricuspid regurgitation has found no clinical application so far. The major limitations of this technique are the common association of residual shunts and other valve regurgitation (especially pulmonary regurgitation) in pediatric patients with tricuspid regurgitation and the difficulty in determining right ventricular volumes accurately with two-dimensional echocardiography.

Tricuspid valve prolapse can be associated with significant tricuspid regurgitation. In the parasternal long-axis apical four-chamber view, systolic bulging of either the anterior or septal leaflet superior to a line drawn through the tricuspid annulus is diagnostic of prolapse. It is important to note the appearance of the leaflets and to determine if any myxomatous changes are present.

Tricuspid valve is considered to be flail if the tip of the leaflet points towards the atrium (Fig. 97.5). Shortened chordal attachments can prevent the valve from closing completely in systole, or small incompletely formed leaflets can be inadequate for complete valve closure. Incomplete closure of leaflets can also be seen in the presence of dilated or hypertensive right ventricle [11].

Cardiac Catheterization and Other Investigations

Cardiac catheterization is performed only in selected cases. Cardiac catheterization is rarely indicated for evaluation of tricuspid valve disease. When catheterization is indicated (e.g., to evaluate coronary anatomy), the hemodynamic findings include a prominent right atrial *c-v* wave during ventricular systole in severe tricuspid regurgitation. Elevated RA pressure with

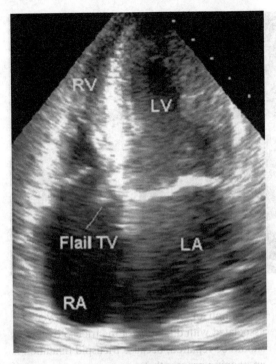

Fig. 97.5 Apical four chamber view showing flail tricuspid valve leaflet. The tip of the cusp is pointing towards the right atrium

Table 97.2 2006 ACC/AHA guidelines pertaining to the surgical management of tricuspid valve disease/ regurgitation

Class I	Tricuspid valve repair is beneficial for severe TR in patients with MV disease requiring MV surgery (Level of Evidence: B)
Class IIa	Tricuspid valve replacement or annuloplasty is reasonable for severe primary TR when symptomatic (Level of Evidence: C)
	Tricuspid valve replacement is reasonable for severe TR secondary to disease/abnormal tricuspid valve leaflets not amenable to annuloplasty or repair (Level of Evidence: C)
Class IIb	Tricuspid annuloplasty may be considered for less than severe TR in patients undergoing MV surgery when there is pulmonary hypertension or tricuspid annular dilatation (Level of Evidence: C)
Class III	Tricuspid valve replacement or annuloplasty is not indicated in asymptomatic patients with TR whose pulmonary artery systolic pressure is less than 60 mmHg in the presence of a normal MV (Level of Evidence: C)
	Tricuspid valve replacement or annuloplasty is not indicated in patients with mild primary TR (Level of Evidence: C)

ACC indicates American College of Cardiology, *AHA* American Heart Association, *TR* tricuspid regurgitation; and *MV*, mitral valve

a slow fall in early diastole and a diastolic pressure gradient across the tricuspid valve is characteristic of tricuspid stenosis.

Other imaging modalities include computerized tomography and cardiac magnetic resonance imaging (cMRI). Cardiac MRI is now the preferred method for evaluating RV size and function.

Management of Tricuspid Valve Disease

Appropriate therapeutic strategy (medical and/or surgical management) may be required depending on the patient's clinical status and the cause of the tricuspid valve abnormality.

Tricuspid Regurgitation

The controversy about the timing and technique of surgical intervention for TR has diminished since the advent of echocardiography for pre- and intraoperative assessment. At present, surgery on the tricuspid valve for TR is performed most commonly at the time of mitral valve (MV) surgery. This situation has been considered a class I indication for TV surgery. As per the recommendations for management of tricuspid valve disease, there is class I indication for tricuspid valve repair for severe TR in patients with MV disease requiring surgery [12] (Table 97.2). TR secondary to damage to the valve by endocarditis and trauma may be considered for cusp and chordal reconstruction instead of replacement [13, 14].

In recent years, although annuloplasty has become an established surgical approach to significant TR, valve replacement is indicated when the valve leaflets themselves are diseased, abnormal, or destroyed. In case of valve replacement, bioprosthesis may be preferred than mechanical prosthesis because of the high rate of thromboembolic complications within the tricuspid position. In patients with associated conduction defects,

Fig. 97.6 Apical four chamber view two dimensional and color Doppler imaging showing significant tricuspid regurgitation following Mitral valve replacement

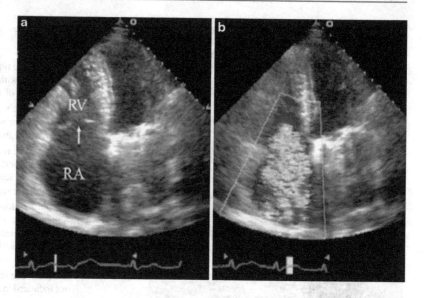

insertion of a permanent epicardial pacing electrode at the time of valve replacement is recommended to avoid later need to pass a transvenous lead across the prosthetic valve [12].

Tricuspid Stenosis

Medical therapy is used to relieve symptoms of heart failure and fluid retention. Tricuspid valve balloon valvotomy has been advocated for tricuspid stenosis of various causes [15–17]. However, severe TR is a common consequence of this procedure, and long-term results are poor when severe TR develops because of RV dysfunction and/or systemic venous congestion. Commissurotomy or valve replacement is recommended in cases with hemodynamically significant tricuspid stenosis.

Functional Tricuspid Regurgitation

Functional tricuspid regurgitation (FTR) may resolve with treatment of underlying cause; for example, in the patient with severe mitral stenosis and pulmonary hypertension with resulting right ventricular dilatation and TR, relief of mitral stenosis and the resulting decrease in pulmonary artery pressure may result in substantial

diminution of the degree of TR. However, TR associated with dilatation of the tricuspid annulus should be repaired, because tricuspid dilatation is an ongoing process that may progress to severe if left untreated (Fig. 97.6). Survival of patients with moderate or severe FTR was significantly reduced compared with the survival of patients without or with only mild FTR [18]. Studies have shown that even less than mild FTR, if left untreated, can worsen by 2 grades after close to 5 years postoperatively [19]. The ACC/AHA guidelines [12] recommend tricuspid annuloplasty for less than severe TR in patients undergoing MV surgery when there is pulmonary hypertension or tricuspid annular dilatation (Class IIb). An aggressive treatment strategy for FTR in patients undergoing mitral valve (MV) surgery, according to the echocardiographic systolic dimension of the tricuspid annulus, was recommended by Calafiore et al. [20]. Correction of FTR when the systolic tricuspid annulus dimension is in the higher normal range (>24 mm) was found to be helpful in reducing the FTR grade in the midterm.

Surgical Management

In children, acquired tricuspid insufficiency is usually functional in origin, due to the dilatation of the native tricuspid annulus following exposure to pulmonary hypertension secondary to concomitant mitral valve disease. The organic involvement of the tricuspid valve by rheumatic fever and endocarditis constitutes the other etiologies. In rheumatic tricuspid valve dysfunction, pure insufficiency is due to the retraction of the tricuspid leaflets as well as fibrosis of the subvalvular apparatus. Mixed stenotic and regurgitant lesions are due to the commissural fusion and lack of coaptation of the leaflets by progressive fibrosis and retraction with time. Pure rheumatic tricuspid stenosis is rare. Contrary to rheumatic mitral valve disease, restricted movement of the valve leaflets is seldom seen in rheumatic tricuspid valve disease. In almost all cases of organic rheumatic tricuspid valve diseases, the mechanism of tricuspid insufficiency is similar to type III rheumatic mitral valve disease. As in mitral valve repair, commissurotomy, resection of the retracted primary chordae tendineae, shaving of the retracted leaflet tissue, and concomitant annuloplasty are usually sufficient to correct the tricuspid valve dysfunction and ensure some degree of functional longevity of the affected tricuspid valves. In the authors' experience, 15 % of the repaired organic rheumatic tricuspid valves require replacement over a period of 20 years postoperatively, due to progressive retraction and calcification. In case of tricuspid valve replacement, a valvular substitute of first choice is either a mitral homograft [21] or biological prosthesis, in order to avoid the problems related to anticoagulation.

In case of FTR, tricuspid annuloplasty alone is effective in majority of the cases in correcting the insufficiency, except for cases in which the leaflets tethering due to a grossly dilated right ventricle are too significant (with a tenting depth above 1 cm).

In cases of tricuspid valve endocarditis, resection of the vegetations and abscesses and the use of pericardial patch to fill up the resected leaflet area are considered the main techniques. After the resection of the infected tissue, the prolapsing segments of the anterior and septal leaflets can be repaired by septal or posterior leaflet chordal transposition to the free edge of the anterior leaflet or by using artificial cords. Concomitant

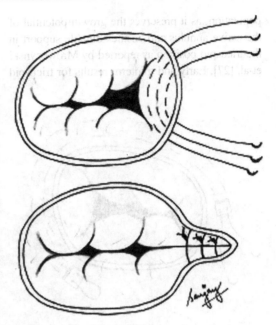

Fig. 97.7 Kay annuloplasty

annuloplasty with a ring becomes mandatory in case of annular dilatation or for reducing the tension applied on the free edge of the leaflet onto which the chordae were transposed or an artificial cord was fixed (by increasing the coaptation surface between leaflets).

Bicuspidalization of the tricuspid valve (Kay annuloplasty) (Fig. 97.7), De Vega (Fig. 97.8), annuloplasty using rigid ring (Fig. 97.9), and flexible, semiflexible, and biodegradable rings (Fig. 97.10) constitute the different surgical annuloplasty techniques.

Although Carrier et al. reported similar low failure rates and good long-term survival benefit with De Vega, Bey flexible linear reducer, and Carpentier-Edwards ring annuloplasties [22], many clinical studies have obtained superior repair durability and long-term survival using a ring, as compared with De Vega annuloplasty or suture bicuspidalization of the tricuspid valve [23–26].

The tricuspid biodegradable ring is available in pediatric and adult sizes ranging from 16 to 36, just as for the mitral version. The biodegradable ring may be especially advantageous in the pediatric population, as it preserves the growth potential of the native annulus and ensures durable support in the tricuspid position as reported by Mrowczynski et al. [27]. Early and midterm results for tricuspid

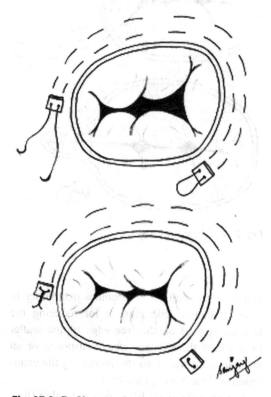

Fig. 97.8 De Vega annuloplasty

annuloplasty using the biodegradable ring in comparison to the De Vega annuloplasty have been published [28, 29]. The nondegradable component in the central portion of the ring prevents redilatation of the tricuspid annulus by providing permanent resistance against tensile stretch, thus playing an essential role in the low rate of recurrent tricuspid regurgitation over time, as reported by Basel et al. [29] and as observed in these authors' unpublished experience.

Postoperative Management

The postoperative monitoring of patients following tricuspid valve surgery should include continuous monitoring of heart rate, rhythm, central venous pressure, systemic arterial pressure, and in some cases pulmonary artery pressure and urine output. Follow-up of markers of tissue perfusion (lactate level, mixed venous saturation, near infrared spectroscopy) remains paramount in titrating cardiovascular support. Serial echocardiographic assessment may be needed especially in the setting of infective endocarditis and severely compromised ventricular function. Caregivers ought to very carefully identify cardiopulmonary interactions and aim to wean patients towards extubation as soon as deemed safe; interventricular interactions, systolic but

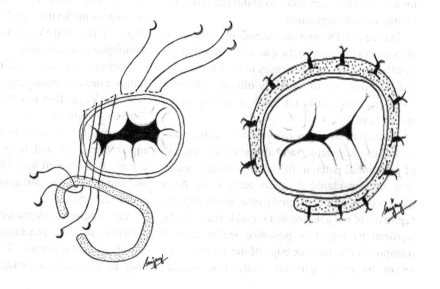

Fig. 97.9 Rigid ring annuloplasty

Fig. 97.10 Biodegradable
annuloplasty ring
implantation

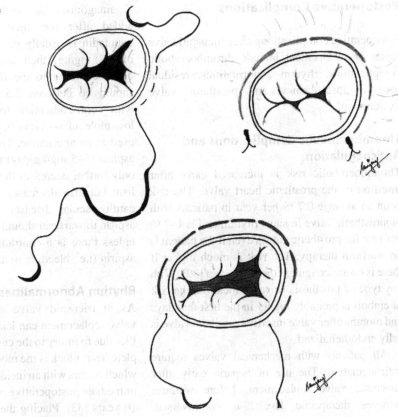

also – and very importantly – diastolic dysfunction, also deserve careful assessment and management. Cardiovascular support is often based on the use of milrinone for its inotropic, pulmonary, and systemic vasodilator, and lusitropic effects while remaining aware of the potential disproportion between these effects and the degree of systemic vasodilation that may require the association of vasoconstrictors. Decreasing right ventricular afterload is important and some patients will benefit from ventilator strategies to maintain pH between 7.40 and 7.45 and eventually the use of nitric oxide to achieve such goal. Severe right ventricular dysfunction and pulmonary hypertension require very specific management that is discussed in more detail elsewhere in this textbook. Management of the latter conditions shall not be successful unless triggers (i.e., acidosis, pain, volume overload, sepsis, atelectasis, or pleural effusions) are avoided and aggressively managed. Arrhythmias and conductive disorders

also require energetic management adapted to the specific diagnosis, and atrioventricular and interventricular synchronization should be considered in patients with persistent low cardiac output. Persistent right ventricular dysfunction with high filling pressures and impending multiorgan dysfunction requires a comprehensive reevaluation of hemodynamics; some patients may benefit from decompression of the right-sided heart by creating a "pop-off" at the atrial level. Caregivers should keep a low threshold to insert a peritoneal catheter in patients with progressing ascites. Careful serial assessment of multiorgan function and rectification of identified anomalies are vital. Last but not least, patients – and mostly those with chronic cardiac failure – need nutritional support in order to promote an anabolic state. Anticoagulation protocols are very institutional dependent. Details about anticoagulation are further discussed below and in another chapter in this textbook.

Postoperative Complications

Postoperative complications after tricuspid valve repair or replacement include thromboembolic complications, rhythm abnormalities, residual tricuspid insufficiency, and prosthetic valve dysfunction.

Thromboembolic Complications and Anticoagulation

Thromboembolic risk is increased early after insertion of the prosthetic heart valve. The risk is on an average 0.7 % per year in patients with bioprosthetic valve in sinus rhythm and is 1–2 % per year for prosthetic valves even if the patient is on warfarin therapy. The risk is much higher if there is no anticoagulant therapy given [30]. With any type of prosthesis or valve location, the risk of emboli is probably higher in the first few days and months after valve insertion, until the valve is fully endothelialized.

All patients with mechanical valves require anticoagulation. The use of heparin early after prosthetic valve replacement, before warfarin achieves therapeutic levels, is controversial. Many centers start heparin as soon as the risk of increased surgical bleeding is reduced (usually within 24–48 h), with maintenance of activated prothrombin time (aPTT) between 55 s and 70 s. After an overlap of heparin and warfarin for 3–5 days, heparin is discontinued when an INR of 2.5–3.5 is achieved. In some patients, achievement of therapeutic INR must be delayed several days after surgery because of possible complications.

Guidelines for anticoagulation therapy and target coagulation profile following tricuspid valve replacement are similar to those recommended following mitral valve replacement. Children with biological prosthetic valves are usually provided with antiplatelet agent like acetylsalicylic acid (3–5 mg/kg/day). For children with mechanical prosthetic valves, heparin infusion is usually started when postoperative bleeding reduces to a minimum. A heparin bolus (75 U/kg over 10 min) followed by an infusion rate (28 U/kg/h for <1 year old and 20 U/kg/h for >1 year old) targeting an aPTT of 60–85 s is recommended [31]. Antivitamin K antagonists like oral coumadin is usually added after the chest drainage stops. Oral coumadin is usually given with a loading dose of 0.2 mg/kg, then adjusting the subsequent dose according to the INR. The targeted INR should be between 2.5 and 3.5. For patients with contraindication to oral anticoagulation, low-molecular-weight heparin (LMWH) can be used as an alternative. The addition of low-dose aspirin (3–5 mg/kg/day) to warfarin therapy not only further decreases the risk of thromboembolism but also decreases mortality due to other cardiovascular diseases [32]. The addition of aspirin to warfarin should be strongly considered unless there is a contraindication to the use of aspirin (i.e., bleeding or aspirin intolerance).

Rhythm Abnormalities

As in tricuspid valve annuloplasty, tricuspid valve replacement can lead to rhythm abnormalities due to injury to the conduction system. Complete heart block is the most serious complication which occurs with an incidence of up to 5 % in the immediate postoperative period and up to 25 % in 10 years [33]. Placing the sutures at the base of the septal leaflet rather than in the annulus would prevent injury to the conduction system. Pacemaker implantation is indicated in such cases if the ventricular escape rate remains less for the child's age.

Residual Tricuspid Insufficiency and Prosthetic Valve Dysfunction

Significant residual tricuspid regurgitation occurs in case of persistent severe pulmonary arterial hypertension or mitral valve disease. Control of these comorbidities will prevent and control this complication. Prosthetic valve dysfunction can occur as a result of fibrocalcific degeneration or functional stenosis. The latter condition is characterized by high transvalvar gradient and elevated right atrial pressure. The best preventive strategy for this complication is implantation of a larger prosthesis at the time of surgery. Reoperation for residual tricuspid insufficiency or prosthetic valve dysfunction is indicated only in the presence of significant symptoms and clinical deterioration.

Conclusions

Acquired tricuspid valve abnormalities in children are most often due to functional annular dilatation causing regurgitation, infective endocarditis, or rheumatic heart disease. The tricuspid valve dysfunction can be identified as predominant stenosis or purely regurgitant condition with the aid of various investigations. Medical management often fails in hemodynamically significant lesions and repair or replacement of the valve will be needed. There are many surgical repair techniques in practice obviating the need for replacement. Thromboembolism and complete heart block are the dreaded post-repair/replacement complications.

References

1. Silver MD, Lam JHC, Ranganathan N et al (1971) Morphology of the human tricuspid valve. Circulation 43:33–48
2. Skwarek M, Hreczecha J, Dudziak M et al (2007) The morphology and distribution of the tendinous chords and their relation to the papillary muscles in the tricuspid valve of the human heart. Folia Morphol 66(4):314–322
3. Bruce F, Waller JH, Fess S (1995) Pathology of tricuspid valve stenosis and pure tricuspid regurgitation-part I. Clin Cardiol 18:97–102
4. Bruce F, Waller JH, Fess S (1995) Pathology of tricuspid valve stenosis and pure tricuspid regurgitation-part II. Clin Cardiol 18:167–174
5. Hauck AJ, Freeman DP, Ackermann DM et al (1988) Surgical pathology of the tricuspid valve. A study of 363 cases spanning 25 years. Mayo Clinic Proc 63:851–863
6. Shore DF, Rigby ML, Lincoln C (1982) Severe tricuspid stenosis presenting as tricuspid atresia: echocardiographic diagnosis and surgical management. Br Heart J 40:404–406
7. Seibert KA, Rettenmier CW, Waller BF et al (1982) Osteogenic sarcoma of the heart. Ani J Med 73:136–141
8. Hollman A (1957) The anatomical appearance in rheumatic tricuspid valve disease. Br Heart J 19(2):211–216
9. Hauck AJ, Freeman DP, Ackermann DM (1998) Surgical pathology of the tricuspid valve: a study of 363 cases spanning 25 years. Mayo Clin Proc 63(9):851–863
10. Pellikka PA, Tajik AJ, Khandheria BK (1993) Carcinoid heart disease. Clinical and echocardiographic spectrum in 74 patients. Circulation 87:1188–1196
11. Rebecca Snider A, Gerald A, Ritter SB (1997) Methods for obtaining quantitative information from the echocardiographic examination. In: De Young L (ed) Echocardiography in pediatric heart disease, 2nd edn. Mosby, St. Louis, MO
12. Carabello BA, Chatterjee K, de Leon AC et al (2006) ACC/AHA 2006 guidelines for the management of patients with valvular heart disease a report of the American College of Cardiology/American Heart Association Task Force on Practice Guidelines (Writing Committee to Revise the 1998 Guidelines for the Management of Patients With Valvular Heart Disease). J Am Coll Cardiol 48(3):e1–e148
13. Lange R, De Simone R, Bauernschmitt R (1996) Tricuspid valve reconstruction, a treatment option in acute endocarditis. Eur J Cardiothorac Surg 10:320–326
14. Sutlic Z, Schmid C, Borst HG (1990) Repair of flail anterior leaflets of tricuspid and mitral valves by cusp remodeling. Ann Thorac Surg 50:927–930
15. Orbe LC, Sobrino N, Arcas R et al (1993) Initial outcome of percutaneous balloon valvuloplasty in rheumatic tricuspid valve stenosis. Am J Cardiol 71:353–354
16. Kratz J (1991) Evaluation and management of tricuspid valve disease. Cardiol Clin 9:397–407
17. Onate A, Alcibar J, Inguanzo R (1993) Balloon dilation of tricuspid and pulmonary valves in carcinoid heart disease. Tex Heart Inst J 20:115–119
18. Atiq M, Lai L, Lee KJ (2005) Transcatheter closure of atrial septal defects in children with a hypoplastic right ventricle. Catheter Cardiovasc Interv 64:112–116
19. Nath J, Foster E, Heidenreich PA (2004) Impact of tricuspid regurgitation on long-term survival. J Am Coll Cardiol 43:405–409
20. Calafiore AM, Iacò AL, Romeo A et al (2011) Echocardiographic-based treatment of functional tricuspid regurgitation. J Thorac Cardiovasc Surg 142:308–313
21. Kalangos A, Sierra J, Beghetti M (2004) Tricuspid valve replacement with a mitral homograft in children with rheumatic tricuspid valvulopathy. J Thorac Cardiovasc Surg 127:1682–1687
22. Carrier M, Pellerin M, Guertin MC et al (2004) Twenty-five years' clinical experience with repair of tricuspid insufficiency. J Heart Valve Dis 13:952–956
23. Matsuyama K, Matsumoto M, Sugita T et al (2001) De Vega annuloplasty and Carpentier Edwards ring annuloplasty for secondary tricuspid regurgitation. J Heart Valve Dis 10:520–524
24. Tang GH, David TE, Singh SK (2006) Tricuspid valve repair with an annuloplasty ring results in improved long-term outcomes. Circulation 114(1 suppl):I577–I581
25. Rivera R, Duran E, Ajuria M (1985) Carpentier's flexible ring versus De Vega's annuloplasty:

a prospective randomized study. J Thorac Cardiovasc Surg 89:196–203

26. Ghanta RK, Chen R, Narayanasamy N (2007) Suture bicuspidalization of the tricuspid valve versus ring annuloplasty for repair of functional tricuspid regurgitation: midterm results of 237 consecutive patients. J Thorac Cardiovasc Surg 133:117–126

27. Mrowczynski W, Mrozinski B, Kalangos A et al (2011) Biodegradable ring enables growth of the native tricuspid annulus. J Heart Valve Dis 20: 205–215

28. Burma O, Ustunsoy H, Davutoglu V et al (2007) Initial clinical experience with a novel biodegradable ring in patients with functional tricuspid insufficiency: Kalangos biodegradable tricuspid ring. Thorac Cardiovasc Surg 55:284–287

29. Basel H, Aydin U, Kutlu H et al (2010) Outcomes of De Vega versus biodegradable ring annuloplasty in

the surgical treatment of tricuspid regurgitation (midterm results). Heart Surg Forum 13(4): E233–E237

30. Vongpatanasin W, Hillis LD, Lange RA (1996) Prosthetic heart valves. N Engl J Med 335:407–416

31. Monagle P, Chalmers E, Chan A et al (2008) Antithrombotic therapy in neonates and children: American College of Chest Physicians Evidence-Based Clinical Practice Guidelines (8th Edition). Chest 133:887S–968S

32. Turpie AG, Gent M, Laupacias A et al (1993) A comparison of Aspirin with placebo in patients with warfarin after heart valve replacement. N Engl J Med 329:524–529

33. Gordon RS, Ivanov J, Cohen G et al (1998) Permanent cardiac pacing after a cardiac operation: predicting the use of permanent pacemakers. Ann Thorac Surg 66: 1698–1704

Ebstein Malformation of the Tricuspid Valve: Early Presentation

98

Christopher J. Knott-Craig and Steven P. Goldberg

Abstract

Ebstein malformation of the tricuspid valve is a downward, apical displacement of the posterior and septal leaflets, with a broad, sail-like anterior leaflet, which is tethered to a variable degree. Presentation in the neonatal period is one of high mortality, and there is a spectrum of surgical options ranging from a complete biventricular repair to single-ventricle palliation. This chapter focuses on Ebstein malformation of the tricuspid valve or Ebstein anomaly in the neonatal period; another chapter in this textbook further discusses this disease in later life.

Keywords

Ebstein anomaly • Neonate • Infant • Tricuspid valve • Surgery

Brief Historical Background

Wilhelm Ebstein, born in 1836 in Poland, was a pupil of eminent pathologist Rudolph Virchow, having moved to Berlin for his medical training [1]. In 1864, he had the opportunity to perform an autopsy on a 19-year-old man who had suffered from symptoms of both cyanosis and congestive heart failure, wherein he described a severe malformation of the tricuspid valve: "A membrane originated from a normally developed annulus...and was related to both the anterior and posterior walls of the right ventricle, and blended with the posterior half of the endocardium." He goes on in great detail to describe the displaced and adherent leaflets that characterize the defect [2]. It was not until the 1950s when Ebstein anomaly (EA) – as it was known since the 1920s – was reported in a live patient, a 34-year-old woman who presented with peripheral edema and a retinal hemorrhage [3]. Helen Taussig reported the first case in a child in 1960 [4].

C.J. Knott-Craig (✉) • S.P. Goldberg
Pediatric Cardiothoracic Surgery, University of Tennessee Health Science Center, Le Bonheur Children's Hospital, Memphis, TN, USA
e-mail: cknottcr@uthsc.edu;
Steven.Goldberg@lebonheur.org;
sgoldberg17@yahoo.com

Introduction

Ebstein anomaly (EA) is a rare disease (1–5/200,000 live births, 1 % of congenital heart disease [5]), characterized by spiral downward

E.M. da Cruz et al. (eds.), *Pediatric and Congenital Cardiology, Cardiac Surgery and Intensive Care*,
DOI 10.1007/978-1-4471-4619-3_34, © Springer-Verlag London 2014

(apical) displacement of the septal and posterior leaflets of the tricuspid valve, leaving a broad, "sail-like" anterior leaflet. The now "supravalvular" portion of the right ventricle is thinned, compliant, effectively becoming "atrialized," and the remaining "functional" right ventricle and outflow tract can be quite diminutive. This leads often to severe tricuspid insufficiency, right ventricular failure, and cyanosis [6]. Patients that present with EA in the neonatal period are an exceptionally high-risk group, with mortality rates described as high as 100 %, with 18 % of those deaths occurring in the newborn period [7–9]. In a series of 46 neonates with EA, Yetman et al. demonstrated the increased mortality with the presence of cyanosis (70 % vs. 14 % for acyanotic, $p < 0.0001$) [8]. In an effort to quantitatively stratify risk, Celermajer et al. developed an echocardiography-based scoring system (GOSE score: Great Ormond Street Echo score) in 1992, wherein the ratio of the areas of the cardiac chambers are combined according to the following formula: (right atrium + "atrialized" right ventricle) ÷ (functional right ventricle + left atrium + left ventricle) [9]. A score is assigned (I–IV) based on the ratio, and then a mortality estimate can be derived; for example, a grade IV (ratio ≥1.5) carries an expected mortality of 100 % [10].

Given this, there is a stark absence of consensus regarding the optimal management, especially surgical, in this extremely high-risk patient population. In a recent broad survey of the Pediatric Health Information System (PHIS) database, of 415 neonates identified with Ebstein anomaly, 62 % were managed medically, with 24 % mortality; 15 % underwent palliative shunting; 9 % went down a single-ventricle palliative route; 4 % underwent a complete biventricular repair; and 1 % were transplanted [11].

Anatomy

The anatomic hallmarks of Ebstein anomaly are as follows:

(a) Downward (apical) displacement of the tricuspid leaflets (septal > posterior > anterior)
(b) Broad, "sail-like" anterior leaflet
(c) Adherence ("failure of delamination") of the leaflets to the underlying endocardium, including multiple points of tethering of the anterior leaflet
(d) Massive dilation of the "atrialized" portion of the right ventricle
(e) Dilation of the anatomic tricuspid annulus
(f) Commonly associated cardiac defects (e.g., right ventricular outflow tract obstruction, atrial septal defect) [12]

In addition to the varying degree of size to the "functional" right ventricle, there is very often hypoplasia or atresia of the pulmonary artery. This can take on the form of true anatomical atresia (24 %) or a "functional" pulmonary atresia (54 %) in which the diminutive right ventricle is unable to generate antegrade pulmonary blood flow [8]. In congenitally corrected transposition of the great arteries, 15–50 % of left-sided (i.e., systemic) tricuspid valves are "Ebsteinoid" in nature [6]. The conduction system in Ebstein anomaly is frequently abnormal, with accessory pathways yielding a 14–20 % incidence of Wolff-Parkinson-White syndrome in older patients [13].

Physiology and Pathophysiology

Symptomatic neonates with EA present predominantly with cyanosis and severe congestive cardiac failure. This is the result of severe tricuspid regurgitation and marked cardiomegaly from massive enlargement of the right atrium and atrialized right ventricle (Fig. 98.1) [14]. Cyanosis is often a prominent feature given multiple factors: (a) the lack of effective antegrade pulmonary blood flow in anatomic or functional pulmonary atresia, (b) the severe tricuspid regurgitation creating a large right-to-left shunt through an atrial septal defect, and (c) the extrinsic compression of lungs by the space-occupying mass of the dilated right heart. In the neonate,

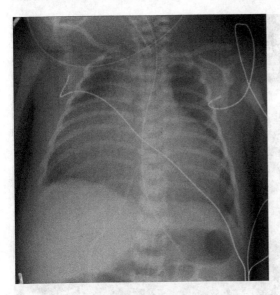

Fig. 98.1 Chest radiograph demonstrating massive cardiomegaly

these factors are amplified by the elevated pulmonary resistances. The ventricular septum may bow into the left, causing inadequate left ventricular filling and a low cardiac output. All of these factors conspire to create a situation of hemodynamic instability coupled with hypoxemia and metabolic acidosis that may portend a dismal prognosis [15].

Diagnosis

Clinical

The neonate with EA is often critically ill, and if the functional right ventricle is either too small to generate a forward cardiac output, or unable to overcome the elevated pulmonary vascular resistances, then a ductal-dependent circulation may result, combined with features of congestive heart failure [16]. Tachyarrhythmia may complicate the presentation, and supraventricular arrhythmia occurs in 5–10 % of neonates [17]. In less symptomatic infants, physical findings include the holosystolic murmur of tricuspid insufficiency

and possibly an ejection-type systolic murmur over the right ventricular outflow tract. The degree of malformation of the tricuspid valve determines the intensity of the murmur [18].

ECG

Up to 20 % of EA patients will have accessory pathways and/or Wolff-Parkinson-White (WPW) syndrome. In those cases, the electrocardiogram may demonstrate the typical preexcitation delta wave and shortened PR segment. In those without WPW, the predominant ECG findings are those of diminished amplitude of the right-sided QRS complex, a right bundle branch block, and variable orientation of the electrical axis. The ECG is also essential in detecting other supraventricular arrhythmias such as atrial flutter or fibrillation, having their origin in the massive right atrial dilation [18].

Imaging

The classic radiographic appearance of EA is massive "wall-to-wall" cardiomegaly, with severely symptomatic neonates having cardiothoracic ratios exceeding 80 % (Fig. 98.1) [19]. It is echocardiography that is most useful in the diagnosis of EA, however. The precise anatomical detail of the leaflets can be determined (Fig. 98.2), as well as assessment of the severity of the valvular insufficiency by color-flow Doppler. The remainder of the intracardiac anatomy can be delineated (e.g., atrial septum, right ventricular outflow tract). The sonographic hallmark of EA is an apical displacement of the septal leaflet a distance of ≥ 8 mm/m^2 [20].

Laboratory

There are no specific laboratory markers for neonatal EA, but serial measurements of serum

Fig. 98.2 Echocardiogram demonstrating apical displacement of the tricuspid leaflets

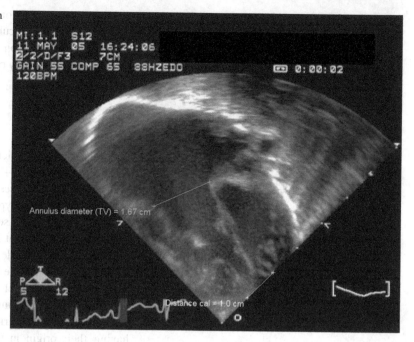

lactate in the intensive care unit can aid in evaluating the adequacy of cardiac output and tissue oxygen delivery.

Decision Making

There is currently no consensus opinion regarding the optimal management of EA in the neonate and young infant [11]. Various permutations on repair of the valve by means of a reduction tricuspid annuloplasty and utilization of the broad anterior leaflet as a "monocuspid" valve have had long-standing and durable results in patients from infancy to adults, as has valve replacement in suitably sized patients [21]. In very severely ill neonates with severe tricuspid insufficiency and right ventricular outflow tract obstruction, single-ventricle palliation has been recommended by Starnes and colleagues, who first reported a right ventricular exclusion procedure – effectively creating tricuspid atresia – with subsequent progress down a Glenn and Fontan pathway [22]. By 2000, however, Knott-Craig et al.

reported the first successful series of neonates with EA who underwent a complete two-ventricle repair, including repair of the valve and all other associated cardiac lesions [23].

Current indications for surgery in the neonatal period [9, 10, 23, 24]:

1. Relatively asymptomatic neonates
   (a) GOSE score grade IV
   (b) Cardiothoracic ratio ≥ 0.8
   (c) Severe tricuspid regurgitation
2. Symptomatic neonates
   (a) Severe cyanosis
   (b) GOSE score grade III–IV
   (c) Cardiothoracic ratio ≥ 0.8
   (d) Severe tricuspid regurgitation
   (e) Associated cardiac defects [23]
3. Other indications
   (a) Persistent ventilator dependency
   (b) Persistent need for inotropic support
   (c) Persistent   prostaglandin-dependent circulation
   (d) Congestive heart failure [25]
   (e) Rising serum lactate levels despite inotropic support

Special mention should be made of the fact that the above indications for tricuspid valve repair apply only in the setting of a normal *left* ventricle. If the left ventricle is hypoplastic, or morphologically normal with decreased function, then transplantation as the primary therapy should be considered.

Medical Management

In the immediate postnatal period, patients that are reasonably *stable* are given an initial trial of medical therapy. This includes (1) supplemental oxygen, (2) observation for adequate cardiac output, and (3) prostaglandin E_1 as required. In an *unstable* patient, immediate therapy may involve (1) intubation and paralysis (as required), (2) inotropic support (e.g., dopamine 5–10 mcg/kg/min with or without isoproterenol), (3) inhaled nitric oxide (iNO) if pulmonary resistances remain elevated, and (4) prostaglandin E_1, if deemed ductal-dependent. In cases of associated "functional" pulmonary atresia (e.g., no prograde pulmonary blood flow), the patient is closely observed in a cardiac intensive care unit with repeated echocardiograms. About half the neonates will stabilize and improve over a few days as the pulmonary vascular resistance decreases. During that time, echocardiograms will often demonstrate increasing prograde blood flow through the pulmonary valve. Initial paralysis with mechanical ventilation may be helpful in minimizing the effects on cardiac output of the gross cardiomegaly which is usually present [23, 24]. If improvement occurs, the prostaglandin infusion is weaned, and the oxygen saturations and serum lactates are carefully monitored, and an attempt is made to wean the positive pressure ventilation. The prostaglandin infusion is weaned over a few days, carefully observing the oxygen saturations clinically, as well as the serial echocardiograms, for evidence of progressive forward flow through the pulmonary valve. If their condition deteriorates or oxygen saturations fall below 75–80 %, surgical therapy is indicated and depends upon the morphologic parameters described above. Those with associated anatomic pulmonary atresia will require early surgical intervention [24].

A particularly lethal situation develops when the right ventricle is unable to eject any blood through the pulmonary valve (physiologic pulmonary atresia) and there is significant pulmonary regurgitation present. When this occurs and there is severe tricuspid regurgitation present, a "circular shunt" develops: blood ejected into the aorta returns to the right atrium through a patent ductus arteriosus and incompetent pulmonary valve, thereby stealing blood from both the systemic and pulmonary circulations and resulting in a rapidly decompensating neonate. In these circumstances, ECMO is singularly unhelpful. In these circumstances, stopping the PGE_1 infusion is indicated in the hope that this would cease the circular shunt. Ventilatory strategies and the use of iNO may be helpful in further decreasing pulmonary resistances, thus promoting more anterograde flow toward the pulmonary arteries. If therapeutic failure occurs, then the main pulmonary artery may need to be ligated emergently and a modified Blalock-Taussig shunt performed, with or without simultaneous ECMO initiation.

Surgical and Interventional Management

The fundamentals of a complete biventricular repair are as follows:
(a) Tricuspid valve repair
(b) Plication of the atrialized right ventricle
(c) Reduction atrioplasty of the dilated right atrium
(d) Fenestrated closure of the atrial septal defect
(e) Correction of other associated cardiac lesions (e.g., pulmonary atresia)

The repair is performed with full cardiopulmonary bypass, using either moderate systemic

Fig. 98.3 Tricuspid
annuloplasty stitch placed
in coronary sinus and at
location of anteroposterior
commissure. *ASD* atrial
septal defect

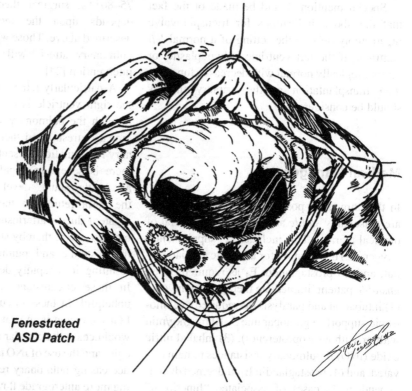

**Fenestrated
ASD Patch**

hypothermia or deep hypothermic circulatory
arrest. It is critical to identify the course of the
right coronary artery so as not to injure it during
atrial reduction. The free wall of the enlarged
right atrium is widely excised. The atrial septal
defect is closed with a patch, leaving a 3–4 mm
fenestration behind as a "pop-off" to help accommodate impaired right ventricular function in the
postoperative period. The basis of the valve repair
is the creation of a "monocuspid" valve in which
the anterior leaflet will coapt with the septum after
annuloplasty, as the septal and posterior leaflets
are displaced apically and nonfunctional. The
annuloplasty stitch is placed with one pledgetted
end in the coronary sinus and the other at
the expected location of the anteroposterior
commissure (Fig. 98.3). Approximation of the
annuloplasty stitch effectively partitions the tricuspid valve orifice into two openings – the more
"caudal" of the two representing the atrialized

right ventricle (Fig. 98.4a). Closure of this orifice
then plicates the atrialized portion of the ventricle
(Fig. 98.4b). Tethering of the anterior leaflet can
be overcome by taking it down from the tricuspid
annulus and either fenestrating or dividing some
of the subvalvular attachments (Fig. 98.5)
followed by resuspension of the valve to the
plicated and reduced annulus (Fig. 98.6). Often
the use of a pledgetted suture placed through the
base of a major papillary muscle to the anterior
leaflet which is then sutured to the interventricular
septum – a Sebening stitch – helps stabilize
the tricuspid valve repair. Once the intra-atrial
repair is completed, other associated lesions
such as anatomic pulmonary atresia can be
addressed – either with small transannular patch
opening of the right ventricular outflow tract to
create a 7–8 mm outflow tract, or with the insertion of a small valved conduit which is our current
preference (Fig. 98.7) [26].

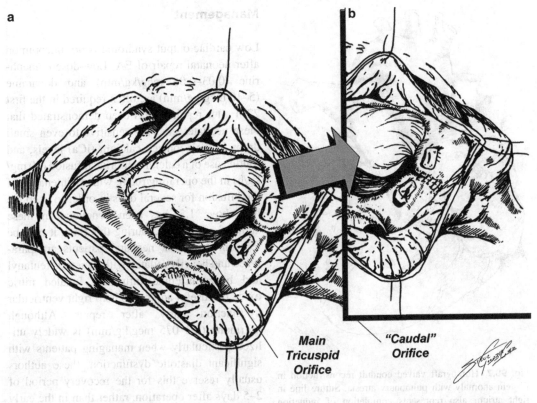

Fig. 98.4 (a) Approximation of annuloplasty stitch creates two openings, the "caudal" orifice containing the entrance to the atrialized right ventricle, (b) Closure of the caudal opening plicates the atrialized right ventricle and creates a competent monocuspid valve

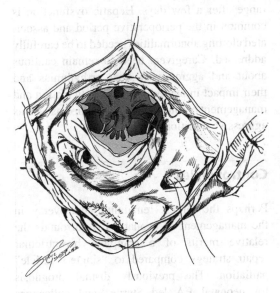

Fig. 98.5 Detachment of anterior leaflet from tricuspid annulus. Subvalvular attachments are mobilized

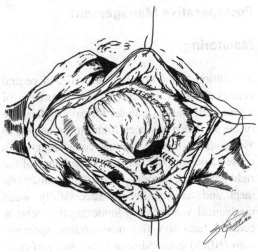

Fig. 98.6 Annuloplasty stitch with reattachment of anterior leaflet

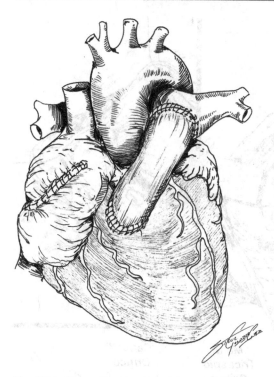

Fig. 98.7 Homograft valved conduit reconstruction in Ebstein anomaly with pulmonary atresia. Suture line in right atrium also represents completion of reduction atrioplasty

Postoperative Management

Monitoring

In addition to the standard arterial and central venous catheters, placement intraoperatively of a peritoneal dialysis catheter for passive drainage of the abdomen has been found to be useful, as ascites from hepatic venous congestion (as a consequence of poor diastolic compliance of the right heart) can introduce respiratory embarrassment and an inability to successfully wean mechanical ventilation. Monitoring the trend in cerebral (and somatic) near-infrared spectroscopy (NIRS) as an indicator of adequacy of cerebral oxygen delivery has become a standard part of many intensive care units' protocols.

Management

Low cardiac output syndrome is not uncommon after neonatal repair of EA. Low-dose epinephrine (0.03–0.06 mcg/kg/min) and dopamine (5–10 mcg/kg/min) are often required in the first 72 h after repair. It has been demonstrated that these neonates are very sensitive to even small drops in their ionized calcium (iCa) levels, and routine use of a calcium chloride infusion (10 mg/kg/h) in the operating room, with maintenance of the infusion for several days in order to keep the iCa above 1.5, has been beneficial in these authors' experience. During this time, it may be recommended that neonatal patients are paralyzed and heavily sedated with generous fentanyl and benzodiazepine infusions. Inhaled nitric oxide is a useful adjunct to help right ventricular dysfunction early after repair. Although milrinone (0.3–075 mcg/kg/min) is widely utilized particularly when managing patients with significant diastolic dysfunction, these authors usually reserve this for the recovery period of 2–5 days after operation, rather than in the early postoperative period. Frequently, the oxygen saturations are 65–80 % in the early postoperative period, but they gradually improve to the 90 % range after a few days. Hepatic dysfunction is common in the perioperative period and associated clotting abnormalities needed to be carefully addressed. Caregivers need to remain cautious about and aggressively treat arrhythmias and their impact in hemodynamics. Anticipation and management of multiorgan dysfunction as well as aggressive nutrition are also vital.

Controversies

Perhaps the largest remaining controversy in the management of neonatal EA surrounds the relative merits of a complete biventricular repair strategy compared to "single-ventricle" palliation. The previously dismal prognosis for neonatal EA led Starnes and colleagues to introduce a univentricular strategy [22].

With this approach, the true tricuspid annulus is closed subtotally with a 3–4 mm fenestration in the patch. This results in exclusion of the right ventricle, and pulmonary blood flow is established with creation of a systemic-to-pulmonary shunt. While their initial survival was just under 70 % without fenestration, the addition of the fenestration improved the outcomes in that subgroup to 80 % (8/10) in the report of their first 16 patients [27]. The complete two-ventricle repair strategy, with correction of all associated cardiac defects in addition to restoring a competent tricuspid valve, was begun in 1994 by Knott-Craig et al. with the first series reported in 2000 [23, 28]. By 2007, he demonstrated 74 % inhospital survival (20/27 patients) [26], which compared favorably with the 69 % early survival from Starnes' group [22]. Other RV exclusion procedures have been introduced in the meantime, including a novel technique from Sano [29], and the centers that have adopted such strategies do so based upon the fragility of the leaflet tissue and complexity of the repair, the uncertainty of the competency of the repaired valve, and the high-risk nature of complex surgery on a critically ill newborn with poor right ventricular function [30]. Those who believe strongly in a complete repair promote the benefit of *not* committing the patient to subsequent Fontan physiology, retaining the possible advantages of biventricular function. If, after the neonatal period, the right ventricle is on the borderline of acceptability, and/or the tricuspid repair has greater than mild-moderate insufficiency, the addition of a bidirectional Glenn – the so-called 1½-ventricle repair – can help to "unload" the right heart [31].

Occasionally, neonates with EA have poorly functioning diminutive right ventricles and little tricuspid regurgitation, and they remain cyanotic when the prostaglandin is weaned. These neonates may be best served by simply placing a modified Blalock-Taussig shunt and *not* addressing any of the other defects during their initial operation. At a later stage (e.g., 4–8 months of age), a more formal repair can be contemplated, with possibly adding a bidirectional Glenn anastomosis to unload the small RV [31].

Outcomes and Long-Term Follow-Ups

In a 16-year follow-up of biventricular repair in 32 patients with EA (neonates, n = 23; infants < 4 months, n = 9), Knott-Craig and colleagues demonstrated a 90.6 % ability to complete a total repair, with 78.1 % early survival and 74 % ± 8 % late survival, with the lone late mortality from respiratory syncytial virus pneumonia 2 years after surgery. In the subgroup of patients *without* pulmonary atresia, the 15-year Kaplan-Meier survival estimate was 79 % ± 13 % (compared to 40 % ± 15 %, p = 0.03, for those *with* pulmonary atresia). Additionally, there was a statistically significant reduction in tricuspid regurgitation (p = 0.01). Excluding replacement of the valved pulmonary conduit, freedom from reoperation (i.e., tricuspid valve) was estimated to be 74 % ±10 % at 15 years by Kaplan-Meier method, in contrast to patients palliated with right ventricle exclusion procedures, all of whom require subsequent staged surgical procedures. All patients in the series are in New York Heart Association functional class I or II, and only one patient is on antiarrhythmic medications at last follow-up [25]. This is in contrast to recent reports of decreased survival with patients undergoing repair (versus univentricular palliation) by the University of Michigan group, although in their series of 24 neonates with Ebstein anomaly over a 20-year span, only four patients underwent tricuspid repair [32].

Future Developments

An important recent addition to the surgical options for EA is the "cone" repair described by da Silva (see ▶ Chap. 99, "Ebstein Malformation of the Tricuspid Valve in Children, Adolescents and Young Adults"), in which all subvalvular attachments save for the leading edge chordae are freed up and mobilized, and all three tricuspid leaflets are sewn together into a conical shape [33]. While the cone repair had traditionally been applied to adolescents and adults, the series with the youngest patients (n = 30, median age 60 months, range 2–192 months) demonstrated that the addition of a bidirectional Glenn (in non-neonates) improved the competency of the tricuspid repair at median follow-up time of 22 months, with theoretical longer-term benefit to maintenance of right ventricular function [34]. It remains to be seen to what degree the cone repair will be applicable to neonatal patients.

With advances in critical care pre- and postoperative management, the hope – and expectation – is that the mortality from the neonatal presentation of Ebstein anomaly will decline in the near future.

References

1. Jacques AM, Kostantinov IE, Zimmerman V (2001) Wilhelm Ebstein and Ebstein's malformation. Eur J Cardiothorac Surg 20:1082–1085
2. Ebstein W (1866) Ueber einen sehr seltenen fall von insufficienz der valvula tricuspidalis, bedingt durch eine angeborene hochgradige missbildung derselben. Arch Anat Physiol 7:238–254
3. Soloff LA, Stauffer HM, Zatuchni J (1951) Ebstein's disease: report of the first case diagnosed during life. Am J Med Sci 222:554–561
4. Taussig HB (1960) Congenital malformations of the heart, 2nd edn. Harvard University Press, Cambridge, MA
5. Dearani J, Danielson GK (2000) Congenital heart surgery nomenclature and database project: Ebstein's anomaly and tricuspid valve disease. Ann Thorac Surg 69(4 Suppl):S106–S117
6. Anderson KR, Zuberbuhler JR, Anderson RH, Becker AE, Lie JT (1979) Morphologic spectrum of Ebstein's anomaly of the heart: a review. Mayo Clin Proc 54:174–180
7. Celermajer DS, Dodd SM, Greenwald SE, Wyse RK, Deanfield JE (1992) Morbid anatomy in neonates with Ebstein's anomaly of the tricuspid valve: pathophysiologic and clinical implications. J Am Caoll Cardiol 19:1049–1053
8. Yetman AT, Freedom RM, McCrindle BW (1998) Outcome in cyanotic neonates with Ebstein's anomaly. Am J Cardiol 81:749–754
9. Celermajer DS, Cullen S, Sullivan ID, Spiegelhalter DJ, Wyse RK, Deanfield JE (1992) Outcomes in neonates with Ebstein's anomaly. J Am Coll Cardiol 19:1041–1046

10. Celermajer DS, Bull C, Till JA, Cullen S, Vasisillikos VP, Sullivan ID, Allan L, Nihoyannopoulos P, Somerville J, Deanfield JE (1994) Ebstein's anomaly: presentation and outcome from fetus to adult. J Am Coll Cardiol 23:170–176
11. Goldberg SP, Jones RC, Boston US, Haddad LM, Wetzel GT, Chin TK, Knott-Craig CJ (2011) Current Trends in the Management of Neonates with Ebstein's Anomaly. World J Pediatr Congenital Heart Surg 2(4):554–557
12. Dearani J, Danielson GK (2003) Ebstein's anomaly of the tricuspid valve. In: Mavroudis C, Backer CL (eds) Pediatric cardiac surgery, 3rd edn. Mosby, Philadelphia
13. Danielson GK, Driscoll DJ, Mair DD, Warnes CA, Oliver WC (1992) Operative treatment of Ebstein's anomaly. J Thorac Cardiovasc Surg 104:1195–1202
14. Roberson DA, Silverman NH (1989) Ebstein's anomaly: echocardiographic and clinical features in the fetus and neonate. J Am Coll Cardiol 14:1300–1307
15. Knott-Craig CJ, Goldberg SP (2007) Management of neonatal Ebstein's anomaly. Semin Thorac Cardiovasc Surg Pediatr Card Surg Ann 10(1):112–116
16. Newfeld EA, Cole RB, Paul MH (1967) Ebstein's malformation of the tricuspid valve in the neonate: functional and anatomic pulmonary outflow tract obstruction. Am J Cardiol 19:727–731
17. Oh JK, Holmes DR Jr, Hayes DL, Porter CB, Danielson GK (1985) Cardiac arrhythmias in patients with surgical repair of Ebstein's anomaly. J Am Coll Cardiol 6:1351–1371
18. Kumar AE, Fyler DC, Miettinen OS, Nadas AS (1971) Ebstein anomaly: clinical profile and natural history. Am J Cardiol 28:84–95
19. Amplaz K, Lester RG, Scheibler GL, Adams P Jr, Anderson RC (1959) The roentgenologic features of Ebstein anomaly of the tricuspid valve. Am J Roentgenol 81:788–794
20. Seward JB (1993) Ebstein's anomaly: ultrasound imaging and hemodynamic evaluation. Echocardiography 10(6):641–664
21. Boston US, Dearani JA, O'Leary PW, Driscoll DJ, Danielson GK (2006) Tricuspid valve repair for Ebstein's anomaly in young children: a 30-yar experience. Ann Thorac Surg 81:690–696
22. Starnes VA, Pitclick PT, Bernstein D, Griffin ML, Choy M, Shumway NE (1991) Ebstein's anomaly appearing in the neonate. J Thorac Cardiovasc Surg 101:1082–1087
23. Knott-Craig CJ, Overholt ED, Ward KE, Razook JD (2000) Neonatal repair of Ebstein's anomaly: indications, surgical technique, and medium-term follow-up. Ann Thorac Surg 69:1505–1510
24. Knott-Craig CJ, Goldberg SP, Ballweg JA, Boston US (2012) Surgical decision making in neonatal Ebstein's anomaly: an algorithmic approach based on 48 consecutive neonates. World J Pediatr Congenital Heart Surg 3:16–20

25. Boston US, Goldberg SP, Ward KE, Overholt ED, Spentzas T, Chin TK, Knott-Craig CJ (2011) Complete repair of Ebstein's anomaly in neonates and young infants: a 16-year follow-up. J Thorac Cardiovasc Surg 141:1163–1169

26. Knott-Craig CJ, Goldberg SP, Overholt ED, Colvin EV, Kirklin JK (2007) Repair of neonates and young infants with Ebstein's anomaly and related disorders. Ann Thorac Surg 84:587–593

27. Reemsten BL, Fagan BT, Wells WJ, Starnes VA (2006) Current surgical therapy for Ebstein anomaly in neonates. J Thorac Cardiovasc Surg 132:1285–1290

28. Knott-Craig CJ, Overholt ED, Ward KE, Ringewald JM, Baker SS, Razoook JD (2002) Repair of Ebstein's anomaly in the symptomatic neonate: an evolution of technique with 7-year follow-up. Ann Thorac Surg 73:1786–1793

29. Sano S, Ishino K, Kawada M, Kasahara S, Kohmotot T, Takeuchi M, Ohtsuki S (2002) Total right ventricular exclusion procedure: an operation for isolated congestive right ventricular failure. J Thorac Cardiovasc Surg 123:640–647

30. Bove EL, Hirsch JC, Ohye RG, Devaney EJ (2009) How I manage neonatal Ebstein's anomaly. Semin Thorac Cardiovasc Surg Pediatr Card Surg Ann 12:63–65

31. Malhotra SP, Petrossian E, Reddy VM, Qiu M, Maeda K, Suleman S, MacDonald M, Reinhartz O, Hanley FL (2009) Selective right ventricular unloading and novel technical concepts in Ebstein's anomaly. Ann Thorac Surg 88:1975–1981

32. Shinkawa T, Polimenkanos AC, Gomez-Fifer CA, Charpie JR, Hirsch JC, Devaney EJ, Bove EL, Ohye RG (2010) Management and long-term outcome of neonatal Ebstein anomaly. J Thorac Cardiovasc Surg 139:354–358

33. Da Silva JP, Baumgratz JF, da Fonseca L, Franchi SM, Mopes LM, Tavares GM, Soares AM, Moreira LF, Barbero-Marcial M (2007) The cone reconstruction of the tricuspid valve in Ebstein's anomaly. The operation: early and midterm results. J Thorac Cardiovasc Surg 133:215–223

34. Liu J, Qiu L, Zhu Z, Chen H, Hong H (2011) Cone reconstruction of the tricuspid valve in Ebstein anomaly with or without one and a half ventricle repair. J Thorac Cardiovasc Surg 141:1178–1183